International Handbooks of Quality-of-Life

Aims and Scope

The International Handbooks of Quality-of-Life Research offer extensive bibliographic resources. They present literature reviews of the many subdisciplines and areas of study within the growing field of quality of life research. Handbooks in the series focus on capturing and reviewing the quality of life research literature in specific life domains, on specific populations, or in relation to specific disciplines or sectors of industry. In addition, the Handbooks cover measures of quality of life and well-being, providing annotated bibliographies of well-established measures, methods, and scales.

More information about this series at http://www.springer.com/series/8365

Irma Eloff
Editor

Handbook of Quality of Life in African Societies

Springer

Editor
Irma Eloff
Faculty of Education
University of Pretoria
Pretoria, South Africa

ISSN 2468-7227 ISSN 2468-7235 (electronic)
International Handbooks of Quality-of-Life
ISBN 978-3-030-15366-3 ISBN 978-3-030-15367-0 (eBook)
https://doi.org/10.1007/978-3-030-15367-0

This Springer imprint is published by the registered company Springer Nature Switzerland AG.
The registered company address is: Gewerbestrasse 11, 6330 Cham, Switzerland

Foreword

Quality of Life in African Societies explores the many possibilities for achieving optimal levels of well-being for the diverse people living in countries south of the Sahara. The book adopts a positive view of quality of life looking through the lens of *eudaimonia*, with its focus on the capability to draw on commonplace resources to make the most of life.

There is always 'something new coming out of Africa'.[1] The collection of 25 chapters in *Quality of Life in African Societies* offers a fresh perspective on African well-being that captures the many positive attributes of family and community life. Importantly, the contributors to the volume are 'insiders' who know first-hand what matters for life quality in the local situation – many earlier reports on the state of African societies have been compiled by 'outsiders'. Too often such reports by 'outsiders' have tended to focus exclusively on the 'objective' aspects of quality of life that are captured in facts and figures. Here we are asked to look beyond the present state of 'objective' quality of life to take a more holistic view of African well-being: to consider how best people living in African societies can realise their life goals, and those of their families and communities, using their own resources. Lastly, the scope of the volume extends to the whole of the sub-Saharan region in contrast to earlier ones that concentrated on quality of life on the southern tip of the continent.[2]

Not only do the contributors to *Quality of Life in African Societies* address the many challenges facing Africa, they also offer imaginative suggestions for solutions. Societal-level concerns include the need for economic growth and development in Africa, food security, and the elimination of malaria. At the community level, we are introduced to positive changes brought about by, among other, health and adult literacy campaigns, innovative school well-being and teacher-training programmes. At the individual level, we hear accounts of personal experiences of living with HIV/AIDs, the dividends of expressing gratitude, the need for strong women to serve as role models, and the importance of a positive cultural identity. The format of contributions are varied and include critical reflections on the literature, introductions to theory

[1] A saying attributed to Pliny the Elder (Møller and Roberts, 2017, p. 173)

[2] 'South African Quality of Life' was published in 1997 as volume 1 in the Springer Social Indicators Research Series as well as in *Social Indicators Research*. The follow-up volume on 'Quality of life in South Africa ten years into democracy' was published as a special issue in *Social Indicators Research* in 2007.

and practice, evaluations of interventions to promote well-being, as well as elegant essays and narratives that resonate with African voices.

Many of the chapters speak of the traditional strengths found in Africa that have assisted societies to withstand adversity over millennia, such as community cohesiveness, resourcefulness, and resilience. Culture is considered as an essential ingredient of the good life. We learn that projects and initiatives work best when they are either home-grown or are adapted carefully to meet local conditions, as in the case of theory-based interventions and ones informed by international practice. As one author notes, community-driven participatory programmes that are based on indigenous knowledge and local ethics will have a better chance of sustainability in the longer term. Culturally sensitive tools used in research and interventions draw on a rich African repertoire of conversations, story-telling, metaphors, and indigenous games. On the other hand, we hear that positive outcomes are also achieved using twenty-first-century digital and mobile technology. For example, chapters grouped under the heading of *environment and technology* report digital devices and 'serious games' are used to disseminate health messages and assist youth to better assess their risk behaviour.

Readers are invited to share both the joys and tribulations faced by African action researchers when carrying out community projects and programmes aimed at promoting the personal growth and resilience of participants. The enthusiasm generated by community-driven projects is often tangible – as when a teacher-training project takes on 'a life of its own'! Although the reporting on such programmes is inspiring, we are warned that not all interventions are successful. There are lessons to be learnt about what works and what does not in collectivist societies. Interventions that are insensitive to local customs and mores may fail, whereas culturally relevant approaches seem to work best.

The volume is divided into five parts. The introductory section reviews the quality-of-life literature with emphasis on the eudaimonic and positive psychology perspective, and introduces key concepts related to the social aspects of quality of life. In the second, third, and fourth parts, initiatives aimed at meeting Sustainable Development Goals for Africa are reported under the headings of development in *health* and *education* and *environment and technology*. Chapters grouped under the heading of *family* in the fifth part review the importance of belief in ancestors and spirituality, satisfactory family functioning, and child well-being.

One of the last chapters in the volume, this time written by a sympathetic 'outsider', reflects on how a visiting scholar based outside the continent understands the African ethic of *ubuntu*, a concept that is seen as key to advancing quality of life among the diverse peoples of Africa. This essay might be regarded as a timely 'reality check' to chart the way forward for future scholars of African quality of life.

Possibly the most important message from this collection of papers is that African societies are future-oriented. The final contribution to the volume written by the editor showcases the optimism and hope that inspire confidence that things will get better in the future.[3] Contributors note that Africa is a youthful continent. Promoting the well-being of the next generation is a winning strategy – the youth represent the future of society. Much will depend on how African societies provide opportunities for youth to gain not only skills but also dignity, self-respect and self-confidence to cope with the demands of a changing world. Many of the initiatives documented in this volume seek pathways to realising what is often referred to as the continent's demographic dividend.

To sum up, here is a book that offers a wealth of fresh ideas on what will make a difference for the well-being of the people living south of the Sahara. We learn there is enough energy and positivity at hand to make 'Africa work'[4] towards achieving a better quality of life in future. Best of all, *Quality of Life in African Societies* provides evidence that individuals and communities, working in concert, *can* advance well-being in Africa.

Emeritus Professor, Quality of Life Studies, Valerie Møller
Institute of Social and Economic Research
Rhodes University
Grahamstown, South Africa

References

Mills, G., Obasanjo, O., Herbst, J., & Davis, D. (2017). *Making Africa work: A handbook for economic success*. Cape Town, South Africa: Tafelberg.

Møller, V. (Ed.) (1997). *Quality of life in South Africa* (Social Indicators Research Series, Vol. 1). Dordrecht/Boston/London: Kluwer Academic Publishers. (Reprinted from *Social Indicators Research* 41(1–3)).

Møller V. (Ed.) (2007). Quality of life in South Africa – Ten years into democracy. *Social Indicators Research, 81*(2), 181–454.

Møller, V., & Roberts, B. (2017). New beginnings in an ancient region: Well-being in sub-Saharan Africa. In R. J. Estes & M. J. Sirgy (Eds.), *The pursuit of human well-being: The untold global history* (pp. 161–215). Cham, Switzerland: International Handbooks of Quality-of-Life Research/Springer.

[3]The concluding chapters in both the 1997 and 2007 South African reports on quality of life focus on social optimism for the future. The first chapter on Africa to appear in the World Happiness Report picks up on the theme of hope for the future (Møller et al., 2017).

[4]Referring to the evocative title of a new technical handbook for Africa compiled by African scholars and leaders (Mills et al., 2017).

Contents

Part III Health

Part IV Education

About the Editor

Irma Eloff is a professor of Educational Psychology at the University of Pretoria. She is also the Chairperson of the Council of *'Die Suid-Afrikaanse Akademie vir Wetenskap en Kuns'*. She is a member of the Academy of Science of South Africa (ASSAf) and a founding member of the South African Positive Psychology Association (SAPPA). In 2012, she was chosen amongst the top three Most Influential Women in Business and Government in South Africa in the Education category. She is a former dean of Education at the University of Pretoria. She was the seventh dean and the first woman to hold the position. During her term, Education at the University of Pretoria achieved a ranking in the top 150–200 of the world on the *World QS World university rankings* for five consecutive years.

She is the founder of the African Deans of Education Forum (ADEF), which is a focal point of the UNESCO International Teacher Task Force. The Teacher Task Force works to support the Sustainable Development Goals. Irma is an NRF-rated researcher and a registered psychologist in South Africa.

Irma Eloff is an editor of the books *Understanding Educational Psychology*, *Insigte uit Opvoedkundige Sielkunde* and *Keys to Educational Psychology*. She is the co-author of the book *Life Skills & Assets*.

She has held visiting professorships at Yale University, Rhodes University, the University of Wisconsin-Milwaukee, CPUT Wellington, Bath Spa University, UK, and Fordham University in New York. In 2018 she was awarded a Förderkreis 1669 Wissenschafft Gesellschaft professorship at the Universität Innsbruck.

Irma is an alumnus of the Universities of Pretoria, Stellenbosch, Northwest and the GIBS Business School.

Part I

Social Context, Culture and Community

1 Cultures of Positivity: Interconnectedness as a Way of Being

Marié P. Wissing, Lusilda Schutte, and Angelina Wilson Fadiji

Abstract

In this chapter we argued that a good quality of life and well-being is manifested in a culture of positivity emerging from meanings made in people's embeddedness in relationships and life contexts. Interconnectedness is a fundamental quality of being human, and to a great extent determines people's quality of life and meaning experiences. We adopted a broad conceptualization of quality of life including a eudaimonic well-being perspective in which meaning and positive relationships play a core role. We described a Meaning and Relatedness Well-being model (M&RW) comprising of meaning and relatedness as core facets, with assumed dynamic interactions between intrapersonal, interpersonal, social, community and ecosystem levels within the intertwinedness of biological and cultural situatedness. We used the M&RW model as backdrop to illustrate interconnectedness as a way of being well particularly in African contexts as manifested in lay people's experiences drawing from previous empirical research.

M. P. Wissing (✉) · L. Schutte
Africa Unit for Transdisciplinary Health Research, North-West University, Potchefstroom, South Africa
e-mail: Marie.Wissing@nwu.ac.za; Lusilda.Schutte@nwu.ac.za

A. Wilson Fadiji
Africa Unit for Transdisciplinary Health Research, North-West University, Potchefstroom, South Africa

Education and Skills Development Unit, Human Sciences Research Council, Cape Town, South Africa

In the so-called the third wave of positive psychology it is noted that the understanding of well-being focuses increasingly on relatedness and interconnectedness among people, highlighting the embeddedness of people in their socio-demographic, economic, environmental and cultural contexts (Wissing, 2018 – see also Delle Fave, 2014; Delle Fave et al., 2017; Demirci & Ekşi, 2018; Fowers & Anderson, 2018; Harrell, 2015, 2018; Helne & Hirvilammi, 2015; Warren & Donaldson, 2018). Being in relationships/interconnectedness with people (living or deceased), social and ecological contexts, and with spiritual powers, is strongly assumed as a way of being and giving meaning to life in most African contexts, and to a great extent in other (non-)individualistic contexts (e.g., Baloyi & Mokobe-Rabothata, 2014; Delle Fave & Soosai-Nathan, 2014; Harrell, 2018; Nwoye, 2017; Ogbonnaya, 1994; Selvam, 2013, 2015; Selvam & Collicutt, 2013; Urata, 2015; Wang, Wong, & Yeh, 2016; Warren & Donaldson, 2018).

In this chapter, we propose that well-being is manifested in a specific quality (culture of positivity) of meanings made in people's embeddedness in relationships and contexts. Meanings are

I. Eloff (ed.), *Handbook of Quality of Life in African Societies*, International Handbooks of Quality-of-Life, https://doi.org/10.1007/978-3-030-15367-0_1

made in the dynamic interactions between intrapersonal, interpersonal, social, community and ecosystem levels within the intertwinedness of biological and cultural situatedness. Interconnectedness is a fundamental quality of being human, and to a great extent determines people's quality of life. Although "quality of life" is mostly conceptualized and explored in terms of satisfaction with life, GDP and socio-economic variables in traditional quality of life studies (cf., Rojas, 2004, 2014, 2018), we adopt a broader conceptualization including a eudaimonic well-being perspective in which meaning and positive relationships play a core role – meanings are made in relatedness. In this chapter we will firstly clarify some notions expressed in our title. Then we will describe and use the Meaning and Relatedness Well-being model (M&RW) of interconnectedness (Wissing, 2016) as backdrop to illustrate interconnectedness as a way of being well particularly in African contexts.

1.1 Cultures of Positivity/Well-Being

1.1.1 Culture

Many definitions of culture can be found in existing literature, and a common trend is the reference to meaning and relational and contextual embeddedness. For example, the notion of shared meaning and relational functioning features in Triandis's description of culture as a climate of shared meaning systems that provides norms or standards for perceiving, believing, evaluating, communicating, and behaving among the people sharing a language, historical period or location (Triandis, 1996). Chiu and Chen (2004) defined 'culture' as "a network of knowledge that is produced, distributed and reproduced among a collection of interconnected people" (p. 173). Accentuated here is the notion of *interconnectedness/relatedness* in which cognitions (knowledge/meaning) are made and shared.

Harrell (2015) provided an encompassing definition of culture in her analysis of culture and well-being as part of her proposed PEaCE theory. She described culture as "*the multiple historical, sociopolitically-situated, and organizing systems of meaning, knowledge, and daily living that involve* ***patterns of being, believing, bonding, belonging, behaving, and becoming*** *which provide foundational frames for developing worldview, interpreting reality, and acting in the world for a group of people who share common ancestry, social location, group identity, or defining experiential context; but for whom, as individuals or intersectional subgroups, particular elements of a cultural system may be embraced, internalized, and expressed differently. Cultural systems emerge and transform over time through cumulative and adaptation-oriented person-environment transactions, and are maintained and transmitted through collective memory, narrative, and socialization processes*" (Harrell, 2015, p. 18) (emphasis original). Harrell (2015) opined that cultural systems are dynamic and simultaneously embedded in institutional and social contexts. Such cultural systems are patterns of meaning and identity, which are reflected in actions and relationships. Similar ideas that individual functioning is interdependent with the meanings and practices of specific socio-cultural contexts were expressed by others, for example Cruz and Sonn (2011) who noted that culture (in a traditional sense – but it is also true for culture in a broad sense) is inseparable from who we are as persons and how we function as social beings, but also that culture is shaped by socio-historical and political processes.

In this chapter the construct "culture/cultures" is broadly used as referring to climates/atmospheres/breathing spaces as existing in a broader network/system or in a niche or node within a broader system with shared norms, processes and behaviour among the collection of interconnected people; it can also refer to internal states or individual climates and processes, and to culture in the narrow more traditional sense. Cultures or climates in a psychosocial sense are thus distinguished on individual, group, community, and larger societal, national and broader levels.

1.1.2 Positivity/Well-Being: The Positives and Negatives of Life

In this chapter we use the terms positivity and well-being interchangeably to indicate the functioning well quality of psychosocial health. Positive and negative feelings, experiences and events are part of life and need to be recognized as such even if the focus is on the positive /functioning well aspects. The positives and negatives of life as constructs refer in many perspectives to two polarities or to two separate dimensions of human experience (e.g., Seligman & Csikszentmihalyi, 2000), but they can also be deeply intertwined in human experiences (cf., Held, 2017; Johnson & Wood, 2015; Lomas, 2018; Lomas & Ivtzan, 2015). In general positive psychology and wider psychological literature, these constructs mainly refer to: affect (positive and negative affect); life-events (positive/good and negative/bad); mental health versus mental ill-health; specific qualities on individual, group/social and institutional levels (positive qualities such as satisfaction, happiness, hope, optimism, perspective, capacity for joy, work-ethic; and negative qualities such as depression, anxiety, lack of self-regulation, aggression, etc.); value connotations of the good versus the bad (is the good the same as the right, the prudent as the moral, is the bad also wrong?); and what is preferred (sustainably preferred) versus not-preferred. The idea of the positive as what is preferred and the negative what is not-preferred was indicated by Seligman (2002) and elaborated by Pawelski (2016a, 2016b) who added the idea that the positive is what is sustainably preferred over time. Tamir and Gross (2011) stressed that the definition of the positive and negative should not only be in terms of how they (the emotions) feel (pleasantness), but also whether they promote positive functioning or not. King, Heintzelman, and Ward (2016) indicated that positive feelings can indeed promote the experience of meaning and functioning well.

What is positive and what is negative also depend on the *context* in which this evaluation is made, i.e. how it is interpreted taking the contextual aspects into account (Held, 2016, 2017). This point was initially strongly made by McNulty and Fincham (2012) who challenged the assumption that specific psychological processes or characteristics are inherently beneficial for well-being and that the conditions in which constructs referring to these processes are investigated should be taken into account. They illustrated their position with reference to forgiveness, which may in the long run harm the well-being (and even survival) of women who are in abusive relationships. The importance of context to determine the meaning of 'positive' constructs or the quality of experiences as desirable or not-desirable, or understanding the intertwinedness is increasingly being emphasized (e.g., Harrell, 2018; Held, 2017; Kimhi, 2016; Lomas, 2016, 2018; Lomas & Ivtzan, 2015). The importance of worldviews (that may differ in various cultural contexts) for the understanding and evaluation of what is seen as good or bad, or as positive or negative in a particular life context, had been indicated by amongst others Held (2017) and Slife, O'Grady, and Kosits (2017).

Kuppens, Realo, and Diener (2008) found in an empirical study that positive and negative emotional experiences are differentially emphasized in various cultural contexts and that these are less negatively associated in collectivist than individualist cultural contexts. Very little research exists in this regard in the African relatively collectivist context. In the literature emotional or affective complexity is viewed as instances when positive and negative emotions can co-occur and have a low correlation (positive or negative). Hershfield, Scheibe, Sims, and Carstensen (2013) contended that a weak negative or a positive correlation between positive and negative affect shows a relative independence of positive and negative emotions, and that it is associated with greater emotional complexity. Such correlations were found to be lower in relatively collectivist Asian cultural contexts than in non-Asian western contexts (Schimmack, Oishi, & Diener, 2002). In a South African context, Wissing (2016) showed that positive and negative emotions as measured with the Positive and Negative Affect subscales of the Affectometer 2 displayed smaller positive correlations in various African, relatively more collectivist groups, than in multicultural or white relatively more individualist groups, indicating a more natural co-existence of the positives and negatives of life in African collectivist contexts.

In understanding "positivity", we discuss an interconnectedness model of well-being with meaning and relatedness as core facets. We propose that the dynamics of the positives and negatives in life are manifested in the quality of processes and experienced relatedness and connectedness (to others, the environment, the physical context and the mental and emotional context) and are expressed in the meanings detected and construed in these (cf., Wissing, 2016). If the quality of experiences and meanings construed or detected are characterized by harmony rather than disharmony, a culture of positivity/well-being/functioning well exists (cf., Dambrun, 2017; Dambrun et al., 2012; Delle Fave, 2014, 2017; Delle Fave et al., 2016; Wang, Wong, Yeh, & Wang, 2018). The idea that the quality of experiences on the individual level is reciprocally influenced by processes and climates of the broader interpersonal, social, political, and cultural systems, all seamlessly connecting to each other, links with that of Kashima (2014) who contended that cultural and social dynamics are in fact about changes in *meanings* over time within these processes and *relations*. This notion also resonates with White's (2017) perspective on relational well-being and relational ontology.

The notion of "cultures of positivity" is thus used in this chapter in a broad sense and refers to niches or nodes of well-being/positivity among a collection or 'family' of processes/intrapersonal facets (e.g., emotion, cognition and behavior) or interconnected people in a network. The reference to the climate or atmosphere in a niche of facets/processes/interconnected people – be it a small node or a larger system – can be characterized by a relatively harmonious resonance among elements, relatively high levels of positive affect, a 'healthy' positive-negative affect ratio, complex affect and cognition, as well as other characteristics of functioning well such as the experience of meaning, gratitude, hope, etc. Both hedonic and eudaimonic features are part of broader well-being. Keyes (1998) described *social well-being* (associated with a culture of positivity) as characterized by the experiences and perceptions of coherence, integration, actualization, contribution and adaptation in a social context. These characteristics will also be markers of cultures of positivity in smaller social niches or nodes of connectedness. Cultures of positivity thus not only refers to affect, emotions and satisfaction with life, but is also about meaning and values and group enabling processes and behaviors, i.e. well-being in a broad sense. A 'culture of positivity' is conceptualized to be found on various levels from the intrapersonal to interpersonal to the social or community levels. Manifestations and processes on the various levels can influence each other reciprocally.

In this chapter it is argued that the quality of experienced relatedness and connectedness (to others, the environment, the physical context and the mental and emotional context) and the meanings detected and construed in these determine the overall level of experienced well-being and broader culture of positivity. We will describe and illustrate manifestations of cultures of positivity and quality of life as expressed in lay people's experiences of meaning and relatedness in various African communities.

1.2 The Meaning and Relatedness Well-Being Model (M&RW)

Specific components of the M&RW model will be argued, described, and illustrated with empirical examples in an African context, reflecting the quality of life described here as a culture of positivity.

1.2.1 Meaning

Meaning as a main construct in the proposed M&RW model (Wissing, 2016) share some notions with the philosophical views of Metz

(2015) and theoretical perspectives of Wong (2011, 2016) but also differs from these in so far as that meaning in the M&RW model is conceptualized as emerging from qualities and processes in relationships and connections. We concur with Metz's (2015) view of the fundamental conditions of human existence namely, human personhood, human sociality, and human environmental situatedness. He, however, also contended that life is meaningful in so far as that reason (in a wide sense including emotion, behaviour, etc.) is directed at, and positively engaged with the basic conditions (deep facets) of human existence, and posited that his model captures the intuitions about the good, the true and the beautiful better than any other theory (he only took cognisance of theories in Western contexts). Our perspective differs from his in that, amongst others, his naturalist fundamentality theory of meaning sees it as solely playing out in a physical world (he rejected all 'supernaturalist' views), whereas the M&RW model proposed here includes also a spiritual or transcendental component – highly applicable also in an African context. In this regard our notion of meaning is closer to that of Urata's (2015) nested model taking cognisance of both philosophical and psychological literature and also including a transcendental system. The notion of meaning in the proposed M&RW model shares some ideas with those in Wong's (2011, 2016) meaning model and meaning orientated research trying to answer the question of how is it possible for people to live meaningful and fulfilling lives despite the dark side of life such as suffering, death, disaster, and negative affect eliciting experiences. He contended also that meaning is based on values and cultural norms.

Our view also dovetails with that of Heine, Proulx, and Vohs (2006) who contended that meaning in life refers to understanding who we are, our place in the world and how we fit into the grand scheme of things; and to that of Martela and Steger (2016) who argued that evaluations of the presence of meaning involve the extent to which an individual deems life as purposeful, coherent and significant. Other researchers also considered meaning as a holistic phenomenon at the core of human existence and well-being: It is linked to the core of the self (Schlegel & Hicks, 2016; Schlegel, Hicks, King, & Arndt, 2011) and need to be explored not only quantitatively, but specifically also qualitatively in a bottom up manner (George & Park, 2016). In order to tap into the extent to which individuals experience meaning in their lives, researchers typically explore subjective evaluation of how meaningful an individual estimates his or her life is (Lambert et al., 2013).

Meaning as proposed in the M&RW interconnectedness model does not only refer to the understanding of meaning in the sense of cognition, purpose, emotion and behavior, but also to a bodily felt preverbal sense as implied in attachment theory and hypothesized in Gendlin's (1996) description of a preverbal felt sense as part of his focused oriented psychotherapy. In her adaptation of the felt sense hypothesis Ann Weiser Cornell developed a view of the felt sense as mainly relational, and extended the view of the focusing process, which she called Inner Relationship Focusing, to discovering of meaning via the bodily felt sense in relationship with and among all the parts of the self (cf., Cornell & McGavin, 2008). This bodily, biological component in which meaning is anchored is also highlighted in Delle Fave and Massimini's (2015) description of the interplay between culture and biology. Czekierda, Banik, Park, and Luszczynska (2017) found in a systematic review of empirical studies that the experience of meaning in life and physical health are significantly (albeit weak to moderately) associated, and that this association is stronger when measures of meaning were combined with items referring to a sense of harmony and peace – thus positive relational qualities.

Notions of the main components of meaning in the literature differ, but also evolve further over time: Steger, Oishi, and Kashdan (2009) proposed a meaning model with two main components: (i) coherence/cognitive understanding, and (ii) purpose/motivation/aims and aspirations. Martela and Steger (2016) opined that meaning has three main components as found in their literature review, namely coherence, purpose and significance (the latter described in terms of affective evaluation). They view relatedness as a source of meaning rather than a component. The components identified by Martela and Steger (2016) link to some degree with those proposed by George and Park (2016), namely cognitive, motivational and affective/existential mattering. The transcendental aspect of meaning is noted by various researchers such as Delle Fave and Soosai-Nathan (2014) and King, Hicks, Krull, and Del Gaiso (2006).

Meaning in life is linked to well-being in a variety of cultural contexts and life stages. For example, Ho, Cheung, and Cheung (2010) showed that meaning in life is significantly associated with multidimensional life satisfaction in a Korean sample of adolescents; Rathi and Rastogi (2007) established that meaning in life is linked to well-being in an Indian sample of adolescents; and Reker and Wong (2012) established that personal meaning is associated with positive psychosocial adaptation in later years. Reflecting on meaning in life and life stages, Awasthi, Chauhan, and Verma (2016) revealed that adolescents were found to be deeply involved in the search for meaning whereas the elderly participants showed greater levels of presence of meaning. In a South African and broader African context an important source of meaning is found in horizontal and vertical relationships (e.g., Baloyi & Mokobe-Rabothata, 2014; Mason, 2013; White, 2017; Wissing, Khumalo, & Chigeza, 2014). In explaining meaning within an African context, Mason (2013) argued that African metaphors, which encapsulate unique cultural beliefs and worldviews, were embedded in the knowledge or experiences of meaning. Based on this, he concluded that appreciating the concepts of ubuntu and Batho Pele might be a breakthrough in understanding meaning in an African context.

Some empirical examples will now be provided from different African samples where interconnectedness and relatedness was implied as the core of the experience of meaning, illustrating the interwovenness of these constructs in the manifestation of cultures of positivity.

When asked what the most important meaningful things for a person are and why these are meaningful, participants in a South African context typically referred to 'children', 'family', 'church', 'God', 'life' but also 'life stock', 'house' (PURE-FORT3, Ganyesa; see Wilson, Wissing, Schutte, & Kruger, 2018a; Wissing, Schutte, & Kruger, 2018b for a description of context and general method). They thus referred to close horizontal and vertical relationships, but also to contextual material things. Interestingly when motivating the reasons for material things to be sources of meaning they typically referred to relational aspects such as wanting to provide for children or family, or, for example, when mentioning a 'life stock' as a source of meaning the reason was to be able to contribute to a funeral in the community, pointing strongly to the importance of context in understanding cultures of positivity.

In making sense of their experiences in a context of poverty and deprivation, adolescents in Northern Ghana capitalized on the sense of connectedness forged in close relationships with family members. These networks provided a source of hope and purpose in the process of meaning-making:

> Our parents bring hope to us. They bring hope to the hopeless. What I am saying is that they sometimes motivate us (19-year old male, Grade 12).

Relatedly, vertical relationships with the supernatural were drawn upon in difficult times. Making sense of the future from the belief that the connection to the supernatural would provide a pathway from the present to a proposed future was common in this context (see also Wilson & Somhlaba, 2016).

> Sometimes I pray to God knowing that one day things will be better. Prayers are the key to any success (19-year- old male, Grade 12).

In Wilson and Mittelmark (2013), female porters in Ghana indicated that understanding God's sovereignty was crucial in making meaning in life. They appreciated that there will be good days and bad days, all dependent on what God decides to give them. Their connection with the spiritual served as an explanatory factor for their lives.

> If today is bad, tomorrow will be better; there will be times where we'll get more money. I'm fine; life is fine. It's better than before. It's not every day good will come. God can be good today and bad tomorrow. This makes life meaningful (20-year old female).

Some lessons that can be gleaned from spirituality and meaning in the African context, is that spiritual relatedness provides some form of comfort and hope in adversity. Its significance lies in enabling individuals to feel that they can comprehend and manage the challenges they encounter. Greeff and Loubser (2008) argued that spirituality as a form of religious expression enabled Xhosa-speaking families in South Africa to resile as a result of the meaning derived from it. Religious expressions such as prayer and fellowships provided hope, outlook and a sense of purpose to the sample of study. In line with this, Copeland-Linder (2006) indicated that religious attributions to God enabled individuals to find meaning in stressful situations because it provided perspective to problems and a sense of purpose in life. Religion seems to be able to provide clear and definite frameworks of meaning that address life's existential concerns (Newton & McIntosh, 2013) and thus contribute to a positive quality of life in everyday living.

Horizontal relationships also appeared to be crucial in making sense of living life on the streets among female porters in Ghana. These women who were migrants from the Northern part of Ghana, forged close relationships with other women in the context of unsafe physical spaces where they were at risk for rape and other forms of harm (Wilson & Mittelmark, 2013). Within these physical spaces, social spaces of connectedness were created in order to sustain one another and fulfil their goals.

In illustrating, the cultures of positivity as being ingrained in eudaimonic aspects of well-being such as meaning-making and goal-setting, research in Ghana revealed that satisfaction in life was embedded in the experience of purpose and achievement of goals.

> To be satisfied in life means to achieve the goals that you have set (20-year-old male, Grade 11).

Also noteworthy is the manifestation of the interconnectedness of well-being in niches of positivity grounded in consideration of interpersonal evaluation. Adolescents in Ghana related their experience of life satisfaction to positive perceptions from significant others as seen below.

> ...Sometimes it is [about how] people see you. For instance, if people talk about you in a good [way] it makes you say you are satisfied with your behaviour. ... But if they think of you negatively then you [have to] strive towards redeeming your image (17-year old male, Grade 11; Wilson & Somhlaba, 2016).

1.2.2 Relatedness

"Relatedness" in the M&RW model refers to links and interactions among the various intrapersonal, interpersonal, and transpersonal components, i.e. the links facilitating interactions within facets of the self and between the individual and their physical and spiritual environments in space and time including other people, the physical, cultural and historical contexts. Relatedness in the M&RW model refers to all connections in which an individual is situated. These connections are conduits through which interpretations and meanings are made or discovered. They are the channels in which the dynamics of processes take place which determine the quality of the experiences and balance between the positives and negatives.

Integration or interconnectedness among affect, cognition and other facets on an intrapersonal level is linked to functioning well as noted in research on self-compassion (e.g., Neff & Costigan, 2014) and self-regulation (Van Tongeren et al., 2018). With regard to interpersonal connectedness, Nafstad, Blakar, Carlquist, Phelps, and Rand-Hendriksen (2009) remarked that main stream psychology has greatly ignored the very important reality of life, namely that each of us is dependent on other people in many ways, and that we are by nature prosocial beings. Prilleltensky and Prilleltensky (2007) stressed from a social psychology perspective the interconnectedness of individual, interpersonal and collective well-being, and Helne and Hirvilammi (2015) as well as Harrell (2015) argued from a sustainable developmental perspective that human well-being and the ecosystem are interrelated and interdependent on each other for health and well-being on the long term. White (2010) argued that relationships are not possessed but people become who they are through these relationships. People are better understood within a specific social and cultural context (White, 2010). Wissing et al. (2014) indicated that relational well-being is viewed as an important marker of psychosocial well-being in many theories, but that its nature, dynamics, measurement and manifestation in various contexts are not well-explored, explicated and captured in comprehensive theories and is actually a seriously neglected topic in positive psychology. O'Connell, O'Shea, and Gallagher (2016) indicated the paucity of research on interventions to enhance social relationships.

It is well known to all of us how important our close relationships are as they are the sources of our joy and experiences of meaningfulness, but also sometimes the sources of pain and great sadness. In the literature various positive qualities and experiences are associated with positive relationships, for example, positive affect, intimacy, caring, sharing, loving, interest, minding, excitement, self-disclosure, curiosity, wonder, gratitude, forgiveness – mostly studied as intrapersonal processes (e.g., Fincham & Beach, 2010; Gable & Gosnell, 2011; Gable & Reis, 2010; Gere & Macdonald, 2013; Majors, 2012; Meunier & Baker, 2012; Wissing, 2014). Some typical features of positive relationships are (i) *Knowing the other and letting yourself be known* – i.e., reciprocal self-disclosure, mutual understanding and deeper connectedness; (ii) *Mutual trust* – i.e., self-disclosure which assumes safety and trust, and expects that no harm will be done and confidences will be respected; (iii) *Intertwined lives* – i.e., interdependence and mutual influence in thinking, feeling and acting; (iv) *Concern and caring* – i.e., mindfulness expressed in a genuine concern for the other, monitoring how the other is doing, and relationship maintenance; (v) *We-ness and mutuality* – i.e., closeness expressed in using "we" or "us", and a sense of overlap between lives (however not "enmeshed"); (vi) *Commitment* – i.e., the intention to continue the relationship despite the ups and downs that may occur and to spend energy on maintaining and building the relationship.

Several empirical studies indicated the important link between positive relationships and well-being. The centrality of relationships in human life for the experience of meaningfulness was long ago already argued in Baumeister's classical work on meaning in life (Baumeister, 1991), and the strength of the "belongingness hypothesis" was demonstrated in a review of empirical findings by Baumeister and Leary (1995). They argued with reference to empirical findings that when the need for belongingness is not fulfilled, it has detrimental effects on adjustment, health and well-being, whereas satisfaction of needs for relatedness contributes to greater satisfaction with life, happiness and a sense of meaning and purpose in life. This need for social relationships is grounded in the biological need to belong that offer a symbolic promise of continuity and immortality (Lifton, 1979). This also linked to the opportunity for procreation (Mikulincer, Florian, & Hirschberger, 2004) and the feeling of being part of larger than transcends the limitations of an entity (Aron & Aron, 1996). Ryff and Singer (1998, 2000) reviewed empirical findings showing that the experience of loving relationships and purposeful living is linked to better recovery from illnesses, and also operates as a protective and promotive mechanism for health and well-being. These findings were further substantiated by Ryff and Singer (2008) in a review of empirical findings suggesting that living a life of purpose and meaning and high quality bonds with others are associated with psychological well-being and better physical health. Ryff, Singer, and Love (2004) showed that eudaimonic well-being, that includes positive relationships and purpose and meaning in life, contributed to better health as illustrated by lower cortisol levels, lower cardiovascular risk, lower pro-inflammatory cytokines and longer REM sleep. Relationships are deeply linked to meaning, but also to other markers of well-being such as happiness. For example, Delle Fave et al. (2016) showed the primacy of harmony and relational connectedness as core characteristics of happiness as experienced by lay people in various countries. Gable and colleagues (e.g., Algoe, Gable, & Maisel, 2010; Gable, Gonzaga, & Strachman, 2006) showed the importance of the quality of interactions between partners and the importance of sharing positive experiences. Gable and Reis (2010) reported extensively on empirical evidence for the intrapersonal and interpersonal salubrious effects of capitalization (including perceived partner responsiveness referred to above) as defined in their model. The centrality of interconnectedness for well-being on and among various system levels and in various contexts were also highlighted by Delle Fave (2017), Dambrun (2017), Fowers and Anderson (2018), Harrell (2018), and Warren and Donaldson (2018).

The role of spiritual well-being and its intertwinedness with individual and interpersonal relatedness and well-being is neglected in current research and theory. There is an existing, but relatively small body of empirical evidence showing that meaning in life is associated with spirituality, transcendence and a connection to something larger than the self and sacred (vertical relatedness). Steger (2012) reviewed evidence that experienced meaning in life is associated with general spiritual experiences, intrinsic religiosity, religious activity, and connectedness with what is deemed sacred and transcendent. Joshanloo (2010) showed that both spirituality and religiosity are significantly associated with well-being defined and operationalized hedonically and eudaimonically (the latter included meaning facets as in Ryff's and Keyes's scales) in an Iranian sample. These studies thus showed that relatedness to facets of the self, others, society and the transendent is associated with the experience of meaning in life and various other indicators of well-being. However, there seems to be a gap in the existing western empirical studies on the relationship between spiritual connectedness and connection in human bonds, and on the way in which meaning, spirituality and relational well-being hang together, except for findings that both relationships and spirituality were deemed the most important sources of meaning in some studies referred to above. In an African context, the connection between vertical, horizontal and intrapsychic dimensions of functioning are very prominent. In this regard, Wissing et al. (2014) noted that interpersonal and spiritual relatedness are intertwined in relational well-being and meaning in an African group.

Our M&RW interconnectedness model dovetails with African worldviews. Some of the characteristics of this worldview is that it is grounded in interdependence, collectivism, harmony with nature, and spirituality (Baloyi & Mokobe-Rabothata, 2014; Gyekye, 1995; Nwoye, 2015). Accordingly, "Africans understand their being-in-the-world as a qualitative tapestry of connected systems which deal with life issues collectively and collaboratively" (Baloyi & Mokobe-Rabothata, 2014, p. 265). This inclusive connectedness even extends beyond the visible world of the senses to the spiritual realm (Nwoye, 2015). The spiritualist perspective is dominant in understanding human functioning in an African context (Nwoye, 2015). The spiritual and/or ancestral background of an individual is as important as their intrapersonal, interpersonal, bodily, and social dimensions (Nwoye, 2015). Other scholars have linked the well-being of the individual and even future generations with the sense of communality (Dandala, 2009). In the Eastern Cape of South Africa, life satisfaction was determined by not only financial status but the ability to live well with others (Cramm, Møller, & Nieboer, 2010). The emphasis on harmony and stability in these studies link also with a collectivist orientation and worldview which often underlies relationships in the African context.

Some empirical examples will now be provided from different African datasets where the importance of interconnectedness and relatedness on the various levels of human functioning, and the associations thereof with well-being, as manifestations of cultures of positivity are demonstrated.

In an older South African Setswana-speaking sample, participants were asked what their most important relationships were together with the reasons for the importance of these relationships. Horizontal relationships (such as with family, parents, children, spouses friends, and neighbours) were very commonly mentioned, and the reasons often reflected provided, enacted, and mutual support (Wilson, Wissing, & Schutte, 2018b). The associations between horizontal relationships, meaning in life and well-being were also often expressed.

> Neighbours…… Is the first person to respond in good or bad times, and also looks after my house when I am not there (Rural participant 5, 63-year old female).
> Cooperating with children…to send them to run errands and they should be willing to do that (Rural participant 1, 60-year old female).
> Family….We help each other" (Urban participant 8, 61-year old female)
> "Children … My children to have purpose (Rural participant, 93-year old female).
> Wife … We live happy and I love her" (Urban participant, 76-year old male).

However, the impact of interpersonal relationships on well-being could take different forms and might include both positive and negative experiences depending on the context. For instance, Wilson and Somhlaba (2016) found that, although some adolescents in poor regions of Northern Ghana experienced quality social interactions from members of extended families, others were faced with neglect and lack of provision for their basic needs. In some cases, peers were preferred when in need for material support, while others experienced adequate care from the family. Although social exchanges across both family and peers were necessary for relational well-being, not all of these enhanced overall well-being.

> I always have problem with my step-mother. I always think that if you ask something from my father she will always ask my father not to give you. I think so because she always talks about us badly. These things make me unhappy most of the time (20-year old male, Grade 12).
> I relate well with my family most especially my mother (20-year old male, Grade 11).
> Yes they [family] always try their best, even though it is not enough they try their best for me (20-year old male, Grade 11).

Apart from interpersonal relationships emerging as important relationships in African contexts, there is also an emphasis on the transcendental. In a study among older Setswana-speaking participants in South Africa, God and spiritual organizations emerged as important relationships, because they offered support, spiritual guidance, meaning, and pleasure. A sense of connectedness with the supernatural afforded the experience of a sense of identity and answers to difficulties posed by life's difficult circumstances (see also Wilson et al., 2018b).

> Church … It makes my feelings to be right (Urban participant, 58-year old female).
> Church … It's the one that supports me and teaches me purpose (Rural participant, 87-year old male).
> Church…..It builds me spiritually (Rural participant 25, 74-year old female).
> God….. Because when I pray, after a while, I see answers and that life changes for the better (Rural participant 11, 61-year old male).

Among Ghanaian adolescents, spiritual relatedness provided the assurance that needs would be met. Such assurance was needed to make sense of the deprivation that the adolescents were faced with (cf., Wilson & Somhlaba, 2016).

> Yea, like … if I need something and I didn't get it… like for example, I told my parents that I need money and they say they don't have and I will say ok by the grace of Almighty Allah you will get it (18-year old female, Grade 11).

1.2.3 Meaning, Relatedness and Context

Empirical studies showed that close interpersonal and family relationships are the primary sources for the experience of happiness and meaningfulness in various cultural contexts (Baumeister, Vohs, Aaker, & Garbinsky, 2013; Delle Fave, Wissing, Brdar, Vella-Brodrick, & Freire, 2013). It has been empirically indicated that well-being (defined and operationalized from both eudaimonic and hedonic perspectives) is influenced by sociodemographic characteristics such as gender, age, and in particular education, and socioeconomic status (e.g., occupational status, income); and cultural context (Karasawa et al.,

2011; Reker & Woo, 2011; Stroink & DeCicco, 2011; Uchida & Ogihara, 2012; Wissing & Temane, 2013). There is thus an influential relationship between the individual and larger context. In all cultural contexts, relationships and meaningful pursuits are important, but the specific construals of the self, relationships and what is meaningful may differ to a great extent, and thus also the expression thereof in specific behaviors within the parameters of opportunities and boundaries of the specific context. Studies in the African context are scarce, and it cannot be assumed that African collectivist orientations are the same as Asian perspectives (Wissing & Temane, 2013).

Much of the research on well-being overlooked the interplay between individuals and their social and cultural environment, especially in African realities. Such contextual factors are often neglected in western psychology, which primarily focuses on the subjective dimension of well-being and on the level of autonomy individuals experience in determining which goals, values and meanings they prefer. However, both the environment and the individual ceaselessly undergo changes (Slife & Richardson, 2008), and western perspectives ignore the fact that cultural differences in value systems affect the weight and the meaning individuals may attribute to collective norms, daily activities, and social roles (Berry, Segall, & Kagitcibasi, 1997; Triandis, 1994). Even within a geographical boundary, relational experiences and well-being in general could differ. For instance, due to urbanization, older people are increasingly losing their place in rural settings and there is immense social exclusion being experienced in urban settings (Walsh, O'Shea, Scharf, & Shucksmith, 2014). The experience of social exclusion manifested in little concern for others, fewer opportunities for interaction, financial insecurity and changing compositions of localities with the moving away of friends and family (Walsh et al., 2014). Wilson et al. (2018b) indicated that among older adults living in rural areas in South Africa, dependability and trust characterized relational interactions, which was not very apparent in urban settings. Relatedly, Wilson and Somhlaba (2017) found that contextual demographic variables such as gender and religious affiliation determined levels of hope and emotional well-being. Adolescents affiliated with Islam did better on emotional well-being as compared to their Christian counterparts.

The tendency to neglect contextual factors is also found in positive psychology (Christopher & Hickinbottom, 2008; Richardson & Guignon, 2008). This limitation derives from the western individualistic background in which positive psychology was developed, and leads researchers to neglect the impact of cultural norms and beliefs on the subjective interpretation of meaning, well-being and quality of life (Becker & Marecek, 2008). Cultural, economic, and collective rules and norms can expand or restrict the opportunities for action, development and flourishing available to individuals and groups within a society. Although some empirical (mostly western) studies showed connections between the quality of relationships, meaningfulness and well-being, as well as the influence of context, there is gap in the literature on how meaning, relational well-being and context hang together in an African context and quality of life.

Some empirical examples from African studies that stress the importance of context in intra-, inter- and transpersonal functioning, and which include reference to the experience and manifestation of meaning and relatedness, will now be provided. This illustrates how quality of life and cultures of positivity are embedded in context.

A sample of rural Setswana-speaking South African participants from the Ganyesa area were asked the researcher about their community and what was good about their community (PURE-FORT3 project referred to above). Responses included the following:

> The residents of this community are people who have a positive impact in people's lives, they come together and help each other in problems. … They are the kind of people who have good intentions about what they want to do (70-year old female).
>
> They help people when they are in trouble, they are full of love. … I love how they work together if you are in need (47-year old female).
>
> They are good people and they have peace. If you need help they do help you. I love how they operate here in Ganyesa and how people have good hearts (47-year old female).

> People of this community are good people, they help each other when they are in need. … I grew up here this is a village, life here is better than life in the city especially if you are not working (48-year old male).

In exploring the literature, we find that there is a dearth of reference to meaning, relationships and context in psychological well-being research. However, some existing studies on relational well-being tend to implicitly indicate the centrality of social networks for the experience of meaning and other forms of positivity in context. In some deprived contexts in Ghana, research shows that the experience of happiness was tied to the well-being of their children (Wilson & Mittelmark, 2013).

> I'm not happy; my child is sick, and I don't have money. When my child is well, then I can say that I'm happy (20-year old female).

When comparing aged urban and rural Setswana-speaking South African contexts, Wilson et al. (2018b) revealed that manifestations of relational well-being differed between the two groups. In urban contexts, relationships with the family were appreciated because of the strong bonds of identity it provided, while in rural contexts, this was linked mainly to the provision of needs.

> Children……They are my life and I make sure that they fit in the community (Urban participant 1, 60-year old female).
>
> Family…..Because I love them (Urban participant 4, 60-year old female).

1.2.4 The M&R Model Embedded in the Scientific Text

The M&RW model is conceptualized as embedded in the theoretical layer of the scientific text that can be viewed as consisting of empirical, theoretical and meta-theoretical facets or layers differing in abstraction levels but influencing each other reciprocally (cf., Madsen, 1988). This whole scientific text is conceptualized to be situated in time and space. On the empirical side people entertain certain values contributing to their experience of the meaning *of* life, they experience meaning and relatedness *in* various domains and contexts of life, and they will intentionally or non-intentionally act to give meaning *to* their lives as will be manifested in the quality of relatedness to the self, others, the environment, the greater good and the Other. Empirical findings and observations on this level inform the conceptualization of the M&RW model of well-being. From the meta-theoretical perspective, ontological and epistemological assumptions influence model conceptualization. The meta-theoretical layer includes philosophical beliefs about the world (worldview or ontology, specifically also conceptions about the nature of human beings) and about science (philosophy of science or epistemology, specifically with reference to the origin of cognition/knowledge and its relation to reality).

The M&RW model specifically assumes a systems perspective of the world and humans, and a strong relational ontology stance (i.e., assuming the interconnectedness of all things – cf., Nicolescu, 2014a, 2014b, 2015a, 2015b; Richardson, 2012), a virtue ethics perspective (transcending the means-end split – cf., Fowers, 2010, 2012), and is grounded in a eudaimonic philosophical perspective. As far as epistemological assumptions is concerned, it is assumed that the origin of "knowledge" can be empirical, rational or intuitive, and with regard to the issue of the relation between cognition and reality, critical-realist, constructivist and pragmatist positions can be entertained in various substudies to inform theory-building. With regard to methodological assumptions, it is assumed that both quantitative and qualitative methods are acceptable in the production of knowledge, with a preference for a multi- or mixed method-approaches for knowledge generation.

1.2.5 Meaning and Relatedness as Core or DNA of the Model

The inextricable link of meaning and relatedness is visually depicted in the proposed model analogously to the biological DNA-helix or double spiral string (see Fig. 1.1) also symbolizing

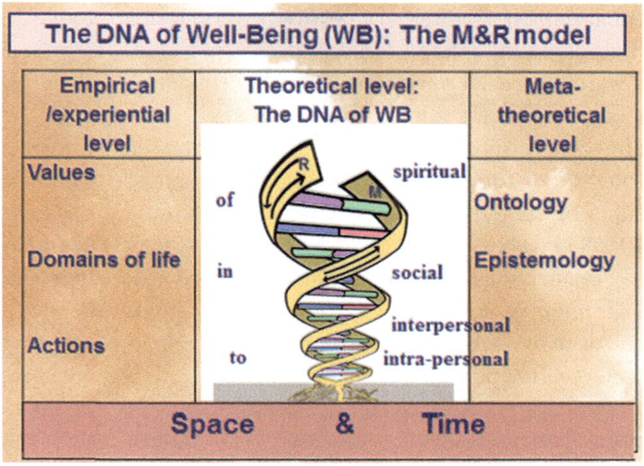

Fig. 1.1 The meaning and relatedness well-being model (Wissing, 2016)

the biological anchoredness of human beings. However, in the visualization of the M&RW model the helix string widens as in a cone, spiraling upwards to include wider and increasing complex systems (from intrapersonal, to interpersonal, social and transcendental) all functioning in space and time. Meaning and relatedness as core components in functioning well are anchored and transmitted in the interplay of biology and culture as two interlinked systems which influence individual development, behavior and social development as described by Delle Fave and Massimini (2015).

The interplay of biology and culture was argued by Delle Fave and Massimini (2015) by showing how biological developments helped individuals to start to manipulate their environments and eventually create norms, rules, and roles which facilitated the development of culture. According to them the development of culture over time can be viewed as a second inheritance system, but with several differences from the biological system. Meanings are made or discovered through *psychological selection* which is the individual processing of bio-cultural information. Psychological selection can be influenced by cultural factors (such as religious beliefs).

The basic unit of information in the cultural system is the *meme* (Delle Fave & Massimini, 2015) analogously with the gene as the replication unit in the biological system. A meme is a unit of cultural meaning, any characteristic of a culture, for example language, which can be transmitted from one generation to the next in a way analogous to the transmission of genetic information. Memes are *carried and stored* in the central nervous system in the form of ideas, knowledge, experiences, learned rules for behavior, and they are also expressed in cultural artefacts (products of human activity such as books, art, music, buildings), i.e. *they are meaning carriers*. Whereas genes cannot *survive its carriers*, memes can. Genes are *coded* in biological structures (DNA), but *memes are expressed in multiple codes* such as language, rituals, dance, and non-verbal behavior. Whereas genes are *passed on* via biological transmission, memes can be communicated and spread in various ways to many people at the same time, for example via words, non-verbal communication, and in writing. Thus, such messages can *spread fast* and to many people at the same time – *via all sorts of connections and relationships* (self-talk, family discussions, group processes, internet, etc.). These ideas resonate with the notion of Baumeister and Landau (2018) that "human use of meaning is inherently collective" (p. 7).

In the cultural system *new information units can be formed* (Delle Fave & Massimini, 2015) which can be beneficial for development and adaptation. Such new units can be deliberately sought to facilitate change – for example the enhancement of cultures of positivity on all levels (intrapersonal, interpersonal and transpersonal) towards a greater good. New memes originating in an individual's mind as a plan, goal or intention can result in a change or transformation sought. For this change to be positive, it should enhance complexity (Delle Fave & Massimini, 2015), i.e. it has to improve, increase or strengthen the connections among its parts, and promote their integration (as viewed from a living systems perspective). A complex system requires the harmonious functioning of all its components.

Differently from the above interpretation of cultural memes as only spreading via connections and relationships, the M&RW model posits that the *meanings and memes are actuality made and experienced within connections and relationships.* This idea is also very poignantly stated by Marujo and Neto (2014) with reference to interpersonal relationships: "Relational goods are goods which cannot be produced, consumed, or acquired by a single individual, because they depend on interaction with others, are enjoyed only if shared, and could not be provided in exchanges where anyone could anonymously supply one or both sides of the bargain. *Relational goods imply therefore a coordination of meanings among the persons in relation, where construction of meaning develops not as individual psychological processes, but arises through specific ways of coordination with others*" (p. 165). To this we add that construction of meaning can develop among various intrapsychological parts, as well as between the individual and broader social systems, and the transpersonal valued Givens. In this sense the M&RW model links to transdisciplinary hermeneutics that allows the distinction of three types of meaning as described by Nicolescu (2014a, 2014b, 2015): *"1. Horizontal meaning – i.e. interconnections at one single level of Reality. This is what most of the academic disciplines do; 2. Vertical meaning – i.e. interconnections involving several levels of Reality. This is what poetry, art or quantum physics do; 3. Meaning of meaning – i.e. interconnections involving all of Reality – the Subject, the Object and the Hidden Third".*

The interwovenness of meaning and relatedness as core facets of well-being is found in various empirical studies in an African context. For example, Theron and Theron (2014) illustrated how the lived experience in an African social context where interpersonal processes play an important role, meaning-making and resilience are deeply influenced by the person-context interactions and culture. Ryff (2014) described three case studies, amongst others that of Mark Mathabane, showing how meaning is made and personal potentials realized, despite serious hardships, through embeddedness in strong social ties in an African context. Wissing et al. (2014) qualitatively explored the most meaningful things in life and why these are meaningful for a Batswana group of African students. Their findings showed that the most important source of meaning is relationships, and in particular the family. The main reasons provided for why these sources of meaning were important were that family provides support, but in particular that family is intrinsically deemed as valuable. Different from the case in many western contexts, interpersonal and spiritual relatedness were deeply intertwined in this African student group. For example, a participant responded: "*because without family you are nothing so yah, they mean a lot to me. And also God that I serve, I thank him to give me this family* (participant 32)" (Wissing et al., 2014, p. 150). The link between meaning/understanding and relationships for a participant in a rural African community is for example also expressed in answers to a question about important goals and reasons therefore: "*Understanding..... to live in peace without anyone holding grudges against one another*" (participant 38, 56-year old female)" (Wilson et al., 2018a, p. 9).

1.3 Summary and Way Forward

In this chapter we described cultures of positivity and quality of life with reference to experienced meaning and relatedness on and among intrapersonal, interpersonal and transpersonal levels. We use the Meaning and Relatedness Well-being model (M&RW) to conceptualize and explain these processes, and illustrated support for main components of this model with references to lay people's experiences of meaning and relational well-being in various African contexts. Further research need to explore and explicate the dynamics of meaning-making in relationships and contextual situatedness in diverse cultural contexts. The theory of self as information agent proposed by Baumeister, Maranges, and Vohs (2018) is a step in the direction of explicating such dynamics. Moving from an analysis of intrapersonal process these authors contend that meaningful information is not only a resource for individual action, but also provides the content for, and is part of the individual's interaction with the social environment. In particular future research should explore the dance of positive and negative affect and experiences, motivational factors, behavior and values in the meaning-making processes within relationships as manifested in various contexts and situatedness in life (e.g., health and illness, poverty and migration, climate change, adversity and flourishing times, etc.), and how these processes contribute to cultures of positivity and a good quality of life. In this regard we anticipate that more multi-, inter- and transdisciplinary research will be necessary to understand the complexity of well-being, cultures of positivity and good quality of life for all. There is in quality of life studies and from various other angles increasingly calls for transdisciplinary research apart from strong disciplinary work, for example in the traditional quality of life approach by Rojas (2018), but also form other disciplines and philosophy of science approaches (e.g., Arcidiacono & Di Martino, 2016; Dieleman, 2015; Finkenthal, 2016; Herzlich, 2018; Nicolescu, 2010, 2012, 2015b; VanderWeele, 2017).

References

Algoe, S. B., Gable, S. L., & Maisel, N. C. (2010). It's the little things: Everyday gratitude as a booster shot for romantic relationships. *Personal Relationships, 17*, 217–233.

Arcidiacono, C., & Di Martino, S. (2016). A critical analysis of happiness and well-being. Where we stand now, where we need to go. *Community Psychology in Global Perspective, 2*(1), 6–35. https://doi.org/10.1285/i24212113v2i1p6

Aron, E. N., & Aron, A. (1996). Love and the expansion of the self: The state of the model. *Personal Relationships, 3*(1), 45–58. https://doi.org/10.1111/j.1475-6811.1996.tb00103.x

Awasthi, P., Chauhan, R., & Verma, S. (2016). Meaningfulness in life span perspectives: An overview. *Purushartha: A Journal of Management Ethics and Spirituality, 7*(2), 98–113.

Baloyi, L., & Mokobe-Rabothata, M. (2014). The African conception of death: A cultural implication. *Proceedings from the 21st International Congress of the International Association for Cross-Cultural Psychology*, 232–241.

Baumeister, R. F. (1991). *Meanings of life*. New York, NY: Guilford Press.

Baumeister, R. F., & Landau, M. J. (2018). Finding the meaning of meaning: Emerging insights on four grand questions. *Review of General Psychology, 22*(1), 1–10. https://doi.org/10.1037/gpr0000145

Baumeister, R. F., & Leary, M. R. (1995). The need to belong: Desire for interpersonal attachments as a fundamental human motivation. *Psychological Bulletin, 117*, 497–529.

Baumeister, R. F., Vohs, K. D., Aaker, J. L., & Garbinsky, E. N. (2013). Some key differences between a happy life and a meaningful life. *The Journal of Positive Psychology, 8*(6), 505–516. https://doi.org/10.1080/17439760.2013.830764

Baumeister, R. F., Maranges, H. M., & Vohs, K. D. (2018). Human self as information agent: Functioning in a social environment based on shared meanings. *Review of General Psychology, 22*(1), 36–47. https://doi.org/10.1037/gpr0000114

Becker, D., & Marecek, J. (2008). Positive psychology. *Theory & Psychology, 18*(5), 591–604. https://doi.org/10.1177/0959354308093397

Berry, J. W., Segall, M. H., & Kagitcibasi, C. (1997). *Handbook of cross-cultural psychology: Social behavior and applications*. Boston, MA: Allyn & Bacon.

Chiu, C., & Chen, J. (2004). Symbols and interactions: Application of the CCC model to culture, language, and social identity. In S. H. Ng, C. N. Candlin, & C. Y. Chiu (Eds.), *Language matters: Communication, culture, and social identity* (pp. 155–182). Hong Kong, China: City University of Hong Kong Press.

Christopher, J. C., & Hickinbottom, S. (2008). Positive psychology, ethnocentrism, and the disguised ideology of individualism. *Theory & Psychology, 18*(5), 563–589. https://doi.org/10.1177/0959354308093396

Copeland-Linder, N. (2006). Stress among black women in a South African township: The protective role of religion. *Journal of Community Psychology, 34*(5), 577–599. https://doi.org/10.1002/jcop.20116

Cornell, A. W., & McGavin, B. (2008). Inner relationship focusing. *The Folio A Journal for Focusing and Experiential Therapy, 21*(1), 21–33.

Cramm, J., Møller, V., & Nieboer, A. (2010). Improving subjective well-being of the poor in the Eastern Cape. *Journal of Health Psychology, 15*(7), 1012–1019. https://doi.org/10.1177/1359105310367833

Cruz, M. R., & Sonn, C. (2011). Decolonizing culture in community psychology. *American Journal of Community Psychology, 47*(1–2), 203–214. https://doi.org/10.1080/17437199.2017.1327325

Czekierda, K., Banik, A., Park, C. L., & Luszczynska, A. (2017). Meaning in life and physical health: Systematic review and meta-analysis. *Health Psychology Revolution, 11*(4), 387–418. https://doi.org/10.1080/17437199.2017.1327325

Dambrun, M. (2017). Self-centeredness and selflessness: Happiness correlates and mediating psychological processes. *PeerJ, 5*, e3306. https://doi.org/10.7717/peerj.3306

Dambrun, M., Ricard, M., Despres, G., Drelon, E., Gibelin, E., Gibelin, M., et al. (2012). Measuring happiness: From fluctuating happiness to authentic-durable happiness. *Frontiers in Psychology, 3*, 16. https://doi.org/10.3389/fpsyg.2012.00016

Dandala, M. H. (2009). Cows never die. Embracing African cosmology in the process of economic growth. In M. F. Murove (Ed.), *African ethics: An anthology of comparative and applied ethics* (pp. 63–84). Scottsville, South Africa: University of Kwazulu-Natal Press.

Delle Fave, A. (2014). Harmony. In A. C. Michalos (Ed.), *Encyclopedia of quality of life and well-being research* (pp. 2695–2697). Dordrecht, The Netherlands: Springer.

Delle Fave, A. (2017). *Happiness lies in the middle: Evidence from theories and empirical findings, Keynote (F. Diener Lecture)*. Paper presented at the ISQOLS2017 Annual Conference on Quality of Life: Towards a better Society, Innsbruck, Austria.

Delle Fave, A., & Massimini, F. (2015). Cultural change and human behaviour: Evolution or development? Crossing the border. *International Journal of Interdisciplinary Studies, 3*(1), 41–52.

Delle Fave, A., & Soosai-Nathan, L. (2014). Meaning as inter-connectedness: Theoretical perspectives and empirical evidence. *Journal of Psychology in Africa, 24*(1), 33–43. https://doi.org/10.1080/14330237.2014.904090

Delle Fave, A., Wissing, M., Brdar, I., Vella-Brodrick, D., & Freire, T. (2013). Cross-cultural perceptions of meaning and goals in adulthood: Their roots and relations with happiness. In A. S. Waterman (Ed.), *The best within us: Positive psychology perspectives on eudaimonia* (pp. 227–248). Washington, DC: American Psychological Association.

Delle Fave, A., Brdar, I., Wissing, M. P., Araujo, U., Castro Solano, A., Freire, T., et al. (2016). Lay definitions of happiness across nations: The primacy of inner harmony and relational connectedness. *Frontiers in Psychology, 7*, 1–23. https://doi.org/10.3389/fpsyg.2016.00030

Delle Fave, A., Bassi, M., Allegri, B., Cilia, S., Falautano, M., Goretti, B., et al. (2017). Beyond disease: Happiness, goals, and meanings among persons with multiple sclerosis and their caregivers. *Frontiers in Psychology, 8*, 2216. https://doi.org/10.3389/fpsyg.2017.02216

Demirci, İ., & Ekşi, H. (2018). Keep calm and be happy: A mixed method study from character strengths to well-being. *Educational Sciences: Theory & Practice, 18*, 303–354. https://doi.org/10.12738/estp.2018.2.0799

Dieleman, H. (2015). Transdisciplinary hermeneutics; working from the inner self, creating ecologies of knowing. *Atlas, Transdisciplinary Journal of Engineering & Science, 6*, 72–85.

Fincham, F. D., & Beach, S. R. H. (2010). Of memes and marriage: Toward a positive relationship science. *Journal of Family Theory and Review, 2*, 4–24. https://doi.org/10.1111/j.1756-2589.2010.00033.x

Finkenthal, M. (2016). Disciplinarian thinking, interdisciplinarity and multi-disciplinarity revisited, with complexity in mind. In M. Micle & C. Mesaros (Eds.), *Communication today: An overview from online journalism to applied philosophy* (pp. 260–265). Budapest, Hungary: Trivent Publishing. https://doi.org/10.22618/TP.PCMS.20164.349024

Fowers, B. J. (2010). Instrumentalism and psychology. *Theory & Psychology, 20*(1), 102–124. https://doi.org/10.1177/0959354309346080

Fowers, B. J. (2012). Placing virtue and the human good in psychology. *Journal of Theoretical and Philosophical Psychology, 32*(1), 1–9. https://doi.org/10.1037/a0025819

Fowers, B. J., & Anderson, A. R. (2018). Aristotelian philia, contemporary friendship and some resources for studying close relationships. In T. Harisson & D. I. Walker (Eds.), *The theory and practice of virtue education* (pp. 184–196). London, UK: Routledge. https://doi.org/10.26385/SG.070218

Gable, S. L., & Gosnell, C. L. (2011). The positive side of close relationships. In K. M. Sheldon, T. B. Kashdan, & M. F. Steger (Eds.), *Designing positive psychology: Taking stock and moving forward* (pp. 265–279). Oxford, UK: Oxford University Press.

Gable, S. L., & Reis, H. T. (2010). Good news! Capitalizing on positive events in an interpersonal context. *Advances in Experimental Social Psychology, 42*, 195–257.

Gable, S. L., Gonzaga, G. C., & Strachman, A. (2006). Will you be there for me when things go right? Supportive responses to positive event disclosures.

Journal of Personality and Social Psychology, 91(5), 904–917. https://doi.org/10.1037/0022-3514.91.5.904

Gendlin, E. T. (1996). *Focusing-oriented psychotherapy: A manual of the experiential method*. New York, NY: Guilford Press.

George, L. S., & Park, C. L. (2016). Meaning in life as comprehension, purpose, and mattering: Toward integration and new research questions. *Review of General Psychology, 20*(3), 205–220. https://doi.org/10.1037/gpr0000077

Gere, J., & Macdonald, G. (2013). Assessing relationship quality across cultures: An examination of measurement equivalence. *Personal Relationships, 20*(3), 422–442. https://doi.org/10.1111/pere.12001

Greeff, A. P., & Loubser, K. (2008). Spirituality as a resiliency quality in Xhosa-speaking families in South Africa. *Journal of Religion and Health, 47*(3), 288–301. https://doi.org/10.1007/s10943-007-9157-7

Gyekye, K. (1995). *An essay on African philosophical thought: The Akan conceptual scheme*. Philadelphia, PA: Temple University Press.

Harrell, S. P. (2015). Culture, wellness, and world "PEaCE": An introduction to person-environment-and-culture-emergence theory. *Community Psychology in Global Perspective, 1*(1), 16–49.

Harrell, S. P. (2018). 'Being human together': Positive relationships in the context of diversity, culture, and collective well-being. In M. A. Warren & S. I. Donaldson (Eds.), *Toward a positive psychology of relationships: New directions in theory and research* (pp. 247–284). Santa Barbara, CA: Praeger.

Heine, S. J., Proulx, T., & Vohs, K. D. (2006). The meaning maintenance model: On the coherence of social motivations. *Personality and Social Psychology Review, 10*(32), 88–110.

Held, B. S. (2016). The negative side of positive psychology. *Journal of Humanistic Psychology, 44*(1), 9–46. https://doi.org/10.1177/0022167803259645

Held, B. S. (2017). Positive psychology's a priori problem. *Journal of Humanistic Psychology, 58*(3), 313–342. https://doi.org/10.1177/0022167817739409

Helne, T., & Hirvilammi, T. (2015). Wellbeing and sustainability: A relational approach. *Sustainable Development, 23*(3), 167–175. https://doi.org/10.1002/sd.1581

Hershfield, H. E., Scheibe, S., Sims, T. L., & Carstensen, L. L. (2013). When feeling bad can be good: Mixed emotions benefit physical health across adulthood. *Social Psychological and Personality Science, 4*(1), 54–61. https://doi.org/10.1177/1948550612444616

Herzlich, C. (2018). A journey in the field of health: From social psychology to multi-disciplinarity. *Journal of Health Psychology, 23*(3), 386–396. https://doi.org/10.1177/1359105317709474

Ho, M., Cheung, F. M., & Cheung, S. F. (2010). The role of meaning in life and optimism in promoting well-being. *Personality and Individual Differences, 48*(5), 658–663. https://doi.org/10.1016/j.paid.2010.01.008

Johnson, J., & Wood, A. M. (2015). Integrating positive and clinical psychology: Viewing human functioning as continua from positive to negative can benefit clinical assessment, interventions and understandings of resilience. *Cognitive Therapy and Research, 41*(3), 335–349. https://doi.org/10.1007/s10608-015-9728-y

Joshanloo, M. (2010). Investigation of the contribution of spirituality and religiousness to hedonic and eudaimonic well-being in Iranian young adults. *Journal of Happiness Studies, 12*(6), 915–930. https://doi.org/10.1007/s10902-010-9236-4

Karasawa, M., Curhan, K. B., Markus, H. R., Kitayama, S. S., Love, G. D., Radler, B. T., et al. (2011). Cultural perspectives on aging and well-being: A comparison of Japan and the United States. *International Journal of Aging & Human Development, 73*(1), 73–98. https://doi.org/10.2190/AG.73.1.d

Kashima, Y. (2014). How can you capture cultural dynamics? *Frontiers in Psychology, 5*, 995. https://doi.org/10.3389/fpsyg.2014.00995

Keyes, C. L. (1998). Social well-being. *Social Psychology Quarterly, 61*(2), 121–140.

Kimhi, S. (2016). Levels of resilience: Associations among individual, community, and national resilience. *Journal of Health Psychology, 21*(2), 164–170. https://doi.org/10.1177/1359105314524009

King, L. A., Hicks, J. A., Krull, J. L., & Del Gaiso, A. K. (2006). Positive affect and the experience of meaning in life. *Journal of Personality and Social Psychology, 90*(1), 179–196. https://doi.org/10.1037/0022-3514.90.1.179

King, L. A., Heintzelman, S. J., & Ward, S. J. (2016). Beyond the search for meaning. *Current Directions in Psychological Science, 25*(4), 211–216. https://doi.org/10.1177/0963721416656354

Kuppens, P., Realo, A., & Diener, E. (2008). The role of positive and negative emotions in life satisfaction judgment across nations. *Journal of Personality and Social Psychology, 95*(1), 66–75. https://doi.org/10.1037/0022-3514.95.1.66

Lambert, N. M., Stillman, T. F., Hicks, J. A., Kamble, S., Baumeister, R. F., & Fincham, F. D. (2013). To belong is to matter: Sense of belonging enhances meaning in life. *Personality and Social Psychology Bulletin, 39*(11), 1418–1427. https://doi.org/10.1177/0146167213499186

Lifton, R. J. (1979). *The broken connection: On death and the continuity of life*. New York, NY: Simon & Schuster.

Lomas, T. (2016). Positive psychology – the second wave. *The Psychologist, 29*, 536–539.

Lomas, T. (2018). The quiet virtues of sadness: A selective theoretical and interpretative appreciation of its potential contribution to wellbeing. *New Ideas in Psychology, 49*, 18–26. https://doi.org/10.1016/j.newideapsych.2018.01.002

Lomas, T., & Ivtzan, I. (2015). Second wave positive psychology: Exploring the positive–negative dialectics of wellbeing. *Journal of Happiness Studies, 17*(4), 1753–1768. https://doi.org/10.1007/s10902-015-9668-y

Madsen, K. B. (1988). *A history of psychology in metascientific perspective*. Amsterdam, The Netherlands: Elsevier.
Majors, K. (2012). Friendships: The power of positive alliance. In S. Roffey (Ed.), *Positive relationships: Evidence based practice across the world* (pp. 127–143). Dotrecht, The Netherlands: Springer.
Martela, F., & Steger, M. F. (2016). The three meanings of meaning in life: Distinguishing coherence, purpose, and significance. *The Journal of Positive Psychology, 11*(5), 531–545. https://doi.org/10.1080/17439760.2015.1137623
Marujo, H. Á., & Neto, L. M. (2014). Felicitas Publica and community well-being: Nourishing relational goods through dialogic conversations between deprived and privileged populations. *Journal of Psychology in Africa, 24*(1), 102–114. https://doi.org/10.1080/14330237.2014.904096
Mason, H. D. (2013). Meaning in life within an African context: A mixed method study. *Journal of Psychology in Africa, 23*(4), 635–638. https://doi.org/10.1080/14330237.2013.10820679
McNulty, J. K., & Fincham, F. D. (2012). Beyond positive psychology? Toward a contextual view of psychological processes and well-being. *American Psychologist, 67*(2), 101–110.
Metz, T. (2015). Précis of meaning in life: An analytic study. *European Journal for Philosophy of Religion, 8*(2), 1–4.
Meunier, V., & Baker, W. (2012). Positive couple relationships: The evidence for long-lasting relationship satisfaction and happiness. In S. Roffey (Ed.), *Positive relationships: Evidence based practice across the world* (pp. 73–89). Dordrecht, The Netherlands: Springer.
Mikulincer, M., Florian, V., & Hirschberger, G. (2004). The terror of death and the quest for love: An existential perspective on close relationships. In J. Greenberg, S. L. Koole, T. Pyszczynski, J. Greenberg, S. L. Koole, & T. Pyszczynski (Eds.), *Handbook of experimental existential psychology* (pp. 287–304). New York, NY: Guilford.
Nafstad, H. E., Blakar, R. M., Carlquist, E., Phelps, J. M., & Rand-Hendriksen, K. (2009). Globalization, neoliberalism and community psychology. *American Journal of Community Psychology, 43*(1–2), 162–175. https://doi.org/10.1007/s10464-008-9216-6
Neff, K. D., & Costigan, A. P. (2014). Self-compassion, wellbeing, and happiness. *Psychologie in Österreich, 2*(3), 113–119.
Newton, T., & McIntosh, D. N. (2013). Unique contributions of religion to meaning. In J. A. Hicks & C. Routledge (Eds.), *The experience of meaning in life* (pp. 257–269). Dordrecht, The Netherlands: Springer. https://doi.org/10.1007/978-94-007-6527-6_20
Nicolescu, B. (2010). Methodology of transdisciplinarity – levels of reality, logic of the included middle and complexity. *Transdisciplinary Journal of Engineering & Science, 1*(1), 19–38.
Nicolescu, B. (2012). Transdisciplinarity: The hidden third, between the subject and the object. *Human & Social Studies, 1*(2), 13–28. https://doi.org/10.2478/v10317-012-0002-5
Nicolescu, B. (2014a). *From modernity to cosmodernity: Science, culture, and spirituality*. Albany, NY: State University of New York Press.
Nicolescu, B. (2014b). Methodology of transdisciplinarity. *World Futures, 70*(3–4), 186–199. https://doi.org/10.1080/02604027.2014.934631
Nicolescu, B. (2015a). The hidden third and the multiple splendor of being. In V. Bazhanov & R. W. Scholz (Eds.), *Transdisciplinarity in philosophy and science: Approaches, problems, prospects* (pp. 62–79). Moscow, Russia: Russia Navigator.
Nicolescu, B. (2015b). Transdisciplinary methodology of the dialogue between people, cultures, and spiritualities. *Human & Social Studies, 4*(2), 15–28. https://doi.org/10.1515/hssr-2015-0011
Nwoye, A. (2015). What is African psychology the psychology of? *Theory & Psychology, 25*(1), 96–116. https://doi.org/10.1177/0959354314565116
Nwoye, A. (2017). An Africentric theory of human personhood. *Psychology in Society, 54*, 42–66.
O'Connell, B. H., O'Shea, D., & Gallagher, S. (2016). Enhancing social relationships through positive psychology activities: A randomised controlled trial. *The Journal of Positive Psychology, 11*(2), 149–162. https://doi.org/10.1080/17439760.2015.1037860
Ogbonnaya, A. O. (1994). Person as community: An African understanding of the person as an intrapsychic community. *Journal of Black Psychology, 20*(1), 75–87. https://doi.org/10.1177/00957984940201007
Pawelski, J. O. (2016a). Defining the 'positive' in positive psychology: Part I. A descriptive analysis. *The Journal of Positive Psychology, 11*(4), 339–356. https://doi.org/10.1080/17439760.2015.1137627
Pawelski, J. O. (2016b). Defining the 'positive' in positive psychology: Part II. A normative analysis. *The Journal of Positive Psychology, 11*(4), 357–365. https://doi.org/10.1080/17439760.2015.1137628
Prilleltensky, I., & Prilleltensky, O. (2007). Webs of well-being: The interdependence of personal, relational, organizational and communal well-being. In J. Haworth & G. Hart (Eds.), *Well-being: Individual, community and social perspectives* (pp. 57–76). London, UK: Palgrave Macmillan.
Rathi, N., & Rastogi, R. (2007). Meaning in life and psychosocial wellbeing in pre adolescents and adolescents. *Journal of the Indian Academy of Applied Psychology, 33*(1), 31–38.
Reker, G. T., & Wong, P. T. P. (2012). Personal meaning in life and psychosocial adaptation in the later years. In P. T. P. Wong (Ed.), *The human quest for meaning: Theories, research, and applications* (pp. 433–456). New York, NY: Routledge.
Reker, G. T., & Woo, L. C. (2011). Personal meaning orientations and psychosocial adaptation in older adults. *SAGE Open, 1*(1), 1–10. https://doi.org/10.1177/2158244011405217

Richardson, F. C. (2012). On psychology and virtue ethics. *Journal of Theoretical and Philosophical Psychology, 32*(1), 24–34. https://doi.org/10.1037/a0026058

Richardson, F. C., & Guignon, C. B. (2008). Positive psychology and philosophy of social science. *Theory & Psychology, 18*(5), 605–627. https://doi.org/10.1177/0959354308093398

Rojas, M. (2004). *The complexity of well-being: A life satisfaction conception and a domains-of-life approach*. Paper presented at the International Workshop on Researching Well-being in Developing Countries, Bremen, Germany.

Rojas, M. (2014). Encyclopedia of quality of life and well-being research. In A. C. Michalos (Ed.), *Encyclopedia of quality of life and well-being research*. Dordrecht, The Netherlands: Springer.

Rojas, M. (2018). Indicators of people's well-being. *Social Indicators Research, 135*(3), 941–950. https://doi.org/10.1007/s11205-016-1507-y

Ryff, C. D. (2014). Self realisation and meaning making in the face of adversity: A eudaimonic approach to human resilience. *Journal of Psychology in Africa, 24*(1), 1–12. https://doi.org/10.1080/14330237.2014.904098

Ryff, C. D., & Singer, B. H. (1998). The contours of positive human health. *Psychological Inquiry, 9*(1), 1–28. https://doi.org/10.1207/s15327965pli0901_1

Ryff, C. D., & Singer, B. H. (2000). Interpersonal flourishing: A positive health agenda for the new millennium. *Personality and Social Psychology Review, 4*(1), 30–44.

Ryff, C. D., & Singer, B. H. (2008). Know thyself and become what you are: A eudaimonic approach to psychological well-being. *Journal of Happiness Studies, 9*, 13–39. https://doi.org/10.1007/s10902-006-9019-0

Ryff, C. D., Singer, B. H., & Love, D. G. (2004). Positive health: Connecting well-being with biology. *Philosophical Transactions of the Royal Society of London B. Biological Sciences, 359*, 1383–1394. https://doi.org/10.1098/rstb.2004.1521

Schimmack, U., Oishi, S., & Diener, E. (2002). Cultural influences on the relation between pleasant emotions and unpleasant emotions: Asian dialectic philosophies or individualism-collectivism? *Cognition & Emotion, 16*(6), 705–719.

Schlegel, R. J., & Hicks, J. A. (2016). Reflections on the scientific study of meaning in life. *Journal of Constructivist Psychology, 30*(1), 26–31. https://doi.org/10.1080/10720537.2015.1119080

Schlegel, R. J., Hicks, J. A., King, L. A., & Arndt, J. (2011). Feeling like you know who you are: Perceived true selfknowledge and meaning in life. *Personality and Social Psychology Bulletin, 37*(6), 745–756.

Seligman, M. E. P. (2002). *Authentic happiness: Using the new positive psychology to realize your potential for lasting fulfillment*. New York, NY: Free Press.

Seligman, M. E. P., & Csikszentmihalyi, M. (2000). Positive psychology: An introduction. *American Psychologist, 55*(1), 5–14.

Selvam, S. G. (2013). Towards religious spirituality. *Journal for the Study of Religions and Ideologies, 12*(36), 129–152.

Selvam, S. G. (2015). *Pastoral care of the family in the light of sound psychology*. Paper presented at the Tangaza Conference on Family Nairobi, Kenya.

Selvam, S. G., & Collicutt, J. (2013). The ubiquity of the character strengths in African traditional religion: A thematic analysis. In H. H. Knoop & A. D. Fave (Eds.), *Well-being and cultures: A positive psychology perspective* (pp. 83–102). Heidelberg, Germany: Springer. https://doi.org/10.1007/978-94-007-4611-4_6

Slife, B. D., & Richardson, F. C. (2008). Problematic ontological underpinnings of positive psychology. *Theory & Psychology, 18*(5), 699–723. https://doi.org/10.1177/0959354308093403

Slife, B. D., O'Grady, K. A., & Kosits, R. D. (2017). *The hidden worldviews of psychology's theory, research, and practice*. New York, NY: Routledge.

Steger, M. F. (2012). Experiencing meaning in life: Optimal functioning at the nexus of well-being, psychopathology, and spirituality. In P. T. P. Wong (Ed.), *The human quest for meaning* (2nd ed., pp. 165–184). New York, NY: Taylor & Francis.

Steger, M. F., Oishi, S., & Kashdan, T. B. (2009). Meaning in life across the life span: Levels and correlates of meaning in life from emerging adulthood to older adulthood. *The Journal of Positive Psychology, 4*(1), 43–52. https://doi.org/10.1080/17439760802303127

Stroink, M., & DeCicco, T. (2011). Culture, religion, and the underlying value dimensions of the metapersonal self-construal. *Mental Health, Religion & Culture, 14*(9), 917–934. https://doi.org/10.1080/13674676.2010.536979

Tamir, M., & Gross, J. J. (2011). Beyond pleasure and pain? Emotion regulation and positive psychology. In K. M. Sheldon, T. B. Kashdan, & M. F. Steger (Eds.), *Designing positive psychology: Taking stock and moving forward* (pp. 89–100). New York, NY: Oxford University Press.

Theron, L. C., & Theron, A. M. C. (2014). Meaning-making and resilience: Case studies of a multifaceted process. *Journal of Psychology in Africa, 24*(1), 24–32. https://doi.org/10.1080/14330237.2014.904099

Triandis, H. C. (1994). *Culture and social behavior*. New York, NY: McGraw-Hill.

Triandis, H. C. (1996). The psychological measurement of cultural syndromes. *American Psychologist, 51*(4), 407–415.

Uchida, Y., & Ogihara, Y. (2012). Personal or interpersonal construal of happiness: A cultural psychological perspective. *International Journal of Wellbeing, 2*(4), 354–369. https://doi.org/10.5502/ijw.v2.i4.5

Urata, Y. (2015). A psychological model to determine meaning in life and meaning of life. *Journal of Philosophy of Life, 5*(3), 215–227.

Van Tongeren, D. R., DeWall, C. N., Green, J. D., Cairo, A. H., Davis, D. E., & Hook, J. N. (2018). Self-regulation facilitates meaning in life. *Review of General Psychology, 22*(1), 95–106. https://doi.org/10.1037/gpr0000121

VanderWeele, T. J. (2017). On the promotion of human flourishing. *Proceedings of the National Academy of Sciences*, 1–9. doi:https://doi.org/10.1073/pnas.1702996114

Walsh, K., O'Shea, E., Scharf, T., & Shucksmith, M. (2014). Exploring the impact of informal practices on social exclusion and age-friendliness for older people in rural communities. *Journal of Community & Applied Social Psychology, 24*(1), 37–49. https://doi.org/10.1002/casp

Wang, S.-Y., Wong, Y. J., & Yeh, K.-H. (2016). Relationship harmony, dialectical coping, and nonattachment: Chinese indigenous well-being and mental health. *The Counseling Psychologist, 44*(1), 78–108. https://doi.org/10.1177/0011000015616463

Wang, S.-Y., Wong, Y. J., Yeh, K.-H., & Wang, L. (2018). What makes a meaningful life? Examining the effects of interpersonal harmony, dialectical coping, and nonattachment. *Asian Journal of Social Psychology*. https://doi.org/10.1111/ajsp.12212

Warren, M. A., & Donaldson, S. I. (2018). *Toward a positive psychology of relationships: New directions in theory and research*. Santa Barbara, CA: Praeger.

White, S. C. (2010). Analysing wellbeing: A framework for development practice. *Development in Practice, 20*(2), 158–172. https://doi.org/10.1080/09614520903564199

White, S. C. (2017). Relational wellbeing: Re-centring the politics of happiness, policy and the self. *Policy & Politics, 45*(2), 121–136. https://doi.org/10.1332/030557317x14866576265970

Wilson, A., & Mittelmark, M. B. (2013). Resources for adjusting well to work migration: Women from northern Ghana working in Head Porterage in Greater Accra. *Africa Today, 59*(4), 25–38.

Wilson, A., & Somhlaba, N. Z. (2016). Dynamics and perceptions of social support and their impact on well-being: A qualitative study of adolescents in Northern Ghana. *International Journal of Mental Health Promotion, 18*(5), 263–275. https://doi.org/10.1080/14623730.2016.1243485

Wilson, A., & Somhlaba, N. Z. (2017). Gender, age, religion and positive mental health among adolescents in a Ghanaian socio-cultural context. *Child Indicators Research*. https://doi.org/10.1007/s12187-017-9495-2

Wilson, A., Wissing, M. P., Schutte, L., & Kruger, I. M. (2018a). Understanding goal motivations in deprived contexts: Perspectives of adults in two rural South African communities. *Applied Research in Quality of Life*. https://doi.org/10.1007/s11482-017-9583-y

Wilson, A., Wissing, M. P., & Schutte, L. (2018b). "We help each other": Relational patterns among older individuals in south African samples. *Applied Research in Quality of Life*, 1–20. https://doi.org/10.1007/s11482-018-9657-5

Wissing, M. P. (2014). Meaning and relational well-being: A reflection on the state of the art and a way forward. *Journal of Psychology in Africa, 24*(1), 115–121. https://doi.org/10.1080/14330237.2014.904100

Wissing, M. P. (2016). The dance of sun and shadow in multicultural well-being: Cultures of positivity in South Africa (Invited keynote). Paper presented at the Italian Positive Psychology Conference Cesena, Italy.

Wissing, M. P. (2018). Embracing well-being in diverse contexts: The Third Wave of positive psychology (Invited speaker). Paper presented at the First Africa Positive Psychology Conference Potchefstroom, South Africa.

Wissing, M. P., & Temane, Q. M. (2013). The prevalence of levels of well-being revisited in an African context. In C. L. M. Keyes (Ed.), *Mental well-being: International contributions to the study of positive mental health* (pp. 71–90). Dordrecht, The Netherlands: Springer. https://doi.org/10.1007/978-94-007-5195-8_4

Wissing, M. P., Khumalo, I. P., & Chigeza, S. C. (2014). Meaning as perceived and experienced by an African student group. *Journal of Psychology in Africa, 24*(1), 92–101. https://doi.org/10.1080/14330237.2014.904101

Wong, P. T. P. (2011). Positive psychology 2.0: Towards a balanced interactive model of the good life. *Canadian Psychology, 52*(2), 69–81.

Wong, P. T. P. (2016). Acceptance, transcendence, and yin-yang dialectics: The three basic tenets of second wave positive psychology. www.drpaulwong.com/inpm-presidents-report-november-2016

Communities in Action: The Participation of Communities in Two South African Literacy Campaigns

2

Veronica McKay

Abstract

This chapter describes two national literacy initiatives to illustrate the way in which literacy interventions can contribute to the enhancement of the quality of life of vulnerable communities. Using a mixed methods research approach, it explores two adult literacy campaigns (the South African Literacy Initiative and the Kha Ri Gude Mass Literacy Campaign) implemented in South Africa and highlights how they targeted their interventions in order to impact positively on the quality of life of the learners, their families and their communities. Written from an insider perspective this chapter outlines the features that contributed to enabling illiterate adults to address some of the many challenges they faced. The author outlines the background to the Kha Ri Gude campaign (which found its roots in the earlier South African Literacy Initiative) and focuses on how the two campaigns jointly impacted on and benefitted the lives of nearly five million learners, their families and communities. The author argues that the social capital and the web of interconnections emerging from the social movement context of the literacy campaigns, this she argues provided a network of agency and resilience to the desperateness faced by communities.

2.1 Introduction

Since 1994, the South African government promulgated a suite of policies and legislative frameworks that support adult basic education and training (ABET), affirming its role in the process of social change and development. There was an acceptance that literacy and basic education were essential for enabling adults with little or no education possibilities to expand their life choices. Literacy and basic education were intended to meet a range of social, economic and developmental needs and were regarded as the foundation for justice and equality, contributing to the core values adopted for South Africa's democracy, enabling adults to participate actively in the social aspects of their lives, empowering them in their personal capacities, and redressing historical imbalances.

Notwithstanding achievements in the field of education since 1994, the system continued to produce and reproduce gender, class, racial and other inequalities. It was not surprising therefore that 12 years after its first democratic election in 1994, South Africa was faced with the decision whether or not to embark on a literacy campaign because the national ABET system had not made any significant impact on reducing the number of adult illiterates. A ministerial committee was established to design the literacy campaign, and after 2 years of research and preparation, the South African

V. McKay (✉)
University of South Africa, Pretoria, South Africa
e-mail: mckayvi@unisa.ac.za

I. Eloff (ed.), *Handbook of Quality of Life in African Societies*, International Handbooks of Quality-of-Life, https://doi.org/10.1007/978-3-030-15367-0_2

Kha Ri Gude[1] Mass Literacy Campaign was launched in 2008. This campaign drew on the human and intellectual capital of the South African National Literacy Initiative (SANLI) that was run on behalf of the national Department of Education by the University of South Africa's Institute for Adult Basic Education from 2002 to 2003. This paper shows how the two large-scale campaigns played a seminal role in building resilience and agency among its target group, offering hope in otherwise hopeless situations. The article also makes indirect reference to the role of the community development workers who were trained by Unisa and who worked as "foot soldiers" alongside the literacy volunteers, ensuring a coherent intervention in the nexus of poverty and despair.

2.2 Campaigning for Literacy

I was privileged enough to lead two government literacy campaigns, and for this chapter I draw on my experience in this regard. The first campaign was SANLI, which served to pilot the large-scale Kha Ri Gude Mass Literacy Campaign. Both afforded me the privilege of working in and with poor communities and witnessing first-hand the contribution that literacy made to building the resilience of communities and catalysing human agency among learners. Jointly the two campaigns reached about five million learners who attended one of the 40,000 classes that were held each year across South Africa over the period 2002–2003 (during which time SANLI was implemented) and from 2008 to 2016 (during which time the Kha Ri Gude campaign was implemented).

While I am writing this chapter, I am also engaged in writing the parliamentary close-out report on the Kha Ri Gude campaign and am acutely aware of the impact made in addressing the many problems of poverty. Research shows how this multiple award winning[2] Kha Ri Gude campaign increased resilience of the groups of learners and communities, resonating with what Paulo Freire (2006) terms a "pedagogy of hope," and akin to what Nobel prize winner Amartya Sen refers to as "Literacy as Freedom." As Sen eloquently states, "illiteracy and innumeracy are forms of insecurity in themselves – not being able to read or write or count or communicate is itself a tremendous deprivation" (UNESCO, 2003, p. 1). Prof. H. S. Bhola, who inspired much of my work in literacy, has referred to illiteracy as "the denial of an essential element of the human heritage and the imposition of an intellectual bondage" (Bhola, 1984, p. 25). It is the freedom that this chapter sets out to explore.

2.2.1 Why Literacy?

The two literacy campaigns specifically targeted marginalised groups (who comprised the majority of South Africa's illiterate adults), including women, the aged, people with disabilities, street children and prisoners. In addition to imparting the skills of literacy, the educators who volunteered to teach literacy were critical in enabling learners to develop a sense of agency and to collectively tackle the many associated problems that poor and vulnerable groups faced.

As evidenced by the research relating to the two campaigns and by the experience that was gained, the learners benefitted both in terms of skills and abilities gained through acquiring literacy and numeracy (McKay, 2015), and the

[1] Kha Ri Gude is Tshivenda for "Let us learn." It was decided to use the Tshivenda terminology as a way of accentuating the minority status of the language.

[2] The *Kha Ri Gude* campaign has won a number of awards, including the Pan South African Language Board (PanSALB) award in 2010, for the excellence of the campaign materials in all 11 official languages; the Government Communication and Information System's Umbungsweti Award (in 2009) for the campaign's developmental communication strategy reaching adults in the most remote and impoverished sites and its efforts to include deaf and blind learners and the Expanded Public Works Programme (EPWP) award (in 2012) for its effective delivery to the poor. In 2016, the International UNESCO Confucius Prize for Literacy for its well-developed campaign that applied scientific research on how illiterate adults read.

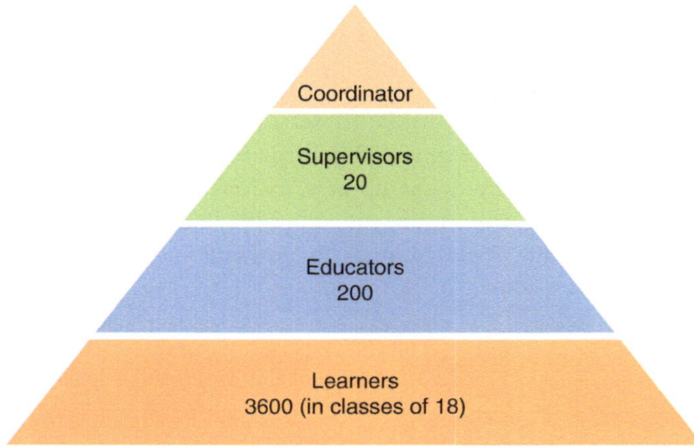

Fig. 2.1 Cascade used for managing the Kha Ri Gude literacy campaign clusters. (Reprinted from McKay, 2012)

campaign's implementation model, which organised illiterate learners into groups of between 15 and 18 learners who were from the same community had similar backgrounds and faced similar challenges. The following figure shows the cascade used to manage the literacy campaigns (Fig. 2.1). I will subsequently show in Fig. 2.3 how the cascade is integrated into the social nexus, which bridges the campaign with various community stakeholders in order to maximise the campaigns' impact.

As shown in the above figure, the learners were taught by a volunteer educator who was from the same geographical location as the learners, and who in turn was supported by a regional supervisor who was managed by one of the provincial coordinators.

In this chapter, I show the critical role the literacy interventions played in fostering community cohesion and peaceful co-existence. In addition, I show that the campaigns' creation of literacy learning groups clustered together people with common problems, enabled them to collectively develop strategies to address challenges.

I have argued elsewhere and with others (McKay, 2007, 2012, 2015, 2018a, b; McKay & Romm, 2015; Singh & McKay, 2004) that the two campaigns impacted on the social and personal development of the learners and that their becoming literate enhanced their confidence, contributed to personal development, and promoted social and political participation. Bhola (1984, p. 24) captures this in his reference to adult literacy as the "initiation into the magical circle of the literate." As he puts it:

> Literacy is truly an initiation into the magical circle of the literate. Literacy is a categorical skill: first the individual is illiterate, then the individual is literate. It is also a demonstrable skill, and thus has built-in social certification. Other forms of non-formal education, regardless of the amount or significance of the information that may be communicated through them, do not have the same aura. Literacy releases the individual from a sense of personal inferiority, from the relationship of dependency and subservience, and allocates a new status and potential.

My role in both the South African campaigns, gave me direct access to the poorest communities across the country, specifically in rural areas and informal settlements where illiteracy and poverty are most acute. I witnessed first-hand how literacy changed the lives of the poor, enabling millions of adults to access the "magical circle."

Sachs (2005, p. 20), in his famous book *The End of Poverty*, identifies three levels of poverty: extreme or absolute, moderate and relative poverty. For the poorest of the poor, he points out, poverty means you are "chronically hungry, unable to access healthcare, lack the amenities of safe drinking water and sanitation, cannot afford education for some or all of the children, and perhaps lack rudimentary shelter." The extreme poor are "caught in the poverty trap, unable on their own to escape from extreme material deprivation."

Sen (1999) describes the cumulative effect of such deprivations as an absence of freedom to function or participate in economic or social life, Bhola (1984, p. 25) portrays illiteracy as the denial of an essential element of human heritage, arguing that literacy opens up new options for the enjoyment of culture since it equips the individual with the skills to read the existential world:

> Reading involves decoding the meanings carried within the linguistic code; and writing involves stating one's meaning in the same linguistic code. This experience of codification and decodification is transferred to the existential world in which the individual lives. The individual learns to decodify the social and political realities as codified (or structured) by others. At the same time, this literate individual is able to codify realities as personally experienced. This might mean conscientization and a possible emergence from a culture of silence.
>
> The literate can use the print to enjoy the cultural forms and creations of peoples and lands far and wide, instead of being limited to the merely oral and local. Finally, literacy has been justified on purely ideological grounds. The Universal Declaration of Human Rights (United Nations, 1967) recognizes ignorance as an obstacle to the self-fulfilment of the individual. As literacy exemplifies one of humankind's paramount achievements—the invention and use of symbolic systems—illiteracy is the denial of an essential element of the human heritage and the imposition of an intellectual bondage.

2.2.2 Working in Poor Communities

Through its classes, Kha Ri Gude (and similarly SANLI) had direct access to the poor and vulnerable, penetrating the poorest areas of the country—the rural areas, informal settlements and urban townships. The two literacy campaigns targeted specifically women (in particular in rural areas), out-of-school youths, the unemployed, prisoners and adults with disabilities.

Given that 74% of poor people in South Africa live in rural areas, it was not surprising that both literacy campaigns concentrated on rural areas, but also on urban townships and informal settlements where poverty was acute and where inhabitants suffered because of poor infrastructure, lack of water, sanitation and electricity, poor health and healthcare, HIV/AIDS, malnutrition, low household income and high migration (Aliber, 2003; Bosworth, 2016; Lehohla, 2017; Lind, 2008).

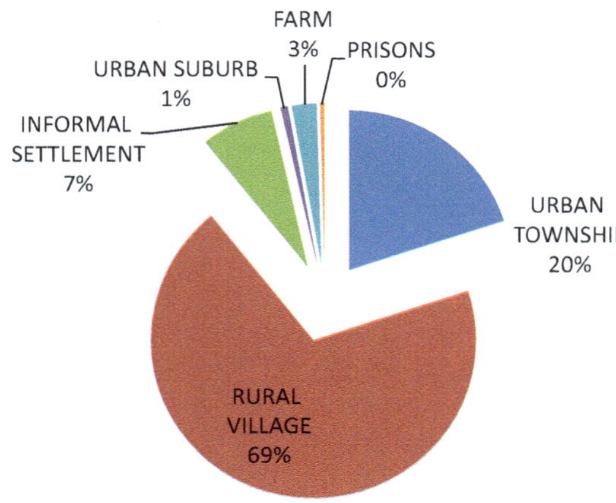

Fig. 2.2 Distribution of learners by residential type

The following figure shows the residential and settlement patterns of the literacy learners (Fig. 2.2).

The remainder of this chapter draws on research into the "the magical circle of literacy," showing its impact on the lives of five million adults and explaining its reach into their families and communities.

2.2.3 Linking Literacy to the Development Agenda

I begin this section with a brief explanation of how, in the interest of directing literacy programmes towards the developmental agenda, the learner materials were thematically informed by local, national and international development agendas. Both the campaigns embedded the teaching of reading, writing and numeracy in development-related themes that were inspired by the United Nations' (UN) millennium development goals and sustainable development goals in order to optimise the social, economic and developmental opportunities afforded by literacy acquisition. Accordingly, the learner workbooks, more specifically for the Kha Ri Gude campaign, were thematically organised to focus on, for example, entrepreneurship, HIV/AIDS, gender, democracy, human rights, and environmental awareness (UN, 2000, 2015). Moreover, there was a deliberate attempt to mainstream social justice and redress issues across the curriculum[3] to encourage learners to think about related matters and make applications in their everyday lives in an endeavour to broaden their choices and opportunities.

In conceptualising the Kha Ri Gude campaign, endeavours were made to design the campaign practices and its core materials to promote progressive democratisation through the dissemination of civic education materials that would improve civic awareness. A major consideration was how literacy and numeracy teaching could address the social needs of the learners and contribute to learner empowerment. A parallel concern was directing the campaign at what Giddens (1991) terms *emancipatory politics* which supplies the foundation for the emergence of *life politics*. As he puts it, "it prepares the stage for life political concerns" (p. 223–225). Life politics is the politics of self-actualisation—it is concerned with questions of rights and obligations (p. 223–225) and how, in an arena which professes to be democratic, *structures* for the exercise of democracy are put in place.[4] This view suggests that social structures (and institutions) are in themselves unable to guarantee democracy in the absence of human participation. In applying Giddens's view of life politics to literacy, McKay and Makhanya (2008) and McKay, 2018b stress that literacy is an essential tool for participation, particularly in developing societies where vast numbers of people lack the skills that enable participation.

[3]The curriculum included mother tongue literacy, English as a first additional language and numeracy. The life skills component was developed via the thematic approach. The themes utilised for the campaign were as follows: I am learning; My family, my home; Living together; Healthy living; World of work; Our country; The world around us.

[4]These may include constitutional rights, human rights, balloting, regular elections, and the availability of social services.

The two campaigns combined aimed to empower close on five million learners to make purposeful choices alongside their acquisition of literacy. Akter et al. (2017, p. 271) refer to the concept of "empowerment as being complex and multidimensional," varying across disciplinary traditions and contexts with the focus on gaining control over decisions and resources that determine one's quality of life and "translating choices into desired actions and outcomes." Thus, being empowered relates to having agency or the ability to make purposeful choices. Agency in this sense is akin to the aspirational element of what Freire (2006) terms the "pedagogy of hope."

2.3 Research Approach

The information used for this chapter emanates from a mixed methods study aimed at reaching an understanding of the role of literacy in contributing to the development of learners' agency and resilience through the development of social capital and community connectedness.

Mixed methods research is often referred to as a "third movement" in the evolution of research methodology, serving as a resolution to quantitative and qualitative paradigm wars. Creswell and Garrett (2008, p. 327) posit that in "mixing" quantitative and qualitative data, consideration is given to *when*, *where* and *why* methods are mixed and *what* the added value of "mixing" methods is. They argue that where the researcher collects "both quantitative and qualitative data, merging, linking, or combining of the sources of data, and then conducting research as a single study … the mixed methods research provides more than quantitative or qualitative research alone." Moreover, in using this research method, consideration is given to the various moments at which the "mixing" may be applied.

The study undertook a "concurrent mixed" or "multi-methodological" approach to gathering qualitative and quantitative data and mixing (and integrating) the data in the same research enterprise (Morse, 2003) to offer a more nuanced understanding of the extent of the impact literacy made on learners' lives and on the enhancement of their agency arising from their learning and their newly established networks. Both the quantitative and qualitative data were obtained from large data sources, and the complementary strengths of these sources were drawn upon to obtain an enriched understanding (Johnson & Onwuegbuzie, 2004); Johnson, Onwuegbuzie, & Turner, 2007; McLafferty & Onwuegbuzi, 2006). These authors refer to the advantages of the "mixed methods contingency theory," which allows for the coexistence of quantitative and qualitative research approaches, suggesting that the variation in data collection makes it possible to answer the research question from a number of perspectives. Moreover, the mixed methods approach has the advantage of limiting gaps in the data collected (i.e. gaps that occur when one methodology does not provide all the information required).

In following a mixed methods research approach, I use the following data sources:

Firstly, I draw on the experience I gained during 2002 to 2003 in which I was charged with establishing and managing the Department of Education's SANLI campaign, and also the experience I gained in my capacity as a chief executive officer in the Department of Basic Education from 2007 to 2012. In the light of my role in both campaigns, the study may be regarded as essentially ethnographic, with my personal role being construed as a participant observer and a coactive researcher. Leading both campaigns gave me opportunities to access letters, e-mails, official data and reports, and also to interact with learners and other field operatives. These data sources provide an important backdrop for this chapter.

Secondly, I draw on the data emanating from an analysis of a sample of 2032 educators' journals ($n = 2032$) that were discussed during educators' monthly communities of practice (COP)[5] meetings. In analysing the journal reports, I coded various categories according to prominent themes that had emerged. In this chapter, I draw mainly on those aspects that refer to the impact that learning made on various aspects of the lives of the learners. In quoting from the sample of journals, this chapter captures the voices of the educators (McKay, 2018a, b).

Thirdly, the chapter draws on focus group discussions conducted with SANLI learners and educators at a random sample of sites across South Africa.

Fourthly, I use the quantitative data gathered to better understand the perceived impact of the literacy programme from the learners' perspective. This data was obtained from the learners' assessment portfolios[6] (LAPs) captured during 1 year (2011)[7] of the Kha Ri Gude campaign and drawn from the responses of a sample of 485,941 learners ($n = 485{,}941$) who completed the campaign in 2011. The data was processed using the SAS statistical package and various statistical procedures, including Spearman's rank correlation coefficient.

Lastly, I draw on the responses the literacy learners gave during exit interviews at the end of their course. To determine which of 24 indicators the learners perceived as having improved as a result of their literacy, the 40,000 educators read out the following statements to the learners in their mother tongues and ticked those aspects with which the learners agreed (Table 2.1):

The 24 indicators that are referred to above (DBE, 2011, p. 2) and are discussed below are

[5]The educators in the campaign were organised into groups of 10, which functioned as communities of practice groups where educators shared problems and solutions. They were required to maintain journals, which they discussed at their meetings. The process is fully discussed in McKay (2017).

[6]The LAPs contained 10 assessment activities for Literacy and 10 for Numeracy, which learners completed at various stages in their programme. At the end of the learning programme the educator administered a survey of 24 items. Learners were required to indicate which items resonated with their perception of the impact of the learning on various areas of their lives. The LAPs provided biographical information on the learners, for example, age, home language, type of residential area (informal settlement, village (as indicated in Fig. 2.2), prior learning, employment status and gender.

[7]The Kha Ri Gude campaign reached 4,386,251 learners in the period 2008–2017. The year 2011 was selected for this study as a stable year with the campaign having overcome initial teething problems or being busy winding down issues, thus providing more reliable data.

Table 2.1 Impacts of literacy assessed in the learners' exit interviews

1	I feel more self-confident	13	I feel that people treat me better
2	My life in my family has improved	14	I feel more respected in my family
3	I feel more respected in the community	15	I have more friends
4	I share what I learn with my family	16	I ask my family to help me with my learning
5	I take part in more community issues	17	I can more easily solve problems
6	I better understand my child's schooling	18	I understand the importance of eating correctly
7	I can help my child with education	19	I have started growing vegetables
8	I attend school or other meetings	20	I have improved my position at work (if he/she works)
9	I better understand health and healthcare	21	I have started some work that helps me to earn
10	I can manage money better	22	I would like to carry on learning
11	I can use a cellphone, or ATM or other device	23	I have encouraged others to join Kha Ri Gude
12	I have more books or magazines in my home	24	Other (fill in)

Department of Basic Education [DBE] (2011, p. 2)

informed by the views that literacy contributes to and promotes the following:

- Self-esteem and empowerment: widening choices and access to other rights
- Political benefits: increased civic participation in community activities, trade unions and local politics
- Cultural benefits: questioning attitudes and norms, improved ability to engage with one's culture
- Social benefits: better knowledge of healthcare, family planning and HIV/AIDS prevention, higher chance of parents educating children
- Economic benefits: increased knowledge about income-generation possibilities (Alidou et al., 2006, p. 16; Street, 1984, 1995/2014; McKay, 2018b).

Mixing the quantitative and qualitative data enabled an understanding of what meanings learners attributed to their becoming literate and to what extent their perceptions of the benefits of literacy resonated with the benefits that UNESCO (2006, p. 136–140) refers to as contributing to the following: protection of human rights and personal liberties, political participation and community action, more tolerant attitudes and democratic values of inclusion, respect for cultural diversity and peace, as well as a range of capabilities for maintaining good health, longevity, learning throughout life, raising healthy children and educating them.

2.4 The Development of Agency and Resilience Through the Development of Social Capital

I now turn to exploring the role of literacy in engendering agency and social capital and discuss how literacy contributes to the development of resilience. I argue that literacy plays a critical role in developing agency and building social capital and that these are essential attributes for building resilience and improving the quality of lives of poor communities. I discuss data from the survey (DBE, 2011) referred to above, and explore the perceptions of new literate learners of the impact of their participation in literacy classes on their lives, their families and their communities. The data, coupled with qualitative sources, shows how the literacy classes contributed to the development of resilience and increased social action which enabled learners, their families and communities to lead more meaningful lives – especially through the social movement learning afforded by a mass campaign.

2.4.1 The Relationship Between Agency, Social Capital and Resilience

Aldrich and Meyer (2015, p. 2) argue that resilience is that feature which enables individuals and communities to face and manage the negative pressures that impact on them, and to successfully cope with and navigate around or through crises. They point out that the development of resilience in situations of despair is always seen to have an "aspirational element."

Preece (2013, p. 304) examines the role that adult basic education plays in impacting on learners in situations of poverty. She refers specifically to its impact on learners' self-esteem and confidence, health, well-being, civic participation and progression to other forms of learning. In focusing on learners' increased confidence, she states that when people have more self-confidence, their ability to take more control over their lives increases—a sentiment also expressed by Fullick (2009, p. 35) who points out that "people in poverty need learning that supports all aspects of their lives and develops capital that enhances personal identity and social solidarity as well as human capital."

While Boughton (2016, p. 161) concurs that literacy plays a critical role in empowering and improving the lot of the poor, he cautions that literacy and basic education are not a panacea for the problems of the poor who live in developing countries. As he states: "For people living in those regions, literacy and education will not provide a path out of poverty unless the process which put them there in the first place are radically altered." Torres (2004, p. 93) shares this sentiment, stating that with the growth of poverty worldwide, adult basic education and literacy have come to be viewed as a key strategy of poverty alleviation and as an essential component for enabling the poor to take control of their lives often under very hostile economic circumstances. She, however, cautions that while literacy can help break the poverty cycle, one must not forget that "poverty is not the result of illiteracy but very much the contrary." Hence she points out that the most effective way to deal with poverty is dealing with the structural economic and political factors that generate it and reproduce it at a national and global scale.

Notwithstanding the aforementioned appeal for structural changes, my experience of leading two literacy campaigns in South Africa showed that learners, through their social networks, were enabled to find some leeway in which they, together, found ways to improve the quality of their lives.

It is for this reason that I contend that the mobilisation and organisation of the mass-based campaigns and the careful selection of thematic learning content had a profound impact on enabling learners to take charge of their lives. The relationship between skills development and the social organisation of learning is referred to by Freire in his *Pedagogy of the oppressed* (2000) and also by other authors (e.g. Botman, 2014; Boughton, 2016; McLaren & Leonard, 1993; Shor, 1993) who highlight how critical pedagogy engenders a critical consciousness through engaging learners in "problematis[ing] generative themes from daily life and other topics relevant to society and academic subject matter" (Botman, 2014, p. 99). It was for this reason that the materials developed for both campaigns were based on generative themes that drew on local, national and international millennium and sustainable development goals. (The themes utilised for the campaign were as follows: I am learning; My family, my home; Living together; Healthy living; World of work; Our country; The world around us).

In addition to including generative themes and developing literacy skills to empower the learners, the campaign stimulated learners to develop social capital networks to enable them to deal with the social issues they faced. They were encouraged to do so collectively by establishing literacy classes and learning groups that were taught by local educators. The organisational arrangement of bringing learners together in classes was seminal in the development of social networks.

During one of my class visits in an informal settlement in Soshanguve, Pretoria, I asked the learners whether they had known each other prior to the start of their classes. Most of the learners indicated that they had not. As one woman pointed out, "I saw them here and there but only got to know them when I joined this class." The class formations and the clusters or groupings of learners (motivated by the learning themes) brought about linkages between the community members resulting in the formation of social capital networks essential for the development of agency and resilience.

McLaren and Leonard (1993, p. 32–33) draw attention to the importance of the organisational arrangements, the generative learning content and the pedagogical approaches of literacy programmes working together to contribute to social action.

The literacy campaigns drew on the theory and practice of critical pedagogy, but being African campaigns they were of necessity imbued with the values of ubuntu. In Table 2.2, I juxtapose McLaren and Leonard's (1993) and Botman's (2014) assumptions about the theory and practice underlying critical education with the beliefs of ubuntu (Bolden, 2014; Chilisa, 2009; Chilisa & Preece, 2005; Gumbo, 2017; Letseka, 2016; Ruele, 2017), showing how the two views of pedagogy are intertwined.

Boughton (2016, p. 151) in fact refers to the social component of literacy classes as being important, arguing that literacy essentially goes beyond economic interests because it is more than an individual cognitive capability. According to him, literacy has a social dimension that leads to other beneficial effects relating to individual and social well-being, effects that are derived from "social movement learning," which is usually associated with mass literacy campaigns. The emergence of social movement learning was found in the two South African literacy campaigns: the large-scale learning movements

Table 2.2 Comparing critical pedagogy with a pedagogy based on ubuntu principles

Critical pedagogy	Pedagogy based on ubuntu
Participatory where learners become actively involved in analysing thematic problems and researching their daily contexts	Ubuntu is collectivist and expresses the values of collaboration, cooperation and community, the ethos of care and respect for others and the importance of solidarity in the face of adversity (Bolden, 2014, p. 3)
Contextualised where the learning is grounded in learners' reality, their language and situations	Ubuntu's "I am because we are" points towards a strongly constructivist ontology in which a person's sense of being cannot be detached from the social context in which they find themselves (Bolden, 2014, p. 2)
Critical where class discussions encourage self- and group reflection	Ubuntu is intersubjective in that it focuses on the *relationship* between the individual and the collective, rather than privileging one over the other
Democratic where classroom practices encourage learners to share their knowledge	Chilisa (2009, p. 13–4) uses proverbs to explain participatory democracy: "Everyone has a right to a say, for even what might appear like a bad suggestion helps people to think of better ideas," and "Everybody throws in a word and every contribution has a value in a gathering"
Dialogical with dialogue structured around learner's problems, leading to action	Ubuntu stresses the importance of the collective and their co-dependence. This is aptly expressed in the African proverb, "you cannot remove fluff with one finger (Setlhodi, 2018, p. 7)
Multicultural with a curriculum that is balanced in terms of race, class and gender, language and ethnicity	Ubuntu has the potential to reach out beyond narrow racial and ethnic identities (Letseka, 2016, p. 144), and classes should be presented with a localised and relevant curriculum (Ruele, 2017, p. 82)

(continued)

Table 2.2 (continued)

Critical pedagogy	Pedagogy based on ubuntu
Activist where the knowledge and skills lead to action	Knowledge is to be used to reflect, question and take action on coloniser/colonised relationships (Chilisa, 2009, p. 28)
Affective where learners are regarded holistically taking into account their feelings and well-being	Ubuntu stresses the importance of a subjective and emotional appreciation of human experience rather than privileging objectivity and rationality (Bolden, 2014, p. 2)
It is de-socialising in the Freirean sense where learners are de-socialised from being passive and authority-dependent to learning to problematise problems and taking action to address problems	It seeks dialogue that invites communities to reflect on the worldviews that inform their practices and to critique and reconcile these with the values of humanness (Chilisa and Preece, 2005, p.49)

gained momentum through the critical mass of participants (educators and learners), leading to the formation of massive, interlinked social networks.

Aldrich and Meyer (2015, p. 2) speak of social capital networks as being essential for enabling resilience and action. They explain that the networks' establishment of norms and trust facilitate relationships that bring about mutual benefits, and they define social capital "as the aggregate of actual or potential resources that are linked to the durable networks of relationships of mutual acquaintance."

Both the SANLI and the Kha Ri Gude campaigns brought together a mass of learners, 413,000 and 4,386,251 learners respectively. The clusters of learners displayed a sense of kinship, reciprocity and strong identification with many of the groups, branding themselves or even creating uniforms to define themselves. The clustering of learners enabled the groups to collectively tackle many day-to-day problems and to cooperate for mutual benefit, with the groups often waiting long for learners to complete their learning programmes. The groups' practice demonstrates adherence to the ubuntu principle of reciprocal responsibility (Bolden, 2014, p. 5) where members of a group support one another and, in so doing, increase their resilience and the likelihood of the group's survival.

Johnston et al. (2009) describe how involvement and participation in groups can have positive consequences for enabling greater individual and community resilience which, according to Aldrich and Meyer (2015, p. 3), refer to the *collective ability* of a community in a geographically defined area to deal with stress and efficiently resume the rhythms of daily life through cooperation. Letseka (2016, p. 113) posits that communal interdependence is rooted in one's community. He explains that ubuntu implies an interactive ethic "in which humanity is shaped by our interaction with others as co-dependent beings, offering key values of group solidarity, compassion, respect and human dignity."

Social networks and social capital are critical for strengthening social infrastructure at a community level and beyond and are essential for developing resilience. All definitions of social capital point out that it is contingent on increased trust and social cohesion. The two South African campaigns relied on the many recognised social capital groupings, including saving or social societies, trade unions, stokvel (rotating credit) groups, burial societies, church communities, associations for the aged or disabled—all of which offer reciprocal support for their members. The campaign utilised networks to mobilise learners and it capitalised on the trust that existed within the groups of learners to strengthen the campaign. It was necessary for the campaigns to ensure that the groups provided safe places for learners to discuss their problems and collectively arrive at solutions. Letseka offers an explanation as to why this was critical in working with the disadvantaged South African. He points out as follows:

> Ubuntu has the potential to foster a shared moral discourse and states that "the struggle for Ubuntu is therefore a struggle for people trying to heal the brutality and desperateness of a society that is deeply ruptured by its past history of segregation and racial discrimination. (2016, p. 114)

2.4.2 Organising for Literacy

My experience of the two South African literacy campaigns showed that through the organisational arrangements of the literacy classes, the campaigns played an important role in developing human agency. Moreover, through clustering learners in interlinking learning groups, the campaign cascade enabled the establishment of the social capital necessary for empowering learners and enabling community resilience and social cohesion.

The findings from the mixed methods research studies refer to a myriad of ways in which the learning groups (and clusters of learning groups) brought about change by putting pressure on local authorities to, for example, build a bridge where children needed to cross a river to go to school, or set up communal gardens to provide food security, or offer home-based care for the aged or those who were ill in their community. In addition, a large majority of the learning groups tackled household insecurity by setting up small businesses such as brickmaking, or craft work such as sewing and beadwork, or starting a bakery. In the face of extreme poverty, there were cases where learners, who themselves were poor, set out to establish development projects to assist others who were less fortunate than themselves such as the aged or people with disabilities. In the following section, I refer to some examples of such cases.

2.4.3 Literacy Within a Social Nexus

Torres (2004, p. 50) refers to the importance of the development of large-scale social networks in literacy campaigns as they mobilise a critical mass of learners. She describes a literacy campaign as a "mass" movement or an "educational movement" engaged in social and political transformative action. She points out that the conditions and outcomes for small-scale programmes are quantitatively and qualitatively different from those of large-scale programmes that draw on the benefits of critical mass as a form of social capital for momentum.

Dale and Newman (2006, p. 17) also talk about the ability of community networks to build social capital as a precursor to the creation of the resilience needed to sustain communities. They argue that the development of social networks is critical in helping marginalised communities to cope with difficulties arising from poverty and to create the community agency necessary to foster change and development.

Social capital has been defined in several ways: Coleman (1988) and Portes (1998) essentially conceptualise social capital as being held by individuals, whereas Putnam (2001) explores the ways in which it operates as a community asset held by all within a social network. Community social capital is distinguished by the norms of reciprocity and trustworthiness, and in this sense it refers to the connections that a group can use to achieve its objectives.

Dale and Newman (2006, p. 19) see agency as integral to social capital, which enables a group to respond to challenges. They refer to the dimensions of agency as the capacity of persons to transform existing states of affairs, plan and initiate action, and respond to events outside of one's immediate sphere of influence to produce a desired effect. They stress the importance of enabling social capital that links with other clusters or groups of people: "a web of diverse interconnections that enable community resilience." Further, they refer to the "bonding ties" that allow internal groups to form and function through establishing norms and internal bonds of trust, and the "bridging ties" that allow groups access to outside resources.[8] Thus they argue that the importance of social capital and network formation include both the *bonding* and the *bridging* abilities that enable local groups to organise themselves and connect with other groups, institutions or organisations in a way that allows a community to extend its reach beyond its bound-

[8]Dale and Newman (2006, p. 19) and Boughton (2016) caution that communities with few economic resources find it difficult to effectively create change within their neighbourhoods. For any action to occur, communities needed to have networks of social capital in place that could mobilise for change, with critical mass being critical for enabling change at a larger scale.

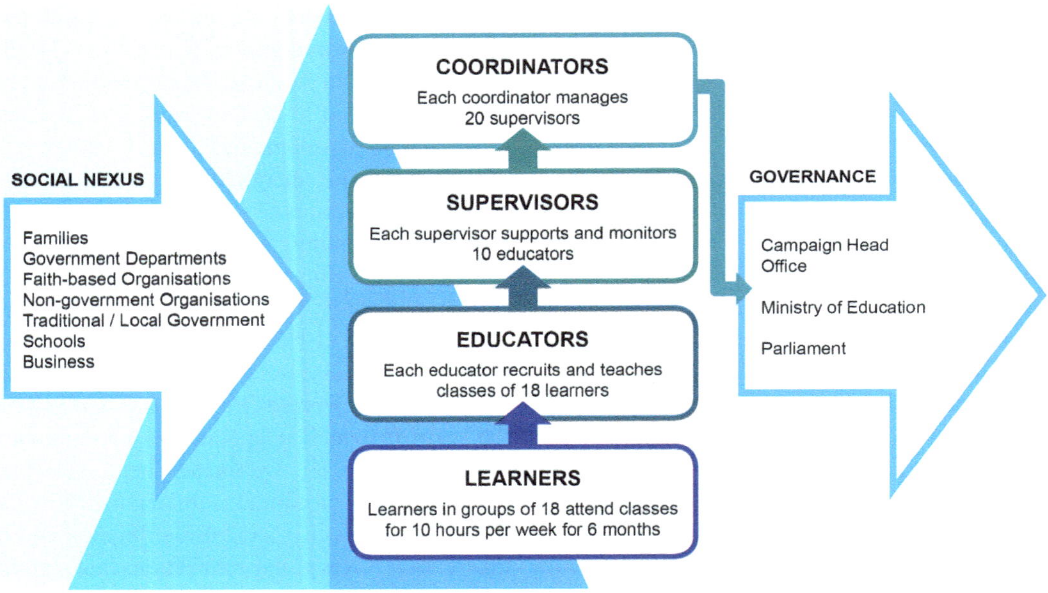

Fig. 2.3 The Kha Ri Gude campaign cascade within a social nexus. (Adapted from McKay 2018a p. 378)

aries. This is essential for effectively engaging with system-scale problems that might stretch far beyond the reach of an individual community (Dale & Newman, 2006, p. 20).

Figure 2.3 above shows how the cascade of the Kha Ri Gude literacy campaign recognised the importance of both bonding within groups and bridging the groups in a broader social nexus. As a mass-based campaign, it relied on volunteerism and community participation, requiring some 40,000 volunteers to form the backbone of the teaching, recruitment, mobilisation and advocacy network.

In terms of its bridging function the campaign relied on interconnections with other supportive stakeholders including chiefs, mayors, local business, a range of community-based and non-government organisations as well as government departments to enable it to make a range of impacts which would go far beyond learning the skills of reading, writing and calculating.

The above diagram portrays the four levels involved in the cascade of the campaign and gives an indication of the roles played by the various levels of the cascade in supporting the campaign. The supervisor had a monitoring function, which included supporting and motivating the ten educators for whom he or she was responsible. The groups of 10 supervisors formed the basis of the educator tier with clusters akin to COP meetings, with each of the 4000 supervisors facilitating a group of 10 educators. The learner and the educator groups played a role in assisting in problem-solving, providing guidance and sharing information (McKay, 2012, 2015, p. 381). As the above figure shows, the literacy campaign operations were located within a social nexus, which provided support and input into the campaign processes specifically for supporting the learners, and which transcended the groups by bridging them with the wider community, ultimately linking the learners with other clusters across the country. McKay (2018a) points out that the COP learning clusters in the South African literacy campaigns aimed to establish a "we relationship" for "we learning" or cooperative learning to encourage knowledge generation and connected action. To this end, the 40,000 educators were organised into 4000 groups and were supported by their respective supervisors.

The COP group formations enabled the educators to think through complex issues, report on and solve learner problems together, and because of the scale of the campaign, the COP groups reaped the benefits of mass mobilisation and the impact of the mass movement.

Drawing on Wenger (1998), Gumbo (2017, p. 317) in fact refers to the relevance of the COP theory, stating that COPs resonate with the principles of ubuntu/botho according to which learning is a "communal event in a social sense" that allows opportunity to share communal resources in order to sustain communal engagements. Communities create environments that encourage discourse about communal set-ups. He points out that "Africans have extended family ties in accordance with COP principles or frameworks" (p. 319).

It was for this reason that the campaign functioned as clusters of COP groupings. Well-functioning COP groupings, according to Ison, Blackmore, Collins, Holwell, & Iaquinto, 2014, p. 111), have a mutual engagement, a shared enthusiasm for the task at hand, and a common commitment to collaborative work in a shared domain. In the case of the campaign, the learning clusters provided support for learners trying to survive under dire circumstances. Wenger (1998) comments on the interest in building communities and the focus on learning systems in order to fully leverage projects through peer-to-peer connections. Figure 2.3 shows how the campaign was able through massification to extend beyond the classroom into the broader social nexus.

2.5 Findings: Learning to Support Development

I begin this section with a discussion of the findings of the learner responses to the 24 survey items listed in Table 2.1 (DBE, 2011) and referred to in McKay, 2018b. The chart shown in Fig. 2.4 pertains to the learners' perceptions of the impact of the literacy campaign on their lives.

The indicators in the above chart were classified as follows:

- The light blue bars refer specifically to learners' increased agency. They show learners' perceptions of increased self-confidence, self-esteem, feelings of being better treated and with more respect, and increased community participation.
- The red bars refer to learners' perceptions of their increased social networks, having more friends, improved family relationships and feeling more respected.
- The green bars refer to learners' perceptions of the utility of their newly acquired skills.
- The two purple bars refer to improved income-generation activities.
- The pale green bars refer to the importance of lifelong learning in supporting children's learning and encouraging others to learn.
- The last bar, marked as "other," refers to additional impacts that are not captured for this study.

In the next sections, I will discuss the significance of the findings.

2.5.1 Increased Agency

As depicted in the blue bars in Fig. 2.4, the survey highlighted learners' perceptions of increased agency. Their perceptions were that they had increased self-esteem and confidence (92.4%), feelings of being better treated (86.79%) and being treated with more respect (88.4%), and consequently their community participation increased (87.5%). In our interactions, learners almost always expressed how much more confident they felt.

The following excerpt, based on a visit to a class in Masionenge Village, draws attention to the important role that literacy learning played in the lives of these rural women who attended a class in the local village primary school:

> The learners welcomed us by singing a song. The lyrics of this particular song are a special feature: they mobilise women to write and work in teams instead of working as isolated individuals. All the women are engaged in subsistence farming for their household's consumption, and learning to work in teams will be very useful to all of them. … The school garden is neatly groomed and [school children] in the classrooms on either side are inquisitive but very quiet.

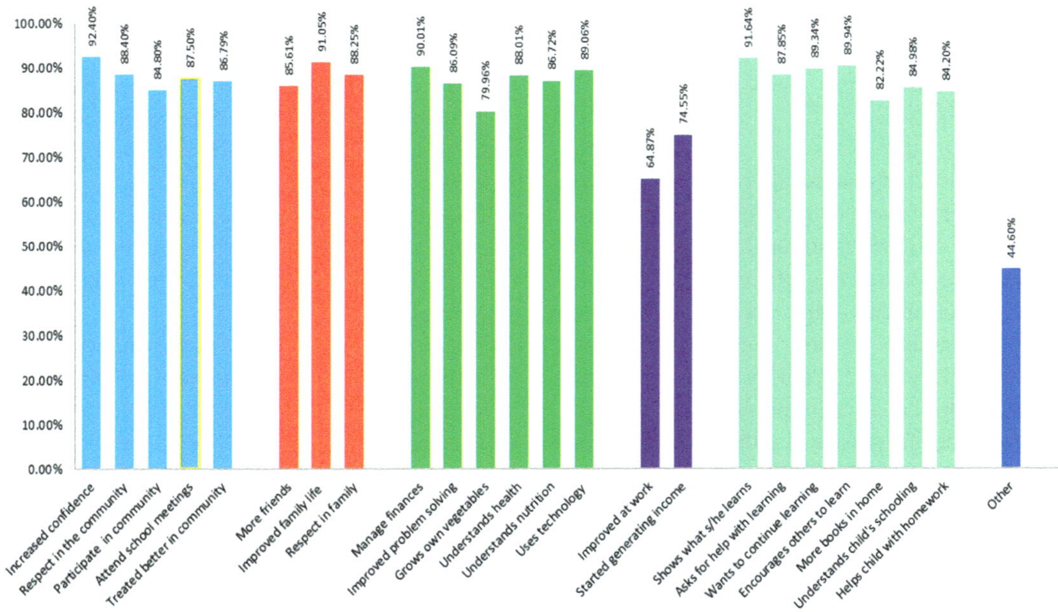

Fig. 2.4 Learners' perceptions (in terms of percentages) of the impact of their learning on various aspects of their lives

> According to Louisa Mkgoholo [their educator], the outstanding feature of this group is the growth they have experienced in self-worth and self-esteem and their discovery of "the self" in late adulthood. Louisa says that since discerning their potential through learning to read and write, they are starting to participate in other activities and are more involved in the community and improving the environment.
>
> The principal of the school, Mr. NM Malatji agrees with Louisa's assessment. He has also seen the effect on the learners, indirectly, through the improvement in their children's performance (their mothers are now able to assist them with their homework). "There is a positive attitude in the community now. People are generally more motivated," he says. (Unisa, 2003, p. 12)

2.5.2 Enhanced Self-Esteem

The above excerpt provides evidence that the learners experienced enhanced self-esteem, showing that their overall subjective estimation of their worth had changed. Engagement in literacy acquisition enabled learners to take control of their lives and deal with the frustrations associated with being illiterate (Unisa, 2003). The findings as depicted in the blue bars in Fig. 2.4 similarly indicate that learners experienced feelings of increased "self-worth and self-esteem" and a discovery of "the self" that arose from their participation in literacy education. These findings provide overwhelming evidence of the value of community-based adult education, described in the literature as being rooted in the personal development of the learners and increasing their self-esteem and confidence levels (Bhola 1984; McKay, 2012, 2018a; Torres 2004).

Learners' remarks about their enhanced confidence as a result of their acquiring literacy were in stark contrast to their remarks about experiencing the frustrations of being illiterate as a result of little or no schooling. This common theme emerged in the responses of learners at the Gaegolewe Centre in a Winterveld informal settlement. They talked about their frustration of being illiterate and explained how learning to read, write and calculate changed their fate:

> I can now sign my name, I can go and collect my pension and work out how much is due.
> There is no more cheating. It is easier when I go to the shops, because I can check that my change is correct.

When asked whether she had ever been cheated, a learner responded poignantly:

> I don't know. I will never know! (Unisa, 2003, p. 17)

The challenges of illiteracy were not limited to learners in the rural areas: learners in the urban areas also expressed their vulnerabilities. During a site visit to a class of domestic workers and gardeners in Centurion, the class discussed how their frustrations of being illiterate were exacerbated by their new (migrant) "urban living." Their inability to write their own names or conduct financial transactions, such as completing bank forms or other official forms, increased the hardships they experienced as migrants in the urban area. They also mentioned their frustrations of not being able to read street names, notices or warnings. As one learner stated:

> It was when I was unable to read notices and warnings, for example, "No Entry," "Beware of the dog," "No jobs!"

She proceeded to tell of a time she was mauled by a dog because she did not know that a circle with a line through it and a picture of a dog meant she had to beware of the dog.

Another learner spoke of the humiliation she experienced when asking for a job at a place that had a "No jobs" sign on display.

The new-found independence of being able to read and write was evidenced by Emah Skosana who said:

> Before I attended the literacy classes I could not write my name and surname, but now I can. I am able to complete a banking slip when I am sending money to my children at home. Before, I had to ask for assistance.

It is noteworthy that, of the 24 indicators referred to in Table 2.1, self-confidence was shown to rank the highest with 92.42% of the learners stating that they felt more confident at the end of the learning programme. Of the learners, 88.4% stated that they felt more "respected by the community," 86.79% felt they were "treated better in the community," and 85.61% indicated that they had expanded their social networks, which is also an extrinsic feature that might contribute to increased confidence.

The enhancement of learners' self-esteem and confidence is aptly shown in an excerpt from a report on a site visit to a prison literacy class. The case cited shows how under extreme circumstances, acquiring literacy impacted on the lives of the inmates and alleviated the pain of incarceration:

> The noise level is very high. A loudspeaker blares, calling inmates to attend to visitors, the big steel gates clang and people shout and hurl abuse at one another. Yet somewhere in the mayhem there is a classroom. ... The volunteer educators who work with the correctional services to bring adult prisoners within the scope of the campaign are used to these conditions. The learners themselves may lack self-worth and have low self-esteem. Some may be experiencing psychological stress as a result of prison gangs, whilst others may be depressed about a sentence that is going to come to an end soon.
>
> In this desperate situation, many men and women, young and old, who are serving a prison sentence, have become literate through the campaign. Many are even happy and enormously proud that they can now make contact with their loved ones via the written medium. In fact, one of the volunteer educators who works with imprisoned adults says that the first thing these learners do when they've acquired the skill of writing is to write a letter home to show what they have learnt and achieved.
>
> Some learners say that their attitudes have changed, and that they now respect other people's rights. One of them comments that he has never seen the purpose of school, but now that he has learnt to write letters to his wife and children, his outlook on education has changed. Another says he now knows the "good way" and that the learning showed him this way. Most of them feel positive that the knowledge, skills and attitudes they have acquired will help them when they are released. (Unisa, 2003, p. 23)

2.5.3 Literacy Relieving the Plight of Poverty

The Kha Ri Gude campaign required a multi-pronged approach to assist its beneficiaries to cope with a range of social problems they encountered on a day-to-day basis. In the face of rising food costs it was necessary to enable people to address food security in vulnerable communities and mitigate hunger and malnutrition.

The classes that were presented and the COP educator groups that were established opened the way for a range of possible interventions. These formations provided hubs that were used as a basis for interventions aimed at improving household food security for the rural and urban poor and enabling communities to improve their access to food and to enhance their own household food security. While most learners targeted by the two campaigns subsisted on a social grant, the interventions that increased their household food security enabled them to make their grants go further as they could produce food for their own households and market the surplus via women's cooperatives. Food security interventions played an important role in the campaigns, offering support to orphans and other vulnerable people. These projects targeted those most vulnerable to malnutrition in communities—infants, young children and the immune compromised—but also improved general family income levels.

2.5.4 Increased Social Networks

The importance of social networks is reflected in Fig. 2.4. The red bars in this figure show that a high number of learners perceived that their social networks had increased since embarking on literacy instruction, with a majority indicating that they had more friends (85.61%), experienced improved family relationships (91.05%) and felt more respected (88.22%). It is noteworthy that, of the 24 indicators, self-confidence was ranked the highest. Although the "feeling" of self-confidence may be considered intrinsic and subjective, the perception was extrinsically reciprocal with learners feeling "respected by the community," and feeling "better treated in the community."

In fact, UNESCO (2016, n.p.) refers to the way in which the Kha Ri Gude literacy campaign fostered community cohesion and peaceful coexistence through its "implementation model that created learners' groups that bring together people with common goals for themselves and their communities." Specific reference is made to the learners' expanded social networks: "besides the actual literacy learning experience, a lot of program participants come for the social aspect. They meet new friends and the learning groups help to overcome loneliness … establish social groupings which cooperate in a range of socioeconomic activities guided by reciprocity." This view was corroborated in one of the educator's journals as follows: "Learners now see school as a social activity that has improved their way of living."

The assessment of the value of literacy initiatives/investments needs to go beyond thinking about the "targets for literacy"—it should be expanded to include "quantitative goals," considering how participation in literacy programmes can "help shape the trajectories of lives" (Hanemann & McKay, 2015, p. 5).

The following quotations from the educators' journals show the increased participation of learners in communal and specifically school matters:

> Mothers are appointed to committees. They can take minutes at meetings and can communicate with others in meetings.
>
> It is especially important to learn English … especially when we have to communicate with teachers.

During class visits, it became apparent how the learners infected one another with their happiness and excitement.

> There is a lot of interaction in this classroom in Mabopane township, with comments flying backwards and forwards. One elderly learner summed up the general transformation that many learners had undergone since joining the literacy campaign when she remarked: I was always sad and depressed. Not anymore! Now I wake up every day and pick up my books and stop complaining. My life feels good. (Unisa, 2003, p. 26)

The following description of a class in the informal settlement of Ivory Park emphasises the social dimension of acquiring literacy and the role it plays in dealing with learner problems:

> The desks are pushed together to form groups and they chat to each other and to the educators about their worries. Small children in the class are being fed by their mothers but this does not disturb the other learners. (Unisa, 2003, p.21)

A similar social benefit was shown during a classroom visit to a learning group in Khayalitsha where evidence was provided of the role the learning groups played in the local community:

> The learners used to meet in a shack which became too cold. One of the learners asked her sister-in-law if the group could meet in her house three times a week. "Luckily," says Nothmbalethu, leaning back against her sister-in-law's fridge, "she said we could use this room."
>
> We all crowd into the room. The learners sit with their books on a bench in front of them. Their volunteer educator, a Unisa ABET [and a BEd] graduate is a seasoned development worker. ... She also happens to teach at the school across the road. In fact, she teaches the children on one side of the road, and the mothers in this class on the other side of the road. She laughs as she tells us that the children often bring their mothers' homework for her to mark at school and "they love it when the others get things wrong!"

The learners reported how the campaign programme had benefitted them:

- "I have opened a spaza shop, I can now count money and I have bought a fridge with the money I have made."
- "I can now read my own letters. I used to hate it when the person reading my letters used to laugh at what the letter said before I knew what was in the letter."
- Another learner confessed that "my husband is scared that now that I have a little education I might call him an illiterate." Another stated that "my husband who is blind loves it when I read to him," and other pointed out that "I can say my own words of love when I write my own letters."

2.5.5 Interrelated Networks

The classes and learning groups served as forums for learners to discuss their problems. Many of the challenges the learners experienced were discussed in class and these discussions, which were captured in the educators' journals, were escalated for further discussion at the educator COP meetings convened by supervisors. In this way the 40,000 classes were networked into the larger campaign network. McKay (2018a) explains how the campaign's organisation linked learner classes and clusters with other classes and clusters. She explains the expanded connectedness of the learning clusters (as depicted in Fig. 2.3) that shows how the campaign delivery model was decentralised across 40,000 learning sites and a range of settings across the country.[9] She also considers the key role the educators and the COP groups played in supporting the national intervention that aimed to reach 4.7 million adults and some 40,000 volunteer educators to provide large-scale literacy services. She (2018a p. 377) draws attention to what she refers to as a "robust system of support that would empower and capacitate campaign operatives to teach and deal with a host of challenges that they might face both in- and outside their classrooms."

While Fig. 2.3 shows how the literacy classes may be regarded as social capital within the broader social nexus, it is clear that the literacy learning classes and the campaign's organisational model impacted on the smallest social institution, namely the family, giving rise to advantages that might accrue to a literate family in terms of their access to more information, their economic survival and their general command of better communication and living skills. Moreover, given the large numbers of women learners in the campaign who in Fig. 2.4, perceived that they came to be "more respected" in the family (91.5%), the campaign offered ways of improving the status of women in their families, enabling them to exercise agency and take control over their lives, including their financial situations.

2.5.6 Survivalist Entrepreneurial Activities

Unemployment in South Africa is a major social challenge, with youth unemployment among the highest on the continent. While progress has been made in addressing poverty over the past decade, the poor in rural areas and the townships face

[9] SANLI utilised a scaled down version of this organisational structure.

challenges relating to the effective delivery of basic economic and social services.

The green bars in Fig. 2.4, which refer to learners' perceptions of the utility of their newly acquired skills, show that learners perceived that they had better problem-solving skills (86.09%), that they had a better understanding of managing their finances and using technology, and understood nutrition better. The educators reported that the increased problem-solving abilities of "groups" of learners enabled them to help not only themselves but also others in their communities, thereby increasing group resilience.

The formation of learning groups, which enhanced learners' resilience, enabled learners to set up small businesses, such as spaza shops, and start bead-making and craft projects. Learners also ventured to learn other skills, from brick- to curtain-making. Another group started making coffins and got the support of a local undertaker who gave them a venue for their literacy classes. Choirs marketed their services at weddings and funerals, and women's groups manufactured school jerseys and set up bakeries with funding from the Department of Trade and Industry.

The following quotation describing a class of learners shows how the classes helped learners to deal with the problems in their day-to-day lives.

> We meet a group of about 30 women at the Lofentse Girls High School. They are mostly unemployed and their ages range from 17–60 years. Kgomotso, the volunteer educator, opens each lesson with a prayer. The learners often have much to say in prayer and praise of the opportunity that have had to learn. The group is remarkable cohesive. The rhythm of the work session is clearly visible as the learners follow their usual pattern. Once they have finished their prayers. They start talking about a newspaper article that caught their eye during the course of the week. Much discussion of the chosen article usually takes place before the lessons begin, aligning the topic to their own lives. Acquiring the art of using the English language is a common goal in the group. Once this is achieved, the learners have their eye on employment opportunities. (Unisa, 2003, p. 13)

The learners in the campaigns consisted mostly of unemployed, poor rural and urban individuals who came from communities that were excluded from social dialogue (McKay & Makhanya, 2008). Moreover, the HIV/AIDS pandemic threatened the livelihoods of these people, with women facing the most severe consequences and older women having to take on a second round of family responsibility to care for orphaned grandchildren, a phenomenon which the International Labour Organisation (2004, p. 32) terms the "feminisation of poverty."

The two purple bars in Fig. 2.4 refer to improved income-generation activities. It was found that 77.55% of the learners "started earning" after enrolling for the Kha Ri Gude programme. While it is recognised that they may not have been referring to jobs in the formal sector (since only 10% were formally employed), "starting to earn" meant that these learners had become engaged in informal/survivalist work activities since the start of their literacy training. Of those who were employed, 64.87% stated that their job positions had improved as a result of their becoming literate.

As the UNESCO Institute for Lifelong Learning points out in respect of the Kha Ri Gude campaign:

> Learners acquire basic literacy skills including basic spoken English. This has enabled hitherto illiterate youth and adults to be more independent in conducting daily business including undertaking shopping errands and travelling. … In addition, programme graduates have also been empowered to engage in more profitable income-generating activities or to improve the profitability of their existing projects. Essentially therefore, the programme enables both employees—most of whom had been unemployed—and learners to be self-reliant and to contribute towards their families' well-being and living standards. (UNESCO, 2016)

The learning materials encouraged learners to seek out entrepreneurial opportunities, and some of the outcomes were reflected in the educators' journals:

> As a group of educators, we will teach all the learners under us the skills that we have for business.
>
> Learners are happy to be able to write. They even have thoughts of opening spaza shops because they can count, read and write.
>
> Learners are now able to participate in community projects like farming.

Learners have learned skills like beadwork and sewing.
Learner started to crochet things that they sell.
The learners in my class started a bead-making project and they sell beads to help themselves.
Learners started to make things with beads that we are going to sell.
The teacher and her learners have a good relationship. Her learners help their family to bake bread, and she taught them how to sew clothes.
She and her learners have set up a vegetable garden and the families get vegetables from this garden.
Her learners help the community by moulding clay posts and sell them to the community.
The class is now planning to buy materials in order to use their shoe-making skills that I taught them.
The group has formed and is growing vegetables together and will take them home and sell them.

2.5.7 Learning to Learn

Lastly, the pale green bars in Fig. 2.4 refer to the importance of lifelong learning in supporting children's learning and encouraging others to learn.

As shown in the figure, 89.34% of the learners expressed a desire to continue learning, suggesting that the campaign had created an "appetite" for learning. Moreover, 84.98% of the learners stated that they "better understand their child's schooling," and 84.2% assisted their children with homework, suggesting that their literacy acquisition positively impacted on the education of their children.

In addition, 82.22% of learners indicated that they had more reading materials, books and magazines in their homes. This is notwithstanding the fact that many of the learners lived in rural and informal settlements where the focus is generally not on literacy enrichment (Shrestha & Krolak, 2015).

In line with the spirit of ubuntu, learners were encouraged to collaborate with their learning peers (Biraimah, 2016; Brock-Utne, 2016; Oviawe, 2016). The educators' journals referred to learners' agency in establishing class committees, taking responsibility for finding convenient learning venues, recruiting new learners and ensuring regular class attendance of their peers. Many of the educators' journals mentioned that learners visited their peers who were absent or assisted disabled learners who had difficulties attending classes without assistance.

The literacy programme aimed at improving parenting techniques and teaching strategies for supervising children's homework. The exit survey showed that 84.2% of the learners assisted children with homework and a further 84.98% indicated that they were more knowledgeable about their children's education.

The learning materials were designed specifically to heighten learners' awareness of parenting techniques and to reinforce strategies for supervising children's homework. The exit survey (see responses in Fig. 2.4) showed that since becoming literate, 84.2% of learners experienced changes in the extent to which they assisted their children with homework, and a further 84.98% indicated that they were more knowledgeable about their children's education.

Osman (2009, p. 34), in her review of the literacy campaign, states that learners felt that the programme was beneficial to them "in that it assisted them to help the children with their homework, and also provided an opportunity for the children to help the older caregivers with theirs."

The following notes taken from the educators' journals revealed the impact that literacy acquisition had on the schooling of learners' children.

> They are now empowered to attend school meetings and to participate in school activities.
>
> They can help their children with their homework because they know how to read.

The converse was also reflected in the educators' journals. It was not unusual for children to visit their parents' literacy classes to obtain information on how they could better assist their parents with their homework. As one educator explained in her journal:

> Children come to class to check on their parents' marks and to check their answers [to the assessment activities] and to find out what homework they have to do. They regularly check on how well their parents are doing.

In similar vein, another educator referred to the inter-generationality of learning:

> Learners are now able to help their children with homework, and their children also help them with their work.

Fullick (2009, p. 45) sums up the importance of community-based learning as effective networks. As she puts it:

> Community-based learning can be effective in promoting networks in deprived areas. This is because community learning often arises from interests shared by groups of people …. Community-based learning can help people to operate effectively in a group: it helps people to listen, reflect and share; it develops understanding and trust of others and the ability to gain support from others. By developing confidence, as well as the "hard" skills of contextual knowledge and practical competencies, such learning can be applied to the social contexts in which people find themselves.

2.6 Conclusion

In this chapter I focused on how programmes for acquiring literacy and the organisation of mass-based campaigns impact on adult learners whose lives are socially, economically and even psychologically impoverished. It shows how campaigning for literacy enables active communities to develop the agency and collective social capital to tackle extremely difficult life circumstances, enhancing the quality of their lives and enabling learners to give meaning to their lives even under dire circumstances.

I conclude by citing Torres (2004, p. 22) who sums up the many ways in which adult basic learning impacts on personal, community and national development, improving the quality of life of people in various domains:

- giving hope, dignity, self-esteem, empowerment, enhanced self-expression and communication skills, positive attitudes, sense of future, better overall objective and subjective conditions for livelihoods and for improving the quality of one's life;
- the achievements of their children where (especially mothers') educational background, provide better conditions, not only educationally but in many other aspects, for their offspring; and
- on the local and the broader community enhancing community and civic participation with adult learners increasing their concern about social and environmental issues, and citizenship.

The learner experiences described in this chapter illustrate as Bhola (1984, p. 24) contends, "that literacy is truly an initiation into the magical circle of the literate, releasing the individual from a sense of personal inferiority, from the relationship of dependency and subservience, and allocates a new status and potential." It is catalytic in improving the quality of life of the learners, their families and communities.

References

Akter, S., Rutsaert, P., Juis, J., Nyo, M., SuSan, B., & Pustikar, A. (2017). Women's empowerment and gender equity in agriculture: A different perspective from Southeast Asia. *Food Policy, 69*, 20–279. https://doi.org/10.1016/j.foodpol.2017.05.003.

Aldrich, D. P., & Meyer, M. A. (2015). Social capital and community resilience. *American Behavioral Scientist, 59*(2), 254–269. https://doi.org/10.1177/0002764214550299.

Aliber, M. (2003). Chronic poverty in South Africa: Incidence, causes and policies. *World Development, 31*(3), 473–490. https://doi.org/10.1016/S0305-750X(02)00219-X.

Alidou, H., Boly, A., Brock-Utne, B., Satina, Y., Diallo, K. H., & Ekkehard Wolff, H. (2006). Optimizing learning and education in Africa – the language factor. Gabon: Working document: Association for the development of education in Africa (ADEA). In *ADEA 2006 Biennial Meeting*.

Bhola, H. S. (1984). *Campaigning for literacy: Eight national experiences of the twentieth century with a memorandum to decision makers*. Paris: UNESCO.

Biraimah, K. L. (2016). Moving beyond a destructive past to a decolonised and inclusive future: The role of ubuntu-style education in providing culturally relevant pedagogy for Namibia. *International Review of Education, 62*, 45–62. https://doi.org/10.1007/s11159-016-9541-1.

Bolden, R. (2014). Ubuntu. In D. Coghlan & M. Brydon-Miller (Eds.), *Sage encyclopedia of action research* (pp. 799–802). Thousand Oaks, CA: Sage.

Bosworth, B. (2016). *South Africa – Key to putting informal settlements on the Habitat III agenda*. Retrieved from https://www.urbanafrica.net/news/south-africa-key-to-putting-informal-settlements-on-the-habitat-iii-agenda/

Botman, B. V. (2014). *Educators, praxis and hope: A philosophical analysis of post-apartheid teacher education policy*. Unpublished PhD dissertation. Stellenbosch University.

Boughton, B. (2016). Popular education and mass literacy campaigns: Beyond "new literacy studies". In K. Yasukawa & S. Black (Eds.), *Beyond economic interests. Critical perspectives on adult literacy and numeracy in a globalised world* (pp. 149–164). Rotterdam, The Netherlands: Sense Publishers. https://doi.org/10.1007/978-94-6300-444-2_10.

Brock-Utne, B. (2016). The Ubuntu paradigm in curriculum work, language of instruction and assessment. *International Review of Education, 62*(1), 29–44. https://doi.org/10.1007/s11159-016-9540-2.

Chilisa, B. (2009). Indigenous African-centered ethics: Contesting and complementing dominant models. In D. M. Mertens & P. E. Ginsberg (Eds.), *The handbook of social research ethics* (pp. 407–426). London, UK: Sage. https://doi.org/10.4135/9781483348971.n26.

Chilisa, B., & Preece, J. (Eds.). (2005). *Research methods for adult educators in Africa*. Cape Town, South Africa: Pearson Education.

Coleman, J. S. (1988). Social capital in the creation of human capital. *American Journal of Sociology, 94*(1988), S95–S120. https://doi.org/10.1086/228943.

Creswell, J., & Garrett, A. (2008). The "movement" of mixed methods research and the role of educators. *South African Journal of Education, 28*(3), 321–333.

Dale, A., & Newman, L. (2006). Sustainable community development, networks and resilience. *Environments, 34*(2), 17–27.

Department of Basic Education. (2011). *"Yes I can": Learner assessment portfolio for the Kha Ri Gude South African literacy campaign*. Pretoria, South Africa: Department of Basic Education.

Freire, P. (2000). *Pedagogy of the oppressed*. New York, NY: Continuum.

Freire, P. (2006). *Pedagogy of hope: Reliving pedagogy of the oppressed*. New York, NY: Continuum.

Fullick, L. (2009). *Poverty reduction and lifelong learning* (IFLL Thematic Paper 6). Leicester, UK: National Institute of Adult Continuing Education.

Giddens, A. (1991). *Modernity and self-identity: Self and society in the late modern age*. Oxford, UK: Polity Press.

Gumbo, M. T. (2017). Botho under siege: Elders voice their unhappiness about children's behaviour. In M. T. Gumbo & V. Msila (Eds.), *African voices on indigenisation of the curriculum: Insights from practice* (pp. 306–333). Wandsbeck, Germany: Reach Publishers.

Hanemann, U., & McKay, V. (2015). Lifelong literacy: Towards a new agenda. *International Review of Education, 61*(3), 265–272. https://doi.org/10.1007/s11159-015-9497-6.

International Labour Organisation. (2004). *Working out of poverty*. Geneva, Switzerland: International Labour Organisation.

Ison, R., Blackmore, C., Collins, K., Holwell, S., & Iaquinto, B. (2014). Insights into operationalizing communities of practice: SSM-based inquiry processes. *Systemic Practice Action Research, 27*, 91–113.

Johnson, R. B., & Onwuegbuzie, A. J. (2004). Mixed methods research: A research paradigm whose time has come. *Educational Researcher, 33*(7), 14–26. https://doi.org/10.3102/0013189X033007014.

Johnson, R. B., Onwuegbuzie, A. J., & Turner, L. A. (2007). Toward a definition of mixed methods research. *Journal of Mixed Methods Research, 1*(2), 112–133. https://doi.org/10.1177/1558689806298224.

Johnston, D., Kaye, K., Becker, J., Leonard, G., Saunders, W., Wright, K., …, Ronan, K. (2009). *Building community resilience through community-based education programmes*. Palmerston North, New Zealand: Massey University.

Lehohla, P. (2017). *Poverty trends in South Africa: An examination of absolute poverty between 2006 and 2015* (Report No. 03-10-06). Pretoria, South Africa: Statistics South Africa.

Letseka, M. (2016). *The amalgamation of traditional African values and liberal democratic values in South Africa: Implications for conceptions of education.* (Unpublished PhD thesis). University of South Africa, Pretoria.

Lind, A. (2008). *Literacy for all: Making a difference* (Series on Fundamentals of Educational Planning). Paris: UNESCO International Institute for Educational Planning.

McKay, V. (2007). Adult basic education and training in South Africa. In Adult Education, J. Comings, B. Garner, & C. Smith (Eds.), *Review of adult learning and literacy* (Vol. 7 (9), pp. 285–310). Mahwah, NJ: Lawrence Erlbaum Associates.

McKay, V. (2012). *Reconfiguring the post-schooling sector: A critical review of adult basic education and training provision in South Africa* (Article prepared for the project: Towards credible institutional mechanisms for skills planning. Department of Higher Education and Training). Pretoria, South Africa: Human Sciences Research Council. Labour Market Intelligence. http://www.lmip.org.za/sites/default/files/documentfiles//18%20Veronica_McKay_A_critical_review_on_ABET_provision_in_SA%20(2).pdf.

McKay, V. (2015). Measuring and monitoring in the South African Kha Ri Gude mass literacy campaign.

International Review of Education, 61(3), 365–397. https://doi.org/10.1007/s11159-015-9495-8.

McKay, V. (2018a). Through the eye of a fly: Action research as a support for the South African national literacy campaign. *Systemic Practice and Action Research, 31*, 375–393. https://doi.org/10.1007/s11213-017-9431-x.

McKay, V. (2018b). Literacy, lifelong learning and sustainable development. *Australian Journal of Adult Learning, 58*(3), 390–425. ISSN: 1443-1394.

McKay, V., & Makhanya, M. (2008). Making it work for the South: Using open and distance learning in the context of development. In T. Evans, M. Haughey, & D. Murphy (Eds.), *International handbook of distance education* (pp. 29–48). Bingley, UK: Emerald.

McKay, V., & Romm, N. (2015). Narratives of agency: The experiences of Braille literacy practitioners in the Kha Ri Gude South African mass literacy campaign. *International Journal of Inclusive Education, 19*(4), 435–456. https://doi.org/10.1080/13603116.2014.940066.

McLafferty, C., & Onwuegbuzie, A. J. (2006, November). *A dimensional resolution of the qualitative-quantitative dichotomy: Implications for theory, praxis, and national research policy.* Paper presented at the annual meeting of the Mid-South Educational Research Association, Birmingham, UK.

McLaren, P., & Leonard, P. (1993). *Paulo Freire: A critical encounter*. London: Routledge. https://doi.org/10.4324/9780203420263.

Morse, J. M. (2003). Principles of mixed methods and multi-method research design. In A. Takashori & C. Teddlie (Eds.), *Handbook of mixed methods in social and behavioural research* (pp. 189–208). Thousand Oaks, CA: Sage.

Osman, A. (2009). *Evaluation of the Kha Ri Gude South African literacy campaign*. New York, NY: United Nations Children's Fund (UNICEF).

Oviawe, O. J. (2016). How to rediscover the ubuntu paradigm in education. *International Review of Education, 62*, 1–10. https://doi.org/10.1007/s11159-016-9545-x.

Portes, A. (1998). Social capital: Its origins and applications in modern society. *Annual Review of Sociology, 24*(1), 1–24. https://doi.org/10.1146/annurev.soc.24.1.1.

Preece, J. (2013). Adult education and poverty reduction. In P. Mayo (Ed.), *Learning with adults. International issues in adult education* (pp. 309–316). Rotterdam, The Netherlands: Sense Publishers. https://doi.org/10.1007/978-94-6209-335-5_24.

Putnam, R. (2001). *Bowling alone: The collapse and revival of American community*. London, UK: Simon and Schuster.

Ruele, V. (2017). Adopting a foreign curriculum in Botwana: Benefits and shortcomings and implications for Africanisation. In M. T. Gumbo & V. Msila (Eds.), *African voices on indigenisation of the curriculum: Insights from practice* (pp. 181–223). Wandsbeck, Germany: Reach Publishers.

Sachs, J. D. (2005). *The end of poverty: Economic possibilities of our time*. New York, NY: Penguin.

Sen, A. (1999). *Development as freedom*. Oxford, UK: Oxford University Press.

Setlhodi, I. (2018). Ubuntu leadership: An African Panacea for improving school performance. *Africa Education Review*, 1–17. https://doi.org/10.1080/18146627.2018.1464885. ISSN: 1753-5921(Online).

Shor, I. (1993). From the pedagogy of the oppressed to a luta continua: The political pedagogy of Paulo Freire. In P. McLaren & P. Leonard (Eds.), *Paulo Freire's critical pedagogy* (pp. 25–35). London, UK: Routledge. https://doi.org/10.4324/9780203420263_chapter_2.

Shrestha, S., & Krolak, L. (2015). The potential of community libraries in supporting literate environments and sustaining literacy skills. *International Review of Education, 61*(3), 399–418. https://doi.org/10.1007/s11159-014-9462-9.

Singh, M., & McKay, V. (2004). Improving the quality of adult basic learning and training adult educators. In M. Singh & V. McKay (Eds.), *Enhancing adult basic learning: Training educators and unlocking the potential of distance and open learning*. Pretoria, South Africa: Unisa Press & UNESCO.

Street, B. V. (1984). *Literacy in theory and practice*. New York, NY: Cambridge University Press.

Street, B. V. (2014). *Social literacies: Critical approaches to literacy in development, ethnography and education*. London, UK: Routledge. Original work published 1995, New York, NY: Longman.

Torres, R. M. (2004). *Lifelong learning in the north and education for all in the south?* Beijing, China: International Conference on Lifelong Learning: Global Perspectives in Education.

UNESCO. (2003). *Literacy as freedom*. Paris, France: UNESCO.

UNESCO. (2006). *Education for all global monitoring report*. Paris, France: UNESCO. Retrieved from unesdoc. https://unesco.org/images/0014/001416/141639e.pdf.

UNESCO. (2016). *Kha Ri Gude (let us learn) adult literacy programme*. Retrieved from http://litbase.uil.unesco.org/?menu=13&=ZA&program=69

UNISA. (2003). *Literacy matters. A commemorative report*. Pretoria: ABET/Unisa.

United Nations. (1967). *Universal declaration of human rights*. Paris: United Nations.

United Nations. (2000). *Millennium development goals*. New York, NY: United Nations. Retrieved from www.un.org/millenniumgoals/bkgd.shtml.

United Nations. (2015). *2030 Agenda for sustainable development*. Retrieved from https://sustainabledevelopment.un.org/content/documents/21252030%20agenda%20for%20Sustainable%20Development%20web.pdf

Wenger, E. (1998). *Communities of practice: Learning as a social system*. https://doi.org/10.1017/CBO9780511803932

3 The Development of an Integrated, Multi-level Process to Facilitate the Promotion of Holistic Wellbeing in School Communities

Ansie Elizabeth Kitching

Abstract

This chapter reports on the development of an integrated, multi-level process to facilitate the promotion of holistic wellbeing, as a basis for enhancing the quality of life in six South African school communities situated in lower socio-economic contexts. Holistic wellbeing is understood as individual, relational and collective wellbeing. The rationale behind the research relating to the development of this process was to address the despondence with the contextual challenges in these school communities. A participatory action learning and action research design was applied to ensure that members of the school communities take ownership of the process. The research revealed several outcomes of the process: the promotion of individual wellbeing through the expansion of opportunities for personal development; the encouragement of value-based behaviour; attention to contextual challenges and support needs; relational wellbeing through the strengthening of connections and the facilitation of an ethos of kindness, empathy and care; collective wellbeing through the enhancement of shared responsibility across all the levels of interconnectedness; and the co-construction of a more conducive environment for all members. The research findings also foregrounded the pivotal role of wellbeing support teams in the sustainable implementation of the process as a basis for the enhancement of quality of life in school contexts.

A. E. Kitching (✉)
COMBER North-West University,
Potchefstroom, South Africa
e-mail: akitching@uwc.ac.za

3.1 Introduction

It is in our hands to create a better world for all who live in it. (Nelson Mandela)

As human beings, our lives are intertwined with the lives of others in a web of interconnectedness. This is entailed in the African communitarian concept of *ubuntu*, as described by the aphorism "a person is a person through relationships with other people" (Shepard & Mhlanga, 2014). The complex, interactive and dynamic interplay between us as human beings and our social contexts deeply impacts the quality of our lives. Quality of life refers to the general wellbeing of individuals and societies (Marujo & Neto, 2017) and implies a dynamic and active state of flourishing, described as "both a positive and desirable state of affairs with life as a whole and with specific domains of life, such as health, economic situation, and relationships" (Prilleltensky & Prilleltensky, 2003).

I. Eloff (ed.), *Handbook of Quality of Life in African Societies*, International Handbooks of Quality-of-Life, https://doi.org/10.1007/978-3-030-15367-0_3

In South Africa, the struggle against injustice and inequality during the Apartheid era was to afford freedom and equal access to rights and resources for all. In the post-Apartheid era, this struggle has been replaced with a struggle for an acceptable quality of life for all (Gaibie & Davids, 2009). A survey by the Human Science Research Council in 2017 revealed that roughly half of South African citizens have good quality of life; the other half, who are less privileged, still experience social division and inequality that affect the quality of their lives (HSRC, 2017). The majority of the South African population, according to the latest census (Statistics South Africa, 2013), is between 5 and 16 years old. The implication is that most South Africans whose quality of life is compromised are of school-going age. Weare and Nind (2011) argue that schools are suitable environments for providing interventions that could enhance quality of life in contexts where it has been compromised. South African schools situated in lower socio-economic contexts should therefore be socially inclusive, humanised and coherent spaces (Florian & Spratt, 2013) in which "the full and ever evolving humanity of people" (Fataar, 2015) is considered.

Since the advent of democracy in 1994, various policies have been formulated and implemented in the health and education sectors, with the aim of addressing the challenges associated with the prevailing inequalities between different school contexts. In 2000, the Department of Health brought forth the National Guidelines for the Development of Health Promoting Schools in South Africa (Department of Health, 2000). The national policy guidelines (Department of Health, 2001, 2008) emphasise the holistic development of schools, with a specific focus on safe and supportive teaching and learning environments, strong school-community partnerships, the pursuit of curriculum interventions that focus on skills development, and the development of accessible educational support services such as preventative and health promotion programmes (Lazarus, 2006). In 2012, the Integrated School Health Policy (ISHP) replaced the Health Promotion Policy and the Health and Wellness in Education framework developed in 2006, as well as the School Health Policy developed in 2003.

The IHSP aims to enhance the growth, health and development of children and the communities they reside in through collaboration between the Department of Basic Education and the Department of Health. Various policies govern and influence the ISHP, including Education White Paper 6 (Special Needs Education): Building an Inclusive Education and Training System (2001), which is aimed at providing access to quality education for all learners through the development of environments in which all learners regardless of differences in ability, culture, gender, language, class and ethnicity can experience a sense of belonging and nurturing and be supported to achieve their optimal potential irrespective of intrinsic and extrinsic barriers to learning (Engelbrecht, Savolainen, Nel, Koskeala, & Okkulin, 2017). The Care and Support for Teaching and Learning (CSTL) programme, in turn, is aimed at operationalising the strategic intent of the above-mentioned policies into practice. The vision of CSTL is to transform schools into inclusive centres, thereby addressing the educational rights of learners, including learners that are deemed vulnerable (Department of Basic Education and MIET Africa, 2010).

The problem observed with reference to the implementation of these policies and programmes in practice is that the focus is almost exclusively on addressing deficits and risks that hinder academic performance and not on the enhancement of wellbeing and quality of life. Academic performance and achievement are prioritised to the extent that it leads to the dehumanising of schools (Fataar, 2016; Haslam & Loughnan, 2014). In these dehumanised school contexts, teachers and learners are objectified into robot-like performance machines who have to produce high test scores, often at the cost of their mental health and wellbeing (Shaughnessy, Galligan, & Hurtardo de Vivas, 2008). Moreover, the promotion of wellbeing is not considered an essential part of schooling. The implication is that instead of integrating everyday interactions, activities and interventions that contribute to the promotion of holistic wellbeing in schools into a cohesive process, wellbeing is promoted in a haphazard and fragmented manner.

Consequently, schools where learners do not perform according to expectations are often labelled as "dysfunctional" due to their poor academic results. The labelling of these schools as dysfunctional is unfortunate and sustains the notion of discrimination. In reality, these schools have limited resources, a scarcity of professional support, fewer opportunities for individual learners to develop optimally, large classes, and limited involvement of parents. All these challenges compromise the co-construction of an environment in which quality of life can be enhanced. Evidently, the deficit focus perpetuates a reactive approach that concentrates on the *welfare* of people, rather than on their *wellbeing* (Roffey, 2013, 2015).

This problem is, at least partially, addressed in the research presented in this chapter. The research was conducted between 2015 and 2017 in six school communities in the Western Cape, one of the nine provinces in South Africa. In this chapter, I present the philosophical and theoretical perspectives that informed the research, contextualise the research, describe the development of the process through the application of a participatory action learning and action research methodology, and interrogate the possible contribution of such a process to enhance the quality of life in schools situated in lower socio-economic contexts. Finally, I consider a way forward for the application of the knowledge obtained in the African context.

3.2 Philosophical and Theoretical Perspectives

The conceptualisation of schools as communities is key to our understanding of the role that schools can play in enhancing people's quality of life. Community, in the context of this project, is understood as a relational phenomenon through which individuals are given opportunities to develop affiliations of support and feelings of attachment (Lewis, Lewis, Daniels, & DÁndrea, 2002). The idea of schools as communities has been promoted for a long time and by various researchers (Dewey, 1957; Saleebey, 2001; Sarason, 1974; Sergiovanni, 1994; Strike, 2000, 2004) who emphasised the importance of the social aspects of schooling. The implication of perceiving schools as communities is that the focus shifts from the "I" to the collective "we", and from an exclusive focus on academic work to the inclusion of opportunities for learners to learn more about themselves, build healthy and supportive relationships, and become part of a community that values them (Joyce, 2013).

Schools as communities are dynamic emergent systems in which the parts are interrelated and influence each other (Foster-Fishman & Behrens, 2007). The promotion of the wellbeing of one person can therefore not exist independently from the rest of the school community. A multi-level approach is required in which the focus is on all members of the school community across various levels of interrelatedness (Ng & Fisher, 2013). For Prilleltensky (2005), such a multifaceted understanding of wellbeing necessitated a shift in focus in health and human services from reactive, linear and individually focussed interventions towards strengths, prevention, and the empowerment of school communities to change conditions. The promotion of wellbeing in school communities cannot therefore only focus on the wellbeing of individual members, but should also encompass a focus on the relational wellbeing and collective wellbeing in these contexts. Individual wellbeing entails self-determination, a sense of control, self-efficacy, physical and mental health, optimism, meaning and spirituality. Relational wellbeing encompasses the enhancement of respect, appreciation of diversity, and a focus on cooperation and democratic participation. Collective wellbeing refers to the equitable allocation of bargaining powers, resources and obligations in a community as an enabling context (Nelson & Prilleltensky, 2010).

Schueller (2009) proposes an integration of community psychology and positive psychology, since both perspectives define mental health as different from the mere absence of illness, and share principles and goals aimed at enhancing community strengths. Positive psychology and community psychology theories also converge on various principles and goals, opting to approach wellness from a strength-based approach (Schueller, 2009). Positive psychology aims to reveal those supportive and strengthening mechanisms that allow individuals as well as communities to flourish and to prosper. In this sense, the strength-based approach is more caring and is about much more than the eradication of ill-being or risk behaviours or of simply being symptom-free (Koller & Lisboa, 2007). Positive psychology does not deny negative human experiences, but aims to balance scientific enquiry through their exploration of positive experience (Gable & Haidt, 2005).

Positive psychology provides a meta-theoretical framework for incorporating theoretical approaches that conceptualise quality of life. Quality of life, according to Efklides and Moraitou (2013), can be conceived of as a generic term that pertains to all people, healthy or not, and encompasses positive emotions that go beyond happiness. It has the advantage that it can be applied to many different domains of life such as interpersonal relations, health-related situations, and professional and educational endeavours. Quality of life is a multidimensional construct with both subjective and objective components, and is influenced by personal and environmental factors (Wang, Schalock, Verdugo, & Jenaro, (2010). The notion of a good life can be measured on a spectrum from the objective to the subjective (Ventegodt, Merrick, & Andersen, 2003). This spectrum incorporates a number of existing quality of life theories referred to as the integrative quality of life (IQOL) theory, which incorporates aspects such as wellbeing, satisfaction with life, happiness, meaning in life, the biological information system ("balance"), realising life potential, fulfilment of needs, and objective factors. Møller (2007) distinguishes between the bottom-up model, which states that one's satisfaction with the various domains in one's life determines overall wellbeing and happiness, and the more recent top-down model, also known as the Multiple Discrepancy Theory, which purports that one's overall satisfaction with life determines how one feels about the various aspects of one's life.

Various frameworks have been developed to identify domains and indicators of wellbeing of this multi-dimensional construct. Schalock, Keith, Verdugo, and Gómez (2010) developed a quality of life conceptual and measurement framework that has been validated in a number of studies by demonstrating the factor structure of the domains and determining the etic (universal) and emic (culture-bound) properties of the domains and indicators. This framework identifies eight domains: emotional wellbeing, interpersonal relationships, material wellbeing, personal development, physical wellbeing, self-determination, social inclusion and rights. Fitz-Gibbon and Kochan (2000) developed a quality of school life model containing seven general domains of school performance indicators, including student numbers and resources, quality of life, affect, behavioural skills and cognitive achievement. Faragher and Van Ommen (2017) conceptualised an educational quality of life model following the process described by Schalock, Verdugo, Gomez, and Reinders (2016). These authors distinguish between five domains, namely learning, curriculum and teaching approaches, school organisation, school community, as well as vision and culture, as indicative of educational wellbeing.

From a complexity theory perspective, wellbeing and the enhancement of quality of life emerge in the complex, dynamic ways of relating and interacting between people and cannot be ascribed to specific factors in a linear, causal way (Stacey, 2007; Shaw, 2002). The theory of complex responsiveness processes of relating provides a radically alternative way of thinking about the interaction between individuals in a social context such as schools, and has been used to understand the interactive dynamics in schools (Kitching, 2010; Morrison, 2002; Radford, 2007). From a complex responsive process of relating perspective, members of a school community are interdependent, and individual minds are formed by the social interactions between them while they, in turn, form the social relations in iterative, non-linear self-organising processes

(Stacey, 2003). Based on Stacey's theory, Jörg (2009) argues that human interaction is a generative process in which not information, but influence is central and therefore encompasses the reciprocal influences each of the persons in interaction may have on the other. The complex interactive relational dynamics in a given context therefore provides the basis for facilitating social change and transformation that goes beyond mere first order change. If a critical mass of diversity and complexity is reached within an environment or system, new properties, behaviour and patterns emerge as continuity and change occur. Suchman (2006) states that an awareness of context and relationships and the fostering of greater receptivity and openness to change help to increase resourcefulness, flexibility and adaptability within a particular context.

Due to the complex nature of the promotion of wellbeing and quality of life, the development of strategies should encompass the deliberate coordination of the process. The application of transactive goal dynamics theory provides a multi-level model of goal systems, and informs the understanding of coordination in various distinct ways. The theory is guided by assumptions regarding the complex web of links in which social actors in social systems are situated (Fitzsimons, Finkel, & Vandellen, 2015; Fitzsimons, Sackett, & Finkel, 2016). The theory also underscores the complex interdependence of members' goals, pursuits and outcomes, and encourages the creation and strengthening of linkages between these goals into a network of mutual goals that are collectively beneficial. Efficient goal coordination also implies that the strengths, skills and interests of members are utilised, positive relational experiences are enhanced to improve group cohesion, and agreement between members is obtained in the pursuit of individual, relational and collective goals and targets.

An integration of these philosophical and theoretical perspectives provides a basis for addressing concerns about the wellbeing and quality of life in schools, understood as communities in which the complex dynamic interactions between people influence how they are together in these contexts.

3.3 Contextualising the Research

During the Apartheid years, education was only compulsory for the dominant white population group, and even in instances where other groups had access to education, the standard of education was regulated through racially exclusive systems. Consequently, the majority of the South African population was deprived of a good education (Fiske & Ladd, 2004a, b). In the advent of the new democracy, the Constitution of South Africa promulgated in December 1996 emphasised the values of "human dignity, the achievement of equality and the advancement of human rights and freedoms" (South African Department of Education, 2001). These values were translated into policies and programmes aimed at ensuring that all learners within the education system receive appropriate support to achieve their full potential. An eco-systemic approach to addressing learning barriers was recommended, veering from individualistic approaches in which the problem is seen as residing within the individual, who then needs adjustment (Johnson & Lazarus, 2003). However, despite these efforts, the disparities that developed over years were still prevalent in lower socio-economic contexts.

The prevailing inequity has been addressed through the development of a system that allocates funding according to the socio-economic status of the families. All South African public ordinary schools utilise a system of five categories, referred to as quintiles. This system enables the categorisation of school communities for funding purposes based on the relative poverty of the communities that surround the school (Western Cape Education Department, 2006). Quintile 1 is deemed the 'least poor' while Quintile 1 is the 'poorest'. School communities in Quintiles 4 and 5 are fee-paying schools, while schools that fall within Quintiles 1, 2 and 3 are 'no-fee' schools (Grant, 2013).

Five of the six schools in this study were previously disadvantaged, while the sixth school was a model C school advantaged by the Apartheid system. The implication post 1994 is that the five schools are classified as Quintile 1 schools, while the sixth school is classified as a Quintile 4 school. Yet the majority of learners who currently attend the Quintile 4 school are from the same low socio-economic contexts as the learners in the other schools. All of these schools continuously experience the impact of contextual challenges including the insufficient availability of housing, the unemployment of parents, social ills such as drug abuse and alcoholism, sexual promiscuity, as well as crime. As a result of the prevailing conditions, the schools struggle with learner absenteeism, limited parental involvement and inadequate support for learners who experience challenges, teacher stress, and a lack of resources. The current situation visibly affects the wellbeing and quality of life of all involved, including staff members, learners and parents.

3.4 Entrée into the School Communities

A year before the commencement of the research, the primary researcher was invited by an Educational Trust to act as a consultant in an initiative to enhance the holistic development of the six schools as part of the Trust's social responsibility outreach. In initial discussions with the school principals and staff members of the six schools, it was evident that the staff at these schools did not necessarily perceive the promotion of wellbeing as part of the core business of schooling. They were instead trapped in a cycle of despondence in which they could only focus on problems, and therefore experienced a sense of despair about the limitations and the challenges they had to deal with on a daily basis. Being trapped in this cycle appeared to limit their ability to accept responsibility for transforming their schools into more enabling environments in which people can experience quality of life.

In an effort to enhance their awareness of the value of the promotion of wellbeing in addressing this sense of despair, a group of teachers was invited to participate in a series of conversations about a more pro-active approach. The conversations were informed by the philosophical and theoretical perspectives discussed above, and aimed at enhancing a more pro-active approach to the problems and concerns that kept the staff in a spiral of despair about their situation. A shift towards a more pro-active approach was facilitated by creating an awareness amongst them of the everyday activities and interventions that already contributed to the wellbeing of members of the school community. These included, for example, the small acts of kindness and care shown by teachers on a daily basis, the care of parents who were concerned about their children, teachers acting as mentors to learners, programmes to address hygiene, feeding schemes, pastoral and counselling services for learners experiencing social and emotional needs, parent evenings, as well as non-profit organisations that provide various forms of support for learners.

The initial scepticism about the proposed change towards a more pro-active approach gradually shifted as the group of teachers began to understand the complex and paradoxical nature of being together in a school community. The challenge was to translate the acceptance of the approach into a practical process that considers the complex, diverse nature of each of the contexts. Being informed by a complexity theory perspective (Cilliers, 1998; Mason, 2008) and the principles of community psychology (Lazarus, 2006; Nelson & Prilleltensky, 2010) implied the development of a process based on broad guidelines that could be adapted according to contextual needs, rather than the development of a blueprinted programme.

In July 2014, the development of such a process was discussed with the group of teachers who had been involved in the conversations. The group agreed to collaborate, and accepted a proposal from the primary researcher to establish wellbeing support teams at the schools that could take responsibility for the development of the process. Each team selected a coordinator to take responsibility for bringing the team together and to steer the development of the process in each of the schools. Between July 2014 and November 2014, the teams were expanded to include parents as well as learners to adhere to the recommendation that transformative interventions should involve members of the school community across all levels of interrelatedness (Evans, Hanlin, & Prilleltensky, 2007).

3.5 The Development of the Process

In 2015, funding was obtained from the South African National Research Foundation* to conduct research on the development of an integrated, multi-level process to facilitate holistic wellbeing (referred to as the IMHWB process) in the six school communities. Since entrée into the schools had already been negotiated and the need for further action with reference to the promotion of wellbeing had been identified and confirmed in the conversations with a representative group of teachers, the research commenced in July 2015.

3.6 Methodology

The research presented here is informed by a combination of the transformative paradigm (Mertens, 2009) and participatory paradigms (Creswell, 2007). The ontological implications of combining these paradigms are: that reality is perceived as constructed through social practices, interactions and experiences; that people's lived experiences are understood as socially constructed in specific contexts and influenced by their historical and cultural experiences; that participants have to work actively with researchers to co-construct spaces in which their voices can be heard; that knowledge and everyday action should not be separated; and that institutional and social structures shape reality, therefore social inequalities and conflict between dominant and subordinate subgroups exist and should be considered in the research process (Butler-Kisber, 2010). The epistemological implication of the combination is that the researchers in this project had to be situated in their work in order to establish close relationships with the participants as a means of understanding their lived experiences through active engagement with them as equal partners. The participants, in turn, had to be acknowledged as capable of thinking critically about practice and creating their own theories of practice (Pedler & Burgoyne, 2005) – of co-constructing their own solutions to the problems they encounter in facilitating holistic wellbeing in their school communities. The research community was therefore valued as a vital part of the research and experts of their own experiences (Grant, Nelson, & Mitchell, 2008).

Aligned with the transformative, participatory paradigm, a participatory action research approach was applied to design the research for this study. Brydon-Miller and Maguire (2009) argue that a participatory research approach provides theory and practice designed to reveal and address broader systems of inequality within our schools and communities and to create settings in which children, teachers, parents, and communities can work together to create positive change. A qualitative multiple case study (Yin, 2013) was embedded in the participatory approach to enable the researchers to obtain an in-depth understanding of how the development of the process could contribute to the promotion of holistic wellbeing in various contexts (Baxter and Jack, 2008). The participatory action learning and action research methodology (PALAR) developed by Zuber-Skerritt (2002) was introduced to facilitate the development of the process. This methodology allows people to work together on complex issues which affect their lives; to learn from their experience and from one another; and to engage in a systematic inquiry into how to address and resolve these issues. The application of this methodology is guided by the development of democratic, authentic, trusting and supportive relationships; continual critical reflection in a collaborative learning context; and recognition of the achievements of all participants (Zuber-Skerritt, 2011). In practice, the PALAR methodology encourages participants' commitment through three key features – the start-up workshop, the creation of action learning sets, and the celebration of achievements and milestones. The aim of applying these key features are to foster relationship, reflection and recognition, and ultimately participant learning and the sustainable success of the research project.

The PALAR process is iterative in nature and does not depict a step-by step method that starts at one point and ends at another. The process instead encompasses various cycles of engagement with the participants. Wood and Zuber-Skerritt (2013) therefore recommend a cyclic design to facilitate the process. The cyclic design for the research in this project encompassed five cycles. In the table below, each of the five cycles is discussed with reference to its aim and the activities of the research team and wellbeing support team.

Cycle 1: Connecting Team Members and Envisioning the Outcomes of the Process

All members of the six wellbeing support teams who were available on the day attended a 4-h workshop (Fig. 3.1). A total of 52 participants were involved in the workshop, including 26 learners, 16 teachers and 10 parents from across the 6 school communities. The rationale for including team members from all six schools was to focus on the facilitation of a sense of connectedness between members of a specific school community as well as between members from different school communities. The workshop was facilitated by the primary researcher, assisted by a PhD student as co-facilitator and encompassed the following: (1) relationship-building exercises that allowed the members of the six teams to get to know one another and to exchange information about shared interests and concerns; (2) the dissemination of information about the basic constructs, values and principles associated with the promotion of holistic wellbeing, concluding with an overview of the framework on which the development of the process had been based; (3) the co-construction of a vision for the promotion of holistic wellbeing in their school – this enabled team members to think and work together to envision the outcomes of the process (Kearney, Wood, & Zuber-Skerritt, 2013). The six visions clearly indicated a shift towards a pro-active approach aimed at creating a more enabling environment rather than merely addressing the problems experienced in their contexts, as illustrated in the example in Fig. 3.2.

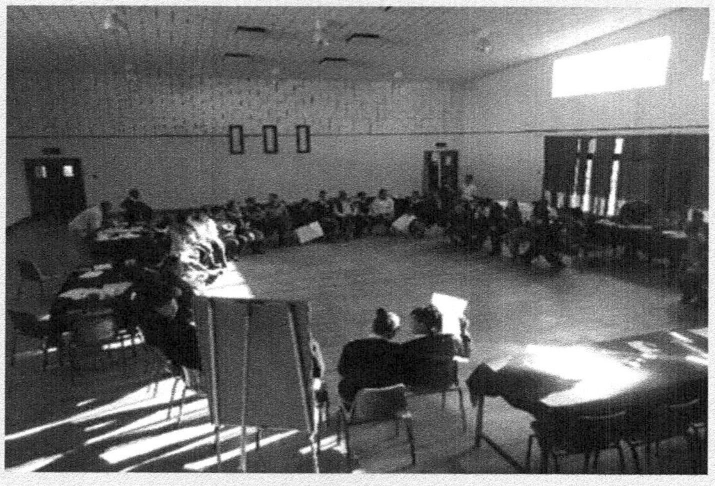

Fig. 3.1 Teams from the six schools in the introductory workshop

(continued)

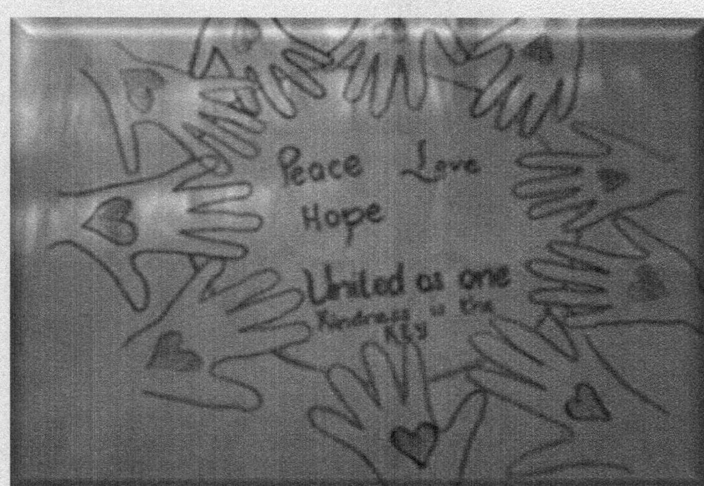

Fig. 3.2 Example of vision

Cycle 2: Initiating the Process in the Respective School Communities

In this cycle, which was spread over two school terms in 2015, the teams initiated the development of the IMHWB process in their respective school communities. A logical first step was to share the vision they had constructed during the workshop with the members of their school communities during meetings and assembly. The schools also used various strategies to make the vision visible to members of the school communities; for example, School E displayed printed posters with the framework and the vision in the staff room, on a wall in the passage close to the Life Orientation classroom, and on a wall next to the entrance to a room allocated to the school's wellbeing support team. School A displayed their vision at the entrance to the school building; close to the pillars on which they painted the core values identified in a character-building session presented by another organisation. Another initiation strategy applied by all six schools was to invite the primary researcher to introduce the process to all the staff members.

Concurrently, monthly action learning set meetings were scheduled. The intention of these meetings was to reflect on the team members' understanding of the process and the responses of other members of the school communities to the initiation of the process. The research team attended these monthly team meetings once a term with the intention of supporting the teams in the initiation of the process. During these meetings, the members of the teams were equipped with relevant knowledge and skills to enhance their confidence about the role that they could play in facilitating the promotion of holistic wellbeing in their school. By the end of 2015, the teams were ready to conceptualise how the process could be sustained in the new academic year. A coordinator confirmed that the initiation of the process *brought a new perspective on their circumstances and gave them hope that some things could be changed.*

Cycle 3: Developing and Implementing Action Plans to Sustain the Process

In this cycle, which started at the beginning of the 2016 academic year, the teams were encouraged to develop and implement action plans to facilitate the ongoing promotion of holistic wellbeing in their schools. At the beginning of the first term, the research team met with the team coordinators from each school to obtain their input for the way forward. The research team emphasised the importance of understanding the promotion of wellbeing as an integrative process in which they incorporate everyday activities, existing actions and interventions, as well as newly-developed actions and interventions, into a cohesive process. The coordinators then led their teams in the development of action plans. These plans were discussed and revisited during an action learning set meeting with the teams at each school. Funding for the plans was obtained from the Educational Trust. The teams then proceeded with the implementation of their action plans. The research team supported them throughout the process. The research team also attended an action learning set meeting once a term to reflect on and revise the action plans with the aim of optimising the teams' role in the promotion of holistic wellbeing in their contexts.

Cycle 4: Reflecting on Progress and Motivating Teams

At the end of 2016, a mid-term celebration was held as part of the PALAR process. During this celebration, the participating schools reported back on the actions, activities and interventions they had introduced while initiating the process. The audience included the school management teams of the six schools, as well as members of the larger community on the process that they established at the schools. The coordinators of the teams insisted that the learners involved be given an opportunity to present on the process to strengthen their voice in this endeavour. The confident manner in which these learners presented illustrated that their contributions should be validated through their inclusion in processes such as these. As part of the celebrations, an international visiting scholar delivered an inspirational address to motivate the wellbeing teams. She specifically emphasised the importance of strengthening relationships between members of the school communities as the essence of facilitating the change that has been envisioned by the teams. She also encouraged the teams to advocate for the recognition of wellbeing promotion as part of the core business of schooling.

Cycle 5: Teams Taking Ownership of the Process

In this cycle, which commenced at the beginning of the 2017 school year, the wellbeing support teams were expected to function independently under the leadership of the coordinators. The responsibility for steering the process had by now been shifted to the coordinators, who were equipped during a work-session to continue with the action learning set meetings to ensure that the process remains transparent and sustainable. Each team developed their own strategic action plans for the new school year in consultation with their research team. The research team had two follow-up action learning set meetings with the coordinators in the first term of 2017.

During this cycle, the wellbeing support teams were also equipped with skills to enhance communication and collaboration between them and the other members of their school communities by another visiting scholar in collaboration with the research team. These training sessions concurrently allowed the teams to share their experiences of the process and to identify the gaps they would need to address as they proceeded. To conclude this cycle, a World Café event was organised to create an opportunity for the wellbeing support teams to reflect on the value of the process, identify challenges and discuss the sustainability of proceeding. The World Café was attended by all the wellbeing support team members who were available as well as the school principals from all the schools. After the World Café, the teams celebrated their achievements with a short feedback session to members of their school communities.

3.7 Data Analysis

The data analysed in this research project included the posters designed during the workshop, the recorded transcriptions of the 18 action learning set meetings, the meeting notes, and reflective journals kept by the researcher, the research assistant and the team coordinators, together with the presentation from the celebration and the data gathered during the World Café event. The process developed by Braun and Clarke (2006) was applied to analyse the data. The process encompasses familiarising oneself with the data, generating codes – classifying or categorising individual fragments of data – searching for themes, reviewing themes, defining and naming themes before interpreting data and drawing conclusions about the process.

The trustworthiness of the findings was ensured through longitudinal involvement in the research contexts, the inclusion of multiple voices and multiple methods to contribute toward in-depth descriptions of the particulars; engagement on a continual basis in reflexive conversations with other researchers to address possible biases and challenges regarding the research process; and member-checking of the findings with the coordinators of the wellbeing support teams, as proposed by Tracey (2010).

3.8 Ethical Considerations

The research was guided by the ethical principles endorsed by the Constitution of South Africa (1996) and the ethical rules of the Health Professions Council of South Africa (HPCSA, 2004), which protect human rights and public safety. Ethical clearance for the study was obtained from the Ethics Committee of the Faculty of Education, North-West University, as well as the Western Cape Department of Education. Goodwill permission was obtained from the School Governing Bodies at each school. The ethical clearance number for the project is NWU-00160-15-A2.

3.9 Findings

The aim of the development of the IMHWB process through the application of a participatory action learning and action research methodology was to provide an integrative basis for incorporating existing as well as newly developed wellbeing-related activities and interventions into a complex, whole-school endeavour to promote wellbeing on individual, relational and collective levels. The wellbeing support teams were equipped to facilitate the promotion of holistic wellbeing based on a framework designed in accordance with the holistic wellbeing model developed by Prilleltensky (2005, 2012).

The findings are reported here with reference to how wellbeing was facilitated on all three levels during the development of the process through the actions, activities and interventions implemented by the wellbeing support teams.

Promoting wellbeing on individual level: The themes identified with reference to the contribution of the process to the promotion of individual wellbeing include (1) the expansion of opportunities for personal development, (2) the encouragement of value-informed behaviour and (3) attention to individual challenges and support needs.

3.10 The Expansion of Opportunities for Personal Development

At the outset of the process, the wellbeing support teams were guided to apply an asset-based approach to identify existing opportunities that have contributed to the personal development of learners in particular. Such opportunities, although limited, included: participation in sports and cultural events presented as part of the functioning of the schools or at sports clubs; going on outings and camps; reading, dance and drama sessions presented by non-profit organisations and well-doers from the communities. A teacher explained the value of the involvement of non-profit groups in the process as follows:

> *They came to our school and helped me to teach the children different ball games. For me it is a tremendous asset, because the children, really... they were part of the group, and the children are in this programme where you can see there is progress, and that for me was a big positive point.*

As part of their intention to expand access to these opportunities, the teams conducted a survey. The aim of the survey was to establish how many children took part in these opportunities, and why some learners used these opportunities while others did not. The survey alerted the teams to the fact that opportunities for personal development were limited across all the schools. In response, they introduced a variety of new opportunities with the assistance of various stakeholders from the community who were already involved in the schools. These opportunities included, for example:

- Excursions to expose learners to places of historical interest (such as museums), venues of scientific importance (such as an aquarium or planetarium), cultural activities (such as significant plays and musicals) or provincial sports events to enable learners to discover and develop their own interests. The value of these excursions for the children was evident during the celebrations when they excitedly reported how these excursions opened up a new world for them.
- Invitations to motivational speakers from various fields to impart life lessons regarding school life, sport, culture, academics, learner and learner-teacher relationships. In many instances, alumni from the schools who served as role models for the learners were invited. At a prize-giving ceremony at School E, a medical doctor in her early thirties encouraged learners to accept responsibility for their choices at an early age. At School B, a teacher invited her husband to share his life journey with the learners, since he had been in the same school many years ago and now has his own business in the community.
- Camps organised by the wellbeing support teams to enhance the self-esteem and confidence of learners by involving them in games and group sessions. School C reported how

they had organised a camp with the specific aim of developing the self-esteem and confidence of learners with low academic performance. In the past, only learners who performed well had been afforded the opportunity to attend these camps. This time, the wellbeing support team who assisted with the organising of the camp insisted that learners with lower academic achievement also be invited. In this way, high-performing learners could develop empathy for those who do not perform as well. The success was evident, as indicated by the statement of a learner who reflected on the experience of the camp: "*The school camp last week was very educational and inspiring in as far as it prepared us for life on many levels.*"

Work-sessions to enhance life skills were conducted. All learners between Grade 4 and 12 in the six schools had the opportunity to attend a 3-h work-session aimed at the development of life skills that enhanced their capacity to understand the importance of wellbeing and how their wellbeing is interconnected with the wellbeing of others, as well as how to take responsibility for their own wellbeing. The learners' feedback on these sessions included statements such as:

> *I feel that it built up my self-confidence and improved how we see and feel about ourselves*
> *I found the session very interesting. She (the presenter) talked to us about how we could find our place in the bigger picture of life. I wish we can attend more sessions like this one. I was so excited about the session that day. I learnt more about wellbeing.*
> *The wellbeing session meant so much to me. I started to see life with a whole new perspective and I truly have a new and more grateful perspective on life.*

Besides the focus on the expansion of opportunities for learners, the wellbeing teams also attended to teachers. In addition to the skills development workshops presented by the Department of Basic Education, often perceived as obligations that they had to fulfil, the wellbeing support teams added opportunities for teachers to actively participate in group discussions, team building sessions and fun activities that reportedly enabled them to deal with stress more effectively. These activities included team building sessions and art-based activities.

The expansion of opportunities for parents was challenging due to the parents' circumstances. However, a group of at least 60 parents were engaged in various opportunities to enhance skills that would enable them to engage more pro-actively with their children and the teachers. The parents indicated that their inclusion in the process opened up opportunities for them to feel valued and appreciated by their community. One parent who had been involved in the wellbeing support team considered her involvement in the wellbeing support teams as the reason for being promoted to mentor for newly appointed staff members at her workplace.

3.11 The Encouragement of Value-Informed Behaviour

Due to the focus of schools on academic performance, learners received recognition for their academic achievements but not for value-informed behaviour, i.e. behaviour that is informed by basic values such as respect, kindness, care and honesty. The focus with reference to behaviour in these schools has instead been on the punishment of misconduct, as evidenced in this statement by one of the teachers:

> *... you are so focussed on the negative, what the child does not do and then you see the positive and realise that is something that can take the child forward.*

In response to this approach, the wellbeing support teams developed various context-specific ways to acknowledge value-informed behaviour. In School A, the names of the learners who displayed value-informed behaviour were mentioned during assembly with a brief appreciation of the behaviour that they displayed. In School E, learners received a lapel pin to wear for a week based on a nomination by their classmates. These learners reported that they felt appreciated and motivated to maintain their good behaviour, and encouraged others to display such behaviour. A system was developed to ensure that as many learners as possible got the opportunity to wear the lapel pin throughout the year. Teachers reported that learners had started to acknowledge one another's value-based behaviour more often. In support of these endeavours in the school context, parents were also encouraged during parent meetings to recognise their children's good behaviour at home, instead of merely focussing on what they do wrong or on their academic failures.

3.12 Pro-active Engagement with Individual Challenges and Support Needs

The teams, through their involvement in the process, gradually shifted from a deficit-based to a strength- and asset-based approach. Based on this shift, they identified pathways to address individual challenges and support needs in a more pro-active manner. Teachers in particular realised that these needs and challenges are closely linked to the poor socio-economic conditions experienced by most families of children who attend these schools. A teacher who has been working in this context for 30 years admitted that she had never realised the extent of the challenges the children experienced due to their circumstances before her involvement in the wellbeing support initiative at the school. She expressed her deepened awareness of the need to care for her learners:

> *I saw a lot of sadness and trauma here and it hit me terribly that young children at the age of 13, 14 had to carry such tremendous responsibilities on their shoulders and that parents will sort of stand at the side and say you are old enough to care of yourself.*

In response, she initiated a project to provide sanitary supplies and toiletries for girls who cannot afford these items. She recognised the importance of maintaining their dignity by ensuring that the girls could have access to the cupboard where it was stored during breaks. The room in which the cupboard was set up also served as a space where wellbeing activities were presented. This contributed to the understanding that the provision of sanitary supplies should be seen as part of the wellbeing initiative and not merely as an act of welfare.

In School C, due to a specific incident between boys and girls during break, a pro-active intervention was developed and implemented to provide sexuality education to all the Grade 5–7 learners. Topics covered puberty, learning about physical changes in the body, the prevention of pregnancy, and addressing ways to prevent and report any kind of sexual abuse. The learners also had the opportunity to ask questions.

A noteworthy outcome of the shift towards a more pro-active approach to dealing with challenges and support needs was that learners who displayed behavioural problems were treated with more dignity due to the development of a more nuanced understanding of the problems they experience. A teacher indicated that being part of the wellbeing support team allows her the opportunity to attend to the children who experience problems and assist them to get support. She also encourages them to strive for a better future and to support others in their community to do so.

The evidence suggests that through their pro-active engagements, the teams no longer perceived the support of learners as the responsibility of professionals who were employed by the Department of Basic Education or non-profit organisations. They were ready to address the challenges and needs in their school communities by combining their own strengths with the resources available in the larger community and the efforts of the Department of Basic Education.

3.13 Promoting Wellbeing on a Relational Level

The themes identified with reference to the contribution of the IMHWB process to the promotion of relational wellbeing were (1) the strengthening of connections across all levels of interrelatedness and (2) the enhancement of an ethos of kindness, empathy and care.

3.14 Strengthening Connections Between People Across All Levels of Interrelatedness

On entrée into the school community, the strict organisational boundaries between teachers, other staff members, learners and parents were evident in the way that schools organised activities only with specific groups in mind. As the development of the process unfolded, this lack of connections across established boundaries urged the teams, to facilitate events that allow the members of the school communities to connect across these boundaries in order to strengthen the relational matrix within the school and beyond. This is in accordance with the principles of community psychology (Lazarus, 2006; Prilleltensky, 2012), which advocate for less hierarchical boundaries.

An excellent example of an action aimed at the strengthening of connections across all levels was a fun day organised by School B. The wellbeing support teams noted the need for bringing learners, teachers and parents together for a fun day. Yet they did not have sufficient money to present such an event outside of the school premises. Instead of perceiving this constraint as a problem, they perceived it as a challenge and decided to get everyone together at the school on a Saturday to eat and play games together. A coordinator reflected as follows on the day:

> *The day was a major success and set a new tone for the interactive dynamics in the school community as a whole.*

At School E, a games day was organised to celebrate the end of examinations with the aim of strengthening the connections between learners in the same class. Each class had to decide which games they would play together and accept responsibility for organising who would provide which games. A teacher who is a member of the wellbeing support team reflected as follows on the event:

> *The children also got to see the teachers in a different light, they saw a different side to the teachers: "Oh X can also make jokes" and "they can also do that" and "that one also". And the appreciation that we had for each other at the end of the day... One would think with the isiXhosa learners (a minority group in this school) you would think... that they would feel excluded. Not at all.*

At School A, the learners on the wellbeing support team, after deliberations with the PhD student who co-facilitated the action learning set meetings, came up with the idea of having games in the hall on Fridays. Their intention was to address bullying behaviour in their school in a pro-active manner. During their discussion with the co-facilitator, they indicated that they did not want to talk about bullying behaviour, but would rather enhance relationships between learners. They proposed that the activity be repeated over a few consecutive Fridays to ensure that all the grades could participate.

The strengthening of connections within these schools also became the focus during camps through the involvement of members of the wellbeing teams. In School B, the camp for Grade 5–7 learners focussed on teamwork as well as communication and conflict management skills. The intention of the workshop was to equip learners with knowledge and skills to collaborate with one another and enhance their communication with one another as a pro-active measure to address disrespectful behaviour and fighting amongst learners. At a camp for secondary school learners, connections were strengthened by deliberately taking learners out of their comfort zones. A learner stated:

> *On the weekend that we went on the camp, we were divided into groups that challenged our comfort zones. Put out of your friendship group in which you feel comfortable into a totally different group... Now X and I we do not like each other but I am forced in her group to communicate so that I can understand her.*

3.15 The Enhancement of an Ethos of Kindness, Empathy and Care

The almost exclusive focus on academic performance in many South African schools does not always allow time to focus on the development of an ethos of kindness, care and empathy in schools. The outcome of this lack of attention to how people relate and interact with one another became evident to the wellbeing support teams when they reflected on the interactive dynamics in their schools during action learning set meetings.

In response to their concerns about the dehumanised nature of their contexts, the wellbeing support teams used every possible opportunity to emphasise the importance of kindness, empathy and care as key to the promotion of wellbeing at various opportunities where members of the school community were together. For example, during assembly, the teachers responsible would explain the meaning of these constructs, give examples of kind and caring interactions and challenge learners and teachers to interact in caring ways through small support interactions. The wellbeing support teams moreover introduced specific actions and activities aimed at the enhancement of an ethos of kindness, care and empathy in their school communities. One way to enhance this ethos was to make use of days earmarked for the celebration of relationships between people, for example Valentine's Day and Mother's Day. The wellbeing support teams ensured that these days were used to reach all the members of the school community though a small gesture of kindness and care. On Valentine's Day, the teams gave all the learners in their schools a small symbol of love that they could share with someone whom they love and appreciate.

As the teams gained more insight into the dynamic nature of the process, they also created their own special days. One such collaborative effort that was implemented in all six school simultaneously was a #HappinessThroughKindness day. It entailed that each learner, at the beginning of the day, received a smiley face sticker with the name of a person in their class. They then had to identify the person, give him or her the sticker, and show acts of kindness to the person and other classmates. As the day developed, the coordinators across the six schools started to share pictures of learners and teachers involved in acts of kindness. Learners reported that the conversations about kindness were carried into the community when learners realised that all the schools were involved in the same activity. The day became a landmark event in terms of connecting the schools in a collaborative process that could impact the whole community. A Kind Kids month was organised across the schools in response to the success of this activity. As part of their commitment to kindness, all 4000 learners received armbands as a symbol of commitment.

The team at School C enhanced an ethos of kindness, empathy and care by organising small groups for parents whose children display challenging behaviour. The team argued that it would be easier for these parents to discuss the challenges in small groups rather than in a full parent meeting. The coordinator stated that *"when we reach out to the parents we will have a better understanding of their needs"*, which indicated her empathetic stance towards these parents.

The impact of the enhancement of an ethos of kindness, empathy and care across the six school contexts is evident in the following statement made by a teacher:

> *We just judge, we never really grasp that empathy for the child and in this project we could. I can listen with more empathy to children...I have a better understanding of things that we don't understand, especially in this community where I teach. (i1)*

3.16 Promoting Wellbeing on a Collective Level

The themes identified with reference to the contribution of the process to the collective wellbeing in the school communities were (1) enhancing awareness of the value of promoting wellbeing within the school context, (2) ensuring shared responsibility for the promotion of wellbeing across all levels of interrelatedness, and (3) co-constructing a supportive, enabling and inclusive environment.

3.17 Enhancing Awareness of the Value of Promoting Holistic Wellbeing in the Schools

The wellbeing support teams cultivated an awareness of the value of promoting holistic wellbeing amongst as many members of the school community as possible by inviting the primary researcher to introduce the framework to all the staff members of each school. The wellbeing framework was used as a discussion tool for facilitating conversations about the need to focus on the promotion of holistic wellbeing in school contexts. A teacher reflected as follows on being informed about the value of promoting holistic wellbeing in school communities:

> *If I think back, before the wellbeing initiative groups came in, we did not think that much about wellbeing. We focussed on the academic side, the child must be able to do this and we still need to do that and the child must come right with this, but we never thought much about... took notice of wellbeing, until you came in with your team and indicated it to us.*

The teachers were challenged to introduce wellbeing to their learners by using the wellbeing wheel. The wellbeing wheel was developed by the New Economics Foundation (2011) and initially included five ways to wellbeing, namely: to take notice; to give; to keep learning; to be active and to connect. A sixth way, namely to care for the planet, was added at a later stage. Each teacher had a wheel of wellbeing poster in their classrooms and was encouraged to apply it in the classroom as part of their conversations with their learners. Feedback obtained from teachers indicated that most teachers have used the six ways of wellbeing as a discussion tool in the classrooms. Some examples of how they have done so include:

By communicating with learners on a daily basis regarding their appearance (neatness), respecting those around them.

I refer to the poster when friends have problems with each other- care about one another, love one another; and also encourage them to participate in sport.

> *Often refer to it when I want to instil certain values in learners. I also try and explain that a person does not have to do extraordinary things to contribute toward a person's wellbeing. I also encourage them to reflect regularly on whether they are still on track.*

With reference to the parents, the team members felt that more awareness should be created amongst parents regarding the holistic wellbeing process, as they felt that this would enhance their involvement. In response, a work-session was organised for parents. The wellbeing approach was explained with reference to how this approach applies to their specific contexts. The parents then engaged in small group discussions about their involvement and the challenges relating to their involvement. Based on these conversations, there were certain elements that stood out in terms of parent involvement. From these elements, suggestions were made as to how some of these challenges could be addressed from a wellbeing approach.

3.18 Enhancing Shared Responsibility for Promoting Holistic Wellbeing

The inclusion of representatives from all levels of interrelatedness on the wellbeing support teams enhanced the shared responsibility for the promotion of holistic wellbeing in these school communities. The teachers who initially volunteered to participate in the conversations indicated that they had always been interested in the psychosocial dimension of schooling and therefore experienced their inclusion on the wellbeing teams as a confirmation of the responsibility they had already taken on. Being part of a team excited them and gave a sense of purpose and meaning.

The initial scepticism about the inclusion of learners was soon replaced with appreciation for the valuable role that learners play in these teams. According to the team coordinator, the learners' involvement allows for vital 'check-ins' on the wellbeing of all learners within the school:

> *... the children initiate ideas, they come up with activities that they think are important, what can be focussed on.../They can also give me input about what else will work for children... I train them, they are our ears.../... The initiative and the stuff comes from the children and they take control and is [sic] very enthusiastic to do stuff, because they know how much it means for the other children.*

In School E, learners were so interested in being part of the wellbeing support team that the coordinator advised them to start a learner support team with their own chairperson and two co-chairs. The learner team has since identified needs that they deem important to address and plan, develop and initiate interventions. The team coordinator will offer practical support and arrange access to resources if necessary. In this way, learners have been empowered to be co-drivers in the wellbeing process. The chairperson of this learner wellbeing support team is still part of teacher-parent team, to ensure that learners are represented on the team and get an opportunity to engage with their school's wellbeing in a more practical and pro-active manner. A learner on the learner team elucidated her involvement:

> *This is actually my main goal, my main duty is basically to be the eyes of the committee and then also to give feedback to the coordinator and then the coordinator will see themselves what happened, but this is not difficult because it is an everyday thing. It is just to be attentive to the manner in which our children speak, the manner in which our children behave, the manner in which our teachers behave.*

In the initial phases of the project, it was challenging to involve parents in the wellbeing support teams. Parents who were invited to join the teams included members of school governing boards and mothers who were already serving their communities as volunteers. The dedication of these parents was evident and they offered their services in a selfless manner based on their care for the children. One of the parents, based on her involvement on the team, expressed her appreciation of this process:

> *I agree, since wellbeing has been here...it is the first time that I am part of something like this. I love working with children. I often go around to the houses, I go to the children and since they've heard about wellbeing they have more respect.*

Another way in which parents were approached to get involved in the teams was during parent evenings or meetings. In the past, these meetings had mainly focussed on discussing academic issues. However, as the wellbeing support teams began to see the value of this process, they decided to allocate time to discuss the holistic wellbeing process with specific reference to how parents can support their child.

Although getting parents on board was a challenge, there is sufficient evidence to indicate that some parents are positive about this process and have experienced their involvement in the wellbeing initiative as a way to contribute to the upliftment of the school community:

> *As a parent, the wellbeing also did something good for me, because at home my child and I can communicate about things that happened at school.*

The data obtained shows that the teams increasingly began to involve other school staff members in making decisions relating to the planning and implementation of wellbeing activities. The coordinators as well as other teachers in the team indicated the importance of everyone being involved, which is why they engaged with the teachers through a process of consulting in terms of shared decision-making relating to wellbeing activities. A coordinator reported:

> *We sit together as a team to discuss our projects and how we are going to move forward. We then take it back to the staff and we take it from there... They also give their ideas.*

The process facilitated by the wellbeing support teams also seems to have encouraged other role-players in the school to synchronise their initiatives with the process. In School C, the head boy and head girl initiated a "Class of the Week" project as part of their training by a non-profit organisation that also supports the schools. The criteria set for the selection of the Class of the Week included learner attendance, the neatness of the learners, the effort made to keep the classroom clean, and participation in extracurricular activities.

3.19 Co-constructing a Supportive, Enabling, Inclusive Environment

The awareness of the important role that the schools play in people's lives, facilitated by the introduction of holistic wellbeing, encouraged the wellbeing support teams to focus on the co-construction of their schools into more supportive and enabling environments. The physical environment as well as the physical needs of children were often foregrounded due to the circumstantial needs of many of the learners. One of the coordinators insisted on painting the staff room and the rest rooms used by the teachers as part of facilitating wellbeing.

The way in which the team coordinator in School B described the establishment of a vegetable garden illustrates the value of the process in facilitating and understanding that whatever happens in the contexts is beneficial for all and should be perceived as a collective asset and not as the work of individual members.

The teams also succeeded in facilitating a wellbeing-conducive climate in the schools by making the wellbeing message more visible and comprehensible for all members of the school community. This was done mainly through the display of posters and the selection of wellbeing-related themes for assembly and follow-up classroom discussions throughout the week. In the process, the language changed from deficit-based to wellbeing-based in discussions across all levels of interrelatedness. The use of wellbeing language seemingly influenced the whole atmosphere in one school, as stated by a learner:

> *... just the word wellbeing on its own has created a positive atmosphere in our school and I think it is important. A positive atmosphere in such a sense that we start to think positively and we can also bring the negative things forward and make everyone aware of it.*

A teacher stated:

> *Wellbeing, I believe for me, is one of the best things that could have happened at our school. The reason being that you no longer think so negatively. You see the positive side of what is here at the school. You experience ... it is not that all is well now but you have hope.*

Currently, each of the schools displays a banner in their foyer to indicate their commitment to being a holistic wellbeing school. The banner confirms their commitment to the ongoing co-construction of a supportive, enabling environment. Below is a picture of the banner and the commitment they pledged.

Our school values the integrated promotion of individual, relational, and collective wellbeing as a way to ensure that everyone in our school community feel connected and supported. We take responsibility for the promotion of wellbeing of our learners, staff and parents by:

- *creating opportunities for all members of our school community to develop and flourish;*
- *establishing and strengthening enabling relationships between staff, learners, parents; co-constructing an enabling, inclusive and equitable environment;*
- *building support networks by reaching out to and collaborate with other school communities and the larger community; integrating all wellbeing enhancing activities to ensure that the promotion of holistic wellbeing becomes a sustainable part of the core business of our school.*

3.20 Discussion

At the start of this chapter, I discussed the poor quality of life experienced by South Africans who attend schools situated in lower socio-economic contexts. Despite policies and programmes developed with the aim of promoting mental health and wellbeing in South African school communities, the problem has not been addressed sufficiently. Consequently, the schools that need the most support are often labelled as dysfunctional – this state of affairs was evident on entrée into the six schools who were involved in the research project. The research was conducted with the aim of supporting these schools to apply a more pro-active approach to dealing with the challenges they face as a result of the socio-economic conditions in which the learners who attend these schools and their families live. In other words to apply a settings approach as proposed by Poland, Krupa, and McCall (2009) by addressing the contexts within which people live, work, and play to increase the likelihood of optimising interventions that is specific to each context and therefore render the school communities more health promoting.

In this chapter, the findings were examined with reference to the contribution that the development of the IMHWB process made to the promotion of wellbeing on individual, relational and collective levels. The question to be addressed here is whether the development of an integrated multi-level process to facilitate the promotion of holistic wellbeing in school communities situated in lower socio-economic contexts can enhance the quality of the life of the members of these school communities.

The contribution of the IMHWB process developed in the six school communities to both subjective and objective dimensions of quality of life seems evident if one considers the correlation between the themes identified with reference to the promotion of holistic wellbeing and the domains and indicators identified in the quality of life conceptual and measurement framework that Schalock et al. (2010) developed. This framework identifies eight domains, with associated indicators for each domain, including:

- Emotional wellbeing: indicated by contentment, self-concept and a lack of stress.
- Interpersonal relationships: indicated by interactions, relationships and support.
- Material wellbeing: indicated by financial status, employment and housing.
- Personal development: indicated by education, personal competence and performance.
- Physical wellbeing: indicated by health and health care, activities of daily living and leisure.
- Self-determination: indicated by personal control, personal goals, values and choices.
- Social inclusion: indicated by community integration and participation, roles and social support.
- Rights: indicated by human respect, dignity and equality as well as legal access.

When applying these domains and indicators to deliberate the possible contribution of the integrated, multi-level process to the enhancement of quality of life in the six school communities in which the research was conducted, the following was noted:

Personal development was enhanced as the process opened up various opportunities to access new experiences that could enhance the development of personal competencies for teachers, parents and learners. Although everyone in the school community had not had opportunities yet, the process certainly paved the way for the development of more opportunities and facilitated an understanding of the important role of school communities in creating such opportunities for personal development in contexts where people might not have the means to create such opportunities for themselves.

Self-determination was enhanced by shifting the focus away from bad behaviour towards value-informed behaviour that served as a basis for the internalisation of the values which enhanced learners' autonomy and personal control over their behaviour. Concurrently, teachers and parents had to accept the role of guide and facilitator of good behaviour, which ensured that the right to human dignity and equality of all involved was respected.

By pro-actively addressing individual challenges and support needs, the physical wellbeing of learners was enhanced through the provision of meals and caring about health issues – the fact that these activities were integrated into the wellbeing process ensured that the dignity of those who received support was maintained. Support initiatives aimed at individual learners, such as mentoring, skills development, support with career choices, and the enhancement of study skills also enhanced self-determination and the pursuit of personal goals and choices.

Interpersonal relationships have evidently been at the core of the process, as indicated by the emphasis placed on social connectedness and an ethos of kindness, care and empathy, which signalled a shift in focus from the individualistic, mechanistic approach that prevailed in these school communities. Marujo and Neto (2017) confirm that relationships and social connectedness are considered sources of meaning in life, as well as being a substantial source of wellbeing. Strong social connection also helps to develop common values and trust in one another at a community level (Kõrreveski, 2011). Moreover, social inclusion was encouraged through the enhancement of an ethos of kindness, care and empathy that facilitated participation for members who might have been excluded previously, including learners who experience serious challenges such as drug addiction and teen pregnancy or who cannot progress academically.

With reference to the promotion of collective wellbeing, the process ensured that all the members of the school community were appreciated and therefore informed about the process, which also enhanced their integration and inclusion into the school community. The members of the school communities also obtained autonomy, which implied that they could gain more control over their circumstances by taking shared responsibility for their wellbeing as well as co-construct spaces that are responsive to their specific needs. The rights of the members of these school communities were now acknowledged as part of the enhancement of their wellbeing, and seemingly became less of a threat and more a matter of respect for and recognition of the other. The emphasis on the voice of the learners as fully-fledged members, as well as the empathetic understanding of the position of the parents, reinforced respect for human dignity and equity.

The process apparently enhanced the humanity of the participants by providing a platform for personal, relational and collective growth in the service of a better life for all. The view of Karatzias, Power, and Swanson (2001) that quality of life in school contexts can be regarded as both a process and an outcome, depending on the context and the design of a particular project, seems applicable here. However, to optimise our understanding of the possible contribution of such a process, it may be valuable to consider the inclusion of quality of life instruments when the development of the process is expanded to more schools.

The pivotal role of wellbeing support teams and team coordinators in the development and implementation of the process should be foregrounded as the basis for the sustainable development and continuation of the IMHWB process. What seems to be critically important is the agential role that these teams play in the promotion of holistic wellbeing in schools. An agential role implies that the teams are not passive recipients of instruction on how to promote holistic wellbeing, but dynamic agents who pro-actively engage with their contexts with the aim of facilitating deep-level social change. In this regard, Marujo and Neto (2017) argue that when people are given the opportunity to reflect on their lives through "*dialogue and mutual interrelatedness and interdependence, in an appreciative, accepting, broad-minded, emotionally exciting, encouraging, inspiring and respectful environment, a new consciousness and revitalization emerges*". The implication is that the teams should continue the conversations as part of this process to promote holistic wellbeing to ensure the sustainability of the process.

Another key aspect in optimising the contribution of the IMHWB process in enhancing quality of life is the understanding that the process is complex and integrative in nature, which means that the wellbeing is not promoted in a sequential manner by implementing specific activities, interventions and programmes. The promotion of wellbeing and the enhancement of quality of life is an organic, ongoing process that needs to be steered deliberately. Elias, Zins, Grazcyk, and Weissberg (2003), concur that initiatives to promote wellbeing should be flexible in nature, even as they are steered. According to these authors, detailed planning rarely works out as envisioned. Therefore, teams need to be flexible in the sense that they should not become despondent when things do not work out as planned. In line with this, research by Forman et al. (2009) indicates that the implementation of evidence-based interventions was hindered to some extent due to teachers' lack of flexibility in their approaches. Henderson and Tilbury (2004) further argue from a whole-school perspective that in order for initiatives to be sustainable, they should have a flexible structure so that they can be applied in other school contexts and can adapt with the school curriculum. In addition, considering the complexity of the process, team members should continuously revisit the process in which they are engaged through regular conversations with all the members of their school communities – allowing them to reflect, to evaluate and to make changes as required. Kielty, Gilligan, and Staton (2017) confirm that adopting a grass-roots approach, in which members of the school community are involved through the unfolding of a natural process instead of imposing a programme from a top-down approach, seems to contribute to members feeling included and motivated and therefore committed to sustaining the efforts.

3.21 Conclusion: Proposing a Way Forward

The development of an integrated, multi-level process to facilitate the promotion of holistic wellbeing in a constructive and pro-active manner in collaboration with members of school communities seems to be a possible strategy to enhance the quality of life for the children and families who are still experiencing limited quality of life in the South African and African contexts. Based on the research presented here, it is recommended that the process should be organic and flexible in nature to accommodate the complex, responsive, interactive and dynamic nature of human interaction. The unique, organic nature of this process can be compared to the African art of basket-weaving – a well-respected skill that is handed down from one generation to the next. Each basket is unique in its style – no two baskets are identical. It is the process of basket-weaving that needs to be mastered. To date, programmes have often been developed and implemented in a top-down and fragmented manner. By contrast, this research indicates that a bottom-up approach that involves the members of school communities in the process enhances their capacity to take responsibility to change their contexts as far as possible within the confines of their circumstances.

The sustainability of a process such as this is enhanced by the establishment of wellbeing support teams. These teams should be well-equipped to facilitate the promotion of holistic wellbeing according to basic principles in a contextually relevant, innovative and creative manner – to continue the metaphor above, to design and weave their own unique baskets in close collaboration with other schools that apply the same principles to design unique baskets in their turn. Once woven, the basket becomes the container that holds all wellbeing-related activities together in a cohesive, integrative whole aimed at the enhancement of quality of life for all.

Acknowledgements The research reported in this chapter was supported by the * National Research Foundation (NRF) of South Africa. I herewith wish to thank the NRF and acknowledge that the opinions, findings and conclusions or recommendations expressed in here are those of the author(s), and that the NRF accepts no liability whatsoever in this regard.

- I also wish to acknowledge the support received from the Rupert Onderwysstigting (Educational Trust) and express my gratitude

to Priscilla Booysen for her willingness to allow me the space to apply my ideas.
- Sincere appreciation is expressed for the commitment and passion with which the coordinators as well as each of the team members from each of the schools engaged in this project. Thank you, Wilma Cyster, Ferentia September, Milly Cyster, Cynthia Hendricks, Ivan Papier, Elmari Hendricks, Robert Carstens and Vuyisa Qobongwana.
- Thank you, Bianke van Rooyen, for acting as co-facilitator and project coordinator.

References

Baxter, P., & Jack, S. (2008). Qualitative case study methodology: Study design and implementation for novice researchers. *The Qualitative Report, 13*, 544–559.

Braun, V., & Clarke, V. (2006). Using thematic analysis in psychology. *Qualitative Research in Psychology, 3*(2), 77–101.

Brydon-Miller, M., & Maguire, P. (2009). Participatory action research: Contributions to the development of practitioner inquiry in education. *Educational Action Research, 17*(1), 79–93. https://doi.org/10.1080/09650790802667469

Butler-Kisber, L. (2010). *Qualitative inquiry: Thematic, narrative and arts-informed perspectives*. London, UK: Sage.

Cilliers, P. (1998). *Complexity and postmodernism: Understanding complex systems*. London, UK: Routledge.

Creswell, J. W. (2007). *Research design: Qualitative, quantitative and mixed methods approaches* (2nd ed.). Thousand Oaks, CA: SAGE.

Dewey, J. (1957). *The school and society*. Chicago, IL: University of Chicago Press.

Efklides, A., & Moraitou, D. (2013). Looking at quality of life and well-being from a positive psychology perspective. In A. Efklides & D. Moraitou (Eds.), *A positive psychology perspective on quality of life* (pp. 1–14). New York, NY: Springer.

Elias, M. J., Zins, J. E., Grazcyk, P. A., & Weissberg, R. P. (2003). Implementation, sustainability, and scaling up of social emotional and academic innovations in public schools. *School Psychology Review, 32*(3), 303–319.

Engelbrecht, P., Savolainen, H., Nel, M., Koskela, T., & Okkolin, M. (2017). Making meaning of inclusive education: Classroom practices in Finnish and South African classrooms. *Compare: A Journal of Comparative and International Education, 47*(5), 684–702. https://doi.org/10.1080/03057925.2016.1266927

Evans, S. D., Hanlin, C. E., & Prillentensky, I. (2007). Blending ameliorative and transformative approaches in human service organizations. *Journal of Community Psychology, 35*(3), 329–346.

Faragher, R., & Van Ommen, M. (2017). Conceptualising educational quality of life to understand school expereinces of students with inteleectual disability. *Journal of Pilicy and Practice in Inteleectual Disabilities, 14*(1).

Fataar, A. (2016). Towards a humanising pedagogy through an engagement with the social-subjective in educational theorising in South Africa. *Educational Research for Social Change, 5*(1), 10–21.

Fiske, E. B., & Ladd, H. F. (2004a). *Illusive equity: Education reform in post-apartheid South Africa*. Cape Town, South Africa: HSRC Press.

Fiske, E. B., & Ladd, H. F. (2004b). *Elusive equity: Education reform in post-apartheid South Africa*. Washington, DC: Brookings Institute Press.

Fitz-Gibbon, C. T., & Kochan, S. (2000). School effectiveness and education indicators. In C. Teddlie & D. Reynolds (Eds.), *The international handbook of school effectiveness research* (pp. 257–282). London, UK: Falmer Press.

Fitzsimons, G., Finkel, E., & Van Dellen, M. (2015). Transactive goal dynamics. *Psychological Review, 122*(4), 648–673. https://doi.org/10.1037/a0039654

Fitzsimons, G., Sackett, E., & Finkel, E. (2016). Transactive goal dynamics theory: A relational goals perspective on work teams and leadership. *Research in Organizational Behavior, 36*, 135–155. https://doi.org/10.1016/j.riob.2016.11.006

Florian, L., & Spratt, J. (2013). Enacting inclusion: A framework for interrogating inclusive practice. *European Journal of Special Needs Education, 28*(2), 119–135.

Foster-Fishman, P. G., & Behrens, T. R. (2007). Systems change reborn: Rethinking our theories, methods, and efforts in human services reform and community-based change. *American Journal of Community Psychology, 39*(3–4), 191–196.

Gable, S., & Haidt, J. (2005). What (and why) is positive psychology? *Review of General Psychology, 19*(2), 103–110.

Gaibie, F., & Davids, Y. D. (2009, July 19–23). *Quality of life among South Africans*. Paper presented at the IX ISQOLS Conference on Quality of Life, Florence, Italy.

Grant, D. (2013). *Background to the national quintile system*. Media release. Retrieved from: http://wced.pgwc.gov.za/comms/press/2013/74. Accessed 21 Jan 2017.

Haslam, N., & Loughnan, S. (2014). Dehumanisation and infrahumanization. *Annual Review of Psychology, 65*, 399–423.

Health Professions Council of South Africa. (2004). *Professional conduct and ethics*. http://www.hpcsa.co.za/Conduct

Henderson, K.. & Tilbury, D. (2004). *Whole-school approaches to sustainability: An international review of whole school sustainability programs*. Report prepared by the Australian Research Institute in Education for Sustainability (ARIES) for The Department of the Environment and Heritage, Australian Government.

Johnson, B., & Lazarus, S. (2003). Building health promoting and inclusive schools in South Africa. *Journal of Prevention & Intervention in the Community, 25*(1), 81–97.

Jörg, T. (2009). Thinking in complexity about learning and education: A programmatic view. *Complicity: An International Journal of Complexity and Education, 6*(1), 1–22.

Joyce, T. M. (2013). School violence: Reimagining schools as safe havens. *Journal of Social Science, 37*(3), 249–258.

Karatzias, A., Power, K. G., & Swanson, V. (2001). Quality of school life: Development and preliminary standardisation of an instrument based on performance indicators in Scottish secondary schools. *School Effectiveness and School Improvement, 12*(3), 265–284.

Kearney, J., Wood, L., & Zuber-Skerritt, O. (2013). Community–university partnerships: Using Participatory Action Learning and Action Research (PALAR). *Gateways: International Journal of Community Research and Engagement, 6*(1), 113–130. https://doi.org/10.5130/ijcre.v6i1.3105

Kielty, M. L., Gilligan, T. D., & Staton, A. R. (2017). Whole school approaches to incorporating mindfulness based interventions: Supporting the capacity for optimal functioning in school settings. *Childhood Education, 93*(2), 128–135.

Kitching, A. E. (2010). *Conceptualising a relationship-focused approached to the co-construction of enabling school communities*. Doctoral thesis. North-West University, Potchefstroom. Retrieved from http://dspace.nwu.ac.za/handle/10394/2/search

Koller, S. H., & Lisboa, C. (2007). Brazilian approaches to understanding and building resilience in at-risk populations. *Child Adolescents Psychiatry, 16*(2), 341–356. viii–ix.

Kõrreveski, K. (2011). *Measuring well-being and quality of life using OECD indicators Quarterly Bulletin of Statistics*. Retrieved from: https://scholar.google.co.za/scholar?hl=enandas_sdt=0%2C5andq=K%C3%B5rreveski%2C+K.+2011+&btnG. Accessed 30 May 2018.

Lazarus, S. (2006). Indigenous approaches to health promotion: Challenges for education support in South Africa. *South African Journal of Psychology, 36*(3), 521–546.

Lewis, J. A., Lewis, M. D., Daniels, J. A., & D'Andrea, M. J. (2002). *Community counseling: Empowerment strategies for a diverse society* (3rd ed.). Pacific Grove, CA: Brooks/Cole.

Marujo, H. À., & Neto, L. M. (2017). Exploring the concept and practices of Felicitas Publica at Lisbon university: A community-based relational approach to well-being. In G. Tonon (Ed.), *Quality of life in communities of Latin countries. Community quality-of-life and well-being*. Cham, Switzerland: Springer.

Mason, M. (2008). What is complexity theory and what are its implications for educational change? *Educational Philosophy and Theory, 40*(1), 35–49. https://doi.org/10.1111/j.1469-5812.2007.00413.x

Mertens, D. M. (2009). *Transformative research and evaluation*. New York, NY: Guildford Press.

Møller, V. (2007). Quality of life in South Africa – The first ten years of democracy. *Social Indicators Research, 81*(2), 181–201. https://doi.org/10.1007/s11205-006-9003-4. Source: OAI.

Morrison, K. (2002). *School leadership and complexity theory*. London, UK: Routledge.

Nelson, G., & Prilleltensky, I. (2010). *Community psychology: In pursuit of liberation and wellbeing* (2nd ed.). New York, NY: Palgrave Macmillan.

New Economics Foundation. (2011). *Five ways to wellbeing: New application, new ways of thinking*. London, UK: New economics foundations. Available online at: http://www.neweconomics.org/publications/entry/five-ways-towell-being-new-applications-new-ways-of-thinking

Ng, E. C. W., & Fisher, A. T. (2013). Understanding well-being in multi-levels: A review. *Health, Culture and Society, 5*(1), 308–323.

Poland, B., Krupa, G., & McCall, D. (2009). Settings for health promotion: An analytic framework to guide intervention design and implementation. *Health Promotion Practice, 10*(4), 505–516.

Prilleltensky, I. (2005). Promoting wellbeing: Time for a paradigm shift in health and human services. *Scandinavian Journal of Public Health, 33*(5), 53–60. https://doi.org/10.1080/14034950510033381

Prilleltensky, I. (2012). Wellness as fairness. *American Journal of Community Psychology, 49*(1–2), 1–21.

Prilleltensky, I., & Prilleltensky, O. (2003). Towards a critical health psychology practice. *Journal of Health Psychology, 8*(2), 197–201. https://doi.org/10.1177/1359105303008002659

Radford, M. (2007). Action research and the challenge of complexity. *Cambridge Journal of Education, 37*(2), 263–278. https://doi.org/10.1080/03057640701372582

Roffey, S. (2013). Inclusive and exclusive belonging: The impact on individual and community wellbeing. *Educational and Child Psychology, 30*(1), 38–49.

Roffey, S. (2015). Becoming an agent of change for school and student well-being. Educational & Child Psychology, 32(1), 21–30. Retrieved from http://www.bps.org.uk/publications/member-network-publications/member-publications/educational-child-psychology. Accessed 5 Nov 2016.

Saleebey, D. (2001). *Human behavior and social environments: A biopsychosocial approach*. New York, NY: Columbia University Press.

Sarason, S. B. (1974). *The psychological sense of community: Prospects for a community psychology*. San Francisco, CA: Jossey-Bass.

Schalock, R. L., Keith, K. D., Verdugo, M. A., & Gómez, L. E. (2010). Quality of life model development and use in the field of intellectual disability. In R. Kober (Ed.), *Enhancing quality of life in people with intellectual disabilities. From theory to practice* (pp. 17–32). New York, NY: Springer.

Schalock, R. L., Verdugo, M. A., Gomez, L. E., & Reinders, H. S. (2016). Moving us toward a theory of individual quality of life. *American Journal on Intellectual and Developmental Disabilities, 121*(1), 1–12.

Schueller, S. M. (2009). Promoting wellness: Integrating community and positive psychology. *Journal of Community Psychology, 37*(7), 922–937. https://doi.org/10.1002/jcop.20334

Sergiovanni, T. J. (1994). *Building communities in schools*. San Francisco, CA: Jossey-Bass.

Shaughnessy, M. F., Galligan, E., & Hurtardo de Vivas, R. (2008). *Pioneers in education: Essays in honour of Paulo Freire*. New York, NY: Nova Publishers.

Shaw, P. (2002). *Changing conversations in organisations. A complexity approach to change*. London, UK: Routledge.

Shepard, N., & Mhlanga, D. (2014). Philosophy for children: A model for Unhu/Ubuntu philosophy. *International Journal of Scientific and Research Publications, 4*(2), 665–684.

South African Department of Education. (2001). *Education white paper 6: Special needs education: Building an inclusive education and training system*. Retrieved from https://wcedonline.westerncape.gov.za/Specialised-ed/documents/WP6.pdf. Accessed 20 Jan 2018.

Stacey, R. D. (2003). *Complexity and group processes: A radically social understanding of individuals*. New York, NY: Brunner-Routledge.

Stacey, R. D. (2007). The challenge of human interdependence. Consequences for thinking about the day to day practice of management in organisations. *European Business Review, 19*(4), 292–302. https://doi.org/10.1108/09555340

Statistics South Africa. (2013). *South African statistics, 2013*. Retrieved from: http://www.statssa.gov.za/publications/SAStatistics/SAStatistics2013.pdf. Accessed 25 Feb 2018.

Strike, K. A. (2000). Schools as communities: Four metaphors, three models, and a dilemma or two. *Journal of Philosophy of Education, 34*(4), 617–642. https://doi.org/10.1111/1467-9752.00198

Strike, K. A. (2004). Community, the missing element of school reform: Why schools should be more like congregations than banks. *American Journal of Education, 110*(3), 215–232. https://doi.org/10.1086/383072

Suchman, A. L. (2006). A new theoretical foundation for relationship-centered care. *Journal of General Internal Medicine, 21*(1), 40–44. https://doi.org/10.1111/j.1525-1497.2006.00308.x710760125

Ventegodt, S., Merrick, J., & Andersen, N. J. (2003). Quality of life theory: An integrative theory of the global quality of life concept. *The Scientific World Journal, 3*, 1030–1040. https://doi.org/10.1100/tsw.2003.82.

Wang, M., Schalock, R. L., Verdugo, M. A., & Jenaro, C. (2010). Analyzing the factor structure and hierarchical nature of the quality of life construct. *American Journal on Intellectual and Developmental Disabilities, 115*, 218–233.

Weare, K., & Nind, M. (2011). Mental health promotion and problem prevention in schools: What does the evidence say? *Health Promotion International, 26*, i29–i69.

Wood, L., & Zuber-Skerrit, O. (2013). PALAR as a methodology for community engagement by faculties of education. *South African Journal of Education, 33*(4), 1–15.

Yin, R. K. (2013). *Case study research: Design and methods*. Thousand Oaks, CA: SAGE.

Zuber-Skerritt, O. (2002). A model for designing action learning and action research programs. *The Learning Organization, 9*(4), 143–149. https://doi.org/10.1108/09696470210428868

Zuber-Skerritt, O. (2011). *Action leadership: Towards a participatory paradigm*. Amsterdam, The Netherlands: Springer.

4 Wellbeing as Positive Outcome of a Social Connectedness Pathway to Resilience: An Indigenous Psychology Perspective

Janna de Gouveia and Liesel Ebersöhn

Abstract
Over a 3-year period, we asked indigenous VhaVhenda and AmaSwati (n = 135, male = 57, female = 78, elders = 53, young people = 82) in two purposively selected, severely challenged remote sites in South Africa to tell us: 'If you go to bed tonight, how do you know this was a good day?' Employing Participatory Reflection and Action, we used an indigenous-appropriate prompt to elicit emic perspectives in home-languages during participatory diagramming. We used thematic analysis for in-case and cross-case analysis of back-translated, verbatim transcriptions of audio-recorded PRA-answers, as well as observation data generated by multiple researchers (visual data, field notes, researcher journals). Several themes of indigenous pathways to resilience with positive wellbeing outcomes became evident – one of which we discuss in this chapter. Similar to findings in other studies from non-western perspectives, participating indigenous South Africans leverage social connectedness in relationships where there is reciprocity and where their valuing of socio-cultural identity exist in social engagement. In times of hardship they leverage social connectedness to flock together for social support in order to resile. Regardless of worldview or harshness of challenges, social connectedness appears to make people happy. Our findings suggest that social connectedness enable eudaimonic wellbeing which reflects positive social functioning and positive psychological functioning.

J. de Gouveia · L. Ebersöhn (✉)
Centre for the Study of Resilience, University of Pretoria, Pretoria, South Africa
e-mail: liesel.ebersohn@up.ac.za

4.1 Introduction

Resilience, wellbeing and social connectedness has relevance for quality of life. With regards to quality of life, in the highly unequal postcolonial South Africa the majority do not report overall life satisfaction (Moller, 2013; Moller & Dickow, 2002). This is understandable given the extreme adversity with which most South Africans live given structural disparity. Resilience implies better than expected outcomes despite such severe challenges. In this chapter we posit that a South African, socio-cultural tendency towards social connectedness bolsters unexpected wellbeing outcomes as indicator of quality of life.

Our intent in this chapter is to share how people with an indigenous heritage in South Africa express wellbeing experiences as they resile given chronic and cumulative adversity characteristic of a highly unequal society. While theoretical understandings of pathways to resilience with positive wellbeing outcomes exist in western and non-

I. Eloff (ed.), *Handbook of Quality of Life in African Societies*, International Handbooks of Quality-of-Life, https://doi.org/10.1007/978-3-030-15367-0_4

western contexts, there is a lack of knowledge on this topic given Afrocentric contexts of indigenous perspectives and adversity associated with structural disparity. Consequently, we frame our study from an indigenous psychology (Yang, 2000) perspective to supplement mostly western-dominant discourses in psychology.

Many differences in the experience of wellbeing are notable within and between countries in western and non-western contexts (Diener, Oishi, & Lucas, 2003; Ryff, 1995; Ryff & Keyes, 1995). However, global knowledge on resilience and wellbeing appears to foreground Eurocentric, global north and western perspectives (Christopher, 1999). By comparison, psychological approaches to resilience and wellbeing in non-western contexts are marginalised (Boyden & Mann, 2005; Ryff, Keyes, & Hughes, 2003; Ungar, 2004, 2005, 2009).

Studies examining western psychology approaches to wellbeing seem to have been conducted primarily in the United States (Carr & Friedman, 2005; Deci et al., 2001; Diener, Gohm, Suh, & Oishi, 2000), the United Kingdom (Dolan, Peasgood, & White, 2008; Ford, Goodman, & Meltzer, 2003) and Europe (Diener et al., 2000; Hammer, 2003; Huppert and So, 2013). Urban settings seem to have dominated the contexts within which these studies were conducted (Lyubomirsky, King, & Diener, 2005). These studies use mainly quantitative and mixed method approaches (Deci & Ryan, 2000; Ryan & Deci, 2001; Ryff, 1989; Ryff & Keyes, 1995; Ryff & Singer, 1998, 2000, 2006; Ryff et al., 2003).

Non-western psychology studies on wellbeing (Hwang, 2004; Ingersoll-Dayton, Saengtienchai, Kespichayawattana, & Aungsuroch, 2004) have been conducted in many emerging economy spaces. Studies conducted in Africa (Cocks & Møller, 2002), South America (Morita, 1998), Asia (Constantine, Myers, Kindaichi, & Moore, 2004) and some parts of Europe (Wallace, 2001) often adopt a qualitative approach to studying wellbeing.

There are South African studies that measure views of 'the other' against standardised western perspectives on wellbeing and how western psychological methods and concepts can be adapted to the South African context (Ebersöhn, 2012; Maree, Ebersöhn, & Molepo, 2006; Matoane, 2012; van Zyl & Rothman, 2012). These South African studies use quantitative and mixed methods approaches (Khumalo, Temane, & Wissing, 2012; Maree et al., 2006; Matoane, 2012; van Zyl & Rothman, 2012). Urban and tertiary education settings have been foregrounded in these South African studies (van Zyl & Rothman, 2012).

As is the case in other countries who do not favour dominant western worldviews, such as Mexico, Japan, China, the Philippines, India and Taiwan (Hwang, 2004), South African scholars recognise the need to develop an indigenous psychology unique to context-specific ways of being (MacLeod, 2004; Mpofu, 2002). This process could result in the production of knowledge that is contextually and culturally relevant and which could facilitate the understanding of psychological phenomena in unique Afrocentric settings (Allwood & Berry, 2006; Evenden & Sandstrom, 2011).

This study thus aligns with Pandey (2011) and De La Rey and Ipser's (2004) belief that it is important to recognise the unique, context-based psychologies of indigenous communities and societies, and that the concepts and ideas specific to the historical and cultural orientations of indigenous groups need to be taken into consideration when researching social theories in these societies. Merely importing, adapting and applying psychological theories generated in the global north to people of indigenous origin without first gaining an authentic understanding of the phenomena which occur in these contexts, may be problematic (Allwood & Berry, 2006; Evenden & Sandstrom, 2011) as conceptualisations may be inappropriate and irrelevant (Evenden & Sandstrom, 2011).

More work is needed to develop psychological concepts that are unique and meaningful to African communities as limited information is available that considers how wellbeing is expressed when studied inductively, rather than deductively (Georgas & Mylonas, 2006; Goduka, 2012; Hwang, 2004).

Our guiding question is therefore: How can insight into indigenous pathways to resilience with positive wellbeing outcomes voiced by inhabitants in two rural, resource-constrained sites in South Africa inform knowledge on well-being? Accordingly the objectives are: to contribute to an indigenous psychology knowledge base on (South African) indigenous pathways to resilience with positive wellbeing outcomes using inductive, qualitative and participatory lenses; to identify indigenous psychology wellbeing themes on indigenous pathways to resilience with positive wellbeing outcomes which emerge when data is generated by participants living in high risk, high need environments who visually map and diagram what they perceive wellbeing to be; to compare indigenous pathways to resilience with positive wellbeing outcomes in relation to existing western and non-western understandings of wellbeing.

One of the benefits of building general psychology on a culturally-indigenous knowledge base is that such a psychology could ultimately be far richer than current Eurocentric models. Science as a knowledge construction process is universal for all societies. However, the images, social representations and forms of logic that are used in the creation of knowledge, originate specifically from the cultural heritages of the scientists who co-create this knowledge (Valsiner, 2007).

4.2 Indigenous Psychology

Indigenous psychology emphasises the examination of psychological phenomena in context and considers social, political, philosophical, religious, cultural and ecological themes which emerge in relation to data as meaningful (Yang, 2000). Indigenous psychology (Yang, 2000) is inclusive of cross-cultural and cultural psychology models. In Table 4.1 we list the main theoretical and methodological features in the first two columns and the dominant features of the model in the third column (Yang, 2000). Indigenous psychology advocates for the use of multiple paradigms or lenses in trying to understand human functioning (Yang, 2000).

Slunecko and Hengl (2006) argue that it may be possible to by-pass the "cultural blinders of one society's heritage" (p. 17) when adopting an indigenous psychology approach to psychological experiences. An indigenous psychology stance could risk relying on stereotypical notions of an indigenous 'other' together with notions of 'culture' as a monolithic, discrete, ahistorical and static whole largely synonymous with 'traditional'. By adopting an indigenous psychology stance, we are cognisant of the challenge of overcoming colonial dichotomies that oppose west and other, modern and traditional, rational and emotional. We do not wish to treat broad categories of people as homogenous and do not wish to homogenise all indigenous people, Africans or South Africans simply because they belong to a broad category based on geography and race.

It is well-known that Ubuntu is a privileged Afrocentric worldview amongst people of indigenous origin in Southern Africa (Chilisa, 2012; Letseka, 2013; Strümpfer, 2013). Ubuntu refers to kinship – affinity for and belonging to a family. Ramose (2002) explains life through an Ubuntu-lens as living in an atmosphere of family. People are viewed as potential members of this clan – an ideal family with friendly and caring relationships (Metz & Gaie, 2010). The implication is that one who appropriates an Ubuntu-identity also appropriates an ethic of care encouraged by relational autonomy and a reliance on empathy (Waghid & Smeyers, 2012).

4.3 Resilience

A resilience framework emerged within a broader transformation in theory and research on psychology that created developmental psychopathology (Masten, 1989; Sroufe & Rutter, 1984). Scholarly attention to resilience in the late twentieth century rekindled interest in positive psychology because these investigators studied, wrote and spoke about the human capacity for positive adaptation and achievement in the face of adversity (Masten, 2001).

Although the understanding of resilience has been broadened to account for community and cultural factors, these are still mainly evaluated from the perspective of Eurocentric scientific discourse (Ungar, 2009). According to Ungar (2009), a coherent definition of resilience that captures the dual focus of the individual and his or her ecology is yet to be presented. Spencer

Table 4.1 Comparison of cross-cultural, cultural and indigenous psychology

Cross-cultural psychology	Cultural psychology	Indigenous psychology
Aim, scope and focus		
To generate a universal psychology by testing, broadening and integrating psychological theories in diverse cultural contexts	To generate a culture-bound knowledge system by developing theories within and across specific cultures	To generate mono-cultural and cross-cultural psychologies and then a universal psychology if possible
A sub-discipline of mainstream psychology	A psychology and anthropology hybrid field	Includes both cross-cultural and cultural psychologies as well as other fields of mainstream and non-mainstream psychologies
Study of psychological and behavioural similarities is emphasised over differences	Study of psychological and behavioural differences is emphasised over similarities	No such preference
Theoretical orientations		
Natural science model	Human science or cultural science model	Both models accepted
Behavioural manifestations are signs of universal psychological processes	Behavioural manifestations have an existence of their own	Both views accepted
Culture and behaviour (or mind) considered distinguishable from each other in terms of independent vs. dependent variable	Culture and behaviour (or mind) considered mutually constitutive and indistinguishable from each other	Both views accepted
Psychological and behavioural processes structures are separate, discrete or even isolated entities	Psychological and behavioural processes structures are grouped together	Both views accepted
Context-free definitions of psychological and behavioural concepts preferred	Context-bound definitions of psychological and behavioural concepts preferred	Both kinds of definitions accepted
Universal explanations more important than local explanations	Local explanations more important than universal explanations	Both kinds of explanations equally important

Adapted from Yang (2000)

et al. (2006) are of the opinion that a "carefully nuanced approach is particularly needed when considering broad ethnic enclaves and, more generally, all humans' normative pursuit of stage-specific life course competencies" (Spencer et al., 2006, p. 627).

In an international resilience study dominant westernised conceptualisations of resilience as an intrapsychic construct were rejected to be replaced with contextually-relevant understanding of resilience (Ungar, 2004). The implication is that both global and culturally or contextually-specific aspects of resilience exist. Culturally-embedded understandings of notions such as wellbeing often challenge traditional standards for behaviours and outcomes (Ungar, 2009). This argument makes an important contribution to the rationale for this study from the perspective of delivering appropriate psychological services. If social researchers and practitioners are guided mostly by one approach over another in their understanding of how people respond to adversity, without recognition and acknowledgement of their specific context, then the interventions that flow from research and assessment practices may be superficial and irrelevant. Macleod (2004) agrees, stating that culture has a profound effect on psychological experiences and should thus not be overlooked.

We conceptualise resilience as a dynamic developmental process whereby an individual is able to achieve or maintain varying levels of positive adaptation despite exposure to significant threat or adversity (Ebersöhn, 2007). We consider resilience as an adaptive process where adversity has a long-term impact on individual functioning and development (Skinner & Zimmer-Gembeck, 2007), suggesting that the way in which people cope with adversity influences the outcomes that they experience – including wellbeing outcomes.

We also understand resilience, in the context of this study, through a lens of chronic and cumulative high risk and need. Ebersöhn (2014) posits resilience processes in poverty as a lifeline chain. Here, uninterrupted incidences of positive adaptation (including positive wellbeing outcomes) are linked one after the other. In this sense, the process of resilience and adaptive coping becomes one which could be characterised as a "cable of nonstop vigilance" (Ebersöhn, 2014, p. 1) where there is neither a concrete beginning to the adversity experience nor an end to positive adaptation. According to Ebersöhn (2014), resilience in high risk, high need settings requires "relentless positive adaptation" (p. 21) which enables individuals and communities to function from day to day in spite of the chronic and cumulative adversity to which they are exposed.

Because resilience is contextual, the culture and context within which individuals and communities function and live, both have a significant influence on decisions that people make in the process of resilience. To this effect, Ebersöhn (2012, 2013) posits the necessity for analytical frameworks informed by indigenous knowledge. Indigenous pathways to resilience refer to embedded socio-cultural systems, beliefs, knowledge and practices used by people from indigenous heritages in response to significant adversity (Ebersöhn, 2013).

4.4 Wellbeing

Embedded in a historical and cultural milieu in which the individual is regarded as a primary attributor to wellbeing, Eurocentric, western orientations regard personal accountability as central to the wellbeing of a given individual. In this light, happiness is regarded as each person's natural and unalienable right; moreover, people are responsible for their own happiness (Ingersoll-Dayton et al., 2004).

Chun, Moos, and Cronkite's (2006) model posits wellbeing as a range of experiences or phenomena which indicate that an individual has successfully appraised and coped with various threats or challenges (Chun et al., 2006) signified by the broader process of resilience. In this sense, Chun et al. (2006) regard wellbeing as one positive adaptation outcome of the resilience process (Chun et al., 2006).

Western psychological studies highlight wellbeing as closely connected with the way in which people perceive themselves (Markus & Kitayama, 1998). Internal traits, values and emotions, as well as autonomy and differentiation are regarded as core to the experience of wellbeing in Western society (Singelis, 1994; Suh, 2009). Personal accountability, as well as independence are emphasised as well (Ingersoll-Dayton et al., 2004). Western research proposes two dominant approaches to wellbeing: hedonism (Diener, 1984) and eudaimonism (Deci, 1976). Within these two approaches several related perspectives exist: psychological wellbeing (Ryff, 1989), social wellbeing (Keyes, 1998), self-determination theory (Ryan & Deci, 2001), orientations to happiness (Seligman, 2002) and flourishing (Keyes, 1998). These perspectives put forward the idea that wellbeing may be regarded as a cluster of behaviours and attitudes encompassing positive emotions, positive psychological and positive social functioning (Ryff et al., 2003).

Non-western psychology theory on wellbeing (Constantine et al., 2004; Houkamau & Sibley, 2011) highlights the idea that individuals exist in relation to their community and environment. This belief extends to the notion that spiritual (Constantine et al., 2004), cultural (Highlen, 1996), racial (Ingersoll-Dayton et al., 2004) and ethnic spheres (Queener & Martin, 2001) also interact and are interdependent role players in the experience of wellbeing. A result of the interdependent nature of life spheres in non-western psychological understandings of wellbeing is the idea that if illness is experienced in one sphere, other spheres may suffer as well (Krippner, 2000; Lee, Oh, & Mountcastle, 1992; Singh, 1999). Thus, it is necessary to establish, maintain or restore harmony and balance to indigenous wellbeing systems (Sue & Sue, 1999; Wing, 1998).

Rice and Steele (2004) found that different cultures produce people with different levels of subjective wellbeing, and that aspects of culture that influence wellbeing do not give way quickly or easily. Neff (2007) found that there appears to be a 'wellbeing hierarchy' in South Africa, due to the legacy of apartheid, which is based on race and ethnicity. Additionally, Neff (2007) found that to a certain extent, there may be cultural differences associated with wellbeing, which exist even between groups in South Africa. Finally, Vorster et al. (2000) found that in South Africa, subjective wellbeing seems to improve relative to the degree of urbanisation that the individual experiences, as well as in relation to one's socio-economic status.

'Cultural identity and capital' refers to the notion that different modes of behaviour, values and attitudes exist that are suited to positive adjustment within a given society (Oishi, 2000; Wilson & Constantine, 1999). The way in which one interprets and makes sense of these cultural elements and assimilates these understandings into an existing self-perceived identity all form part of one's indigenous wellbeing knowledge system (Constantine & Sue, 2006; Neville & Lilly, 2000; Utsey, Ponterotto, Reynolds, & Cancelli, 2000). King, Smith, and Gracey (2009) believe that "cultural identity depends not only on access to culture and heritage but also on opportunities for cultural expression and cultural endorsement within society's institutions" (p.77). In this light, culture, and an individual's understanding of its relevance to life, will affect, inform and filter through to each facet of one's existence. It will also play an integral role in how one navigates and negotiates wellbeing.

According to Houkamau and Sibley (2011), international research on the relationship between culture and identity supports a "culture-as-cure" perspective (p. 379). Such a perspective demonstrates that a positive view of one's own culture is associated with a range of favourable social, psychological and health outcomes. A great deal of international research has reported on the positive relationship between ethnic identity and psychological constructs such as self-esteem, self-efficacy, personal mastery and locus of control. Higher levels of acculturation have also been associated with higher levels of preventative health behaviours among many ethnic minority groups.

Research that focuses on the wellbeing of people from various ethnic groups internationally has focused on enhancing the self-esteem of individual members of groups by encouraging engagement with a group's language and cultural practices (Tucker, 1999; Zimmerman, Israel, Schulz, & Checkoway, 1992). This is because most ethnic groups are endowed with exclusive traditions which enable members to search within and find powerful sources of personal dignity and pride (Hutnik, 1991). Additional research suggests that those individuals who are part of an ethnic minority and choose to accept this aspect of their identity, and who are knowledgeable about the culture of their group, seem to fare better on various measures of psychological wellbeing (Belgrave et al., 1994; Caldwell, Kohn-Wood, Schmeelk-Cone, Chavous, & Zimmerman, 2004).

Crocker, Luhtanen, Blaine, and Broadnax (1994) found that the degree to which individuals positively assessed their ethnic or racial group as collective self-esteem has a significant impact on their health and wellbeing. In instances where individuals were able to acknowledge and separate how they felt from how the rest of society felt about their group, the effects of discrimination (which typically affects wellbeing negatively) were mitigated (Lee, 2003). Furthermore, identifying with one's racial or ethnic group, even when that group forms the minority, increases one's sense of belonging and helps people to feel accepted. The added investment in one's ethnic group and the way that this group makes one feel, appear to be a worthy pathway to wellbeing which affects and directs one's experiences of and responses to other dimensions of life as further pathways to wellbeing (Crocker et al., 1994).

4.5 Social Connectedness

Social connectedness refers to the notion that people live and function in relation to others. In this light, a complex interplay exists between being independent and able to cope on one's own, being dependent but feeling as if one can ask for and accept help where necessary and being willing and feeling able to give assistance to others in their time of need (Constantine et al., 2004; Fozdar and Torezani, 2008a,b; Ingersoll-Dayton et al., 2004; King et al., 2009; Shu & Zhu, 2009). Social connectedness involves a degree of striving for independence because it is important to ensure that others are not burdened to the degree that *they* are not able to cope. This may occur because their perceived sense of responsibility to others in the community exceeds whatever they are realistically able to offer both affectively and instrumentally (Ingersoll-Dayton et al., 2004). Maintaining harmony and equilibrium between 'give-and-take' in the community becomes important, because without this balance, additional stressors in the community may be created (Ingersoll-Dayton et al., 2004).

Various studies have highlighted the role that both affective and instrumental support play (Constantine & Sue, 2006; Cox, 2012; Siu & Phillips, 2002; Suh & Oishi, 2002) in wellbeing. Friends and family both play an important role in providing for the affective and instrumental needs of others. In terms of affective support (Siu & Phillips, 2002), family and friends seem to come together to create an internal support network for people, which functions as a source of personal empowerment and cultural resources for facilitating coping schemata, coping strategies and adaptive coping resources (Constantine & Sue, 2006). These affective support resources enable individuals to adjust their outlook on adversity, as well as their subjective interpretations of their environment when they are faced with various hardships. The term 'provision of instrumental support' refers to the ability to offer or receive practical support strategies: these would typically include having someone to help with the provision of fresh food; looking after another's children while he or she is at work; or helping out around the house, all of which play a role in uplifting morale and the sense of being able to cope with one's day-to-day responsibilities (Siu & Phillips, 2002).

Social harmony refers to the importance of feeling included (sense of belonging) in one's community, living with a sense of safety and experiencing peace. Social harmony is integrally connected to social connectedness, as well as to social mutuality. In order to experience social harmony, people need to be socially connected to and socially engaged (referring to social mutuality) with their social sphere. People must also be able to capitalise on the social resources available within their environment. Social harmony differs from social connectedness because it focusses on the *quality* of relationships with others in one's environment (Fozdar and Torezani, 2008a,b; King et al., 2009; Lu & Gilmour, 2006; Pflug, 2009; Sotgiu, Galati, Manzano, & Rognoni, 2011). For example, Thomas, Cairney, Gunthorpe, Paradies, and Sayers (2010) argue that indigenous perspectives on mental health include being in harmony with one's country, lawfulness, social and kinship relationships. Ingersoll-Dayton et al. (2004) regard the avoidance of conflict, healthy relationships with one's life partner, children and extended family, as well as with friends and neighbours as important to wellbeing. Ingersoll-Dayton et al. (2004) also believe that in maintaining positive relationships with others, individuals are more likely to experience feelings of security and a sense of inclusion in their community. Lu and Gilmour (2006) maintain that the collective welfare of one's community (defined by the health of the social relationships that make up a community) is more important than the interests of individuals living within that community. Therefore, if an individual is to contribute positively to the quality of relationships within a community (so that social harmony may be experienced) then that person may sometimes need to make sacrifices for the good of the village (King et al., 2009).

Social mutuality refers to the notion that in order to experience wellbeing from a non-Western perspective, one must act in accordance with one's cultural group (Diener et al. 2000; Ingersoll-Dayton et al., 2004; Kitayama, Markus, & Kurokawa, 2000; Oishi, 2000). For example, it may be necessary to ensure that one's required roles and responsibilities are performed in line with certain cultural norms and standards. Moreover, it may be necessary to act on the basis of others' needs and expectations when making decisions and engaging in certain behaviours.

Kitayama et al. (2000) argue that in striving for social mutuality, it is important to 'fit in' with one's culture and social group. Individuals may need to adjust the status and nature of their relationships so that they become members of that group. They may also need to constrain, tame or condition their desires and wishes to facilitate interpersonal harmony and unity (Uchida, Norasakkunkit, & Kitayama, 2004).

Acting in line with community-based values such as respect is important in ensuring social mutuality. In most indigenous societies, respect is regarded as fundamental to wellbeing. In the context of Ingersoll-Dayton et al.'s (2004) study, respect is defined as listening to, and following the advice of the others in the community, particularly one's elders. Respect is regarded as important to the experience of wellbeing, because it is seen as a marker of success, as well as an indicator of one's social standing in the community. Moreover, the level of respect which an individual receives is regarded as a reflection of the wisdom which that individual holds. Respect affirms an individual's success as a parent and indicates that the individual's children will care for them in the future. All these markers of respect are also important cultural indicators of social mutuality, and are strived for by most non-Western societies.

The goals which people strive towards also play an important role in the degree of social mutuality which they are able to achieve. According to Oishi (2000), pathways to wellbeing differ across cultures depending on their salient needs and values. The goals which a culture or society strives toward will also be determined by its needs and values. Therefore, if people are to live happily and in relation with others, they must take into account the external standards which their culture, family or village may exert on their lifestyle, and try to live in accordance with these standards. For example, marriage is typically regarded as an important cultural institution which non-Western young men and women strive towards. In pursuing a healthy marriage, many young men and women are able to uphold the traditional values of their culture and realise one of the goals which their parents and community as a whole have set for them (Diener et al., 2000).

Social capital is pertinent to social connectedness. Farid and Lazarus (2008) explain that social capital processes (trust, social support and cooperation) can be accessed and mobilised to enhance relationships and improve the experience of wellbeing. One factor that all of these terms have in common is that they involve a process of mobilising networks of kinship, acquaintances and ties in order to manage and address stress and risk. Germane to this discussion is the indigenous psychology theory relationship resourced resilience (Ebersöhn, 2012, 2014). The theory posits flocking as indigenous pathway to provide social support and manage the distribution of social resources in the face of severe challenges. A central tenet is that individuals view themselves as related to or connected with others via relationships. These relationships imply that individuals are also connected with social resources. Yip et al. (2007), state that cognitive social capital, similar to flocking, denotes collective action (such as trust, reciprocity and sense of belonging) and emotional support to facilitate social networks and support mechanisms with a view to experiencing wellbeing.

4.6 Methodology

The purpose of the Indigenous Pathways to Resilience (IPR) study, Centre for the Study of Resilience, University of Pretoria, is to contribute to psychological resilience knowledge through an indigenous psychology (Yang, 2000) lens. In the longitudinal case study (Stake, 2013), over a 3-year time frame (2012–2014), we investigated the case of indigenous pathways to resilience in severely challenged settings in South Africa. The focus of this chapter is on a section of the Indigenous Pathways to Resilience data, namely the indigenous experiences of positive wellbeing outcomes of resilience pathways. The longitudinal case study design enabled us to not delimit insights to only cross-sectional data as we generated data in three waves of annual 3-day field-visits per site (totalling 9 days in the field per site).

The two remote settings were purposively selected and are indicated in Fig. 4.1. In order to study resilience, the remote Limpopo and Mpumalanga settings met criteria of characteristically chronic and cumulative adversity and consequent high risk and high need synonymous with rural spaces in a highly unequal society with structural disparity. In order to investigate indigenous perspectives, the settings met criteria of populations with many inhabitants of indigenous heritage.

The Vhembe district experiences severe water scarcities, poor water quality, as well as food scarcities (Brooks & Abney, 2013; Rietveld, Haarhoff, & Jagals, 2009). The primary language spoken in the sampled Limpopo site is VhaVhenda (Census, 2011). Table 4.2 summarises census data on the Mutale municipality in the Vhembe district.

Figure 4.2 provides visual data on observations of the Limpopo site indicating the rural infrastructure, lack of access to basic services such as running water and different types of homes.

The selected Mpumalanga site is regarded as agricultural and has a low population density with high proportions of younger children (Aitken, Rangan, & Kull, 2009). The primary home language spoken in the Gert Sibande district is AmaSwati (Census, 2011). Table 4.3 provides additional census data on the Gert Sibande district and the Albert Luthuli municipality.

Figure 4.3 includes contextual photographs of Mpumalanga. Certain aspects of the infrastructure as well as the informal agricultural sector which play an important role in the livelihood of residents in Mpumalanga are also shown in this collage.

The selected sites enabled the inclusion of VhaVhenda and AmaSwati indigenous perspectives (Abrams, 2010). We conveniently sampled (Cohen et al., 2007) VhaVhenda and AmaSwati participants (n = 135, male = 57, female = 78, elders = 53, young people = 82) who live permanently at each research site and hold indigenous

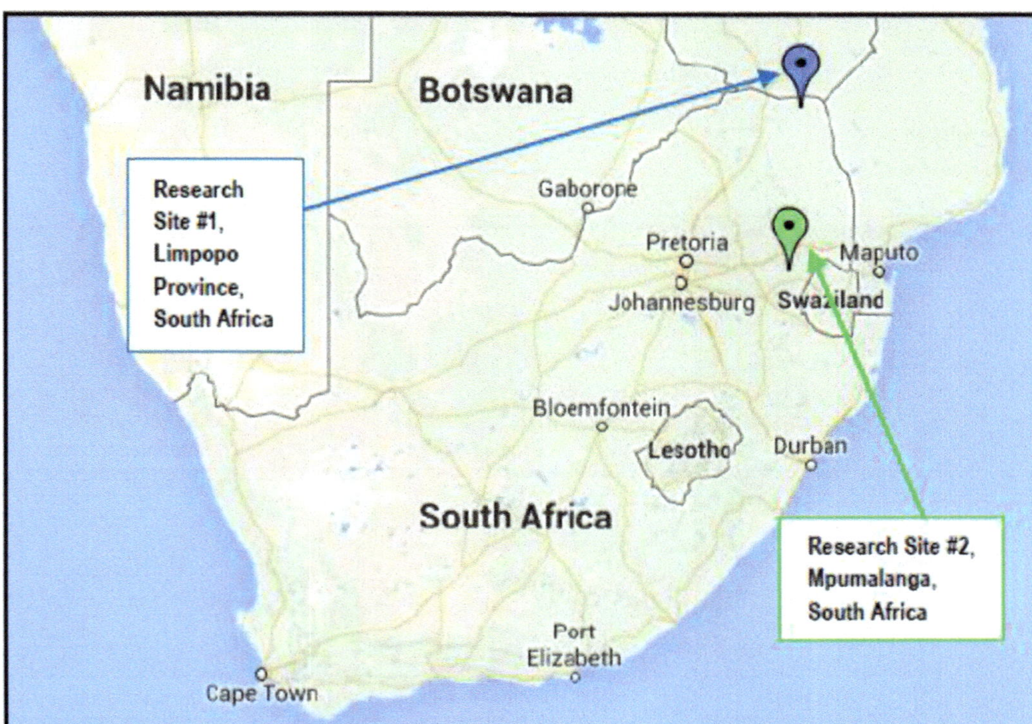

Fig. 4.1 Location of research sites. (Downloaded from Google Maps)

Table 4.2 Census data pertaining to the Vhembe District and Mutale Municipality

Description of profile	Specification of profile	Mutale – local municipality			
		1996		2011	
		Number	Percentage	Number	Percentage
Distribution of functional ages	*0–14 years*	33,067	46.3%	35,086	38.2%
	15–64 years	33,784	47.2%	51,079	55.6%
	65 years and over	4672	6.5%	5705	6.2%
Total		**71,523**	**100%**	**91,870**	**100%**
Education level for 20 years and older	*No schooling*	11,481	39.8%	8301	18.8%
	Some primary	4174	14.5%	6078	13.7%
	Complete primary	1912	6.6%	2341	5.3%
	Some secondary	7188	24.9%	15,720	35.6%
	Gr 12/matric	3118	10.8%	8297	18.8%
	Higher	990	3.4%	3456	7.8%
Total		**28,863**	**100%**	**44,193**	**100%**
School attendance	*Attending*	27,265	76.8%	36,388	85%
	Not attending	8246	23.2%	6386	15%
Total		**35,511**	**100%**	**42,774**	**100%**
Unemployment	*Employed*	4963	32%	9321	51%
	Unemployed	10,561	68%	8953	48%
Total		**15,524**	**100%**	**18,274**	**100%**
Distribution of households by type of dwelling	*Formal*	4795	34.8%	20,726	87.9%
	Informal	28	0.2%	169	0.7%
	Traditional	8955	65%	2693	11.4%
Total		**13,778**	**100%**	**23,588**	**100%**
Distribution of households	*Female-headed*	7507	54%	13,012	54.8%
	Child-headed	398	2.8%	419	1.7%
Total		**13,908**	**NA**	**23,751**	**NA**
Distribution of population groups	*Black African*	72,461	99.6%	91,222	99.3%
	Coloured	65	0.09%	86	0.09%
	Indian/Asian	24	0.03%	69	0.07%
	White	209	0.28%	416	0.54%
Total population		**72,759**	**100%**	**91,793**	**100%**

Adapted from Census (2011)

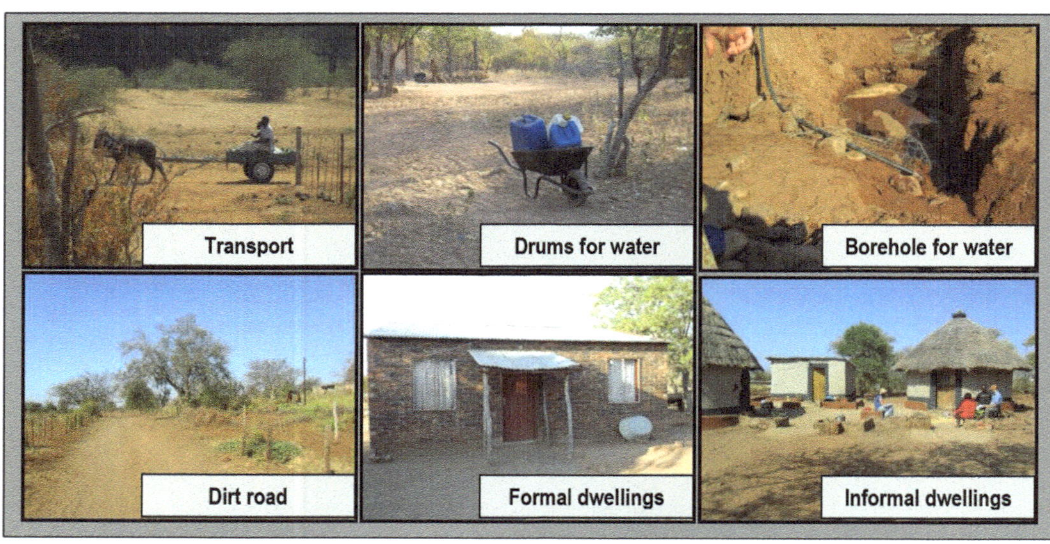

Fig. 4.2 Visual data on observations of the context in the Limpopo site

Table 4.3 Census data pertaining to the Albert Luthuli Municipality in the Gert Sibande District

	Specification of profile	Albert Luthuli – local municipality			
		1996		2011	
Description of profile		Number	Percentage	Number	Percentage
Distribution of functional ages	*0–14 years*	77,348	42.9%	67,801	36.5%
	15–64 years	94,656	52.5%	108,342	58.2%
	65 years and over	8254	4.6%	9868	5.3%
Total		**180,258**	**100%**	**186,010**	**100%**
Education level for 20 years and older	*No schooling*	31,986	40.3%	18,622	19.9%
	Some primary	11,789	14.9%	12,600	13.5%
	Complete primary	5065	6.4%	4146	4.4%
	Some secondary	19,682	24.8%	26,865	28.9%
	Gr 12/matric	8113	10.2%	25,217	27%
	Higher	2715	3.4%	5905	6.3%
Total		**79,350**	**100%**	**93,354**	**100%**
School attendance	*Attending*	68,812	75%	66,700	78.5%
	Not attending	22,871	25%	18,262	21.5%
Total		**91,684**	**100%**	**84,961**	**100%**
Unemployment	*Employed*	20,357	48%	28,593	64.2%
	Unemployed	22,038	52%	15,878	35.8%
Total		**42,395**	**100%**	**44,471**	**100%**
Distribution of households by type of dwelling	*Formal*	17,693	17.7%	36,497	77%
	Informal	39,726	39.8%	2857	6%
	Traditional	42,462	42.5%	7994	17%
Total		**99,881**	**100%**	**47,348**	**100%**
Distribution of households	*Female-headed*	16,828	47%	23,527	49.3%
	Child-headed	692	19.4%	547	11.4%
Total		**35,543**	**NA**	**47,705**	**NA%**
Distribution of population groups	*Black African*	177,862	98%	181,531	98%
	Coloured	240	0.1%	434	0.2%
	Indian/Asian	273	0.1%	755	0.4%
	White	3272	1.8%	2938	1.4%
Total population		**181,647**	**100%**	**185,658**	**100%**

Adapted from Census (2011)

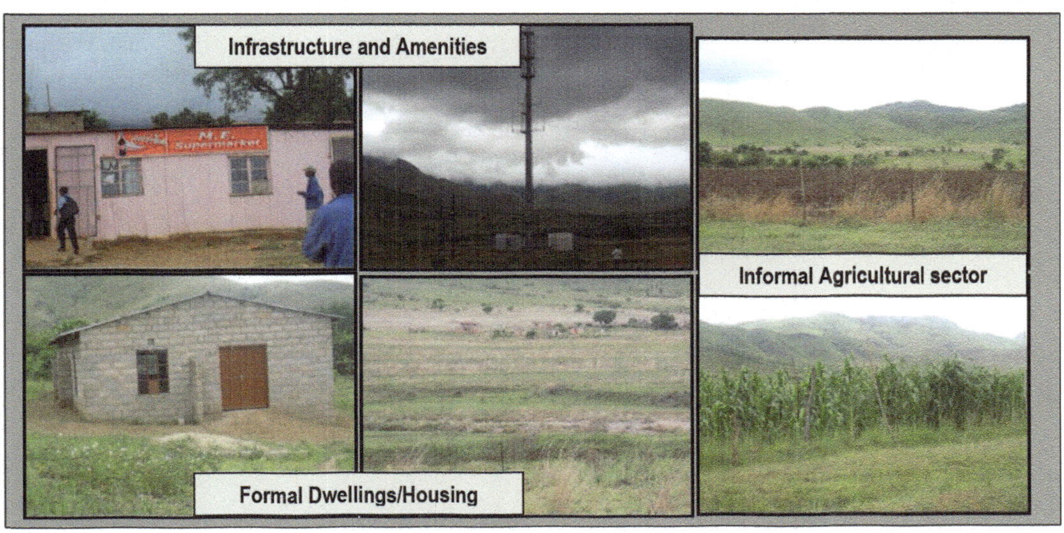

Fig. 4.3 Visual data on observations of the context in the Mpumalanga site

knowledge by virtue of local culture and meaning-making rituals (Odora Hoppers, 2008). We sampled for intergenerational transfer of indigenous knowledge and for gendered perspectives of indigenous experiences – older men (over the age of 35 years), older women (over the age of 35 years), younger men (between the ages of 21 and 35 years) and younger women (between the ages of 21 and 35 years). While studies which compare variables such as age and gender are typically quantitative (such as Khumalo et al., 2012) our decision was informed by Sokoya, Muthukrishna, & Collings (2005) and Arku (2010) who compare age and gender in qualitative studies. We used self-identified indications of home language (VhaVenda and AmaSwati) in a demographic questionnaire to indicate ethnicity.

We opted to use Participatory Reflection and Action (PRA) (Chambers, 2013) to generate data inductively with participants. PRA afforded us the opportunity to create a data generation space where participants could confidently voice their experiences in their home languages in group settings. The power-sharing principle of PRA means participants would not have to feel limited power when answering in written format in a language which is not their own and selecting items from questionnaires in deductive format that match their experiences against an outsider, western profile of resilience.

In Figs. 4.4 and 4.5 we show where the researchers met with participants in communal spaces – a classroom in a local school in Mpumalanga and a community meeting space in Limpopo. Participants worked in groups of older men, older women, younger men and younger women.

As per the PRA-tradition we generated indigenous-relevant prompts with an advisory panel for participatory diagramming activities to elicit PRA-group conversations (Chambers, 2013). We used the metaphor of a mealie as metaphor for wellbeing experiences. Once each group had a poster with a print image of a mealie (as depicted in Fig. 4.6) we verbally posed the following question – which was translated: If you go to bed at night and you close your eyes and go to sleep and you think of everything that happened that day, how do you know that it was a good day?

After consultation within groups participants noted their collective thinking on the posters and then verbally presented their collective answer. These oral presentations were audio-recorded and transcribed verbatim, translated into English, followed by back-translation for verification. We also made use of observation-as-context-of-interaction (Angrosino & Mays de Perez, 2000) which five co-researchers documented as field notes and reflective notes in their researcher diaries. Visual data included photographs of posters, as well as observations of the research sites and the process of data generation.

Translators assisted with explaining PRA-prompts for group discussions. Translators resided in the communities where data was gen-

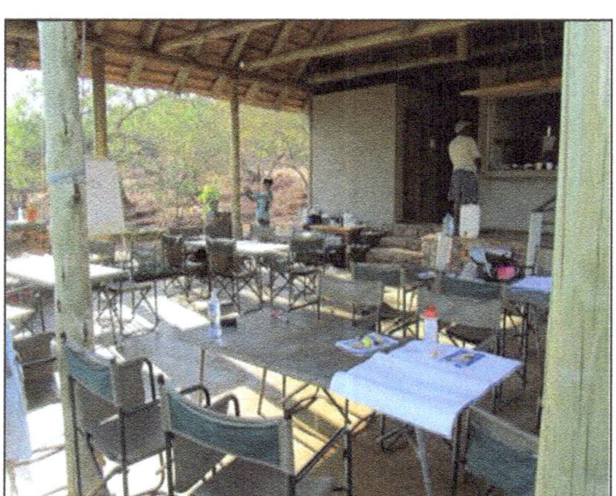

Fig. 4.4 Limpopo Province, July 2013

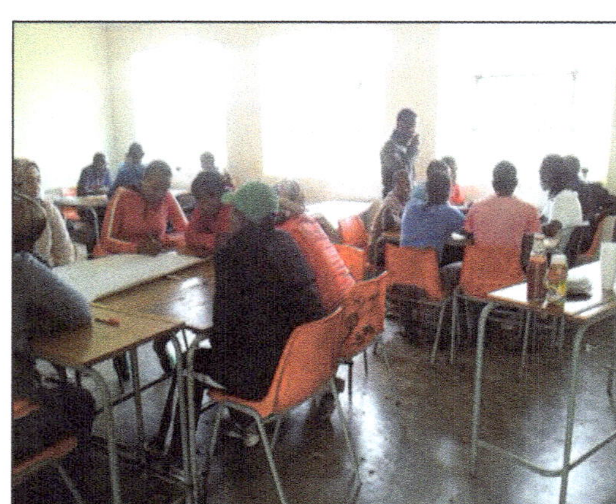

Fig. 4.5 Mpumalanga, November, 2012

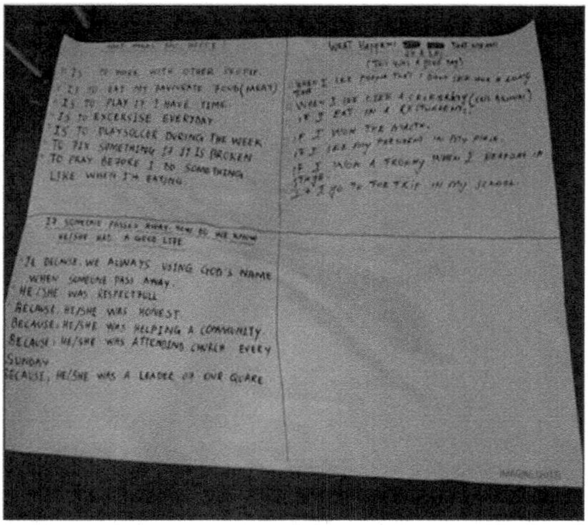

Fig. 4.6 Younger Men, Mpumalanga, November, 2012

erated. In Limpopo translators were native TshiVhenda speakers trained by a local research facility to listen for information in their mother tongue and then reproduce this information in a different language in which they are fluent (English). In Mpumalanga translators were native SiSwati teachers. Translators also assisted with explaining research information during the consent process, as well as the use of cameras and audio recorders (Orb, Eisenhauer, & Wynaden, 2001). In addition, translators assisted with the completion of demographic questionnaires.

Multiple coders were used for thematic in-case and cross-case analysis (Braun & Clarke, 2006) based on iterative processes to generate inclusion and exclusion criteria (Babbie & Mouton, 2001).

In order to ensure trustworthiness we followed the following strategies (Seale, 1999): credibility was enhanced by prolonged engagement in the field, peer debriefing, multiple researchers, multiple perspectives of indigenous experiences (ethnicity, region, gender, age, and different data generation waves), and member checking. Transferability was strengthened by thick descriptions of the cases, purposive sampling of sites, as well as field notes and visual data of observations. We ensured dependability by means of an audit trail, a code-recode strategy and peer examination. Confirmability was addressed by means of researcher reflexivity.

The findings of this study should be read against certain delimitations. Transferability is limited due to the small sample. The convenient sampling of participants resulted in a sample biased towards regional ethnicity, lower socio-economic class, rurality, unemployment, and an oversampling of women and youth. By implication, insights on indigenous pathways to resilience with positive wellbeing outcomes that are excluded are those of people with indigenous roots (i) from other South African ethnic origins, (ii) from different classes, (iii) who live in urban environments, and (iv) who are employed.

4.7 Social Connectedness as Indigenous Pathway to Wellbeing

Following thematic analysis, it was apparent that participants signified social connectedness as a significant indigenous pathway to wellbeing. Social connectedness relates to the wellbeing opportunities implied by social capital and associated social resources to which participants have access because of positive relationships. With regards to wellbeing from a social connectedness perspective two subthemes emerged, namely social reciprocity and valuing socio-cultural identity. Of the total 32 PRA-group discussions, social reciprocity was mentioned in 21, and valuing socio-cultural identity in 22 group discussions.

4.8 Social Reciprocity Character of Social Connectedness as Indigenous Pathway to Wellbeing

Social reciprocity refers to the view that happiness can be achieved when a person receives comfort and support from the community (Constantine et al., 2004; Ingersoll-Dayton et al., 2004; Keyes, 1998; King et al., 2009; Ryff, 1989). Social reciprocity thus includes interdependence and denotes social support as social transactions that are integral to the experience of collective social wellbeing. Aligned social interactions signify being able to ask for and receive support in times of need, as well as being able to offer and provide support to others. Social reciprocity consists of two categories, namely giving social support, and receiving social support.

As part of a social connectedness pathway to wellbeing, social reciprocity was indicated as significant by participants in both sites. Irrespective of age, gender, ethnicity or region participants voiced that giving and receiving social support was significant for a social connectedness pathway to wellbeing.

One of the researchers noted in field-notes that he observed that young men in Limpopo privilege opportunities to enable social support (YM-LP-2012, Lines 53–59):

> They were given a picture of knobkerries and were asked to write how they intend to solve the problem of water in the future. It was evident that communal meetings are a very important way of solving problems. They usually come together with the headman who coordinates activities in the community. The headman brings people together and guides the decision making process until community members are able to vote on the best decision to put into action. This is usually the most acceptable method of making decisions.

Participants referred to instances in the past when they or their neighbours gave social support. When asked "How do others needing help make you happy?" participants responded that they experienced joy when they were able to provide practical assistance to those in need. They specifically mentioned that creating opportunities for others, for example, to earn money, and personally volunteering in the community where help was needed, resulted in opportunities for social engagement and experiencing wellbeing.

The following vignette depicts how older men in Mpumalanga explained giving support as significant to wellbeing (MP-2012, Lines 725–757):

> Johnny (MP-2012; 4): Okay. We considered that question above (referring to the question X wrote on the board: If a loved one pass away. How do you know that he/she had a good life?). We said, maybe the person was successful in running his/her business. The one that has passed away.
>
> Tebogo (MP-2012; 4): Maybe he was helping around the community. Like if someone doesn't have a car.
>
> Johnny (MP-2012; 4): Yes to ask him to take him to the hospital. Yes. So if one of my family has passed away we will ask him to...
>
> Tebogo (MP-2012; 4): Contribute.

Participants also explained how they felt happy when they were able to give each other support to solve community issues that affected the combined quality of life of those living in their village as evident in the vignette below of older women in Limpopo (LP-2013, Lines 258–263):

> Joyce (LP-2013; 1): They got a goat project.
>
> Janna (LP-2013; 1): A goat project?
>
> Joyce (LP-2013; 1): When she have got maybe many goats she can give one, his neighbour so that he can have some. When that goat have got many, he give another one.

Receiving social support was also prominent amongst participants in Mpumalanga. Participants described how others support them in times of need by helping them to solve problems, by providing them with a space to provide and receive psychosocial support – to voice concerns, empathise with hardship and offer guidance on how to cope with adversity. Figures 4.7 and 4.8 capture the prominence of the presence of social support for wellbeing.

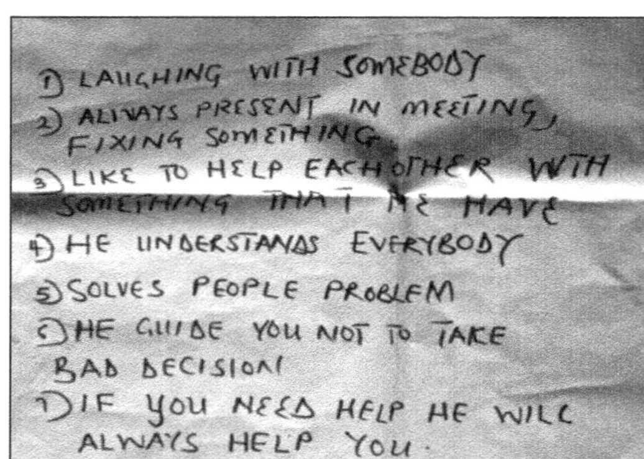

Fig. 4.7 Younger women, Mpumalanga, November, 2013

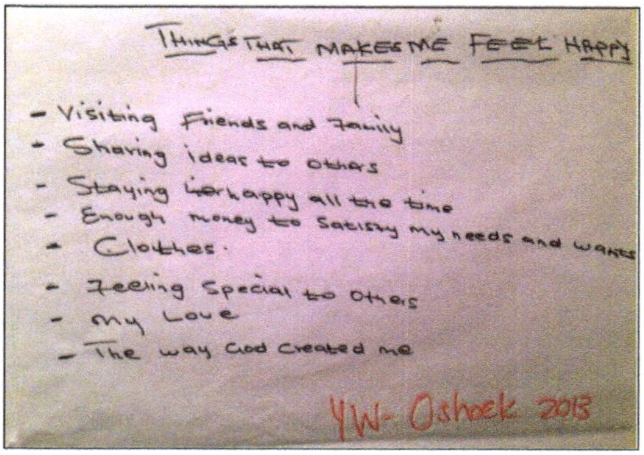

Fig. 4.8 Younger women, Mpumalanga, November, 2013

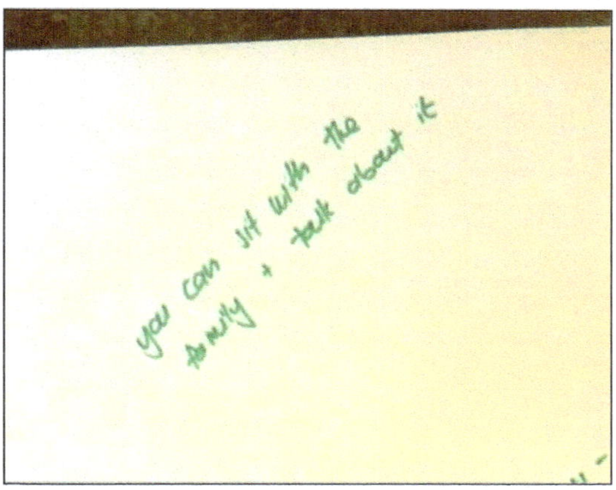

Fig. 4.9 Older women, Limpopo Province, July, 2013

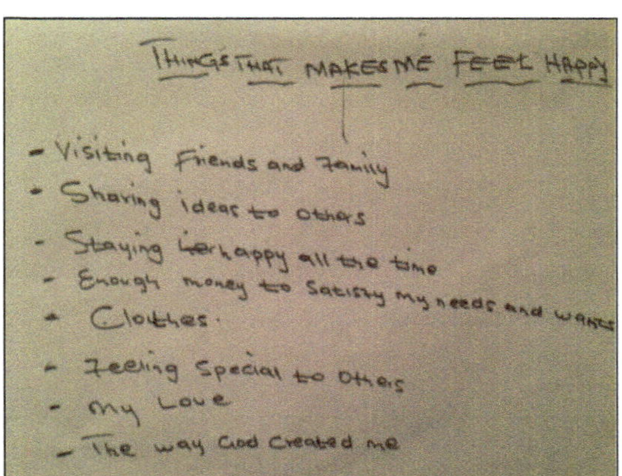

Fig. 4.10 Younger men, Mpumalanga, November, 2012

Figures 4.9 and 4.10 provide examples of where participants reflected on how help from their family contributed to their sense of wellbeing.

Below are two vignettes of PRA-conversations that depict the connection between receiving social support and wellbeing. The first is perspectives of older women in Mpumalanga (MP-2012, Lines 509–511), and the second vignette was provided during member checking in Mpumalanga (MP-2014, MC, Lines 788–795):

Janna (MP-2012; 3): Ok. Is there anything else that you can do to solve a problem?
Suzie (MP-2012; 3): They say you can sit with the family and talk about it.
Tebogo (MP-2012; 4): Maybe they help me with money or something, because I am short of money.
Johnny (MP-2012; 4): Also, sharing minds and ideas.
Obie (MP-2014; MC): I think friends make us happy because there are things you cannot share with your family or your mother. Maybe you can tell your friend.
Marlize (MP-2014; MC): OK so sometimes it's not comfortable to tell close personal things to a family member, but you still need to share with someone?
Obie (MP-2014; MC): Mm.
Marlize (MP-2014; MC): Then your friend can be that extra person that's going to assist you?
Obie (MP-2014; MC): Yes.

The cumulative adversities related to chronic poverty and structural disparity mean that limited basic services severely challenge wellbeing experiences of participants. It was evident that participants used knowledge of social support for their wellbeing to their advantage by mobilising social support to access scarce services – water, electricity and transport. Participants described how they received support via social connectedness pathways from the leaders in their community, village or municipality. The mandate of a culturally-sanctioned intermediary to navigate to and negotiate provision of support (Ungar, 2012) was significant. In this regard the chief or headman (a term used interchangeably in both communities) rallied support to villagers to solve shared problems when they were not able to do so on their own. Additionally, the chief acted as a mediator and negotiator for the village when support was required from the municipality, as evident in an excerpt from a researcher's journal (YM-LP-2012, Lines 60–65):

> The participants emphasised the importance of living as a community by sharing things they have. They also did not rule out the importance of the chiefs and community elders. Hierarchy in the community among leaders was usually spelt [out] in decision-making. Most of the time, when explaining how they took a particular decision in the community, participants mention how they told the head of a household, how the head met the chief, the chief met the municipality etc.

The vignette below explains the expectation of older men in Limpopo that they can depend on receiving social support based on observing protocols of cultural leadership (LP-2013, Lines 131–135):

> Walter (LP-2013; 1): At the head man's yard, that is where they receive motivations and attend their meetings under the control of the head man.
> Marlize (LP-2013; 1): And what happens at the meetings?
> Walter (LP-2013; 1): At the meetings is where they solve issues which is not good in the sense that they have to fix their certain village.

Whereas Figs. 4.9 and 4.10 indicate instances where social support for wellbeing implies receiving social support via traditional governance structures, Figs. 4.11, 4.12, 4.13, 4.14,

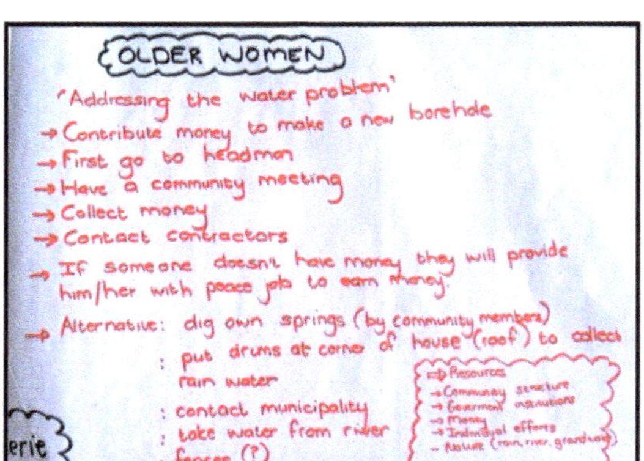

Fig. 4.11 Group analysis, Limpopo Province, June, 2012

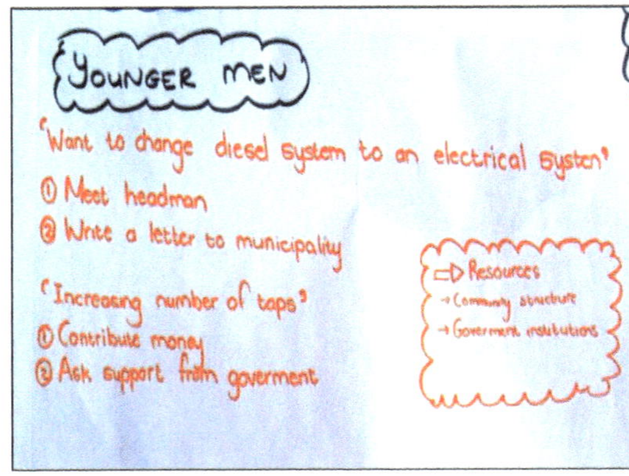

Fig. 4.12 Group analysis, Limpopo Province, June, 2012

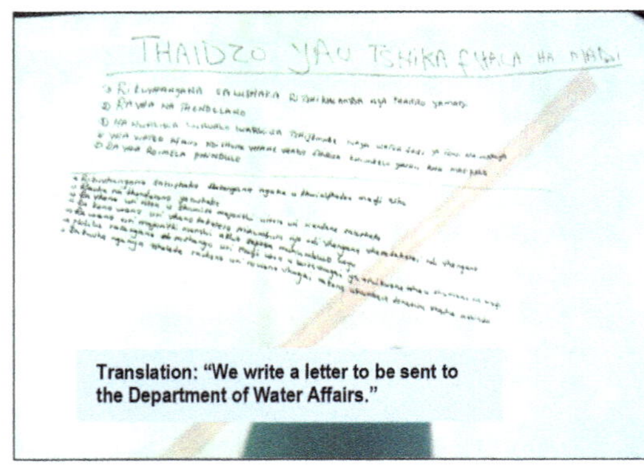

Fig. 4.13 Older men, Limpopo Province, June, 2012

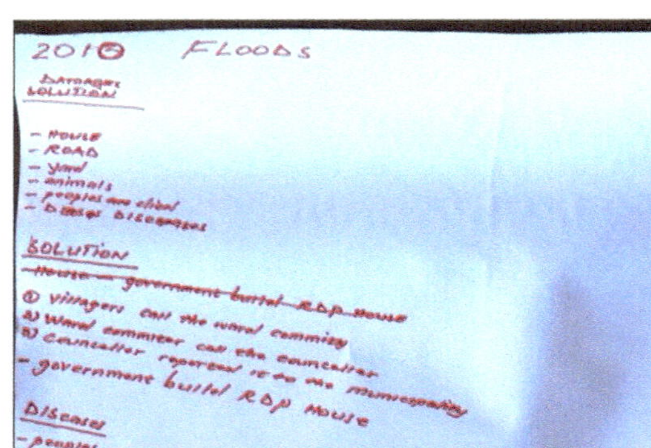

Fig. 4.14 Younger men, Limpopo Province, June, 2012

4.15, and 4.16 show examples of dependence on support from government structures for wellbeing.

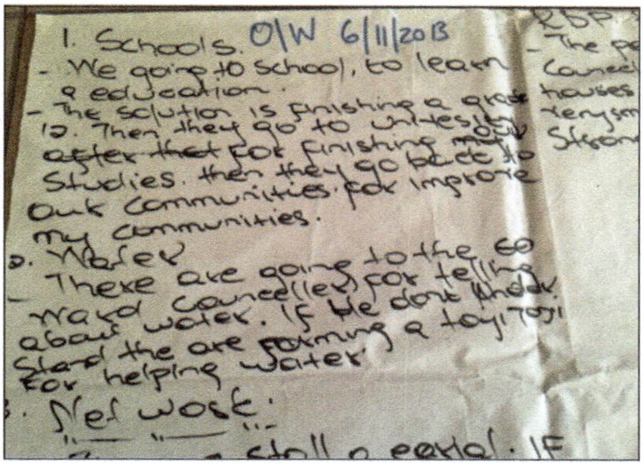

Fig. 4.15 Older women, Mpumalanga, November, 2013

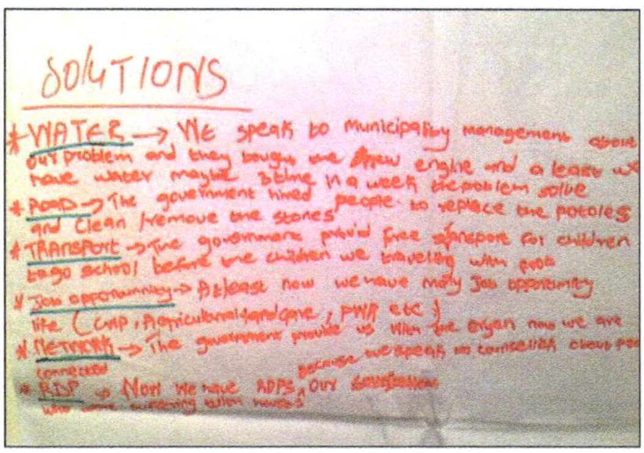

Fig. 4.16 Younger women, Mpumalanga, November, 2013

4.9 Valuing Socio-cultural Identity and Wellbeing

Valuing and conforming to dominant socio-cultural norms was significant for social connectedness as indigenous pathway to wellbeing. Valuing socio-cultural identity is significant for social engagement and refers to feeling a sense of belonging in one's community, as well as experiencing and maintaining harmony in the community (Fozdar and Torezani, 2008a,b; Keyes, 1998; King et al., 2009; Pflug, 2009; Sotgiu et al., 2011). As part of a social connectedness pathway to wellbeing, valuing a socio-cultural identity was indicated as significant by all participants irrespective of age, gender, ethnicity or region.

Participants expressed that they experienced wellbeing when their lives conform to socio-cultural norms. In the following three excerpts, participants explain how wellbeing is possible when people conform to values transferred by elders – including values such as honesty, trust and forgiveness, reducing conflict. The first excerpt is a discussion by younger men in Mpumalanga (MP-2012, Lines 202–205), the second is based on a member-checking discussion in the Limpopo site (LP-2012, Lines 555–562), and the third is an excerpt of older women in Mpumalanga (MP-2012, Lines 630–636):

James (MP-2012; 3): When someone is also respectful and honest then such a person is a good person.
James (MP-2012; 3): When the person greets people, and asks them how they are feeling, say hello. Honest people do not gossip, they say the truth.
Marlize (MP-2014; MC): Why does it make you happy when people have good manners and they have good dignity?
Musi (MP-2014; MC): I think it is important because it shows respect.
Marlize (MP-2014; MC): OK, ja it shows respect and respect is important in your community?
Musi (MP-2014; MC): Yes.
Janna (MP-2012; 4): Caring, loving, honest.
Suzie (MP-2012; 4): A good neighbour.
Janna (MP-2012; 4): A good neighbour.
Suzie (MP-2012; 4): No gossiping.

Acknowledging cultural identity, together with the transfer of socio-cultural knowledge provided opportunities for positive wellbeing experiences. The following member-checking conversations depict how participants denote wellbeing with acknowledging culture (MP-2014, Lines 406–440):

Janna (MP-2014; MC): OK, then you guys told us that you really want to share your culture and you want to teach your culture also, and when you do that then you're happy.
ALL (MP-2014; MC): Yes.
Janna (MP-2014; MC): Tell me, is it sharing your culture only with people from outside or is it also sharing your culture with the little children and other people living in the village?
Obie (MP-2014; MC): Everyone.
Janna (MP-2014; MC): Everyone?
ALL (MP-2014; MC): Yes.

Janna (MP-2014; MC): And why is it important for you to share and teach your culture? Why do you want people to know about Siswati?

Obie (MP-2014; MC): Like most of the time, some white people, when it's come to kill a cow, they use a gun. And us we not use a gun, we use a knife. So like it's very important to know the different culture.

Janna (MP-2014; MC): OK.

Vuyo (MP-2014; MC): We are experiencing a lot of things you know, from culture, from teaching each other. And sometimes I can get... maybe I will have fun with that culture. So, maybe I can teach this guy from... I can teach my culture.

Obie (MP-2014; MC): Especially when it comes to dance, I like to dance. Most of them, the cultures, when it comes to Sunday...

Vuyo (MP-2014; MC): Yo! I love it!

Janna (MP-2014; MC): You said that for you, it's very important to know the history of your community and to know the history of your culture.

ALL (MP-2014; MC): Yes.

Janna (MP-2014; MC): Why do you want to know the history of your village and your culture?

Musi (MP-2014; MC): I think it is important to know our history because it is important that we must know where we are coming from, so that we can tell the next generation about our history.

Vuyo (MP-2014; MC): Like sometimes in our, maybe I've got a dream of becoming an author. Even I can write about my community, the history of my community.

4.10 Discussion

We found similarities between social connectedness and existing knowledge on wellbeing from a western perspective, in particular with regards to eudaimonic wellbeing as positive social and psychological wellbeing. In addition, as pathway to resilience with positive wellbeing outcomes, social connectedness also reflects existing knowledge from other non-Western studies. Like others (Cox, 2012; Delle-Fave et al., 2011; Sotgiu et al., 2011), our findings suggest certain universal pathways to resilience with positive wellbeing outcomes regardless of worldview.

Our findings suggest that social connectedness enables eudaimonic wellbeing. Further study may be necessary to intentionally explore if the positive wellbeing outcomes indicated in this study align with languishing or flourishing (Keyes, 2007). However, the social connectedness pathway to resilience does appear to reflect positive social functioning, positive psychological functioning, as well as positive emotions (Keyes, 2007; Keyes, Shmotkin, & Ryff, 2002; Ryff et al., 2003) – the latter of which is disseminated elsewhere (De Gouveia, 2015).

From our findings it appears that social connectedness enables positive social functioning (Keyes, 1998). Social connectedness affords opportunities for social integration and social acceptance by avowing shared values of a cultural identity for particular protocols of giving and receiving support. Social connectedness links with opportunities for social contribution – to give and receive social support. Social coherence is possible via social connectedness in as much as people are able to belong to a collective that identity in similar cultural ways and for whom expectations of supportive behaviour are similar. Social actualisation is possible within a social connectedness pathway as people can live in accordance with shared cultural identities and buffer each other against shared adversities in ways that are familiar to them.

Our findings suggest that positive wellbeing outcomes (Ryff & Singer, 2006) are possible only when there are positive relations with others within a socially connected network. In addition, such social connectedness provides purpose in life as people are able to provide and receive social support – as scripted in their cultural identity. Social connectedness – and associated social support – also enables them to resile and reflect environmental mastery. Social connectedness also affirms self-acceptance of a cultural identity of collectivism. Individual autonomy is not an aspiration that aligns with an Afrocentric cultural identity. However, collective autonomy is strengthened to respond to collective need and solicit support.

In terms of self-determination theory (Ryan & Deci, 2001), self-actualisation and a fully functioning life appear to be enabled by the relatedness implied by social connectedness enabling social support and affirming cultural identity as a collective phenomenon.

Our findings also differed from the body of existing Western wellbeing knowledge. Western literature on wellbeing suggests that individuals need to live independent, metaphysically separate lives to experience wellbeing (Markus & Kitayama, 1994, 1998). However, in this study, participants reported that it was their interdependence that made them happy. Opportunities to live in ways that demonstrate their interdependence, how they exist in relation to other people in their life-worlds, denoted opportunities to experience positive wellbeing.

Our findings also differ with existing knowledge on wellbeing from a Western worldview regarding the emphasis placed on the value of distinctive internal traits, values and emotions in achieving happiness. Western approaches to wellbeing (Singelis, 1994) highlight the experience of autonomy and differentiation from others as ways of achieving wellbeing. Western psychology's focus on realising one's own goals in order to be happy is related to the idea of autonomy and differentiation. However, participants in this study reported that the welfare and priorities of their community took precedence over their own needs and desires.

Similarities with non-Western wellbeing knowledge are: existence in relation to the community, the role of cultural identity, social connectedness, and social mutuality. Certain non-western pathways to wellbeing were especially evident in this study, namely existence in relation to the community and the role of cultural identity in wellbeing. Non-Western wellbeing literature suggests that individuals should not be regarded as being distinct from or isolated from their community or environment (Constantine et al., 2004; Ingersoll-Dayton et al., 2004; Pflug, 2009). This view is confirmed by the current study as participants in this study reported that their happiness was integrally connected to the welfare of their community.

South African indigenous participants live in terms of relationships. Our findings align with current non-Western knowledge related to social wellbeing. Social connectedness (Constantine et al., 2004) and social mutuality (Ingersoll-Dayton et al., 2004) are related concepts that appear in the non-Western literature on wellbeing. The centrality of relationships for wellbeing experiences is similarly evident in literature on the wellbeing perspectives adopted in African American contexts (Constantine & Sue, 2006; Constantine et al., 2004), as well as Hispanic (Constantine et al., 2004), South African (Cocks & Møller, 2002), Turkish (Gergen, Gulerce, Lock, & Misra, 1996), Indian (Gergen et al., 1996), New Zealand (Gergen et al., 1996), Japanese (Kitayama et al., 2000), Thai (Ingersoll-Dayton et al., 2004), Chinese (Lu & Gilmour, 2006; Shu & Zhu, 2009) and native Australian (Pflug, 2009) contexts.

Like knowledge on wellbeing from Korean (Uchida et al., 2004), Aboriginal (Malin & Maidment, 2003) and Native Hawaiian (McCubbin, 2007) cultural contexts, the South African sample also emphasises the importance of living in accordance with cultural values and cultural heritage for happiness.

As is the case in other studies on wellbeing from a non-western stance, we found that South African people with indigenous roots find wellbeing by rallying together to make use of a variety of resources help individuals to take care of themselves and others (Cohen, Gottlieb, & Underwood, 2000; Cohen, Mermelstein, Kamarck, & Hoberman, 1985; Constantine et al., 2004; Ebersöhn, 2014; Ebersöhn et al., 2014; Ellis, 2007; Farid & Lazarus, 2008; Ingersoll-Dayton et al., 2004; Siu & Phillips, 2002; Stewart, Ware, Sherbourne, & Weels, 1992; Suh & Oishi, 2002; Yip et al., 2007). Access to social resources via social support through one's relationships enhances wellbeing because it provides individuals with a network of resources which can be used to cope with adversity (Cox, 2012; Ingersoll-Dayton et al., 2004; Markus & Kitayama, 1994, 1998). Such access can also buffer stressful events (Berkman & Glass, 2000; Khumalo et al., 2012; Malin & Maidment, 2003; Yip et al., 2007).

The role of cultural identity is highlighted in non-Western studies of wellbeing, as well as in the current study. According to the literature, cultural identity is seen to affect, inform and filter through each facet of an individual's life (King et al., 2009). Likewise, in this study, participants reported that the ways in which they acknowledged and identified with their cultural heritage played an important role in how happy they were. For participants with indigenous, South African heritage wellbeing thus also denotes staying true to the modes of behaviour, values and attitudes specific to one's cultural and historical heritage enhances wellbeing (Constantine & Sue, 2006; Diener et al., 2000; McCubbin, 2007; Oishi, 2000). Participating in activities, rituals and traditions specific to one's own culture fosters a sense of cultural inclusion that may lessen the negative impact of stress through the development of a strong sense of cultural identity, support and association with members of one's own cultural community (Bruchac & Caduto, 1991; Constantine et al., 2004; Constantino, Malgady, & Rogler, 1986; Hamilton, 1985).

Both western characteristics (social integration) and non-western characteristics (mutuality in relationships for social support and valuing socio-cultural identity) of social connectedness were evident in this study. Social connectedness may plausibly be viewed as a **universal characteristic of wellbeing** – irrespective of worldview.

4.11 Conclusion

Despite findings that most South Africans do not report overall quality of life (Moller, 2013; Moller & Dickow, 2002) we found that social connectedness is resilience-enabling to bolster unpredicted wellbeing outcomes. This study shows that social connectedness appears to make people happy – regardless of worldview. The way in which this universal inclination for social connectedness as pathway to wellbeing is manifested amongst some indigenous South Africans echoes pathways of others with dominant non-western views. In particular, South Africans with an indigenous heritage leverage social connectedness in relationships where there is reciprocity and where their valuing of socio-cultural identity can be demonstrated in social engagement. In times of hardship the social connectedness is leveraged to flock together for social support.

Concepts related to social connectedness can be used as indicators of wellbeing during psychological assessment. Similarly, these concepts could inform decisions regarding relevant intervention strategies to enable individuals to mobilise social support during trying times. Health professionals providing services to clients with indigenous-dominant worldviews may benefit from appropriating an indigenous psychology lens in order to reflect on their knowledge and practice.

We gained these insights into indigenous pathways to resilience with positive wellbeing outcomes from co-generating Participatory Reflection and Action data in two South African communities characterised by severe challenges. These insights contribute empirical evidence of South African cultural and contextual views on wellbeing to psychology discourses at large, and to a growing body of indigenous psychology knowledge in South Africa in particular.

References

Abrams, L. (2010). Sampling 'hard to reach' populations in qualitative research: The case of incarcerated youth. *Qualitative Social Work, 9*(4), 536–550.

Aitken, M., Rangan, H., & Kull, C. A. (2009). Living with alien invasives. The political ecology of wattle in the eastern highveld Mpumalanga, South Africa. *Etudes Océan Indien, 42–43*, 115–141.

Allwood, C. M., & Berry, J. W. (2006). Origins and development of indigenous psychologies: An international analysis. *International Journal of Psychology, 41*(4), 243–268.

Angrosino, M. V., & Mays de Perez, K. A. (2000). Rethinking observation: From method to context. In N. K. Denzin & Y. S. Lincoln (Eds.), *Handbook of qualitative research* (2nd ed., pp. 673–702). Thousand Oaks: Sage.

Arku, F. (2010). Time savings from easy access to clean water: Implications for rural men's and women's well-being. *Progress in Development Studies, 10*(3), 233–246.

Babbie, E., & Mouton, J. (2001). *The practice of social research*. Cape Town, South Africa: Oxford University Press.

Belgrave, F. Z., Cherry, V. R., Cunningham, D., Walwyn, S., Letdaka-Rennert, K., & Phillips, F. (1994). The influence of Africentric values, self-esteem, and black identity on drug attitudes among African American fifth graders: A preliminary study. *Journal of Black Psychology, 20*(2), 143–156.

Berkman, L. F., & Glass, T. (2000). Social integration, social networks, social support, and health. *Social Epidemiology, 1*, 137–173.

Boyden, J., & Mann, G. (2005). Children's risk, resilience, and coping in extreme situations. In M. Ungar (Ed.), *Handbook for working with children and youth: Pathways to resilience across cultures and contexts* (pp. 26–48). Canada: Sage, Dalhousie University.

Braun, V., & Clarke, V. (2006). Using thematic analysis in psychology. *Qualitative Research in Psychology, 3*(2), 77–101.

Brooks, D., & Abney, K. (2013). Perceptions of Malaria in Limpopo Province, South Africa.

Bruchac, J., & Caduto, M. (1991). *Native American stories*. Golden, CO: Fulcrum.

Caldwell, C. H., Kohn-Wood, L. P., Schmeelk-Cone, K. H., Chavous, T. M., & Zimmerman, M. A. (2004). Racial discrimination and racial identity as risk or protective factors for violent behaviors in African American young adults. *American Journal of Community Psychology, 33*(1–2), 91–105.

Carr, D., & Friedman, M. A. (2005). Is obesity stigmatizing? Body weight, perceived discrimination, and psychological well-being in the United States. *Journal of Health and Social Behavior, 46*(3), 244–259.

Census Suvery. (2011). *Census 2011 statistical release*. Pretoria, South Africa: Statistics South Africa.

Chambers, R. (2013). From rapid to reflective: 25 years of participatory learning and action. In H. Ashley, N. Kenton, & A. Milligan (Eds.), *Tools for supporting sustainable natural resource management and livelihoods, IIED, Sussex* (pp. 14–164).

Chilisa, B. (2012). *Indigenous research methodologies*. London, UK: Sage.

Christopher, J. C. (1999). Situating psychological well-being: Exploring the cultural roots of its theory and research. *Journal of Counseling and Development, 77*, 141–152.

Chun C, Moos RH, Cronkite RC (2006) Culture: A fundamental context for the stress and coping paradigm. Wong PTP, Wong LCJ Handbook of multicultural perspectives on stress and coping. New York, NY: Springer.

Cocks, M., & Møller, V. (2002). Use of indigenous and indigenised medicines to enhance personal well-being: A South African case study. *Social Science & Medicine, 54*(3), 387–397.

Cohen, L., Manion, L. & Morrison, K. (2007). *Research methods in education* (6th ed.). New York, NY: Routledge.

Cohen, S., Mermelstein, R., Kamarck, T., & Hoberman, H. M. (1985). Measuring the functional components of social support. In I. G. Sarason & B. R. Sarason (Eds.), *Social support: Theory, research and applications*. The Hague, Netherlands: Martinus Nijhoff.

Cohen, S., Gottlieb, B. H., & Underwood, L. G. (2000). Social relationships and health. In S. Cohen, L. G. Underwood, & B. H. Gottlieb (Eds.), *Social support measurement and intervention*. New York, NY: Oxford University Press.

Constantine, M. G., & Sue, D. W. (2006). Factors contributing to optimal human functioning in people of color in the United States. *The Counseling Psychologist, 34*(2), 228–244.

Constantine, M. G., Myers, L. J., Kindaichi, M., & Moore, J. L. (2004). Exploring non-traditional methods of mental health treatment: The roles of indigenous healers and helpers in promoting psychological, physical, and spiritual well-being in people of color. *Counseling and Values, 48*, 110–125.

Constantino, G., Malgady, R. G., & Rogler, L. H. (1986). Cuento therapy: A culturally sensitive modality for Puerto Rican children. *Journal of Counselling and Clinical Psychology, 54*, 639–645.

Cox, K. (2012). Happiness and unhappiness in the developing world: Life satisfaction among sex workers, dump-dwellers, urban poor, and rural peasants in Nicaragua. *Journal of Happiness Studies, 13*(1), 103–128.

Crocker, J., Luhtanen, R., Blaine, B., & Broadnax, S. (1994). Collective self-esteem and psychological well-being among White, Black, and Asian college students. *Personality and Social Psychology Bulletin, 20*(5), 503–513.

De Gouveia, J. M. (2015). Indigenous pathways to well-being as resilience outcome in rural communities. Dissertation, University of Pretoria.

De la Rey, C., & Ipser, J. (2004). The call for relevance: South African psychology ten years into democracy. *South Africa Journal of Psychology, 34*, 544–557.

Deci, E. L. (1976). Notes on the theory and metatheory of intrinsic motivation. *Organizational Behavior and Human Performance, 15*(1), 130–145.

Deci, E. L., & Ryan, R. M. (2000). The "what" and "why" of goal pursuits: Human needs and the self-determination of behavior. *Psychological Inquiry, 11*(4), 227–268.

Deci, E. L., Ryan, R. M., Gagné, M., Leone, D. R., Usunov, J., & Kornazheva, B. P. (2001). Need satisfaction, motivation, and well-being in the work organizations of a former eastern bloc country: A cross-cultural study of self-determination. *Personality and Social Psychology Bulletin, 27*(8), 930–942.

Delle-Fave, A., Brdar, I., Freire, T., Vella-Brodrick, D., & Wissing, M. P. (2011). The eudaimonic and hedonic components of happiness: Qualitative and quantitative findings. *Social Indicators Research, 100*(2), 185–207.

Diener, E. (1984). Subjective well-being. *Psychological Bulletin, 95*(3), 542–575.

Diener, E., Gohm, C. L., Suh, E., & Oishi, S. (2000). Similarity of the relations between marital status and subjective well-being across cultures. *Journal of Cross-Cultural Psychology, 31*(4), 419–436.

Diener, E., Oishi, S., & Lucas, R. E. (2003). Personality, culture, and subjective well-being: Emotional and cognitive evaluations of life. *Annual Review of Psychology, 54*, 403–425.

Dolan, P., Peasgood, T., & White, T. (2008). Do we really know what makes us happy? A review of the economic literature on the factors associated with subjective well-being. *Journal of Economic Psychology, 29*(1), 94–122.

Ebersöhn, L. (2007). Voicing perceptions of risk and protective factors in coping in a HIV & AIDS landscape: Reflecting on capacity for adaptiveness. *Gifted Education International, 23*(2), 149–159.

Ebersöhn, L. (2012). Adding 'flock' to 'fight and flight': A honeycomb of resilience where supply of relationships meets demand for support. *Journal of Psychology in Africa, 22*(1), 29–42.

Ebersöhn, L. (2013). Building generative theory from case work: The relationship-resourced resilience model. In M. P. Wissing (Ed.), *Well-being research in South Africa: Cross-cultural advancements in positive psychology*. Dordrecht, Netherlands: Springer.

Ebersöhn, L. (2014). Teacher resilience: Theorizing resilience and poverty. *Teachers and Teaching, 20*(5), 568–594.

Ebersöhn, L., Sefotho, M., Mampane, R., Loots, T., Omidire, F., Sherman, V., Nxumalo-Tsebe, T. (2014). Imbeleko report: Cultivating resourcefulness, not dependency. Retrieved from http://www.bettercarenetwork.org/sites/default/files/Imbeleko%20Report%20-%20Cultivating%20Resourcefulness,%20Not%20Dependency.pdf.

Ellis, F. (2007). Household strategies and rural livelihood diversification. *The Journal of Development Studies, 35*(1), 1–38.

Evenden, M., & Sandstrom, G. (2011). Calling for scientific revolution in psychology: KK Hwang on indigenous psychologies. *Social Epistemology, 25*(2), 153–166.

Farid, M., & Lazarus, H. (2008). Subjective well-being in rich and poor countries. *Journal of Management Development, 27*(10), 1053–1065.

Ford, T., Goodman, R., & Meltzer, H. (2003). The British child and adolescent mental health survey 1999: The prevalence of DSM-IV disorders. *Journal of the American Academy of Child & Adolescent Psychiatry, 42*(10), 1203–1211.

Fozdar, F., & Torezani, S. (2008a). *Discrimination and well-being: Perceptions of refugees in Western Australia*. New York, NY: Center for Migration Studies of New York.

Fozdar, F., & Torezani, S. (2008b). Discrimination and well-being: Perceptions of refugees in Western Australia. *International Migration Review, 42*(1), 30–63.

Georgas, J., & Mylonas, K. (2006). Cultures are like all other cultures, like some other cultures, like no other culture. In *Indigenous and cultural psychology* (pp. 197–221). Boston, MA: Springer.

Gergen, K. J., Gulerce, A., Lock, A., & Misra, G. (1996). Psychological science in cultural context. *American Psychologist, 51*(5), 496–503.

Goduka, N. (2012). From positivism to indigenous science: A reflection on world views, paradigms and philosophical assumptions. *Africa Insight, 41*(4), 123–138.

Hamilton, V. (1985). *The people could fly: American Black folktales*. New York, NY: Knopf Books for Young Readers.

Hammer, T. (2003). *Youth unemployment and social exclusion in Europe: A comparative study*. Bristol, UK: Policy Press.

Highlen, P. (1996). MCT theory and implications for organizations/systems. In D. W. Sue, A. E. Ivey, & P. B. Pedersen (Eds.), *A theory of multicultural counselling and therapy*. Pacific Grove, CA: Brooks/Cole.

Houkamau, C. A., & Sibley, C. G. (2011). Māori cultural efficacy and subjective well-being: A psychological model and research agenda. *Social Indicators Research, 103*, 379–398.

Huppert, F. A., & So, T. T. (2013). Flourishing across Europe: Application of a new conceptual framework for defining well-being. *Social Indicators Research, 110*(3), 837–861.

Hutnik, N. (1991). *Ethnic minority identity: A social psychological perspective*. New York, NY: Clarendon Press.

Hwang, K. K. (2004). The epistemological goal of indigenous psychology: The perspective of constructive realism. In B. N. Setiadi, A. Supratiknya, W. J. Lonner, & Y. H. Poortinga (Eds.), *Ongoing themes in psychology and culture* (online ed.). Melbourne, FL: International Association for Cross-Cultural Psychology.

Ingersoll-Dayton, B., Saengtienchai, C., Kespichayawattana, J., & Aungsuroch, Y. (2004). Psychological well-being Asian style: The perspective of Thai elders. *Journal of Cross-Cultural Gerontology, 16*, 283–302.

Keyes, C. L. M. (1998). Social well-being. *Social Psychology Quarterly, 61*, 121–140.

Keyes, C. L. M. (2007). Promoting and protecting mental health as flourishing. A complementary strategy for improving national mental health. *American Psychologist, 62*(2), 95–108.

Keyes, C. L., Shmotkin, D., & Ryff, C. D. (2002). Optimizing well-being: The empirical encounter of two traditions. *Journal of Personality and Social Psychology, 82*(6), 1007.

Khumalo, I. P., Temane, Q. M., & Wissing, M. P. (2012). Socio-demographic variables, general psychological well-being and the mental health continuum in an African context. *Social Indicators Research, 105*(3), 419–442.

King, M., Smith, A., & Gracey, M. (2009). Indigenous health part 2: The underlying causes of the health gap. *Lancet, 374*, 76–85.

Kitayama, S., Markus, H. R., & Kurokawa, M. (2000). Culture, emotion, and well-being: Good feelings in Japan and the United States. *Cognition & Emotion, 14*(1), 93–124.

Krippner, S. (2000). The epistemology and technologies of shamanic states of consciousness. *Journal of Consciousness Studies, 7*, 93–118.

Lee, C. M. (2003). Cross-cultural communication theories. In W. B. Gudykunst (Ed.), *Cross-cultural and intercultural communication* (Vol. 5, pp. 7–33). Thousand Oaks: Sage.

Lee, C. C., Oh, M. Y., & Mountcastle, A. R. (1992). Indigenous models of helping in nonwestern countries: Implications for multicultural counselling. *Journal of Multicultural Counseling and Development, 20*(1), 3–10.

Letseka, M. (2013). Education for Ubuntu/Botho: Lessons from Basotho indigenous education. *Open Journal of Philosophy, 3*(2), 337–344.

Lu, L., & Gilmour, R. (2006). Individual-oriented and socially oriented cultural conceptions of subjective well-being: Conceptual analysis and scale development. *Asian Journal of Social Psychology, 9*, 36–49.

Lyubomirsky, S., King, L., & Diener, E. (2005). The benefits of frequent positive affect: Does happiness lead to success? *Psychological Bulletin, 131*(6), 803.

MacLeod, M. L. P. (2004). *The nature of nursing practice in rural and remote Canada*. Ottawa, Canada: Canadian Health Services Research Foundation.

Malin, M., & Maidment, D. (2003). Education, indigenous survival and well-being: Emerging ideas and programs. *The Australian Journal of Indigenous Education, 32*, 85–100.

Maree, K., Ebersöhn, L., & Molepo, M. (2006). Administering narrative career counselling in a diverse setting: Trimming the sails to the wind. *South African Journal of Education, 26*(1), 49–60.

Markus, H., & Kitayama, S. (1994). The cultural construction of self and emotion: Implications for social behavior. In S. Kitayama & H. Markus (Eds.), *Emotion and culture*. Washington, DC: American Psychological Association.

Markus, H. R., & Kitayama, S. (1998). The cultural psychology of personality. *Journal of Cross-Cultural Psychology, 29*, 63–87.

Masten, A. S. (1989). Resilience in development: Implications of the study of successful adaptation for developmental psychopathology. In D. Cicchetti (Ed.), *Rochester symposium on developmental psychopathology* (Vol. 1, pp. 261–294). Rochester: The emergence of a discipline, Lawrence Erlbaum Associates.

Masten, A. S. (2001). Ordinary magic. Resilience processes in development. *American Psychologist, 56*(1), 227–238.

Matoane, M. (2012). Locating context in counselling: The development of indigenous psychology in South Africa. *Psychotherapy and Politics International, 10*(2), 105–115.

McCubbin, L. L. D. (2007). The role of indigenous family ethnic schema on well-being among Native Hawaiian families. *Contemporary Nurse, 23*(2), 170–180.

Metz, T., & Gaie, J. B. R. (2010). The African ethic of Ubuntu/Botho: Implications for research on morality. *Journal of Moral Education, 39*(3), 273–290.

Moller, V. (2013). South African quality of life trends over three decades, 1980–2010. *Social Indicators Research, 113*(3), 915–940.

Moller, V., & Dickow, H. (2002). The role of quality of life surveys in managing change in democratic transitions: The South African case. *Social Indicators Research, 58*, 1–3.

Morita, S. (1998). *Morita therapy and the true nature of anxiety-based disorders (shinkeishitsu)*. Albany, NY: State University of New York.

Mpofu, E. (2002). Indigenization of the psychology of human intelligence in sub-Saharan Africa. In W. Lorner, D. L. Dinnel, S. A. Hayes, & D. N. Sattler (Eds.), *Online readings in psychology and culture*. Washington: Centre for Cross-Cultural Research Western Washington University. Unit 5, Chapter 2.

Neff, D. F. (2007). Subjective well-being, poverty and ethnicity in South Africa: Insights from an exploratory analysis. *Social Indicators Research, 80*, 313–341.

Neville, H. A., & Lilly, R. L. (2000). The relationship between racial identity cluster profiles and psychological distress among African American college students. *Journal of Multicultural Counseling and Development, 28*, 194–207.

Odora Hoppers, C. A. (2008). In the service of humanity: Mapping an agenda for development education. Keynote address at the official launch of the UNISA South African Research Chair in Developmental Education, May, 8.

Oishi, S. (2000). Goals as cornerstones of subjective well-being: Linking individuals and cultures. In E. Diener & E. M. Suh (Eds.), *Culture and subjective well-being*. Cambridge, MA: The MIT Press.

Orb, A., Eisenhauer, L., & Wynaden, D. (2001). Ethics in qualitative research. *Journal of Nursing Scholarship, 33*(1), 93–96.

Pandey, S. (2011). Positive psychology: Blending strengths of western, eastern and other indigenous psychologies. In *1st international conference on "Emerging Paradigms in Business & Social Sciences" (EPBSS-2011), organized by Middlesex University, Dubai*.

Pflug, J. (2009). Folk theories of happiness: A cross-cultural comparison of conceptions of happiness in Germany and South Africa. *Social Indicators Research, 92*, 551–563.

Queener, J. E., & Martin, J. K. (2001). Providing culturally relevant mental health services: Collaboration between psychology and the African American church. *Journal of Black Psychology, 27*, 112–122.

Ramose, M. B. (2002). The philosophy of Ubuntu and Ubuntu as philosophy. In P. H. Coetzee & A. J. P. Roux (Eds.), *Philosophy from Africa: A text with readings*. London, UK: Routledge.

Rice, T. W., & Steele, B. J. (2004). Subjective well-being and culture across time and space. *Journal of Cross-Cultural Psychology, 35*(6), 633–647.

Rietveld, L. C., Haarhoff, J., & Jagals, P. (2009). A tool for technical assessment of rural water supply systems in South Africa. *Physics and Chemistry of the Earth, Parts A/B/C, 34*(1), 43–49.

Ryan, R. M., & Deci, E. L. (2001). On happiness and human potentials: A review of research on hedonic and eudaimonic well-being. *Annual Review of Psychology, 52*(1), 141–166.

Ryff, C. D. (1989). Happiness is everything, or is it? Explorations on the meaning of psychological well-being. *Journal of Personality and Social Psychology, 57*, 1069–1081.

Ryff, C. D. (1995). Psychological Well-being in adult life. *Current Directions in Psychological Science, 4*(4), 99–104.

Ryff, C. D., & Keyes, C. L. M. (1995). The structure of psychological well-being revisited. *Journal of Personality and Social Psychology, 69*, 719–727.

Ryff, C. D., & Singer, B. H. (1998). The contours of positive human health. *Psychological Inquiry, 9*, 1–28.

Ryff, C. D., & Singer, B. H. (2000). Interpersonal flourishing: A positive health agenda for the new millennium. *Personality and Social Psychology Review, 4*(1), 30–44.

Ryff, C. D., & Singer, B. H. (2006). Best news yet on the six-factor model of well-being. *Social Science Research, 35*, 1103–1119.

Ryff, C. D., Keyes, C. L., & Hughes, D. L. (2003). Status inequalities, perceived discrimination, and eudaimonic well-being: Do the challenges of minority life hone purpose and growth? *Journal of Health and Social Behavior, 44*(3), 275–291.

Seale, C. (1999). Quality in qualitative research. *Qualitative Inquiry, 5*(4), 465–478.

Seligman, M. (2002). *Authentic happiness: Using the new positive psychology to realize your potential for lasting fulfillment*. New York, NY: Free Press.

Shu, X., & Zhu, Y. (2009). The quality of life in China. *Social Indicators Research, 92*(2), 191–225.

Singelis, T. M. (1994). The measurement of independent and interdependent self-construals. *Personality and Social Psychology Bulletin, 20*, 580–591.

Singh, A. N. (1999). Shamans, healing, and mental health. *Journal of Child and Family Studies, 8*, 131–134.

Siu, O. L., & Phillips, D. R. (2002). A study of family support, friendship, and psychological well-being among older women in Hong Kong. *The International Journal of Aging and Human Development, 55*(4), 299–319.

Skinner, E. A., & Zimmer-Gembeck, M. J. (2007). The development of coping. *Annual Review of Psychology, 58*, 119–144.

Slunecko, T., & Hengl, S. (2006). Culture and media: A dynamic constitution. *Culture & Psychology, 12*(1), 69–85.

Sokoya, G. O., Muthukrishna, N., & Collings, S. J. (2005). Afrocentric and gendered constructions of psychological well-being in Nigeria: A case study. *Journal of Psychology in Africa, 15*(1), 31–40.

Sotgiu, I., Galati, D., Manzano, M., & Rognoni, E. (2011). Happiness components and their attainment in old age: A cross-cultural comparison between Italy and Cuba. *Journal of Happiness Studies, 12*, 353–371.

Spencer, M. B., Harpalani, V., Cassidy, E., Jacobs, C. Y., Donde, S., Goss, T. N., … Wilson, S. (2006). Understanding vulnerability and resilience from a normative developmental perspective: Implications for racially and ethnically diverse youth. *Development and Psychopathology, 1*, 627–672.

Sroufe, L. A., & Rutter, M. (1984). The domain of developmental psychopathology. *Child Development, 55*, 17–29.

Stake RE (2013) Multiple case study analysis. New York, NY: Guilford Press.

Stewart, A. L., Ware, J. E. J., Sherbourne, C. D., & Wells, K. B. (1992). Psychological distress/well-being and cognitive functioning measures. In A. L. Stewart & J. E. Ware (Eds.), *Measuring functioning and well-being: The medical outcomes study approach*. Durham, NC: Duke University Press.

Strümpfer, D. J. W. (2013). Towards fortigenesis and fortology: An informed essay. In M. P. Wissing (Ed.), *Well-being research in South Africa*. New York, NY: Oxford University Press.

Sue, D. W., & Sue, D. (1999). *Counseling the culturally different* (3rd ed.). New York, NY: Wiley.

Suh, E. M. (2009). Self, the hyphen between culture and subjective well-being. In E. Diener & E. M. Suh (Eds.), *Culture and subjective well-being*. Cambridge, MA: MIT Press.

Suh, E. M., & Oishi, S. (2002). Subjective well-being across cultures. *Online Readings in Psychology and Culture, 10*(1), 1.

Thomas, A., Cairney, S., Gunthorpe, W., Paradies, Y., & Sayers, S. (2010). Strong souls: Development and validation of a culturally appropriate tool for assessment of social and emotional well-being in indigenous youth. *Australian and New Zealand Journal of Psychiatry, 44*(1), 40–48.

Tucker, V. (1999). The myth of development: A critique of a Eurocentric discourse. In R. Munck & D. O'Hearn (Eds.), *Critical development theory: Contributions to a new paradigm*. London, UK: Zed Books.

Uchida, Y., Norasakkunkit, V., & Kitayama, S. (2004). Cultural constructions of happiness: Theory and empirical evidence. *Journal of Happiness Studies, 5*, 223–239.

Ungar, M. (2004). A construction discourse on resilience: Multiple contexts, multiple realities among at-risk children and youth. *Youth and Society, 35*(3), 341–365.

Ungar, M. (Ed.). (2005). *Handbook for working with children and youth: Pathways to resilience across cultures and contexts*. Thousand Oaks, CA: Sage Publications.

Ungar, M. (2009). *Playing at being bad: The hidden resilience of troubled teens*. Toronto, Canada: McClelland & Stewart.

Ungar, M. (2012). Social ecologies and their contribution to resilience. In *The social ecology of resilience* (pp. 13–31). New York, NY: Springer.

Utsey, S. O., Ponterotto, J. G., Reynolds, A. L., & Cancelli, A. A. (2000). Racial discrimination, coping, life satisfaction, and self-esteem among African Americans. *Journal of Counseling & Development, 78*, 72–80.

Valsiner, J. (2007). Culture in minds and societies: Foundations of cultural psychology. *Psychological Studies, 54*, 238–239.

Van Zyl, L., & Rothman, S. (2012). Flourishing of students in a tertiary education institution in South Africa. *Journal of Psychology in Africa, 22*(4), 593–604.

Vorster, H. H., Wissing, M. P., Venter, C. S., Kruger, H. S., Kruger, A., Malan, N. T., & MacIntyre, U. (2000). The impact of urbanization on physical, physiological and mental health of Africans in the North West Province of South Africa: The THUSA study. *South African Journal of Science, 96*, 505–514.

Waghid, Y., & Smeyers, P. (2012). Reconsidering Ubuntu: On the educational potential of a particular ethic of care. *Educational Philosophy and Theory, Supplement, 2*(44), 6–20.

Wallace, B. A. (2001). Intersubjectivity in Indo-Tibetan Buddhism. In E. Thompson (Ed.), *Between ourselves: Second-person issues in the study of consciousness*. Thorveton, UK: Imprint Academic.

Wilson, J. W., & Constantine, M. G. (1999). Racial identity attitudes, self-concept, and perceived family cohesion in Black college students. *Journal of Black Studies, 29*, 354–366.

Wing, D. M. (1998). A comparison of traditional folk healing concepts with contemporary healing concepts. *Journal of Community Health Nursing, 15*, 143–154.

Yang, K. S. (2000). Monocultural and cross-cultural indigenous approaches: The royal road to the development of a balanced global psychology. *Asian Journal of Social Psychology, 3*(3), 241–263.

Yip, W., Subramanian, S. V., Mitchell, A. D., Lee, D. T., Wang, J., & Kawachi, I. (2007). Does social capital enhance health and well-being? Evidence from rural China. *Social Science & Medicine, 64*(1), 35–49.

Zimmerman, M. A., Israel, B. A., Schulz, A., & Checkoway, B. (1992). Further explorations in empowerment theory: An empirical analysis of psychological empowerment. *American Journal of Community Psychology, 20*(6), 7–727.

Adolescent Resilience in the Face of Relentless Adversity: The Role of Strong, Black Women

5

Linda C. Theron and Michael Ungar

Abstract
Apparently intractable adversity (such as structural disadvantage) undermines quality of life for many South Africans, more particularly Black South Africans. Even so, many Black young people are resilient in the face of such risk. Women are prominent in these young people's resilience accounts. To date, however, no study has considered whether/how the Strong Black Woman archetype is implicit in this prominence. The purpose of this chapter is to address the aforementioned gap. To do so, we draw on the Resilient Youth in Stressed Environments Study and report the cases of Thandiwe (a young woman) and Thulani (a young man). A deductive analysis of these critical cases suggests that the resilience of Black South African adolescents is intertwined with being cared for by strong Black women and reciprocating this care. In conclusion, we distil three lessons for stakeholders who are interested in promoting youth resilience.

5.1 Introduction

Harmful events (such as natural disasters, an experience of sexual violence, or armed conflict) and/or adverse circumstances (such as intergenerational poverty or a chronically dysfunctional family) predict negative human outcomes (including poor quality of life) (Rutter, 2013). In South Africa, the Quality of Life (QoL) Trends Study showed that QoL evades many South Africans (Møller, 2013). This trend is racialized and relates largely to adverse life circumstances that are rooted in the Apartheid-era's offensive policies that targeted Black South Africans. Even so, many Black South Africans manage to avoid the negative outcomes that are associated with harmful events and/or adverse circumstances. In their cases, resilience is inferred.

In short, in the face or aftermath of adversity, human resilience is a complex process that facilitates positive outcomes (such as psychological or physical wellbeing) (Masten, 2014). This process regularly draws on commonplace or unremarkable resources (such as caring relatives) or what Masten (2001, 2014) termed 'ordinary magic'. These ordinary resources appear to matter for QoL too. Updated commentaries on QoL have noted that 'small everyday acts' (Møller, 2018, p. 1016) and 'why and how individuals … use their resources and constraints' (Land & Michalos, 2018, p. 861) are important facets of QoL. They are, however, incompletely under-

L. C. Theron (✉)
University of Pretoria, Pretoria, South Africa
e-mail: linda.theron@up.ac.za

M. Ungar
Dalhousie University, Halifax, NS, Canada

I. Eloff (ed.), *Handbook of Quality of Life in African Societies*, International Handbooks of Quality-of-Life, https://doi.org/10.1007/978-3-030-15367-0_5

stood (Land & Michalos, 2018; Møller, 2018). In this chapter we adopt a social ecological approach to resilience and we focus on the resilience of older adolescents (i.e., young people aged 18–24; see Sawyer, Azzopardi, Wickremarathne, & Patton, 2018). In doing so we draw attention to various 'small everyday acts' (Møller, 2018, p. 1016) that enabled and strengthened adolescent resilience and to adolescents' own accounts of 'why and how' (Land & Michalos, 2018, p. 861) these mattered.

From a social ecological perspective, human resilience processes are co-facilitated by individuals (e.g., an adolescent) and stakeholders from the individual's social ecology (e.g., family members, peers, neighbors, service providers, professionals, clergy, policy makers) (Masten, 2014; Ungar, 2015a). To co-facilitate adolescent resilience, stakeholders typically need to supply resilience-supporting resources that adolescents consider valuable (e.g., caring relationships, quality education, or opportunities for employment) and ensure that adolescents have access to these resources. Adolescents co-facilitate their resilience when they appropriate whatever resilience-supporting resources were made available and/or when they advocate for the provision of meaningful supports that are not available or accessible to them (Ungar, 2011).

What counts as meaningful resilience-enabling resources is largely influenced by sociocultural, temporal, and/or contextual variables (Panter-Brick, 2015). In other words, even though specific resources (such as supportive relationships, quality education, enabling spiritual and/or cultural beliefs, or experiences of social justice – see Masten, 2014; Ungar, 2015b) recur across studies of adolescent resilience, it is probable that adolescents living in diverse contexts, or facing disparate risks or different levels of risk, will have differing opinions about the usefulness of a resource which is typically associated with resilience. For instance, a study with 730 rural, school-attending, Sesotho-speaking adolescents, who were challenged by structural disadvantage, showed that access to quality education was integral to the resilience process of these young people (Van Rensburg, Theron, & Rothmann, 2018). They valued education because it potentiated a pathway out of poverty. In comparison, the street-connected, non-school-attending South African adolescents who participated in the study by Hills, Meyer-Weitz, and Kwaku Oppong (2016) considered substances to be a valuable resource as these reduced their awareness of poverty and associated adversities. They did not include education in their explanations of what enabled resilience.

The above examples suggest that in order to optimally understand and promote adolescent resilience (and related outcomes such as QoL), it is important to pay attention to which resources appear to be more meaningful to specific groups of adolescents. In the first author's ongoing resilience-focused research with Black South African adolescents (who were vulnerable because of structural disadvantage), caring women emerged as a particularly meaningful resilience-enabling resource. These young people regularly ascribed their resilience to woman relatives, girl/woman peers, woman teachers, and/or woman service providers (Hall & Theron, 2016; Jefferis & Theron, 2017; Kumpulainen et al., 2016; Theron, 2007, 2013a, 2016, 2017; Theron & Engelbrecht, 2012; Theron & Phasha, 2015; Theron & Theron, 2013, 2014). Mothers are particularly salient in the aforementioned accounts. Most typically, the capacity of mothers and other women to care (practically and/or emotionally) for young people made a difference to the quality of life which these young people reported and was central to why and how these young people coped well with challenging lives. Other South African qualitative studies have also specifically reported that youth resilience is championed by women who facilitate access to resources, provide affective support, pass on cultural heritage, and/or support constructive meaning making (e.g., Casale, 2011; Malindi, 2014; Odendaal & Moletsane, 2011; Phasha, 2010; Zulu, 2018). Similarly, reviews of studies that have focused on the resilience of girls and/or women from South Africa and elsewhere have drawn attention to the resilience-enabling role of women (see Haffejee & Theron, 2017; Jefferis & Theron, 2018).

5.1.1 Purpose of the Chapter

Although men also matter for the resilience of adolescents, including the resilience of South African adolescents (Makusha, Richter, & Bhana, 2012; Theron, 2016), the salience of women as resilience champions invites closer scrutiny. Given that resilience is sensitive to sociocultural, temporal, and/or contextual variables (Panter-Brick, 2015; Ungar, 2011, 2012, 2018), it is possible that the salience of women in the resilience processes of Black South African adolescents reflects Black women's acceptance and enactment of gendered, sociocultural norms, such as that of the Strong Black Woman archetype (Parks, 2010). However, no previous resilience study has explored the intersection of the Strong Black Woman archetype and the salience of women in the resilience accounts of young people. Jefferis and Theron (2018) used stereotypical gender roles and the Strong Black Woman archetype to better understand the resilience of girls and women, but they did not extend this to explaining the prominent role of women in black South African youths' accounts of their resilience.

Accordingly, the purpose of this chapter is threefold. First, it summarizes the stereotypical gender roles that women are typically socialized to enact and explains the Strong Black Woman archetype. Second it introduces the case studies of Thandiwe (a young woman) and Thulane (a young man) and uses them to illustrate how women's facilitation of adolescent resilience reflects the Strong Black Woman archetype. Third, this chapter distils take-home lessons for stakeholders who wish to enable resilience (and related positive outcomes, such as QoL) among young people who are at-risk.

We selected the cases of Thandiwe and Thulani because the biological mothers of both these young people were dead (they had died when Thandiwe and Thulani were children). Given the emphasis on the role of biological mothers in the resilience of South African youth (e.g., Eloff et al., 2014; Malindi, 2014; Odendaal & Moletsane, 2011; Phasha, 2010; Theron, 2013a, 2016, 2017; Theron & Theron, 2013; Zulu, 2018), we were of the opinion that the cases of Thandiwe and Thulani – which do not focus on support from biological mothers – would be "critical" (Yin, 2014, p. 57) to an advanced understanding of the role of Black South African women in the resilience of youth. Yin (2014) argues that a single critical case (i.e., a case which can confirm or challenge current theoretical knowledge) is sufficient. We reported two cases in order to represent the experiences of both a young woman and young man.

5.2 Women's Gendered Roles and the Strong Black Woman Archetype

Gender encompasses the social dimensions of being a man, or woman, and intersects with class, race, ethnicity, cultural values, and other sociocultural determinants (Hammarström & Hensing, 2018). Even though many societies are increasingly questioning and/or purposefully discouraging stereotypical gender roles, conventionally women are still socialized to prioritize the needs of others, affiliate with others (e.g., be warm or show empathy), and downplay their personal emotions or needs (Brody et al., 2014; Jordan, 2013). These traditional roles mean that women are expected to be 'giving, loving, and loyal' (Godsil, Tropp, Goff, Powell, & MacFarlane, 2016, p. 13).

Although these stereotypical roles could potentiate negative outcomes for women (e.g., continuously prioritizing the needs of others over the self could prompt poor quality of life), they have also been associated with resilience. For example, Jordan (2000, 2006, 2008, 2013) proposed a relational-cultural theory that emphasized the capacity to connect with others (i.e., 'relational resilience', Jordan, 2006, p. 82), in culturally relevant ways, as central to how and why people (particularly girls and women) managed to adjust in the face, or aftermath, of adversity. Van Breda (2018) suggested the capacity to connect with others in caring ways was gendered. He based this conclusion on a comparison of the narratives of young men and young women leaving care. He reported that the resilience of the young women was distinguished by their capacity to embrace motherhood and/or assume responsibility for vulnerable others. Such caring was absent from the young men's accounts.

The Strong Black Woman archetype builds on the above mentioned gender roles. Essentially a black woman who is strong is 'resilient, self-contained, and self-sacrificing' (Donovan & West, 2015, p. 384). Women's enactment of these qualities means that the wellbeing and development of others is prioritized; regardless of the adversities that confront her, the woman is "giving, loving, and loyal' (Godsil et al., 2016, p. 13). In other words, the Strong Black Woman archetype values and advocates for women to embrace and embody 'strength and caretaking' (Watson & Hunter, 2016, p. 426). Although the Strong Black Woman archetype is associated with negative physical and mental health effects and has been criticized by feminists, many African-American women (who have historic and first-hand experiences of structural inequities, oppression, and associated adversities) have nevertheless enacted and espoused the archetype (Abrams, Maxwell, Pope, & Belgrave, 2014; Donovan & West, 2015; Watson-Singleton, 2017; Watson & Hunter, 2016).

Similarly, many Black South African women appear to have embraced the Strong Black Woman archetype (Casale, 2011; Ramphele, 2012; Theron, 2016). They had many role models. For example, Black South African women were principal actors in the long struggle against colonial and Apartheid oppression (Booysen & Nkomo, 2010). Also, given the absence of men in Black South African households (particularly in rural areas), Black South African women ensured that their households and communities continued to function and that children were raised well (Casale, Wild, Cluver, & Kuo, 2015). Men were typically absent because of economic migrancy, Apartheid laws which fragmented households, declining rates of marriage, and/or their inability to comply with traditional customs for gaining household access (such as paying 'lobola' [bride price]) (Richter, Chikovore, & Makusha, 2010). A recent study of childcare in South Africa showed that women (particularly Black women) are disproportionately responsible for childcare (physical and financial) (Hatch & Posel, 2018). In other words, despite South Africa's growing attention to gender equity, there is a continued need for Black women to be 'giving, loving, and loyal' (Godsil et al., 2016, p. 13).

Black South African women's commitment to the Strong Black Woman archetype and its valuing of 'strength and caretaking' (Watson & Hunter, 2016, p. 426) is probably also underpinned by the traditional African valuing of interdependence. As interdependent beings, Black South Africans prioritize the collective and accept co-responsibility for the collective's quality of life (Theron & Phasha, 2015). Included in this co-responsibility is a willingness to conform to the expectations of social responsibility that promote taking care of anyone requiring care and doing so in a respectful, enabling manner that signals solidarity and selflessness (Pityana, 1999).

5.3 The Benefits for Adolescent Resilience of the Strong Black Woman Archetype

In this section we apply the essence of the Strong Black Woman archetype, namely the capacity of a Black woman to be 'giving, loving, and loyal' (Godsil et al., 2016, p. 13) even though she herself is challenged by adversity, to the cases of Thandiwe and Thulani. To do this, we focused on the parts of their stories which related to how women enabled and/or constrained how Thandiwe and Thulani adjusted to multiple stressors.

5.3.1 The Resilient Youth in Stressed Environments (RYSE) Study

The cases of Thandiwe and Thulani are drawn from the Resilient Youth in Stressed Environments (RYSE) study, South Africa. RYSE is a multi-year (2017–2021), multi-site study of youth resilience in contexts of environmental and economic stress in Canada and South Africa (see www.ryseproject.org). Its purpose is to better understand the biopsychosocial pathways of youth resilience together with the role which environmental risks and resources play in youth resilience. The RYSE study received ethical clearance from collaborating Canadian and South African institutions.

The South African research site is a township that was originally built to house the blue-collar workers of a large petrochemical plant that manufactures petrochemical products from coal. It is adjacent to the petrochemical plant and close to several coal mines. Like many other townships in South Africa, the township in question is densely populated and characterized by risks that are associated with poor QoL in South Africa (Møller, 2013, 2018). These include violence, crime, communicable disease, and structural disadvantage (including poor infrastructure, widespread poverty, and low-functioning schools). In addition, the township's proximity to the petrochemical plant and coal mines means that its residents are chronically challenged by air and water pollution. Both Thandiwe and Thulani have resided in this township since they were small children.

As in other studies of resilience (e.g., McCubbin & Moniz, 2015; Theron, 2013b), the recruitment of South African RYSE participants was guided by a community-based advisory panel (CAP). The CAP invited voluntary participation from local young people aged 15–24 who believed they could contribute meaningful information about what enabled and constrained the resilience of local young people. A total of 61 South African RYSE participants (including Thandiwe and Thulani) engaged in qualitative work. This included arts-based activities such as draw-and-write (see Mitchell, Theron, Stuart, Smith, & Campbell, 2011) and body-maps (see Ebersöhn, Ferreira, van der Walt, & Moen, 2016), as well as one-on-one unstructured interviews. All of this qualitative work explored young people's lived experiences of what enables and constrains the resilience of local young people. The research team used a variety of prompts and questions to generate reflections and discussions on the aforementioned foci (e.g., What are the biggest challenges youth in your community face? What do the youth do to overcome these challenges? What/who makes it possible for young people to be OK when the petrochemical industry affects their lives in negative ways? How would you explain youth resilience?)

To complete the above-mentioned research activities, Thandiwe and Thulani met with us three times each (August 2017 – March 2018). They both verbalized that they considered themselves to be resilient. Their demographics at the time of participation in the qualitative research are summarized in Table 5.1. Their interviews, as well as their responses to the arts-based activities, were transcribed verbatim. Because both of these young people had been schooled in English, they were comfortable communicating in English and so no translation was necessary.

For the purposes of this chapter, we reviewed how Thandiwe and Thulani explained their resilience with specific focus on those elements which related to how women enabled or constrained resilience processes. Following Creswell's (2009) guidelines for deductive analysis, we coded this data for instances where women enacted the qualities inherent to the Strong Black Woman archetype (i.e., 'giving, loving, and loyal'; Godsil et al., 2016, p. 13).

Table 5.1 Thandiwe and Thulani

	Thandiwe	Thulani
Age	21	20
Mother tongue	isiXhosa	isiZulu
Living arrangements	Together with her son and two biological sisters, Thandiwe lives with her father (a pensioner), his partner and her two daughters	Thulani lives with his grandmother; they are supported by her pension
Employment	Unemployed	Unemployed
Highest education qualification	Grade 12	Grade 11

When we realized that Thandiwe was enacting these same qualities, we revisited the data that Thulani generated and discovered similar instances in his story.

5.3.2 The Hardships of Thandiwe's and Thulani's Lives

Thandiwe and Thulani both reported that their township, with its low levels of employment, inadequate infrastructure, and high levels of violence, did not inspire wellbeing or a sense of safety. In fact, living there did not promote QoL. They spoke at length about the health risks of living adjacent to the petrochemical plant and close to multiple coal mines. For instance, Thandiwe explained:

> Living in this area has affected me in a bad way, coz although it [petrochemical industry] has brought us, uhm, job opportunities ... it has polluted our areas and there is always that bad smell that causes headaches. ... It also causes sinus problems for me. I have been to doctors a lot of times due to that ... having headaches, massive headaches, all the time due to the bad smell. It's quite heart-breaking that, – like I don't know how to call it – but it's [petrochemical industry] helpful né [hey], but then it also destroys our lives. My mom had lung disease and she died from it and its all due to this kind of area. That's what's heart-breaking about this whole thing. Every time whenever I think about it, although I know that I can get a job there [at the petrochemical industry], but then it breaks my heart that I lost someone because of that place, you see. And as I said, it has polluted our areas. Where you walk there are sewages, like it's really bad. And sometimes when you open the water – they tell you that the water will make you sick. Not so long ago, people went to schools telling our little brothers and sisters to boil water first before drinking it .... They even said that a lot of people ended up in hospital because they drank water before boiling them. Yes... it's really sad for me.

As reported in Table 5.1, when they participated in the RYSE qualitative work, both young people were unemployed. In addition to the material insufficiency that this prompted, both young people had experienced that being unemployed meant that it was hard to meaningfully fill so-called working hours. In addition, because the majority of locals were similarly challenged, it was hard to hope that life would improve. Thulani explained these aspects as follows:

> Hey, there's a lot that makes life very hard. Oh there's a lot, you know, it's too much ... unemployment, you know. ... We started in primary and then went to high school, you know. [So] you never had too much time on your hands. So, we grew up and our time was in another person's hands, you know, a person who had an idea of what can I do for your time, what can I make you do in this time, you know? When you come out of that zone and now you have all the time in your hands, that's when you start thinking about stuff like, you know [silence] ... That's why I'm saying that unemployment is a hard thing ... our environment doesn't have a lot of facilities or you know, places where you can do stuff, positive stuff... we're situated around, you know, negativity. Every day you come out of your house, you see like hey, this boy yesterday was stabbed, and this boy died, you know. Everything we hear [is] news of negativity, we never hear news of like people who are going forward and people who are thinking positively.

Thandiwe added that when employment became available, high corruption levels meant that it was hard to access employment opportunities. She said:

> Like when we grew up, you know, our parents used to tell us that maths and science are important to do in school because of the petrol-chemical industry. Most of our parents worked there, so they had this belief that when you have maths and science you will be able to work there, and when you work there you earn a lot of money. Well some of us are not good at maths or science ... some of us failed, some of us didn't get those record marks that they actually want there, and that made most of the youngsters unemployed because they only focused on maths and science, nothing else. ... And on the corruption note, you know when you want a job, you know people usually say that the petrol-chemical industry is like the best place to work you know, and stuff, but then even if you do have those qualifications you don't just get that job unless you have connections inside that place ... so what's the point of having qualifications whilst you won't even be able to get the job. And someone once told me: there's this man who works there [and] he actually confirmed to that person that when we see that your qualifications are better than ours, we just take your CV and throw it away. We throw it away because we think that you will take our job.

Thulani explained further that local residents' dissatisfaction with the high levels of unemployment and poor service delivery, and subsequent strikes, aggravated the risks he and others faced:

> Our lungs are not quite good, inhaling a lot of pollution. And black people are burning a lot of tires.[1] There are a lot of strikes – striking about jobs, houses electricity … [To keep safe,] I usually pray for God to keep me safe and I usually listen to my granny who tells me a lot about life and you know how should I treat myself and how should I behave.

Both Thulani and Thandiwe referred to women who did not enact the ethic of care that is associated with the Strong Black Woman archetype. Their non-caring added to the risks that Thulani and Thandiwe faced. In Thandiwe's case her father's new partner (her 'stepmother') was a stereotypical example. However, less stereotypical, and common to both young people's accounts were references to local women (e.g., neighbors) who gossiped about young people and who begrudged them joy or success. Thulani explained:

> Yo [exclamation that conveys emotion]! You have grannies who act like cameras the whole day you know? [laughter] Just sit outside and act like CCTV you know? Like taking footage of everything, everyone, and then they go indoors, they make tea, you know, and start, 'Hey I saw the other. Did you see that boy? He's reading a lot, he's now crazy, you know?' And you try to live in your space, you try to live on your own energy, because you cannot absorb all that toxicity, you know? The thinking, the toxic vibes. You want to stay in your positive energy and enjoy your own energy, but that's impossible.

Similarly, Thandiwe commented that many women in her neighborhood "will always talk; whether you do something good or bad, they'll always have something to say". She typically experienced this talk as "nasty" because it eroded her self-esteem and quality of life. She said:

> They literally undermine you. Whenever you, like, come around, they always have something negative to say, they never have positive things, they will always want to downgrade you. … I'd get really upset, I'd actually cry myself to sleep sometimes.

[1]In South Africa, tires are typically burnt during strikes. Burning tires produce acrimonious smoke.

5.3.3 Resilience to Hardship

In their accounts of what enabled resilience in the face of the aforementioned challenges, Thandiwe and Thulani both reported personal agency, such as working towards future goals and/or choosing health-promoting behaviors (see Figs. 5.1 and 5.2). Although both Thandiwe and Thulani mentioned their fathers, and although Thandiwe's determination to be different from her father fueled her agency, neither linked their fathers to positive experiences of caregiving. Instead, they linked their experiences of being cared for to Black women (relatives and/or friends) who were 'giving, loving, and loyal' (Godsil et al., 2016, p. 13). This caregiving, along with the strength they drew from witnessing the resilience of Black women (relatives and/or friends), prompted and/or sustained Thandiwe's and Thulani's agency. Further, Thandiwe's and Thulane's personal enactment of the values implicit in the Strong Black Woman archetype (i.e., 'strength and caretaking', Watson & Hunter, 2016, p. 426) facilitated their positive adjustment to the hardships that characterized their lives.

5.3.3.1 The Benefits of Knowing Women Who Are 'Giving, Loving, and Loyal'

In addition to the challenge of having lost her mother when she was 10 years old, Thandiwe did not have a positive experience of family life ("I don't come from a loving, happy family"). Although she experienced her two younger sisters (aged 20 and 14) as loyal ("When I need their help, I know they will be there"), her strongest experience of generosity and care was the acceptance by, and warmth of, her lifelong friend and this friend's family. As emphasized by Thandiwe's words below, the major benefit of having a 'giving, loving, and loyal' friend lay in the sense of belonging and access to food and shelter that this engendered:

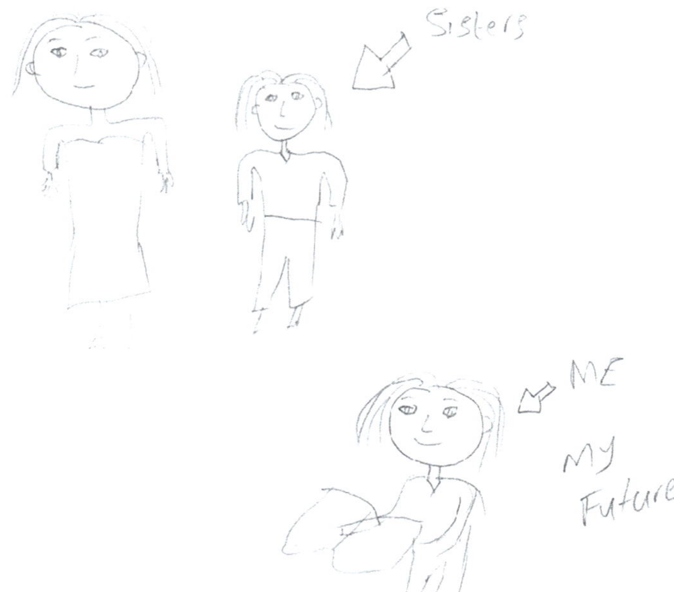

Fig. 5.1 Thandiwe's drawn explanation of who/what supports her resilience

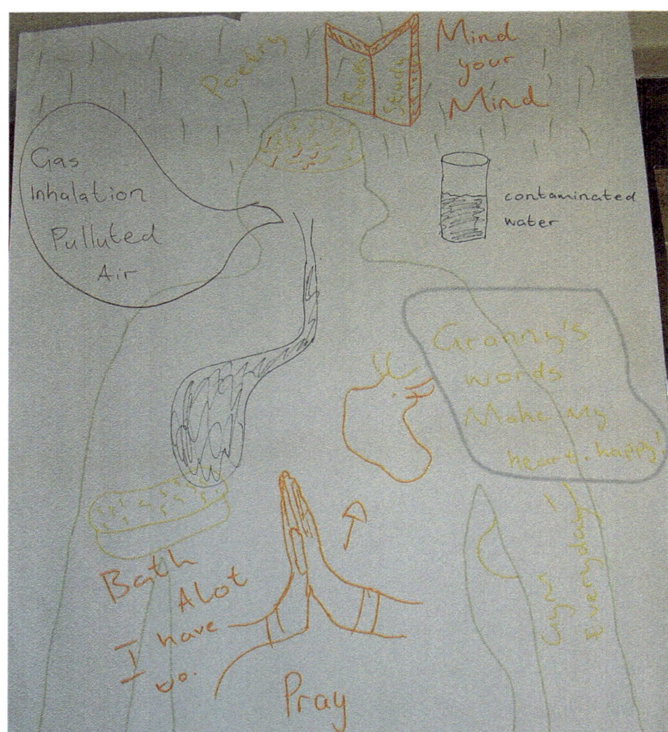

Fig. 5.2 Thulani's body map of what puts him at risk and supports his resilience

> I have one best friend and we've been through school together, and she's been there through thick and thin, you know. She's like my rock [laugher]. She's helped me with everything, with the situation at home. I used to cry like almost all the time at school because of the situation at home. From when my mom died in 2006 (I was in Grade 4) … when my friend came to hug me I just stood there, I felt lost. Life is not easy without a mom. I would not wish that for even my enemy, I would not. It's really hard. … [but, Friend] helped me a lot. In everything. I've even – my friend's family has even actually accepted us (Thandiwe and her younger sisters) as their own kids, you know? Whenever we visit them they'll be like – you know when you're a visitor at a house, they always do things for you? – they'll be like okay bread is somewhere, and the butter is in the cupboard, and they would, uh, you feel welcomed, you know. I actually then feel the love, you know, from them. It actually does make me happy, like I'm actually, I'm accepted somewhere, you know? It actually feels great.

Thulani attached different benefits to the experience of a 'giving, loving, and loyal' woman, namely his grandmother. Unlike Thandiwe, Thulani did not disclose how old he was when his biological mother died. He mentioned her death in passing when he was commenting on his network of relatives ("my mother passed away; I do have a lot of relatives, cousins and aunties"). His maternal grandmother raised him and he repeatedly credited his resilience to her care. Through her care, he learned to value himself and to be true to himself. For instance when he described himself, Thulani used the metaphor of a sponge. He said:

> I'm absorbing growth … my granny used to tell me that everything you think you are, you attract … Mostly only soft things can absorb something … you're going to choose when you see that [one], you know, this one I take in … But you know, in the community we live in, being soft is not part of, it's not in our nature you know. You always want to be appear strong … Black people just want to appear hard, you know … [but] having the courage to be different [is important because] only when you're soft you can absorb, attract …

Thulani valued his grandmother's contribution to his development. She was generous with her life-lessons (including life-lessons about the "past, our heritage, family stuff"). In particular, she modelled qualities (such as kindness and self-discipline] that had the potential to promote a positive attitude and wellbeing, and that eased his life in a resource-constrained, dangerous community. Thulani experienced her example as "contagious". He explained:

> Even though she [grandmother] didn't teach us to be kind, it kind of grew in us that we have to be kind. We saw her being kind, you know? Some people didn't grow up in that environment. Even though their parents taught them no, be kind, you know, they didn't see that in their parents so they didn't believe in that attitude, you know?
> She's always strict, just she's strict in a polite way. She can really discipline herself you know, which makes it easier for us to be disciplined. She doesn't hit us, you know, she doesn't even touch us. We [are] just around her, you know. Just being around her, in a way you will soon align yourself, you know, teach yourself that no, no, no. Because, you see her do it and it's working for her, you know? Because the gym thing you know [he prioritized daily exercise; see Fig. 5.2], me waking up in the morning, going to the gym in the morning, was caused by her waking us in the morning, every day, [with] it's a new day, go do something. You know, eish [exclamation that conveys emotion]! How can I explain my time, because we have nothing to do here, you know? So, let's start a day with, you know, some gym, some exercising, you know, yes that's where it started, that's how it started …

However, Thulani's grandmother's pragmatic caring was not all via example. For instance, she instilled respect for knowledge and a love of reading (which Thulani described as an opportunity to "renew our minds and get more knowledge about how we can take care of ourselves") by purposefully prompting him to read:

> In our house we have a coal stove. So, we use papers [newspapers] to [light it]… I'm usually the one who does it, you know… my granny told me if I'm going to burn a paper I have to make sure that I know what's written on that paper. So you know every paper that I threw in the stove, I made sure that I know the information in that paper. She sometimes asked me questions about that paper [laughter]. And I was like, no ways she won't see me, you know, but she was always [asking], what is that paper you threw in? So that was the thing that kept me reading the papers.

5.3.3.2 The Benefits of Being Someone Who Is 'Giving, Loving, and Loyal'

Thandiwe's account of her resilience included her care for her younger sisters. She spoke about being "like their mom and their dad" (meaning that she had to care for them emotionally and "make means" to feed and clothe them). This role was foisted on her when she was 13:

> He [her father] brought another woman home. When he did, everything changed. Like literally everything changed. My siblings [brothers] left, and I was left alone as the older one. I had to be a mom [to her two younger, biological sisters] at a young age. She came with her kids. It was terrible, because they got everything they wanted, but when we asked for something, it was either we're not going to get it, or we'll get it at their own time. I felt like she was controlling my dad, you know? And I used to think, you know, I actually thought the whole thing that stepmothers are horrible was just made up, but I could see at the time it's true, they're horrible.

Despite her discomfort with how she and her biological sisters were treated, Thandiwe embraced her new role. She accepted responsibility for her biological sisters and put their needs beyond her own. She said that she remembered how her biological mother had done that for her and she wanted them to experience the same. She used her responsibility for them as additional motivation to become well qualified and find employment that would support them all to lead a better life:

> When they need me, they know that I'm there. Like without them, I know that my life would be incomplete. That's why I've always told myself that wherever I go, I'll take them with me. Yes, wherever life would take me, I'd take them, I would never leave them, because I don't want them to suffer. They've suffered enough, you know? I have to like get them out of the current situation that we're facing, that's just like my other goal, to just get them out of that situation.

Thandiwe also had a 2 year old son. He was her sole responsibility as his father had chosen to be absent from his life. Although she was initially angry and hurt about this absence, Thandiwe contained her emotion and focused on caring for her son. She described this as resilience-enabling:

> But when I got him, everything changed. When I saw him for the first time – when I saw him I couldn't believe that I'm actually a mom, because this tiny little person! I was actually scared, but then at the same time I felt the love. Oh, God! I actually have this little human being in my hands right now. It was weird, scary, but it's actually a great feeling, you know, and it changed a lot. It changed my way of thinking. You know, when things were bad I would think of, you know, maybe it would be better if I kill myself or something. I would have those kinds of thoughts. Then when he came, it all changed. Like, okay, yes, I have to do this. He's here and he needs me, I have to do everything for him and my sisters.

Similarly, Thulani's account of his resilience spoke of his intention to care for others. He longed to make a positive difference in the lives of his family, peers, and more broadly, his community.

> Thulani: I do think I'm resilient. Actually a lot of people around here are resilient. A lot of people, you know. Seeing a person smile and looking at the conditions they have, you know, you just wonder how do they smile, or how do they do that? … What makes me resilient is I want to give back you know, I feel like I'm an instrument of giving back. I want to give back hope, you know, faith, and believing.
> Linda: Who gave you the hope and faith and believing that you want to give back?
> Thulani: I think it's my grandmother, you know, because looking back at the circumstances, and the situations we came through, you know it's really hard, it has been really hard. But, she always gives you that feeling of, you know, tomorrow's a new day. She tries again. The same way you know she smiles again tomorrow. You also feel that sense that it's a new day. It is a new day, you know, things are different than yesterday.

In particular he cared about his grandmother's happiness, and the sacrifices she had made for him, and this directed the choices he made:

> Hey, what keeps me going now, you know, I would say it's just to see my grandmother happy. You know? After that I might try to see my community members also happy. But at this very point, you know, I want to see my grandmother happy. I think that's the thing that makes me want to take part in positive things. It will bring joy to her. You know, I think there's a lot of stuff we don't understand. I'm speaking on behalf of youth in the community, we don't understand the hardships our grandmothers and great grandmothers went through, you know, for us...

5.4 Learning from the Cases of Thandiwe and Thulani

Before we detail the three take-home lessons that are implicit in the accounts of Thandiwe and Thulani, it is important to acknowledge that their accounts (as reported in this chapter) reflected how they explained their resilience at three points in time (August 2017 – April 2018). Although these three accounts (facilitated via body-maps, drawings, and interviews) triangulated well, they could change over time. Also, English was not their first language. Even though both of these young people were willing to communicate in English, their accounts of their resilience might have been more expansive had they communicated in their mother-tongue. Despite these limitations, we believe that stakeholders who wish to promote the resilience of the young people can learn from Thandiwe and Thulani. These lessons follow next. In essence, these lessons speak to the resilience-enabling value of so-called 'small everyday acts' (Møller, 2018, p. 1016).

5.4.1 Strong, Caring Women, Who Are Accessible and Available, Matter for Youth Resilience

In 2006 Luthar asserted that caring connections to other people are foundational to resilience. Similarly, Masten (2014, p. 150) reported that the 'central significance of close relationships for resilience has been noted in virtually every review on resilience in development over the past half-century'. Indeed, this centrality is evident in South African resilience studies too; a recent review of 61 South African child and youth resilience studies published between 2009 and 2017 noted that affective support was the most frequently reported resilience-enabler across all of these studies (Van Breda & Theron, 2018). Relationships which facilitated young people's growth and development was the second most frequently reported resource. These affective and developmental supports were often facilitated by caring women, particularly mothers (e.g., Eloff et al., 2014; Malindi, 2014; Odendaal & Moletsane, 2011; Ogina, 2012; Phasha, 2010; Theron, 2013a, 2016, 2017; Theron & Theron, 2013; Zulu, 2018). Thandiwe and Thulani reported similar supports, except they were provided by women who were not their biological mothers (as noted earlier their mothers were dead). In Thandiwe's case the memory of her mother's selflessness shaped her own selflessness. The ages of the women who supported them (Thandiwe's friend was also 21; Thulani's grandmother was 80) suggest that neither youth nor old age is a barrier to women's championship of resilience.

Previous studies of South African child and youth resilience have occasionally reported that Black women resilience champions were both caring and strong (e.g., Casale, 2011; Phasha, 2010; Theron, 2016; Zulu, 2018). These studies have theorized that the prominence and strength of these women related, in part, to the physical absence of fathers. Because Thandiwe's and Thulani's fathers were not physically absent, their cases suggest that strong, caring Black women could be prominent because of their capacity to connect meaningfully with young people. This capacity echoes Jordan's (2000, 2006, 2008, 2013) gendered relational-cultural theory and resonates with the traditional African valuing of interdependence (Pityana, 1999; Theron & Phasha, 2015). Whatever the reason, stakeholders who serve youth have a particular responsibility to sustain the strong, caring women with whom these young people interact.

The above-mentioned studies did not consider how women's enactment of behaviors that do not fit with the Strong Black Woman archetype have the potential to constrain the resilience of young people. Thandiwe's and Thulani's negative experiences of women who slandered them and their peers, or diminished their self-worth, are a reminder that adults have the power to shape the resilience of young people via their everyday actions. Stakeholders need to remind adults of this power and supported adults to embrace those everyday actions (e.g., modeling strength; being caring) that are likely to advance resilience.

Lastly, the women with whom Thandiwe and Thulani had caring connections were Black.

When the isiZulu-speaking participants in Dass-Brailsford's (2005) study reported that their Black teachers supported their resilience, Dass-Brailsford cautioned that this probably related more to these teachers' capacity to understand the participants' lives (having had similar lives themselves), and less to do with race. Similarly, the Black women with whom Thandiwe and Thulani connected shared their daily lives and were intimately acquainted with the hardships of township life. These commonalities probably gave them an intuitive understanding of the caring which Thandiwe and Thulani needed/wanted. Nevertheless, it is interesting that almost 25 years after the official demise of Apartheid, neither Thandiwe nor Thulani mentioned a person whose race was different from theirs and whose caring had supported them to cope well in life. Implicit in the above is the importance of enabling young people's access to caring, strong women who understand their life-circumstances and who are willing and able to be regularly accessible and available.

5.4.2 Caring for Others Matters for Resilience

Thandiwe and Thulani both demonstrated the desire to pay their experiences of caregiving forward (to the next generation, to the community in general) and back (to those who had cared for them and/or been loyal to them). They both verbalized that their resilience was intertwined with such caring (enacted and intended). The desire by youth to make a positive difference to others who have been enabling and/or to others who are in need of support is seldom mentioned in the resilience literature. Exceptions in the South African literature include the studies by Mosavel, Ahmed, Ports, and Simon (2015), Ogina (2012), Phasha (2010), and Theron (2016, 2017). In all of these studies, the youth participants were Black. It is possible that African valuing of interdependence, and how this translates into a deep sense of social responsibility (Phasha, 2010), shaped the selfless caring which the Black participants in the above-mentioned studies reported. Flowing from the cases of Thandiwe and Thulani, it is also possible that caring for others and/or prioritizing others' needs is intertwined with experiences of being well cared for by strong, Black women. Although we do not make causal claims, we thought it significant that both Thandiwe and Thulani reported strong Black women who cared for them and that they both cared about and were strong for others. Further, Thulani's caring concern for his grandmother, peers and community differs from Van Breda's (2018) conclusion that caring/mothering roles are a gender-specific pathway of resilience. It would, therefore, be useful if future large-scale resilience studies investigated whether/how caring/mothering roles support the resilience of both young men and women, and whether a willingness to take care of others relates to lived experiences of being cared for by strong, caring women.

In the interim, stakeholders may want to vary popular intervention agendas (e.g., teaching vulnerable young people to be mindful, see systematic reviews by Felver, Celis-de Hoyos, Tezanos, & Singh, (2016), Hedman-Lagerlöf, Hedman-Lagerlöf, & Öst, (2018), Zenner, Herrnleben-Kurz, & Walach, (2014)). When stakeholders work with Black youth, Thandiwe's and Thulani's cases suggest that an alternative would be to explore the possible resilience benefits of caring for those who are vulnerable and of reciprocating caring interactions. In addition, it would be useful for stakeholders and youth to explore, and challenge, gender stereotypes relating to caring.

5.4.3 There Are Potential Costs to Caring and Being Strong

Many studies associate the enactment of the Strong Black Woman archetype with costs (e.g., mental and/or physical illness) to the women who embrace this archetype (e.g., Abrams et al., 2014; Donovan & West, 2015; Watson & Hunter, 2016; Watson-Singleton, 2017). However, Thandiwe and Thulani benefitted from strong Black women. Certainly Thulani was aware that his grandmother had sacrificed much for him, but we cannot comment definitively on what caring for Thandiwe and Thulani cost the women in their lives. Thandiwe and Thulani also associated resilience with their personal enactment of the selfless caring which is related to the Strong Black Woman archetype – caring and being determined to make a positive difference gave them a sense of purpose and hope. The tension between the documented costs of the Strong Black Woman archetype and the value of the enactment of this archetype to Thandiwe and Thulani fits with resilience scholars' recent attention to the trade-offs that are inherent to processes of adaptation (e.g., Masten, 2016). This tension also calls for resilience studies to follow young people – and their caregivers – over time to better understand the long-term costs and benefits of resilience processes (Wright & Masten, 2015). In the mean time, stakeholders will need to carefully monitor this tension and intervene as necessary.

5.5 Conclusion

At the time of writing this chapter, the township where Thandiwe and Thulani live suffered further setbacks when locals, who were incensed by continued unemployment, corruption, and poor service delivery, blocked all entrance and exits to the township and razed the local mall and post office. Neither Thandiwe, nor Thulani, nor the women who were important to them, were hurt, but their QoL deteriorated further. Against the backdrop of such apparently intractable adversity, the capacity of women and young people to engage in 'everyday acts' (Møller, 2018, p. 1016) that matter for QoL and resilience is anything but 'small'. Instead, their capacity to continue to care for one another and be strong, is extraordinary. Although it is possible that this capacity will have health and wellbeing trade-offs, it is important to acknowledge the immediate resilience benefits that accrue to young people who are cared for by strong Black women and who pay these women's strength and caring forward and back.

References

Abrams, J. A., Maxwell, M., Pope, M., & Belgrave, F. Z. (2014). Carrying the world with the grace of a lady and the grit of a warrior: Deepening our understanding of the "Strong Black Woman" schema. *Psychology of Women Quarterly, 38*(4), 503–518.

Booysen, L. A., & Nkomo, S. M. (2010). Gender role stereotypes and requisite management characteristics: The case of South Africa. *Gender in Management: An International Journal, 25*(4), 285–300.

Brody, L. R., Stokes, L. R., Kelso, G. A., Dale, S. K., Cruise, R. C., Weber, K. M., … Cohen, M. H. (2014). Gender role behaviors of high affiliation and low self-silencing predict better adherence to antiretroviral therapy in women with HIV. *AIDS Patient Care and STDs, 28*(9), 459–461.

Casale, M. (2011). 'I am living a peaceful life with my grandchildren. Nothing else.' Stories of adversity and 'resilience' of older women caring for children in the context of HIV/AIDS and other stressors. *Ageing & Society, 31*, 1265–1288.

Casale, M., Wild, L., Cluver, L., & Kuo, C. (2015). Social support as a protective factor for depression among women caring for children in HIV-endemic South Africa. *Journal of Behavioral Medicine, 38*(1), 17–27.

Creswell, J. W. (2009). *Research design: Qualitative, quantitative, and mixed methods approaches* (3rd ed., p. 251). London, UK: Sage.

Dass-Brailsford, P. (2005). Exploring resilience: Academic achievement among disadvantaged black youth in South Africa. *South Africa Journal of Psychology, 35*(3), 574–591.

Donovan, R. A., & West, L. M. (2015). Stress and mental health: Moderating role of the strong black woman stereotype. *Journal of Black Psychology, 41*(4), 384–396.

Ebersöhn, L., Ferreira, R., van der Walt, A., & Moen, M. (2016). Bodymapping to step into your future: Life design in a context of high risk and high diversity. In R. Ferreira (Ed.), *Thinking innovatively about psychological assessment in a context of diversity* (pp. 228–241). Cape Town, South Africa: Juta.

Eloff, I., Finestone, M., Makin, J. D., Boeving-Allen, A., Visser, M., Ebersöhn, L., … Forsyth, B. W. C. (2014). A randomized clinical trial of an intervention to promote resilience in young children of HIV-positive mothers in South Africa. *Aids, 28*, S347–S357.

Felver, J. C., Celis-de Hoyos, C. E., Tezanos, K., & Singh, N. N. (2016). A systematic review of mindfulness-based interventions for youth in school settings. *Mindfulness, 7*(1), 34–45.

Godsil, R. D., Tropp, L. R., Goff, P. A., Powell, J. A., & MacFarlane, J. (2016). The effects of gender roles, implicit bias, and stereotype threat on the lives of women and girls. *The Science of Equality, 2*. https://equity.ucla.edu/wp-content/uploads/2016/11/Science-of-Equality-Volume-2.pdf. Accessed 22 June 2018.

Haffejee, S., & Theron, L. C. (2017). Resilience processes in sexually abused adolescent girls: A scoping review of the literature. *South African Journal of Science, 113*(9/10), 1–9. https://doi.org/10.17159/sajs.2017/20160318

Hammarström, A., & Hensing, G. (2018). How gender theories are used in contemporary public health research. *International Journal for Equity in Health, 17*(1), 34.

Hall, A.-M., & Theron, L. C. (2016). Resilience processes supporting adolescents with intellectual disability: A multiple case study. *Intellectual and Developmental Disabilities, 54*(1), 45–62.

Hatch, M., & Posel, D. (2018). Who cares for children? A quantitative study of childcare in South Africa. *Development Southern Africa, 35*, 1–16.

Hedman-Lagerlöf, M., Hedman-Lagerlöf, E., & Öst, L. G. (2018). The empirical support for mindfulness-based interventions for common psychiatric disorders: A systematic review and meta-analysis. *Psychological Medicine, 48*, 2116–2129. https://doi.org/10.1017/S0033291718000259

Hills, F., Meyer-Weitz, A., & Kwaku Oppong, A. (2016). The lived experiences of street children in Durban, South Africa: Violence, substance use, and resilience. *International Journal of Qualitative Studies on Health & Well-Being, 11*, 1–12.

Jefferis, T. C., & Theron, L. C. (2017). Promoting resilience among Sesotho-speaking adolescent girls: Lessons for South African teachers. *South African Journal of Education, 37*(3), 1–11.

Jefferis, T., & Theron, L. C. (2018). Explanations of resilience in women and girls: How applicable to black South African girls. *Women's Studies International Forum*. https://doi.org/10.1016/j.wsif.2018.03.006

Jordan, J. V. (2000). The role of mutual empathy in relational/cultural therapy. *JCLP/In Session: Psychotherapy in Practice, 56*(8), 1005–1016.

Jordan, J. V. (2006). Relational resilience in girls. In S. Goldstein & R. Brooks (Eds.), *Handbook of resilience in children* (pp. 79–89). New York, NY: Springer.

Jordan, J. V. (2008). Recent developments in relational-cultural theory. *Women & Therapy, 31*(2–4), 1–4. https://doi.org/10.1080/02703140802145540

Jordan, J. V. (2013). Relational resilience in girls. In S. Goldstein & R. Brooks (Eds.), *Handbook of resilience in children* (2nd ed., pp. 73–86). New York, NY: Springer.

Kumpulainen, K., Theron, L., Kahl, C., Bezuidenhout, C., Mikkola, A., Salmi, S., … Uusitalo-Malmivaara, L. (2016). Children's positive adjustment to first grade in risk-filled communities: A case study of the role of school ecologies in South Africa and Finland. *School Psychology International, 37*(2), 121–139.

Land, K. C., & Michalos, A. C. (2018). Fifty years after the social indicators movement: Has the promise been fulfilled? *Social Indicators Research, 135*(3), 835–868.

Luthar, S. (2006). Resilience in development: A synthesis of research across five decades. In D. Cicchetti & D. Cohen (Eds.), *Developmental psychopathology: Risk, disorder, and adaptation* (Vol. 3, 2nd ed., pp. 739–795). Hoboken, NJ: Wiley.

Makusha, T., Richter, L., & Bhana, D. (2012). Children's experiences of support received from men in rural KwaZulu-Natal. *Africa Development, 37*(3), 127–152.

Malindi, M. J. (2014). Exploring the roots of resilience among female street-involved children in South Africa. *Journal of Psychology, 5*(1), 35–45.

Masten, A. S. (2001). Ordinary magic: Resilience processes in development. *American Psychologist, 56*(3), 227–238.

Masten, A. S. (2014). *Ordinary magic: Resilience in development*. New York, NY: Guilford Publications.

Masten, A. S. (2016). Resilience in developing systems: The promise of integrated approaches. *European Journal of Developmental Psychology, 13*(3), 297–312.

McCubbin, L. D., & Moniz, J. (2015). Ethical principles in resilience research: Respect, relevance, reciprocity and responsibility. In L. C. Theron, L. Liebenberg, & M. Ungar (Eds.), *Youth resilience and culture: Commonalities and complexities* (pp. 217–229). Dordrecht, The Netherlands: Springer.

Mitchell, C., Theron, L. C., Stuart, J., Smith, A., & Campbell, Z. (2011). Drawings as research method. In L. C. Theron, C. Mitchell, A. Smith, & J. Stuart (Eds.), *Picturing research: Drawings as visual methodology* (pp. 19–36). Rotterdam, The Netherlands: Sense.

Møller, V. (2013). South African quality of life trends over three decades, 1980–2010. *Social Indicators Research, 113*(3), 915–940.

Møller, V. (2018). Whatever happened to social indicators in Africa? Whatever happened indeed! A developing world perspective on the Kenneth C. Land and Alex C. Michalos report on 'Fifty years after the social indicators movement'. *Social Indicators Research, 135*(3), 1009–1019.

Mosavel, M., Ahmed, R., Ports, K. A., & Simon, C. (2015). South African, urban youth narratives: Resilience within community. *International Journal of Adolescence and Youth, 20*(2), 245–255.

Odendaal, N. D., & Moletsane, M. (2011). Use of indigenous stone play in child psychological assessment. *Journal of Psychology in Africa, 21*(4), 623–626.

Ogina, T. A. (2012). The use of drawings to facilitate interviews with orphaned children in Mpumalanga province, South Africa. *South African Journal of Education, 32*(4), 428–438.

Panter-Brick, C. (2015). Culture and resilience: Next steps for theory and practice. In L. C. Theron, L. Liebenberg, & M. Ungar (Eds.), *Youth resilience and culture: Commonalities and complexities* (pp. 233–244). Dordrecht, The Netherlands: Springer.

Parks, S. (2010). *Fierce angels: The strong Black woman in American life and culture*. New York, NY: One World/Ballantine Books.

Phasha, T. N. (2010). Educational resilience among African survivors of child sexual abuse in South Africa. *Journal of Black Studies, 40*(6), 1234–1253.

Pityana, B. (1999). The renewal of African moral values. In M. Makgoba (Ed.), *African renaissance* (pp. 137–148). Cape Town, South Africa: Tafelberg.

Ramphele, M. (2012). *Conversations with my sons and daughters*. Johannesburg, South Africa: Penguin UK.

Richter, L., Chikovore, J., & Makusha, T. (2010). The status of fatherhood and fathering in South Africa. *Childhood Education, 86*(6), 360–365.

Rutter, M. (2013). Annual research review: Resilience-clinical implications. *Journal of Child Psychology and Psychiatry, 54*(4), 474–487. https://doi.org/10.1111/jcpp.12057

Sawyer, S. M., Azzopardi, P. S., Wickremarathne, D., & Patton, G. C. (2018). The age of adolescence. *The Lancet Child & Adolescent Health, 2*(3), 223–228.

Theron, L. C. (2007). Uphenyo ngokwazi kwentsha yasemalokishini ukumelana nesimo esinzima: A South African study of resilience among township youth. *Child and Adolescent Psychiatric Clinics of North America.*, 2007, *16*(2), 357–375. https://doi.org/10.1016/j.chc.2006.12.005

Theron, L. C. (2013a). Black students' recollections of pathways to resilience: Lessons for school psychologists. *School Psychology International, 34*(5), 527–539.

Theron, L. C. (2013b). Community-researcher liaisons: The Pathways to Resilience Project advisory panel. *South African Journal of Education, 33*(4), 1–19.

Theron, L. C. (2016). Toward a culturally and contextually sensitive understanding of resilience: Privileging the voices of black, South African young people. *Journal of Adolescent Research, 31*(6), 635–670.

Theron, L. C. (2017). Adolescent versus adult explanations of resilience enablers: A South African study. *Youth & Society*. https://doi.org/10.1177/0044118X17731032

Theron, L. C., & Engelbrecht, P. (2012). Caring teachers: Teacher-youth transactions to promote resilience. In M. Ungar (Ed.), *The social ecology of resilience: Culture, context, resources and meaning* (pp. 265–280). New York, NY: Springer.

Theron, L. C., & Phasha, N. (2015). Cultural pathways to resilience: Opportunities and obstacles as recalled by black South African students. In L. C. Theron, L. Liebenberg, & M. Ungar (Eds.), *Youth resilience and culture: Commonalities and complexities* (pp. 51–66). Dordrecht, The Netherlands: Springer.

Theron, L. C., & Theron, A. M. C. (2013). Positive adjustment to poverty: How family communities encourage resilience in traditional African contexts. *Culture & Psychology, 19*(3), 391–413.

Theron, L. C., & Theron, A. M. C. (2014). Education services and resilience processes: Resilient black South African students' experiences. *Child and Youth Services Review*. https://doi.org/10.1016/j.childyouth.2014.10.003

Ungar, M. (2011). The social ecology of resilience: Addressing contextual and cultural ambiguity of a nascent construct. *American Journal of Orthopsychiatry, 81*(1), 1–17.

Ungar, M. (2012). Social ecologies and their contribution to resilience. In M. Ungar (Ed.), *The social ecology of resilience: A handbook of theory and practice* (pp. 13–31). New York, NY: Springer.

Ungar, M. (2015a). Practitioner review: Diagnosing childhood resilience – a systemic approach to the diagnosis of adaptation in adverse social and physical ecologies. *Journal of Child Psychology and Psychiatry, 56*(1), 4–17.

Ungar, M. (2015b). Resilience and culture: The diversity of protective processes and positive adaptation. In L. C. Theron, L. Liebenberg, & M. Ungar (Eds.), *Youth resilience and culture: Commonalities and complexities* (pp. 37–49). Dordrecht, The Netherlands: Springer.

Ungar, M. (2018). The differential impact of social services on young people's resilience. *Child Abuse & Neglect, 78*, 4–12.

Van Breda, A. D. (2018). 'We are who we are through other people': The interactional foundation of the resilience of youth leaving care in South Africa. *Professorial Inaugural Lecture, 28*(February).

Van Breda, A. D., & Theron, L. C. (2018). A critical review of South African child and youth resilience studies, 2009–2017. *Children and Youth Services Review, 91*, 237–247.

Van Rensburg, A., Theron, L., & Rothmann, S. (2018). A social ecological modeled explanation of the resilience processes of a sample of Black Sesotho-speaking adolescents. *Psychological Reports*. https://doi.org/10.1177/0033294118784538

Watson, N. N., & Hunter, C. D. (2016). "I had to be strong" tensions in the strong black woman schema. *Journal of Black Psychology, 42*(5), 424–452.

Watson-Singleton, N. N. (2017). Strong black woman schema and psychological distress: The mediating role of perceived emotional support. *Journal of Black Psychology, 43*(8), 778–788.

Wright, M. O., & Masten, A. S. (2015). Pathways to resilience in context. In L. C. Theron, L. Liebenberg, & M. Ungar (Eds.), *Resilience and culture. Commonalities and complexities* (pp. 3–22). Dordrecht, The Netherlands: Springer.

Yin, R. K. (2014). *Case study research: Design and methods* (5th ed.). Thousand Oaks, CA: Sage.

Zenner, C., Herrnleben-Kurz, S., & Walach, H. (2014). Mindfulness-based interventions in schools—a systematic review and meta-analysis. *Frontiers in Psychology, 5*, 603. https://doi.org/10.3389/fpsyg.2014.00603

Zulu, N. T. (2018). Resilience in Black women who do not have fathers: A qualitative inquiry. *South African Journal of Psychology, 35*, 574–591. 0081246318782187.

Conversations as Carriers of Meaning to a Common Good

6

H. Á. Marujo, L. M. Neto, and M. P. Wissing

Abstract

In this chapter we argue that wellbeing and quality of life should be addressed at the public sphere, not only at an intra-personal level, with attention to a communal meaning which include more than economic indicators. We advocate for relational wellbeing through conversations among individuals, societies and cultures against the backdrop of a strong relational ontology and making meaning in relatedness on an empirical level as is in particular important in an African context. We consider conversations as carriers of meanings on intra-personal, interpersonal and social levels through interconnectedness and coordination of worldviews. We in particular argue for the social foundations of a common wellbeing, and indicate what meaningful conversations at the community level entails. Finally, we argue the importance of conversations as carriers of meaning to enhance quality of life and facilitation of global peace – one of the most esteemed goals of humanity. This is one of the ways to realize collective meaning.

6.1 Relational Wellbeing and Fundamental Human Rights

> The importance of a sense of global community have real-world implications for policymakers, the advocacy community, and human rights practitioners, and it is up to us to ensure that our work does not end with a publication, but that we do all that we can to extend our research beyond the ivory tower of academia. (Twose & Cohrs, 2015, p. 8)

Wellbeing scholarship is undoubtedly rich and diverse, with many years of dazzling development and a strong scientific basis. A similar upward curve is noticed in human rights activism (https://en.wikipedia.org/wiki/Human_rights_movement). Taking into account the agency of human beings and their potential, the field of positive psychology has helped to recognize the relevance of wellbeing, including amongst others, satisfaction with life, happiness, and meaningful activities, as universal goals and aspirations in the lives of human beings around the world. It also helped to confirm that currently used development indicators, that do not incorporate human values, seem to neglect important aspects in life which are of relevance for people's well-being (Bruni &

H. Á. Marujo · L. M. Neto (✉)
Instituto Superior de Ciências Sociais e Politicas (ISCSP), University of Lisbon, Lisbon, Portugal
e-mail: hmarujo@iscsp.ulisboa.pt; lneto@iscsp.ulisboa.pt

M. P. Wissing
Africa Unit for Transdisciplinary Health Research, North-West University, Potchefstroom, South Africa
e-mail: Marie.Wissing@nwu.ac.za

I. Eloff (ed.), *Handbook of Quality of Life in African Societies*, International Handbooks of Quality-of-Life, https://doi.org/10.1007/978-3-030-15367-0_6

Porta, 2016; Rojas, 2018; Wong, 2017). In so doing, positive psychology underscored the recognition of wellbeing indicators, in particular subjective well-being indicators, in public policy objectives and measurements (subjective well-being indicators mainly included measures of happiness and satisfaction with life – cf. World Happiness Report, 2018). Hence, subjective well-being assessments, and associated research data, became highly relevant in addressing development debates and strategies, as much as more recently, in informing policy makers to assume policies by pioneering a more sensible, balanced and comprehensive view of societies and human beings (Eid & Diener, 2006). Nonetheless, as Diener proposed in (2000, p. 41), "To create a better society where happiness is ubiquitous, a major scientific effort to understand quality of life is needed". This is reiterated Diener et al. (2017).

Historically, the studies centered on *who* is happy, with later on also a focus on *when* and *why* people are happy and the processes that influence their happiness (Diener, op. cit.). Additionally, research has grown around the creation of measures and indexes, namely to assess happiness at the level of nations and to create a world hierarchy of happiness in countries (e.g., Veenhoven, 2017b), with occasional proposals imbedded in a collectivistic cosmology (e.g., Biswas-Diener, 2011; Biswas-Diener & Patterson, 2011; Inglehart, Foa, Peterson, & Welzel, 2008; Marujo & Neto, 2013, 2017a, 2017b; Wissing, 2013).

Still, individualistic formulations of wellbeing have colonized the field of positive psychology until recently. Mimicking the traditional approaches inside the science of psychology, they have been missing a more communitarian and global approach as may also be more applicable in several developing countries in the global south, and Africa in particular (cf. Mahali et al., 2018). Considering the person as an individualistic being, and viewing autonomy (or self-sufficiency) as the absolute value, psychology in general, and positive psychology in particular, rests on a representation of the person as a separate being, with a unique personal point of view, and tendency to pursue his or her own notion of the good (Etzioni, 2018; Gergen, 2009).

Sensitive to this need, more voices are being heard from scholars affirming the need to move away from individualist formulations towards a relational, collectivistic and global approach, acknowledging the significance of social relationships, sense of belonging and prosocial action for the wellbeing of all (Biswas-Diener, 2011; Etzioni, 2018; Rojas, 2018; White, 2017; Wissing, 2014). Consequently, the discourse on the self has been complemented, when not substituted, by a discourse on the relational and the community.

The approach on relational wellbeing is one important tactic to bring community and a global perspective into the forefront of positive psychology and quality of life studies. As asserted by White (2017, p. 128), "Relational wellbeing is understood as arising from the common life, the shared enterprise of living in community – in whatever sense – with others. Relationships thus form a central focus, as both the means through which (psychological, symbolic, social and material) goods are distributed and needs are met, and as intrinsic to the constitution and experience of wellbeing". This type of wellbeing is based in a multiple and open relational horizon that views social ties as plausibly prior to individuals (White, 2017). An example of the importance of relationships for a good quality of life in an African context is illustrated by Wilson et al. (2018) in a study on important relationships as experienced by older Setswana speaking people in South Africa. The reasons participants indicated for the importance of mentioned relationships far out weighted pure instrumental benefits. They specifically mentioned the need for harmony and respect across various relational networks, and expressed appreciation for working and living well and with peace together with friends, family and community.

A further step for positive psychology, debated in this chapter, is to root the current actions inside the field in a relational and community realm that will also be more inclusive to appreciate quality of life issues in an African context, while incorporating concepts and processes related to complex and global humanitarian and societal problems, as an ultimate pathway to common wellbeing and public happiness (Bruni, 2013; Bruni & Porta, 2003, 2016; Castiglioni & Bennett, 2018;

Helliwell, Huang, & Wang, 2017; Helliwell, Layard, & Sachs, 2018; Marujo & Neto, 2014, 2017b; Sachs, 2018; White, 2017; Wissing, 2013). We have a threatened future in front of us, with common challenges for the species and the ecosystems, and positive psychology has a contribution to make. Indeed, the so-called Second Wave of positive psychology (Lomas, 2016; Lomas & Ivtzan, 2015) which accentuates that both the positives and negatives of life should be taken into account for the understanding of well-being, opened the path for positive psychology to make an important contribution to a better understanding of quality of life. The fine-tuning of the Second Wave means appreciatively including collective human struggles and pains – with its consequent dialogue between the positive and the negative – while simultaneously tackling the most intricate societal problems through affirmative and benign, relational and conversational, solution-oriented processes.

Recognizing that positive psychology has already contributed to explain the relationship between subjective wellbeing, and global political and social issues - such as the role of corruption, income levels, unemployment, good governance, strong political institutions, quality of natural environment, democratic participation, social trust, sustainable behavior, migration, among others (e.g. Biswas-Diener & Patterson, 2011; Curral-Verdugo, Navas, Goméz, & Schalock, 2012; Diener & Diener, 2011; Helliwell, Huang & Wang, 2016; Helliwell et al., 2018; Kasser, 2011; Layard, 2005; Veenhoven, 2016, 2017a), the field is already prepared to more explicitly and decisively embrace social issues and common goals such as universal human rights, equality, global peace, intercultural citizenship, ecological protection, and other universal and inalienable human and environmental entitlements.

Universal human rights may be understood as "basic rights protecting fundamental freedoms and human dignity, to which we are all entitled, regardless of nationality, gender, ethnicity, religion, language, or other status" (Twose & Cohrs, 2015, p. 3). Environmental human rights are now tentatively being added to the debate. If the major responsibility for their implementation lies with governments, who must fulfill, respect and safeguard them to the best of their capability (Keita, 2012), it is also at the fundamental relational, organizational and community level that they may be operationalized. Furthermore, an emphasis on collective, peoples' rights has to be added to the individualist Western focus, and a better balance between individual and collective rights is needed for the human rights to serve as a world foundation (Galtung, 2017). As examples, we have "the right of villages to survive as human habitats, the right of traditional crafts to survive, and the rights of clans and tribes to be recognized as collective actors" (Galtung, 2017, p. 7).

However, it is not only about human rights, but also about ethics. According to Velasquez, Andre, Shanks, Meyer, and Meyer (2014) contemporary ethicists defined the common good as general conditions that are equally to everyone's advantage, or as as "the sum of those conditions of social life which allow social groups and their individual members relatively thorough and ready access to their own fulfillment" (Velasquez et al., 2014: p. 1). The common good refers thus to the functioning of social systems, organizations, and environments in a way that all people can depend on them and benefit from them. For example "accessible and affordable public health care system, and effective system of public safety and security, peace among the nations of the world, a just legal and political system, and unpolluted natural environment, and a flourishing economic system" (Velasquez et al., 2014: p. 2). The common good, however, does not happen by itself: it requires the efforts and cooperation of people which can sometimes have different ideas about what is important, what the good life for humans constitutes, or some taking a free-ride while others carry the burden of sacrifices. Even if people agree upon what is valuable, they may differ about the relative values of things. Despite possible obstacles, a focus on the common good helps us to reflect on questions about the kind of society we want to have, how we may achieve it, and what our own and joint roles in these processes can be. We propose that one way is through meaningful conversations.

Research on human rights from the point of view of psychology has long been scarce, as defended in July of 2012 by Ms. Navi Pillay (2012), United Nations High Commissioner for Human Rights, in her keynote speech at the International Congress of Psychology in Cape Town, South Africa. She admitted that psychology and human rights have long been separate grounds, expecting and wishing more cooperation among them. That is unfortunate, since some data from the scant research on the topic is indeed interesting, namely showing that people cognitively represent human rights similarly across cultures (Doise, 2004; Doise, Spini, & Clémence, 1999), and that the more knowledge people have of human rights, and the more imperative they consider them, the more they report behavioural tendencies – intentions and effective behaviour – aimed at human rights endorsement (Cohrs & Boehnke, 2008). Amid other repercussions, these outcomes support the identification of the approaches that human rights education and policies can use to increase constructive results on individuals' behavioural support for human rights (Cohrs, Maes, Kielmann, & Moschner, 2007). For instance, Stellmacher, Sommer, and Brähler (2005) showed that even four or five sessions of human rights education can serve to expand individuals' knowledge of, and attitudes to, human rights. They highlight the importance of human rights education – which itself is a human right – for the expansion of cultures of harmony, wellbeing and peace.

In positive psychology, in particular, human rights, environmental rights, and the UN Sustainable Development Goals (SDGs) have not been present or are disarticulated. Nonetheless, those topics can be found in worldwide contemporary research such as the Global Happiness Policy Report (2018) and the World Happiness Report (2018). We can also find a few publications aiming for social change, marginalized populations, and peace (i.e., Biswas-Diener, 2011; Biswas-Diener, Linley, Govindji, & Woolston, 2011; Castiglioni & Bennett, 2018; Cohrs, Christie, White, & Das, 2013; Diener & Tov, 2007; Marujo & Neto, 2014; Shapiro, Bilali, & Vollhardt, 2009).

For the authors of this chapter, the Second Wave in positive psychology means taking the positives and negatives of life into account, and thereby contributing to high human sustainable development objectives, and doing so through conversations. Language is therefore considered social action, and particular conversations are seen as carriers of meanings that are constitutive of our worlds. During conversations, people create a co-propriety – with the ones in conversation and the context in which they relate – and develop a communal rationality (Delgado-Raak, in press). Social change is therefore recognized as a relational process of co-construction that allows for the emergence of a socially creative process.

Consequently, there is a relational responsibility emerging (McNamee & Gergen, 1998), which should, skillfully, create empowering environments, with "high-strengths density and a prospective, future forming power" (Cooperrider, 2018, p. 9). Featuring the idea that communication is a systemic process of making meaning in social interaction through coordination, quality conversations surface as a way of participating in the creation of better social worlds (Rascon & Littlejohn, 2017). To live a good and just life is not to step outside of relationships, but to participate and contribute totally within them.

Hence, this chapter argues that wellbeing must be addressed at the public sphere, and not only at an intra-personal and self-scrutiny level, advocating for relational wellbeing through conversations among individuals, societies and cultures, and considering them as carriers of meanings through coordination of world views.

6.2 The Social Foundations of Our Common Wellbeing: When Relationships Come First

> To bother to engage with problematic culture, and problematic people within that culture, is an act of love. Alexande (2007, online)

Although recognizing that positive psychology is in itself a force for good, advocates and critics of the celebration of the individual, or a self-centered wellbeing, assert that the intense increase of focus on happiness is a response to emotional capitalism and distant intimacies, with its particular individualized tendencies to satisfy the self (White, 2017). When we look at the individual in isolation, we suppress the other. Several social pathologies and diversified conflicts can be a consequence of this individualized way of looking at humanity. This inclination brings a consequent divide among citizens and the feebleness of the civil society, due to market capitalism, and the result is the corrosion of the social drapery (Bruni & Porta, 2016; Bruni & Stanca, 2008). Individual views on people, their actions and techniques can bring dehumanization (McNamee, 2015), since they endorse a divisive approach among people. Some governments and social structures may make people happier, but not better persons (Etzioni, 2018). The reason why Etzioni (2018) defends that satisfaction is the wrong metric, unless it is combined with an evaluation of the magnitude to which those structures and regimes additionally promote a good life for the commons.

The affirming of the self-development and self-care movements, also entrenched in an individualistic perspective, reinforced a non-relational, individualistic view, and eventually, positive psychology and the happiness studies had their share on the promotion of this ideology (White, 2017). The "I-First" mentality, that reinforces individual control and the perfection of the being, can also contribute to alienation and domination, identifying relationships with other human beings and the planet as secondary and instrumental (Gergen, 2011). The future of our planet and of humanity may be dependent of the caring that we dedicate to relational processes (Gergen, op. cit.).

These objections with the individualistic view are being currently complemented by a rising body of scholarship investigating the communal basis of a life with quality. Offering fresh ways of examining positive human social life, some authors propose solutions that include the renaissance of the community and its strong social belongings, and the emphasis on the common good as a way to plan and live a different type of wellbeing - where justice, fraternity, peace, freedom, intercultural citizenship and meaningful social engagement build connections and generate positive and transformational change (Bruni, 2016; Castiglioni & Bennett, 2018; Etzioni, 2013, 2018; Nelson & Prilleltensky, 2010; Prilleltensky, 2012; White, 2017). So, the idea of happiness moves gradually in the direction of a relational and dynamic process – something we do with, and for, other human creatures and the Common Home – and less for "what we feel", "who we are" or "what we have", thereby experiencing meaning in life and giving meaning to life. Delle Fave and Soosai-Nathan (2014) argued that meanings are made in inter-connectedness. The move in positive psychology towards a focus on relational well-being, interconnectedness and context is also becoming a hallmark of the emerging Third Wave of positive psychology (Wissing, 2018) characterized by a strong relational ontology and acceptance of plurality of worldviews (cf., Slife, O'Grady, and Kosits, 2017), and a cosmological metatheoretical perspective as described by Nicolesco (2010, 2012, 2014, 2015a, 2015b) from a philosophy of science perspective.

In the words of Bok (2011, p. 19) "several researchers have concluded that human relationships and connections of all kinds contribute more to happiness than anything else." The "social capital" concept – that some use to refer to bonding and communal relationships – has been clearly linked with satisfaction with life (e.g., Etzioni, 2018; Putnam, 2000). Occupying time with others with whom one shares ties of kinship – in the context of family, work, church, volunteer work, neighborhoods, and communities – has repeatedly been associated with making people happier (Putnam, 1995; Sugden, 2005). Researchers who examined the effect of community participation (contrasting to purely socializing with friends or family) also found a strong association with happiness. Helliwell (2003, pp. 331–360) evaluated survey data from 49 nations, and found that membership in organizations has a significant positive correlation with happiness (but only non-church). Simply attending monthly club gatherings or volunteering – once a month – is associated with a variation in well-being equivalent to a doubling of income (Bok, 2011, p. 20). Research on meaning in life also found that the most important source for the experience of meaning in life is interpersonal relationships (e.g. Delle Fave, Brdar, Wissing, & Vella-Brodrick, 2013; Delle Fave et al., 2016; Lambert et al., 2013).

There is growing alertness for the fact that social connections may be moulded by contextual characteristics (Duany, Plater-Zyberk, & Speck, 2001; Harrel, 2018; Helne & Hirvilammi, 2015; Warren & Donaldson, 2018). Those social connections, in turn, may help to guard against environmental perils like delinquency, criminality, lawbreaking…that could weaken social cohesion, as much as the community's wellbeing (Cloutier & Pfeiffer, 2015). Recognition and appreciation by others to whom a person is attached seems to be the main source of fondness and self-value (Etzioni, 2018). But more than making the ego happy, social bonds are based on reciprocity and mutuality. It is the mutual enrichment that maintain satisfying and lasting, meaningful, affective relationships (Etzioni, op. cit.). Therefore, happiness is also a community characteristic (Adams, 1992; Cloutier & Pfeiffer; Hagerty, 2000), reinforcing the individual wellbeing, but mainly exceedingly contingent on cohesion and social relations (Cloutier & Pfeiffer; Diener & Seligman, 2002).

White (2017, op. cit., p. 131) advocates several indicators to bridge relational wellbeing with policy and politics. We list them bellow, adapting her proposal, from the point of view of what needs to be accentuated if we want to fully embrace implications of wellbeing from a relational perspective. The emphasis should be:

1. On societal structures. Its political importance is associated with resisting the tendency to shift responsibility from the collective to the individual;
2. On local context and inclusive conversation to promote broad-ranging debate. The aim is to foster a different kind of engagement, which seeks common ground and mutual interest, although not silencing wider and more profound global issues;
3. On providing a more encompassing political vision, as exemplified by indigenous *Buen Vivir* (Living well together) of some countries in South America or *Ubuntu* (I am because we are; behaving well towards others and acting in a way that benefits the community) in Africa (cf. Oviawe, 2016). Although being difficult to run away from the power and impact of global markets and worldwide economic structures, the traditional knowledge of the local people (cf. also Nwoye, 2015; Ratele, 2017; Segalo & Cakata, 2017) can be formally recognized and included in new state constitutions.
4. On re-building policies that support social relations and deepen social recognition, in particular "relational goods" – non instrumental relations with positive outcomes which 'belong' to the relationship itself, rather than to any particular party within it. Relational goods can only be produced through collaboration, and in conditions that permit real engagement with one's partners and reflexivity concerning this engagement. The proposal is that the current accommodation between the market representing the value of freedom and the state representing equality must be tempered by a strong civil society upholding the values of subsidiarity and solidarity.
5. On encouraging a more inclusive social vision. This is grounded not in the idea that people 'have' rights on the basis of which they receive a 'share', but that the share is itself rightful – that is, something that should be done 'because it is right'.

In our view, the pathways towards social transformation arise – with implications for policies, politics and quality of life – from the conversational procedures, considered the most vital mechanism for wellbeing (Cooperrider, 2018; Delgado-Raak, in press; Stavros & Torres, 2018). This can bring us to a movement of "civic maturity" (Pearce, 2001) focusing on the quality of public conversations. Processes of public dialogues tend to be moments in which the communities can find ways of moving forward together, in particular around difficult issues. Working together in dialogic communication is implanted on processes of participatory democracy (Spano,

2001). This author defines participatory democracy taking into consideration that it implies: cooperative activities to determine what the choices for us are; inclusive systems of opportunities for pursuing the public's interest and the common good; solutions developed by citizens in collaboration with governments and technical experts; the use of dialogue, deliberation and discussion to achieve an action-oriented consensus; and active citizen involvement (Spano, op. cit., p. 24). Therefore, focusing on systemic processes, social relationships and patterns of interaction, while relying on "participant" knowledge, come together with a world view of communication as a process by which we collectively make our social worlds and resolve their complexities (Pearce, 1994, 2001). It is in the multiverse of community – with all its complex tapestry – that meaningful and transformational conversations arise. Having meaningful and collaborative conversations as the norm in our communities, as a way to deal with public issues, might enhance public happiness, meaningful experiences and more harmonic ways of relating. Conversations are performative acts, and can constitute a way to create a new breed of citizenry. Therefore, the focus must prioritize a community-first approach, acknowledging the needs and concerns of local communities and inviting for grass roots engagement – where the quality of the dialogue will make the difference. Building and enriching capacities for coordinated relationships are needed for the profound transformations in the world we live in.

6.3 Embracing Meaningful Conversations at the Community Level

> It is necessary to share meaning. A society is a link of relationships among people and institutions, so that we can live together. But it only works if we have a *culture* – which implies that we share meaning; i.e., significance, purpose, and value. Otherwise it falls apart. Our society is incoherent, and doesn't do that very well; it hasn't for a long time, if it ever did. The different assumptions that people have are *tacitly* affecting the whole meaning of what we are doing. (Bohm, 1996, pp. 15–16)

Humanity is rooted in relational and dialogical processes (Anderson, 2013) and conversations lie at the heart of how we interact (Stavros & Torres, 2018). Living into our potential initiates with meaningful conversations. We are almost always engaged in internal dialogues or external interactions; hence our experiences of solitude and communion, of peace and conflict, of moral decisions and courses of actions, of research and intervention, are all imbedded in our relational and conversational selves.

The accent on the social dimensions of contemporary life are substantiated in the idea that "one becomes human in and through relationship" (Bhengu, 2006; Williams, 2003, cit. in White, 2017, p. 123), specifically within the realm of communication (Anderson, 2013). As Harré put it, "The primary human reality is persons in conversation" (Harré, 1983, p. 58). As individuals, we can see ourselves as the intersection of our relationships, which are embedded in conversations (Gergen, 2009). Conversations are the spontaneous, expressive-responsiveness of our living bodies and give us the 'background glue' that holds us together in all our relationships (Shotter, 2010) as well as on an intrapersonal level from where we react, for example, among thinking, feeling, valuing and doing). Therefore, we believe that the alchemy and quality of human communication is foundational for wellbeing and quality of life as a whole.

Etymologically, "communication ... is founded on the Latin *commun* and the suffix "ie", which is similar to "fie," in that it means "to make or to do." So one meaning of "to communicate" is "to make something common," i.e., to convey information or knowledge from one person to another in as accurate a way as possible (Nepal, 2011). According to the Online Etymology Dictionary, in 1520s communication meant, "to impart (information, etc.); to give or transmit (a quality, feeling, etc.) to another". The word comes from the Latin *communicatus*, past participle of *communicare* and means "to share, communicate, impart, inform," literally "to make common". It is the sharing of something – information, knowledge, and meaning. It is related to *communis*, meaning "common, public, general".

The meaning "to share, transmit" (diseases, etc.) is from later on, in the 1530s. The intransitive sense of "to open into each other" is from 1731.

The notion of "conversations" hence refers to reciprocal processes in relationships – that can be within an individual, between individuals, between an individual and society or/and cultural and ecosystem contexts, among individuals and groups, and between an individual and the Sacred. This is highly relevant in the African context where the traditional African worldview and spirituality is based on assumptions of interconnectedness among all things including a relationship with living people, ancestors, God and the environment. All these connections are viewed as necessary for the experience of a balanced and harmonious quality of life (Nwoye, 2017; Ogbonnaya, 1994). The alchemy of a meaningful conversation is to decrement of what is keeping us from listening to one another, and transcends those barriers to mutual understanding.

As David Bohm puts it (1996, p. 18): "In dialogue, when we have a very high energy of coherence, it might bring us beyond just being a group that could solve social problems. Possibly it could make a new change in the individual and a change in the relation to the cosmic. Such an energy has been called 'communion'." Baumeister, Maranges, and Vohs (2018) accentuated the individual as an information agent who functions based on shared meanings in a specific social environment. They opine that people use meaning to connect with others, and that being part of the social group involves learning the group's shared meanings and realities. People interact with other members in the group based on these shared meanings.

Every conversation is – should be – a polyphonic process, where multiple voices are present. Moments of dialogue remind us of how rich and complex conversations are (Delgado-Raak, in press) and how human beings depend on them to construct meaning of their worlds. We all know how unpredictable a conversation is. This unpredictability emerges from the constant process of meaning-making that characterizes it. Indeed, way beyond the standard and simplified views of dialogue as sharing information, the procedure of dialogue, that comes from the Greek word dialogos, and means "to construct the meaning of the word (logos) through (dia)" (Bohm, 1996), implies it. As such, it encompasses a post-modern way of describing dialogical conversations (Stewart & Zediker, 2000). Dialogue in different forms (political, philosophical, and dramatic) historically emerged in Ancient Greece in the context of the polis as a community of actively participating citizens (Dafermos, 2018). A well-known example in the African context is the lekgotla, which refers in South Africa to consultative process between groups pursuing a common goal. The word is from Sesotho and Setswana where it originally had the meaning of courtyard or court, or a meeting place where people will participate in village assemblies. In Botswana this public meeting place is called Kgotla, and it can be held under a tree shade or in formal building. It is viewed as one of the historically first democratic processes. In such a lekgotla the idea is that everyone is allowed a turn to speak and that no interruption may take place while a person is "having his/her say". However, it should be remembered that relationships in the traditional African context are highly hierarchical (Rugira & Sampson, 2017) and that consultative processes and meaning-making conversations mostly take place in in-group discussions where in-group versus out-group favoritism plays a role (Krueger & DiDonato, 2008).

If, as people, we understand ourselves as the intersection of our relationships (Gergen, 2009), every positive intervention could well be understood as a unique product, the result of the relationships-in-conversation that built it. Shotter, in his book "Getting it" (2011) defends that when two or more of us gather in conversations, and we interweave our actions, something unique emerges, what he calls an "it". Shotter (op. cit.) describes it as an amalgamated whole that is generated between the ones involved. Any conversation, therefore, transcends the polarity between self and others. Even talking about relationships is hard, since our language is individualistic in itself. As Bateson and Bateson proposed in 1987, western languages – or culturally dominant languages – do not predispose for debating relationships. We talk about parts, and only afterwards we talk about how they relate. Communicating coherently in truth is challenging.

In his book titled the "Pedagogy of the Oppressed" (2018), the Brazilian educator Paulo Freire defines *dialogue* as the encounter between men, mediated by the word, in order to name the world. Therefore, as he defends, dialogue cannot occur between those who want to name the world and those who do not wish this naming, nor between those who deny others the right to speak their word and those whose right has been denied them. The scarcity of a commitment with the other in our present culture is the reason why we continue to find ourselves cleaved by confrontation and paralyzed by the acrimony of "us vs. them" narratives. However, there is also a clear generative quality of relationality, which is critical to societal change and engenders a socially inclusive political vision as described by White (2017).

Being agents of personal and collective change, human beings are meaning-makers (Prilleltensky, 2012). This author suggests that those processes orbit mainly around mattering and prospering, considered dependent, correspondingly, of fairness and wellness (Prilleltensky, op. cit.). There is a lot of evidence that people will go to great lengths to pursue fairness for themselves, their loved ones, their communities, and their countries (Etzioni, 2018).

According to Bohm (1990, 1996), true dialogue must be aimed not at some immediate or practical solution but at the higher-order objective of meaning. Meaningful conversations had been shown to energize groups and communities, and engender creative opportunities and engagement (Stavros & Torres, 2018). We all know the fulfillment experienced in meaningful conversations where the spaces of self and that of others overlap in a real dialogue. Meaningful conversations inspire cooperative action that can have a positive influence for persons and all kind of systems, from friendships and enterprises to neighborhoods and nations. The metaphor behind conversational dialogues is of a flowing stream of meaning among and through persons (Bohm, 1996), which may allow for the emergence of a new kind of common reality and understanding – that might not be there from the beginning, but is given birth by the conversation itself. It is a shared meaning that holds communities and nations together. "As we talk together the question of what, if anything, its purpose is keeps arising (…) None of the purposes is fixed because we find that as we go further into it the purpose begins to change; we discover a new purpose, and so on. So really, when we set a purpose, we set it only as a beginning, as a point of departure, not as a purpose we hold to. This is the crucial point (…). Purpose flows out of significance and value and that's what we're exploring. We expect that meaning is going to change through our learning as we go along and therefore purpose changes naturally" (Bohm, 1990, p. 1). Communication is itself the reciprocal construction of meaning (Von Glasersfeld, 2003), paving the way for people to coordinate targets with clarification (Castiglioni & Bennett, 2018).

Political participation yields the fertility of connecting with the richness of meaningful activities, in particular when the political climate is perceived as fair (Etzioni, 2013, 2018). In the words of Frey and Stutzer (2000, p. 82), "Citizens do not only gain utility from the outcome of the political process and its material consequences but also from the democratic process itself". This means being duty-bound and acting in a universalistic way, acts that need trusting relationships with others, what Wong (1988, p. 327) calls "particularistic relations". It follows that the more people build new communities, consolidate or renovate their bonds to a community, in particular in the post-affluent societies, the more reallocation of abundance can be expected; and the more the communitarian beliefs are encompassed, the more social justice one can anticipate (Etzioni, 2018). A shift from a prosperous society to a communitarian one will enable major gains in social justice.

6.4 Coordinated Meaningful Conversations for Global Peace: Unpacking the Collective Meaning

> Peace and dialogue are fundamentally interdependent. Audrey Azoulay, Director-General of UNESCO (2018, p. 8)

In light of the above observations, it is our conviction that positive psychology has the potential to offer comprehensive theoretical foundations to questions of peace. Additionally, we believe that all the work done so far on peace studies can enrich the field of positive psychology. We hope to assist in showing that positive psychology can indeed venture, and does well, to deal with such socially important topics.

6.4.1 But Why Peace?

Peace is anybody's agenda, and it is hard to be all out against peace (Galtung, 1969). The idea of peace has long been proposed as one of the most esteemed goals of humanity, a fundamental requirement to accomplishing its potential for stable and thriving societies (Puyana et al., 2018) and dearly needed in the African context. Being a continuous and hard process, the aim of living together in harmony has been at the core of the mandate of the United Nations system for more than 70 years (Azoulay, 2018). Creating actions, structures and institutions for peace is therefore a social driving force that requires constant attention and effort, even if and when peace seems an intangible and impossible goal.

Notwithstanding its universal charm, the complexity and dynamism of peace, and its context-driven imperative, has been defying a common definition (Anderson, 2004). The most currently used definitions show that peace is not only about war and large-scale violence, but also about poverty alleviation, women's empowering, endorsing the potential of younger generations, social justice and equality (Puyana et al., 2018). It is about environmental, cultural and health affairs, where the arts, humanities, sports, legacy, have a place (Puyana, op. cit.). The current concept of "sustainable peace" is interrelated organically with the United Nations Sustainable Development Goals (SDGs), offering a holistic approach where prevention of negative peace and promotion of positive peace are vital.

The development of the peace concept progressed from the universal spectrum of liberal theories to national or local ownership (Puyana et al., 2018), discounting the narrow application of a singular notion of peace and defending "many and plural *peaces*" (Dietrich, 2012). Hence, it is not surprising that its trajectory of definitions has long been complex. According to the conceptualization of Johan Galtung, the father of the peace studies, we can talk about two distinct types of peace. The first one is the absence of direct, or explicit, violence between states and between social groups. This somewhat narrow conception of peace has been entitled "negative peace" (Galtung, 1969). However, a society can still be violent, and thus not peaceful, without manifest violence, if it is structurally oppressive and does not provide fair and good conditions of living (Cohrs & Boehnke, 2008). So, inspired in Mahatma Gandhi's vision of active non-violence, and on concepts such as "just peace", "quality of peace", "local turn", "development and human security", and conflict transformation, coined by several authors (Puyana et al., 2018), a broader meaning of peace emerged later on. It underscored the absence of structural violence, namely systematic oppression – that inhibits people from attaining the accomplishment of all their potentials – and the manifestation of social justice (Galtung, 1969). This type of peace is called "positive peace" (Cohrs & Boehnke, 2008).

Consequently, albeit the contradictions and the limitations in finding universally accepted definitions, and valid ontologies and methodologies, specialists tend to consider that we can emphasize either the obstacles to peace (the ones accountable for direct, overt or structural violence) or the facilitators of peace (the features encouraging nonviolence and social fairness). In psychology, research falling into these classes has emerged, a large portion of which relevant to the impediments to negative peace and therefore concentrating on the causes, intermediaries, and courses of aggression, both at the interpersonal level and at the intergroup level (Cohrs & Boehnke, 2008). This is exemplified by studying the support for military interventions as an obstacle to negative peace. Catalysts of negative peace mainly deal with approaches and methods intended at decreasing violence and aggression. Again, this includes the interpersonal and the intergroup levels, and anti-war activism is an example. The research on obstacles to positive peace have been mainly focused on the ailments and courses accountable for the establishment and upholding of different forms of social inequality and injustice, an example of which is understanding ideologies legitimizing those practices. This research also helps to inform strategies for the reduction of structural violence and the development of positive peace. Such strategies and processes can lead to the advancement of social justice, like the commitment to human rights, liberation psychology with its aim of social transformation and emancipation, interventions on moral emotions (for instance, courage), and prosocial commitments (Cohrs & Boehnke, 2008).

To enrich the fields of positive psychology and quality of life studies, and to contribute to broader community efforts, the authors of this chapter have been interested in the concept of positive peace, in particular in its catalysts. There is a need to work around conversational interventions that can bring forward quality of life facilitators, at the subjective and objective levels, and therefore much more is needed in an African context to enhance quality of life. Thus far focus has been on identifying context-specific participative methods as a starting point for sustaining positive peace, making it primarily a local process, best undertaken through national and cultural policies, and local actors (MacNair, 2006; Marujo & Neto, 2017b; Puyana et al., 2018). We need critical and emancipatory discourses on peace, in particular around the "local turn", that is, the imperative of local ownership of building peace, through a multi-dimensional contribution. Varied areas – human rights protection, environment preservation, sustainable development, gender equality, justice – are currently identified as peace work, and lie at the fore of emerging discourses on peace (Puyana et al., 2018, p. 25) and positive psychology should become one of them, to help broaden and deepen the approach to global peace and also the deeply needed positive quality of life in African contexts. It is our opinion that we can contribute to positive and harmonious microcultures through community conversational interventions. Language serves relationships, and meaning is fabricated in the to-and-fro process in which together we name, define, qualify, and embed lives in other individual and collective stories.

Conversations are not always benign and transformative – they can ignite the worst of human experience – and behaviour that is prosocial is not necessary moral (Etzioni, 2018). Moral dialogues are dialogues that permit to form new common moral considerations to the common good. Characteristically, these social procedures may be vehement, anarchic, and do not have a well-defined beginning, nor an end. Yet, they regularly do promote deep and thoughtful transformations in the moral views – not in values – of the ones who are involved in them (Etzioni, 2018). They change the moral positions of an adequate amount of people so that activities, policies and programs that formerly had little or no backing (e.g. alternative energies, anti-corruption laws), and agendas contemplated as morally inadequate by numerous (e.g. same-sex marriage) profit with pervasive moral endorsement (Etzioni, op. cit.).

Further understanding meaningful conversations on a social and community level that will be to the greater good and a high quality of life in an African context is an open area for further research.

6.5 Conclusion

Positive psychology is inescapably a social force, and is now being asked to take its social vision to a whole new level, reaching larger groups of people, progressing towards higher forms of social accountability, committing to the collective liability to create conditions for nurturing the strengths of everyone, and to harness those strengths for the subsidy of the wider society (Marques, 2015). Such endeavors should include attention from material and environmental aspects of quality of life to subjective wellbeing, values and what is to the greater good.

We continue to over-consume the resources of the world, to create inequality and injustice, and to generate power struggles and anger. We are frequently living without soul and substance in our homes, classrooms, and offices. All these jeopardies are a call-for-action in the direction of a cohesive, compassionate and caring society. Let's not be overwhelmed by the state of our world. Instead, it is time to get together in conversations that matter, considering the loci of change and responsibility from within the individual towards community well-being, empowering populations, and developing positive reciprocal relationships, therefore renewing possibilities to enhance the quality of our conjoint lives, especially in the diverse African contexts.

As asserted by Pearce and Pearce (2000, p. 423), "The reconstruction of contexts, and most other things worth doing, cannot be done unilaterally or in a single act. Social change, just like its apparent opposite social order, is co-constructed in a recursive process that re-constructs us as persons, relationships, and institutions." The protection of human rights in general, and of peace in particular, may contribute to the advancement of wellbeing, so much more research is needed on the quality of life as experienced in communal meaning-making. For historical, cultural and social reasons, Africa can undoubtedly be a privileged territory to explore and innovate on this realm, and inspire new ways to put positive psychology serving humanity.

References

Adams, R. E. (1992). Is happiness a home in the suburbs? The influence of urban versus suburban neighborhoods on psychological health. *Journal of Community Psychology, 20*(4), 353–372.

Alexander, E. (2007). *Power and possibility: Essays, reviews, and interviews*. Ann Arbor, MI: University of Michigan Press. Quoted by M. Popova in: *Elizabeth Alexander on Writing, the Ethic of Love, Language as a Vehicle for the Self, and the Inherent Poetry of Personhood*. https://www.brainpickings.org/2016/05/24/elizabeth-alexander-power-and-possibility-writing/

Anderson, R. (2004). A definition of peace. *Journal of Peace Psychology, 10*, 101–116.

Anderson, H. (2013). Listening, hearing and speaking: *Brief thoughts on collaborative-dialogue. Ways of being "with" ourselves and others*. Non published publication. Retrieved from https://www.taosinstitute.net/Websites/taos/files/Content/5692909/Listen,_Hear_and_Speak_for_Opinions_-_Anderson,_H.pdf

Azoulay, A. (2018). Foreword. In D. F. Puyana et al. (Eds.),. (Coordination, Editorial and Review Team) *Long walk to peace: Towards a culture of prevention*. Paris, France: United Nations Educational, Scientific and Cultural Organization.

Bateson, G., & Bateson, M. C. (1987). *Angels fear: Towards and epistemology of the sacred*. New York, NY: Macmillan Publishing.

Baumeister, R. F., Maranges, H. M., & Vohs, K. D. (2018). Human self as information agent: Functioning in a social environment based on shared meanings. *Review of General Psychology, 22*(1), 36–47. https://doi.org/10.1037/gpr0000114

Bhengu, M. J. (2006). *Ubuntu: The global philosophy for humankind*. Cape Town, South Africa: Lotsha Publication.

Biswas-Diener, R. (2011). Positive psychology as social change. Positive psychology and poverty. R. Biswas-Diener, Positive psychology as social change (125–140). New York, NY: Springer.

Biswas-Diener, R., & Patterson, L. (2011). An experiential approach to teaching positive psychology to undergraduates. *The Journal of Positive Psychology, 6*(6), 477–481. https://doi.org/10.1080/17439760.2011.634818

Biswas-Diener, R., Linley, P. A., Govindji, R., & Woolston, L. (2011). Positive psychology as a force for social change. In K. M. Sheldon, T. B. Kashdan, & M. M. F. Steger (Eds.), *Designing positive psychology: Taking stock and moving forward* (pp. 410–418). New York, NY: Oxford.

Bohm, D. (1990). *On meaning, purpose, and exploration in dialogue*. Retrieved from http://www.david-bohm.net/dialogue/dialogue_exploration.html

Bohm, D. (1996). *On dialogue*. New York, NY: Routledge.

Bok, D. (2011). *The politics of happiness: What government can learn from the new research on well-being*. Princeton, NY: Princeton University Press.

Bruni, L. (2013). Relational goods: A new tool for an old issue. *Estudos Contemporâneos da Subjetividade—ECOS, Thematic Issue on Positive Psychology and Public Happiness, 3*(2), 173–178.

Bruni, L. (2016). Economics, well-being and happiness: History and protagonists. In L. Bruni & P. L. Porta (Eds.), *Handbook of research methods and applications in happiness and quality of life* (pp. 334–348). Cheltenham, UK: Edward Elgar Publishing.

Bruni, L., & Porta, L. (2003). Economia civile and Pubblica felicità in the Italian Enlightnment. *History of Political Economy, 35*(Supplement 1), 361–385.

Bruni, L., & Porta, P. L. (2016). Happiness and quality of life reconciled. In L. Bruni & P. L. Porta (Eds.), *Handbook of research methods and applications in happiness and quality of life* (pp. 1–19). Cheltenham, UK: Edward Elgar Publishing.

Bruni, L., & Stanca, L. (2008). Watching alone: Relational goods, television and happiness. *Journal of Economic Behavior & Organization, 65*(3–4), 506–528.

Castiglioni, I., & Bennett, M. J. (2018). Building capacity for intercultural citizenship. *Open Journal of Social Sciences, 6*, 229–241.

Cloutier, S & Pfeiffer, D. (2015, September/October). Sustainability through happiness: A framework for sustainable development. Sustainable Development, 23(5), 317–327.

Cohrs, J. C., & Boehnke, K. (2008). Social psychology and peace: An introductory overview. *Social Psychology, 39*(1), 4–11.

Cohrs, J. C., Maes, J., Kielmann, S., & Moschner, B. (2007). Determinants of human rights attitudes and behavior: A comparison and integration of psychological perspectives. *Political Psychology, 28*, 441–469.

Cohrs, J. C., Christie, D. J., White, M. P., & Das, C. (2013). Contributes of positive psychology to peace: Toward global well-being and resilience. *American Psychological Association, 68*(7), 590–600.

Cooperrider, D. (2018). Introduction. In J. Stravos & C. Torres (Eds.), *Conversations worth having: Using appreciative inquiry to fuel productive and meaningful engagement* (pp. 1–11). Oakland, CA: Berrett-Koehler.

Curral-Verdugo, M. A., Navas, P., Goméz, L. E., & Schalock, R. L. (2012). The concept of quality of life and its role in enhancing human rights in the field of intellectual disability. *Journal of Intellectual Disabilities Research, 56*(11), 1036–1045.

Dafermos, M. (2018). *Relating dialogue and dialectics: A philosophical perspective*. Retrieved from: https://www.researchgate.net/publication/322256241_Relating_dialogue_and_dialectics_a_philosophical_perspective

Delgado-Raak, G. (in press). *Relaciones pasadas: Explorando sus potencialidades. Conversaciones sobre el impacto de nuestras relaciones passadas em el yo relacional.* Tese apresentada para a obtenção do Grau de Doutoramento na Universitat Ramon Llull, Espanha.

Delle Fave, A., & Soosai-Nathan, L. (2014). Meaning as inter-connectedness: Theoretical perspectives and empirical evidence. *Journal of Psychology in Africa. Special Issue: Meaning and Relational Well-Being, 24*(1), 33–43. https://doi.org/10.1080/14330237.2014.904090

Delle Fave, A., Brdar, I., Wissing, M. P., & Vella-Brodrick, D. A. (2013). Sources and motives for personal meaning in adulthood. *Journal of Positive Psychology, 8*(6), 517–529. https://doi.org/10.1080/17439760.2013.830761

Delle Fave, A., Brdar, I., Wissing, M. P., Araujo, U., Castro Solano, A., Freire, T., … Soosai-Nathan, L. (2016). Lay definitions of happiness across nations: The primacy of inner harmony and relational connectedness. *Frontiers in Psychology, 7*, 30. doi:https://doi.org/10.3389/fpsyg.2016.00030

Diener, E. (2000). Subjective well-being: The science of happiness and a proposal for a national index. *American Psychologist, 55*(1), 34.

Diener, E., & Diener, C. (2011). Monitoring psychosocial prosperity for social change. In R. Biswas-Diener (Ed.), *Positive psychology as social change* (pp. 53–72). Dordrecht, The Netherlands: Springer.

Diener, E., & Seligman, M. E. (2002). Very happy people. *Psychological Science, 13*, 81–84.

Diener, E., & Tov, W. (2007). Subjective well-being and peace. *Journal of Social Issues, 63*, 421–440.

Diener, E., Heintzelman, S. J., Kushlev, K., Tay, L., Wirtz, D., Lutes, L. D., & Oishi, S. (2017). Findings all psychologists should know from the new science on subjective well-being. *Canadian Psychology/Psychologie Canadienne, 58*(2), 87–104.

Dietrich, W. (2012). *Interpretations of peace in history and culture* (Many Places, 1). London, UK: Palgrave Macmillan.

Doise, W. (2004). *Human rights as social representations*. London, UK: Taylor & Francis.

Doise, W., Spini, D., & Clémence, A. (1999). Human rights studied as social representations in a cross-national context. *European Journal of Social Psychology, 29*(1), 1–29.

Duany, A., Plater-Zyberk, E., & Speck, J. (2001). *Suburban nation: The rise of sprawl and the decline of the American Dream*. New York, NY: Macmillan.

Eid, M., & Diener, E. (2006). *Handbook of multimethod measurement in psychology*. Washington, DC: American Psychological Association.

Etzioni, A. (2013). The bankruptcy of liberalism and conservatism. *Political Science Quarterly, 128*(1), 39–65.

Etzioni, A. (2018). *Happiness is the wrong metric: A liberal communitarian response to populism*. Dordrecht, The Netherlands: Springer.

Freire, P. (2018). Pedagogy of the oppressed. *Economic Journal, 110*(466), 918–938.

Frey, B., & Stutzer, A. (2000). *Happiness, economy and institutions* (CESifo Working Paper Series 246). Munich, Germany: CESifo Group.

Galtung, J. (1969). Violence, peace, and peace research. *Journal of Peace Research, 6*(3), 167–191.

Galtung, J. (2017). *Peace: A peace practitioner's guide*. University for Peace. Retrieved from https://www.upeace.org/uploads/file/Ideas%20for%20Peace%20Vol.%2013.pdf

Gergen, K. J. (2009). *Relational being; beyond self and community*. Oxford, UK: Oxford University Press.

Gergen, K. J. (2011). Relational being: A brief introduction. *Journal of Constructivist Psychology, 24*, 280–282.

Global Happiness Policy Report. (2018). Accessed 3 Aug 2018. http://digitallibrary.unic.org.in/TempPdfFiles/986_1.pdf

Hagerty, M. R. (2000). Social comparisons of income in one's community: Evidence from national surveys of income and happiness. *Journal of Personality and Social Psychology, 78*(4), 764.

Harré, R. (1983). *The self as a theoretical concept. Relativism: Interpretation and confrontation* (pp. 387–417). Notre Dame, IN: University of Notre Dame Press.

Harrell, S. (2018). "Being human together": Positive relationships in the context of diversity, culture, and collective well-being. In M. A. Warren & S. I. Donaldson (Eds.), *Toward a positive psychology of relationships:*

New directions in theory and research. Santa Barbara, CA: Preager.
Helliwell, J. F. (2003). How's life? Combining individual and national variables to explain subjective well-being. *Economic Modelling, 20*, 331–360.
Helliwell, J. F., Huang, H., & Wang, S. (2016). *New evidence on trust and well-being* (NBER Working Paper no. 22450). Cambridge, MA: National Bureau of Economic Research.
Helliwell, J., Huang, H., & Wang, S. (2017). Social foundations of world happiness. In J. Helliwell, R. Layard, & J. Sachs (Eds.), *World happiness report 2017* (pp. 8–47). New York, NY: UN Sustainable Development Solutions Network.
Helliwell, J., Layard, R., & Sachs, J. (2018). *World happiness report*. New York, NY: UN Sustainable Development Solutions Network.
Helne, T., & Hirvilammi, T. (2015). Wellbeing and sustainability: A relational approach. *Sustainable Development, 23*(3), 167–175.
Inglehart, R., Foa, R., Peterson, C., & Welzel, C. (2008). Development, freedom, and rising happiness. *Perspectives on Psychological Science, 3*, 264–285.
Kasser, T. (2011). Ecological challenges, materialistic values, and social change. In R. Biswas-Diener (Ed.), *Positive psychology as social change* (pp. 89–108). New York, NY: Springer.
Keita, G. (2012). *An effective champion: APA public interest human rights initiatives*. Paper presented at the Society for the Psychological Study of Social Issues Conference, Charlotte, NC.
Krueger, J. I., & Di Donato, T. E. (2008). Social categorization and the perception of groups and group differences. *Social and Personality Psychology Compass, 2*, 733–750.
Lambert, N. M., Stillman, T. F., Hicks, J. A., Kamble, S., Baumeister, R. E., & Fincham, F. D. (2013). To belong is to matter: Sense of belonging enhances meaning in life. *Personality and Social Psychology Bulletin, 39*(11), 1418–1427. https://doi.org/10.1177/0146167213499186
Layard, R. (2005). *Happiness: Lessons from a new science*. London, UK: Allen Lane.
Lomas, T. (2016). Positive psychology – the second wave. *The Psychologist, 29*, 536–539.
Lomas, T., & Ivtzan, I. (2015). Second wave positive psychology: Exploring the positive-negative dialectics of wellbeing. *Journal of Happiness Studies, 16*, 1–16. https://doi.org/10.1007/s10902-015-9668-y
MacNair, R. M. (2006). *Working for peace: A handbook of practical and other tools*. California, CA: Impact Publishers.
Mahali, A., Lynch, L., Wilson Fadiji, A., Tolla, T., Khumalo, S., & Naicker, S. (2018). Networks of well-being in the Global South: A critical review of current scholarship. *Journal of Developing Societies, 25*, 1–28. https://doi.org/10.1177/0169796X18786137
Marques, A. (2015). *Social change and positive psychology*. Retrieved from http://www.thepositivepsychologypeople.com/social-change-and-positive-psychology/
Marujo, H. Á., & Neto, L. M. (2013). *Positive nations and communities: Collective, qualitative and cultural sensitive processes in positive psychology*. Dordrecht, The Netherlands: Springer.
Marujo, H. Á., & Neto, L. M. (2014). Felicitas Publica and community well-being: Nourishing relational goods through dialogic conversations between deprived and privileged populations. *Journal of Psychology in Africa, 24*(1), 161–181.
Marujo, H. Á., & Neto, L. M. (2017a). Exploring the concept and practices of Felicitas Publica at Lisbon University: A community and relational approach to well-being. In G. Tonon (Ed.), *Community quality of life and well-being in Latin countries* (pp. 67–89). Dordrecht, The Netherlands: Springer.
Marujo, H. Á., & Neto, L. M. (2017b). Creating peace: The education for global peace sustainability project. *Gaudium Sciendi, 12*, Junho. Retrieved from http://www2.ucp.pt/resources/Documentos/SCUCP/GaudiumSciendi/GaudiumSciendi_N12/08.%20Education%20for%20Global%20Peace.pdf
McNamee, S. (2015). *Abup talks: Radical presence*. Retrieved from http://www.abup.no/sheila-mcnamee/
McNamee, S., & Gergen, K. J. (1998). *Relational responsibility*. Thousand Oaks, CA: Sage.
Nelson, G. B., & Prilleltensky, I. (2010). *Community psychology: In pursuit of liberation and well-being* (2nd ed.). New York, NY: Palgrave Macmillan.
Nepal, A. (2011). *Communication*. Retrieved from http://nepalicommunication.blogspot.com/2011/01/origin-of-word.html
Nicolescu, B. (2010). Methodology of transdisciplinarity – levels of reality, logic of the included middle and complexity. *Transdisciplinary Journal of Engineering & Science, 1*(1), 19–38.
Nicolescu, B. (2012). Transdisciplinarity: The hidden third, between the subject and the object. *Human & Social Studies, 1*(2), 13–28. https://doi.org/10.2478/v10317-012-0002-5
Nicolescu, B. (2014). *From modernity to cosmodernity: Science, culture, and spirituality*. Albany, NY: State University of New York Press.
Nicolescu, B. (2015a). The hidden third and the multiple splendor of being. V. Bazhanov, R. W. Scholz, Transdisciplinarity in philosophy and science: Approaches, problems, prospects (62–79). Moscow, Russia, Russia Navigator.
Nicolescu, B. (2015b). Transdisciplinary methodology of the dialogue between people, cultures, and spiritualities. *Human & Social Studies, 4*(2), 15–28. https://doi.org/10.1515/hssr-2015-0011
Nwoye, A. (2015). What is African psychology the psychology of? *Theory & Psychology, 25*(1), 96–116. https://doi.org/10.1177/0959354314565116
Nwoye, A. (2017). An Africentric theory of human personhood. *Psychology in Society, 54*, 42–66.
Ogbonnaya, A. O. (1994). *On communitarian divinity an African interpretation of the Trinity*. New York, NY: Paragon House.

Oviawe, J. (2016). How to rediscover the Ubuntu paradigm in education. *International Review of Education, 62*(1), 1–10. https://doi.org/10.1007/s11159-016-9545-x

Pearce, W. B. (1994). *Interpersonal communication: Making social words*. New York, NY: HarperCollins.

Pearce, W. B. (2001). *Civic maturity: Musings about a metaphor.* Proceedings Fielding Graduate Institute, Action Research Symposium, Alexandria, VA.

Pearce, W. B., & Pearce, K. A. (2000). Extending the theory of the coordinated management of meaning ("CMM") through a community dialogue process. *Communication Theory, 10*, 405–423.

Pillay, N. (2012). Nexus of human rights and psychology: How they serve humanity. *Keynote address* presented at the 30th International Congress of Psychology, Cape Town, South Africa. Retrieved from https://www.div52.org/images/PDF/D52-IPB/ipb_2012-16-4-fall.pdf

Prilleltensky, I. (2012). Wellness as fairness. *American Journal of Community Psychology, 49*, 1–21.

Putnam, R. D. (1995). Bowling alone: America's declining social capital. *Journal of Democracy, 6*(1), 65–78.

Putnam, R. D. (2000). *Bowling alone: The collapse and revival of American community*. New York, NY: Simon & Schuster.

Puyana, D. F., et al.. (Coordination, Editorial and Review Team)(2018). *Long walk to peace: Towards a culture of prevention*. Paris, France: United Nations Educational, Scientific and Cultural Organization, UNESCO.

Rascon, N. A., & Littlejohn, S. (2017). *Coordinated Management of Meaning (CMM): A research manual*. New Mexico, TX: Taos Institute Publications.

Ratele, K. (2017). Frequently asked questions about African psychology. *South Africa Journal of Psychology, 47*(3), 273–227. https://doi.org/10.1177/0081246317703249

Rojas, M. (2018). *Happiness in Latin America has social foundations*. Retrieved from https://s3.amazonaws.com/happiness-report/2018/CH6-WHR-lr.pdf

Rugira, J., & Sampson, S. (2017). The Relationship between family values and ethnonationalism in relation to East Africa (Sub-Saharan). *Acta Psychopathologica, 3*, 35. https://doi.org/10.4172/2469-6676.100107

Sachs, J. (2018). Good governance in the 21st century. In *Global happiness policy report 2018*. New York, NY: Sustainable Development Solutions Network.

Segalo, P., & Cakata, Z. (2017). A psychology in our own language: Redefining psychology in an African context. *PINS, 54*, 29–41. https://doi.org/10.17159/2309-8708/2017/n54a3

Shapiro, I., Bilali, R., & Vollhardt, J. (2009). Peace. In S. J. Lopez (Ed.), *The encyclopedia of positive psychology* (Vol. 2, pp. 672–676). Malden, MA: Wiley-Blackwell.

Shotter, J. (2010). *Social constructionism on the edge: "Witness"-thinking and embodiment*. Chagrin Falls, OH: Taos Institute Publications.

Shotter, J. (2011). *Getting it: Witness-thinking and the dialogical…in practice*. New York, NY: Hampton Press.

Slife, B. D., O'Grady, K. A., & Kosits, R. D. (2017). *The hidden worldviews of psychology's theory, research, and practice*. New York, NY: Routledge.

Spano, S. (2001). *Public dialogue and participatory democracy: The Cupertino community project*. Cresskill, NJ: Hamptom Pres.

Stavros, J., & Torres, C. (2018). *Conversations worth having: Using appreciative inquiry to fuel productive and meaningful engagement*. Oakland, CA: Berrett-Koehler Publishers.

Stellmacher, J., Sommer, G., & Brahler, E. (2005). The cognitive representation of human rights: Knowledge, importance, and commitment. *Peace and Conflict, 11*, 267–292.

Stewart, J., & Zediker, K. (2000). Dialogue and tensional, ethical practices. *Southern Communication Journal, 65*, 224–242.

Sugden, R. (2005). Correspondence of sentiments: An explanation of the pleasure of social interaction. In L. Bruni & P. L. Porta (Eds.), *Economics and happiness: Framing the analysis* (pp. 97–98). New York, NY: Oxford University Press.

Twose, G., & Cohrs, J. C. (2015). Psychology and human rights: Introduction to the special issue. *Peace and Conflict: Journal of Peace Psychology, 21*(1), 3–9.

Veenhoven, R. (2016). Quality of life and happiness: Concepts and measures. In L. Bruni & P. L. Porta (Eds.), *Handbook of research methods and applications on happiness and quality of life* (pp. 309–333). Cheltenham, UK: Edward Elgar Publising.

Veenhoven, R. (2017a). Measures of happiness: Which to choose? In G. Brulé & F. Maggino (Eds.), *Metrics of subjective well-being: Limits and improvements*. Dordrecht, The Netherlands: Springer.

Veenhoven, R. (2017b). *World database of Happiness: Archive of research findings on subjective enjoyment of life Erasmus University Rotterdam, Netherlands*. Available at https://worlddatabaseofhappiness.eur.nl

Velasquez, M., Andre, C., Shanks, T., Meyer, S. J., Meyer, M. J. (2014). *The common good.* https://www.scu.edu/ethics/ethics-resources/ethical-decision-making/the-common-good/

Von Glasersfeld, E. (2003). The constructivist view of communication. In A. Müller & K. H. Müller (Eds.), *An unfinished revolution* (pp. 351–360). Vienna, Austria: Edition Echoraum.

Warren, M. A., & Donaldson, S. I. (2018). *Toward a positive psychology of relationships: New directions in theory and research*. Santa Barbara, CA: Preager.

White, S. C. (2017). Relational wellbeing: Re-centering the politics of happiness, policy and the self. *Policy & Politics, 45*(2), 121–136.

Williams, R. (2003). *Lost icons: Reflections on cultural bereavement*. London, UK: Morehouse.

Wilson, A. C., Mackintosh, K., Power, K., & Chan, S. W. Y. (2018). Effectiveness of self-compassion related therapies: A systematic review and meta-analysis. *Mindfulness*. https://doi.org/10.1007/s12671-018-1037-6

Wissing, M. (2013). Wellbeing research in South Africa. Meaning and relational well-being: A reflection on the state of the art and a way forward. *Journal of Psychology in Africa, 24*(1), 115–121.

Wissing, M. P. (2014). Meaning and relational well-being: A reflection on the state of art and a way forward. *Journal of Psychology in Africa, 24*(1), 183–192.

Wissing, M. P. (2018). Embracing well-being in diverse contexts: The third wave of positive psychology. Invited paper at the First Africa Positive Psychology Conference, 4–7 April 2018, Potchefstroom, South Africa.

Wong, D. B. (1988). On flourishing and finding one's identity in community. *Midwest Studies in Philosophy, 13*(1), 324–341.

Wong, P. T. P. (2017). Meaning-centered approach to research and therapy, second wave positive psychology, and the future of humanistic psychology. *The Humanistic Psychologist, 45*(3), 207–216.

World Happiness Report. (2018). Accessed 3 Aug 2018 from http://worldhappiness.report/

Part II

Environment and Technology

Economic Growth and *Quality of Life* in Africa

7

Carolyn Chisadza and Elsabé Loots

Abstract
Economic growth is an important instrument for reducing poverty and improving quality of life. Having spent a long time in sluggish growth territory, Africa's surge in economic growth since the mid- to late 1990s was indeed worth celebrating. The question is: to what extent was this improvement in growth inclusive and thus shared, by benefitting the quality of life of the broader population? This chapter analyses the growth performance in Africa between 1960 and 2016 and its effect on various quality of life measures. We analyse the full period as well as splitting it into two subperiods, in order to separate the lost decade-era and the era of high growth in Africa. We find that, contrary to expectation, the period of high growth appears not to have significant positive growth spill-over effects on either the average wealth per person, or the quality of life measures. This is in contrast with the improvements in selected quality of life indicators, as measured by the performance in the Millennium Development Goals. The implications highlighted by this analysis suggest that the recent growth in Africa was not inclusive, as it failed to contribute to the improvement in the quality of life of its citizens, thus putting the sustainability of the improvement in jeopardy.

7.1 Introduction

The improvement in the quality of life on the African continent has received much attention in academic literature, as well as from various multilateral organisations over many decades. The attention to the improvement in the quality of life formed the major building block of the paradigm shift in the study of and approach to development, a concept that has evolved since the early 1950s. In this evolution in the thinking on development and how the process impacts on the quality of life, the views on the role of economic growth as a source of funding for the improvement of the quality of life have also changed considerably.

It has been well established in the literature that economic growth can have positive spillover effects on poverty reduction through improved health, increased education and better employment opportunities (Rodrik, 2007). As such, countries with strong economic growth have higher quality of life, which in turn promotes economic growth, and thus the cycle of prosperity is supported. Furthermore, the

C. Chisadza · E. Loots (✉)
Department of Economics, University of Pretoria, Pretoria, South Africa
e-mail: carolyn.chisadza@up.ac.za; elsabe.loots@up.ac.za

I. Eloff (ed.), *Handbook of Quality of Life in African Societies*, International Handbooks of Quality-of-Life, https://doi.org/10.1007/978-3-030-15367-0_7

growth rate in combination with the structure of the growth makes a difference for reducing poverty. If the growth is not inclusive and does not allow the marginalised to share in the proceeds, then future growth may not be sustainable.

This chapter aims to look at the relationship between economic growth and quality of life in Africa. The methodology followed will be from a macroeconomic perspective where we will analyse the impact of growth in African countries on a selected number of proxies measuring the quality of life, covering the 1960s to 2016. Since a broad range of detailed analysis on various dimensions of the quality of life such as health, education and many more, are covered in the chapters in this book, we trust that this chapter will supplement the knowledge and thinking on this multidimensional and important challenge on the continent.

The chapter is structured as follows: the evolution in the thinking on development is discussed by highlighting the various debates surrounding the relationship between quality of life and economic growth. This is followed by an analysis of the growth performance in Africa; the performance of the continent on selected Millennium Development Goals (MDGs); a correlation analysis between economic growth and selected quality of life indicators and the performance of Africa in the Human Development Index over time. The chapter concludes with a summary of the most important findings and possible implications on the challenges for the continent to reach the Sustainable Development Goals.

7.2 Evolution of the Development Thinking and the Role of Economic Growth in Improving the Quality of Life

After the World War II and the subsequent successes of the implementation of the Marshall Plan in developed economies in the 1950s, the idea took hold that this plan could be duplicated to address the problems of poverty and underdevelopment in the developing countries in Africa, Asia and Latin America. The idea, embedded in neo-classical economic theory, was that should countries improve their economic growth performance, the benefits of growth would automatically trickle down to all levels of society and the problems of poverty and underdevelopment would be solved. This neo-classical thinking contended that an improvement in gross national product (GNP) or gross domestic product (GDP) per capita was both necessary and sufficient, in order to address the challenges of poverty, inequality and unemployment.

During the 1980s, Africa and the rest of the developing world were exposed to excessive high oil prices, a decline in commodity prices, low growth, the subsequent external debt crises and the negative impact of the structural adjustment programmes of the International Monetary Fund. These unfortunate events led to the 1980s being labelled as the so-called *lost decade* for the growth and development of the vast majority of African countries. The idea started to take root that economic growth per se and the improvement in per capita income, in other words economic development, could not on its own solve the challenges of poverty, inequality and unemployment.

This led to three important changes in the approach to underdevelopment, with the United Nations through the United Nations Development Programme (UNDP) taking the lead. The first initiative was with the major shift in emphasis on the design and implementation of the first Human Development Index (HDI), as reflected in the first Human Development Report in 1990 (UNDP, 1990). The HDI still includes per capita income as a HDI variable, but added variables on education and health to represent a broader measure of quality of life, known as the level of human development. With the HDI, it was formally acknowledged that economic growth and the implied associated improvement in per capita income could in isolation not address the challenges of poverty, inequality and unemployment. The report emphasized how the process of development should enlarge the choices of people beyond improvement in income. This shift in the thinking of the UN was shortly afterwards followed by the World Bank, which as an institution in the 1980s promulgated economic growth as the ultimate development goal. After the 1990 World Development Report (World Bank, 1990) focussed on poverty, the 1991 World Development Report (World Bank, 1991, p. 4) stated for the first time that the challenge of development is to improve the quality of life. With this statement, the World Bank for the first time acknowledged that an improvement in the quality of life involves more than simply an increase in income, but that improved education, nutrition and health are, amongst others, crucial in the development process.

The third major shift was the announcement of the First Decade of Poverty in 1997 by the United Nations, through its Department of Economic and Social Affairs. The collective decision was taken to monitor poverty for the next decade (1997–2006) and to suggest and support policy changes to alleviate the impact of poverty, and therefore the quality of life, in developing countries.

This paradigm shift in development thinking started to spill over to the wider international development debates, the allocation of donor funding and into the policy spaces, not only in the developing world, but also in the developed world. However, in all these debates and in the literature, it is still acknowledged that economic growth remains a necessary, although not a sufficient condition on its own, for development and thus improvements in the quality of life. Without receiving the benefits of economic growth, financial limitations would stifle development initiatives over the medium to long term. Countries can simply not maintain and sustain the provision of essential services such as education, health, fresh drinking water and others, while only depending on official development assistance or bilateral aid from other countries. The necessity of generating income to sustain basic services through economic growth is thus well-understood in the literature.

Several studies highlight the positive link between economic growth and poverty reduction. Lin (2003) finds that the rapid economic growth experienced in China between 1985 and 2001 contributed significantly to poverty reduction. Similarly, India's decrease in poverty in the 1990s was on the back of accelerated growth rates over this period (Bhanumurthy & Mitra, 2004). However, this increased growth also leads to rising inequality which sometimes negates the growth effects. Besley and Cord (2007) find evidence that the proportion of poor people in Uganda would have been much lower, had growth not widened the income distribution between 1992 and 2002.

Economic growth is also associated with broader measures of human development. Growth not only generates employment opportunities, but also improves general living standards through health and education. Higher levels of economic growth reduce infant mortality (Pritchett & Summers, 1993), increase life expectancy (Barro & Sala-i-Martin, 1995), improve educational outcomes (Barro & Lee, 1997), and lower gender inequalities (Boone, 1996).

The positive effects of economic growth on quality of life are also often encouraged by policy choices. Poor policy formulation can delay or even harm growth, such as increased costs of doing business and insecure property rights that divert foreign investment, or trade restrictions that impede technology transfer and competition.

Coupled with the still central role of economic growth in the broader development debate, is the debate around the structure of growth, i.e. does it trickle down to the wider population and does the wider population share in the benefits of growth, as is evident in the improvement in the quality of life. The question is: to what extent is the structure of growth inclusive.

The next section will examine the growth performance of African countries for the period 1960–2016, and will also discuss the quality of life performance on the continent and analyse the growth spill over effects.

7.3 Growth Performance, MDG Progress and Quality of Life in Africa

7.3.1 Economic Growth in Africa

Africa is the second largest and most populous continent in the world with over 1.2 billion people (World Population Review, 2017). The continent hosts 54 countries with diverse ethnicities, cultures and languages. Although Africa is blessed with an abundance of natural resources, it remains the poorest and most underdeveloped continent in relation to the rest of the world. Several reasons for the continent's delay in reducing poverty include colonization, conflict, delayed democratic transitions, government maladministration, high illiteracy rates, low skills development and lack of capacity to cater for growing populations.

These negatives, however, did not stop Africa from experiencing unprecedented growth during the late 1990s to early 2000s (see Fig. 7.1), driven largely by favourable prices received for primary commodities and China's increased demand for natural resources (Rodrik, 2016). Furthermore, Young (2012) finds that between 1990 and 2006, the real material consumption in Africa was on the rise and relatively close to the growth taking place in other regions of the world. Overall, the continent achieved an average real annual GDP growth of 4% between 1960 and 2016.

In Fig. 7.2, we disaggregate the overall growth into decades, in order to achieve a better understanding of the long-term trend. Initially, African economies enjoyed an economic boom during the 1960s and early 1970s, supported by demand for minerals and agricultural products in the global market (Jerven, 2017), as well as investment and total factor productivity growth (Fosu, 2013). However, this growth was reversed during the mid-1970s and 1980s (the *lost decade* in Africa) as a result of oil price shocks, declining terms of trade, increasing interest rates (Olamosu & Wynne, 2015) and ongoing civil wars which left several countries impoverished.

Since the mid-1990s, a reversal of the declining growth trend is evident: Africa's real annual GDP growth rate jumped to an average of 5.1%

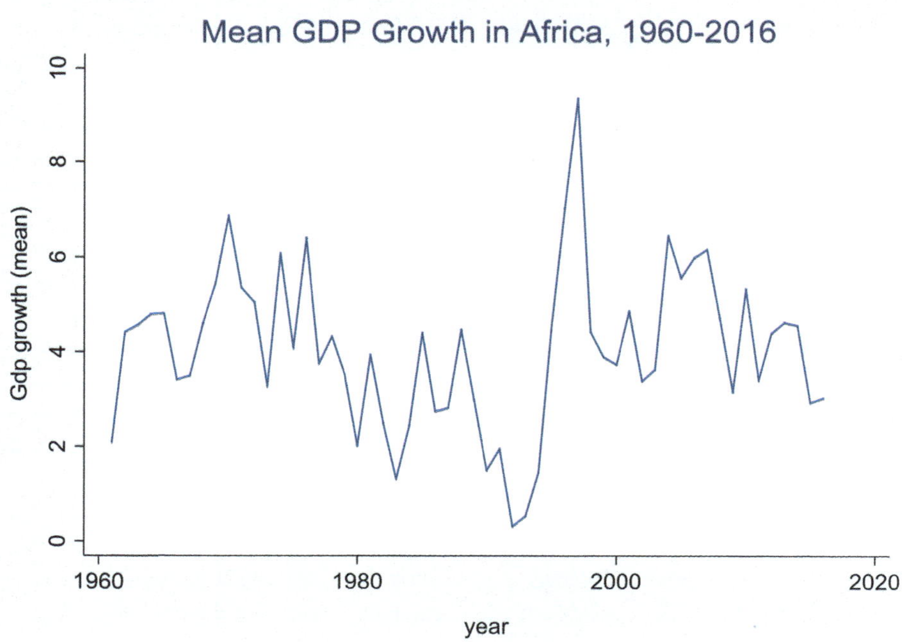

Fig. 7.1 GDP Growth 1960–2016
Notes: Variable is the annual percentage growth rate of GDP. (Source: World Development Indicators)

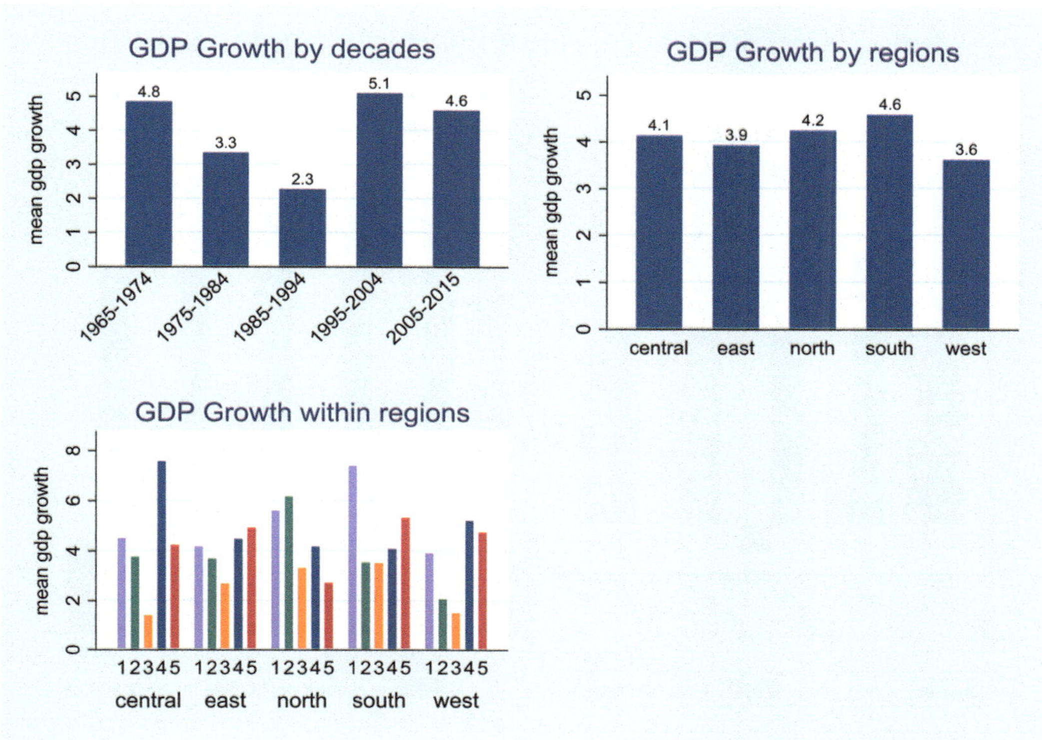

Fig. 7.2 GDP Growth in Africa, disaggregated by decades and regions
Notes: Variable is the annual percentage growth rate of GDP. The periods represent 1 = 1965–1974, 2 = 1975–1984, 3 = 1985–1994, 4 = 1995–2004, 5 = 2005–2015. (Source: World Development Indicators)

between 1995 and 2004, higher than most Asian and Latin American economies. Again, this growth performance is largely attributed to the benefits of high global commodity prices, increased demand for Africa's primary exports, an increase in foreign direct investment flows to the continent and macroeconomic policy reforms.

Due to the larger integration into the world economy, the onset of the 2008 Global Financial Crises was impossible to escape. This is evident in the impact on economic growth on the continent since 2010. This was on the back of several additional shocks: the decline in demand for raw materials from the European and American markets (Olamosu & Wynne, 2015), reduced productivity growth in the oil exporting countries (Algeria, Angola, Nigeria and Sudan) and subsequent decline in the oil price, and increased conflicts (Leke & Barton, 2016). According to Rodrik (2016), the economic decline in the last decade has left several African economies poorer than they were in 1960.

Furthermore, we disaggregate the growth by regions[1] and find that Southern Africa was driv-

[1]We split the regions based on the African Union classification:

Central Africa – Burundi, Cameroon, Central African Republic, Chad, Republic of Congo, Democratic Republic of Congo, Equatorial Guinea, Gabon and Sao Tome and Principe.
Eastern Africa – Comoros, Djibouti, Ethiopia, Eritrea, Ethiopia, Kenya, Madagascar, Mauritius, Rwanda, the Seychelles, Somalia, South Sudan, Sudan, Tanzania and Uganda.
West Africa – Benin, Burkina Faso, Cape Verde, Ivory Coast, Gambia, Ghana, Guinea, Guinea-Bissau, Liberia, Mali, Mauritania, Niger, Nigeria, Senegal, Sierra Leone and Togo.
Northern Africa – Algeria, Egypt, Libya, Morocco and Tunisia.
Southern Africa – Angola, Botswana, Lesotho, Malawi, Mozambique, Namibia, South Africa, Swaziland, Zambia and Zimbabwe.

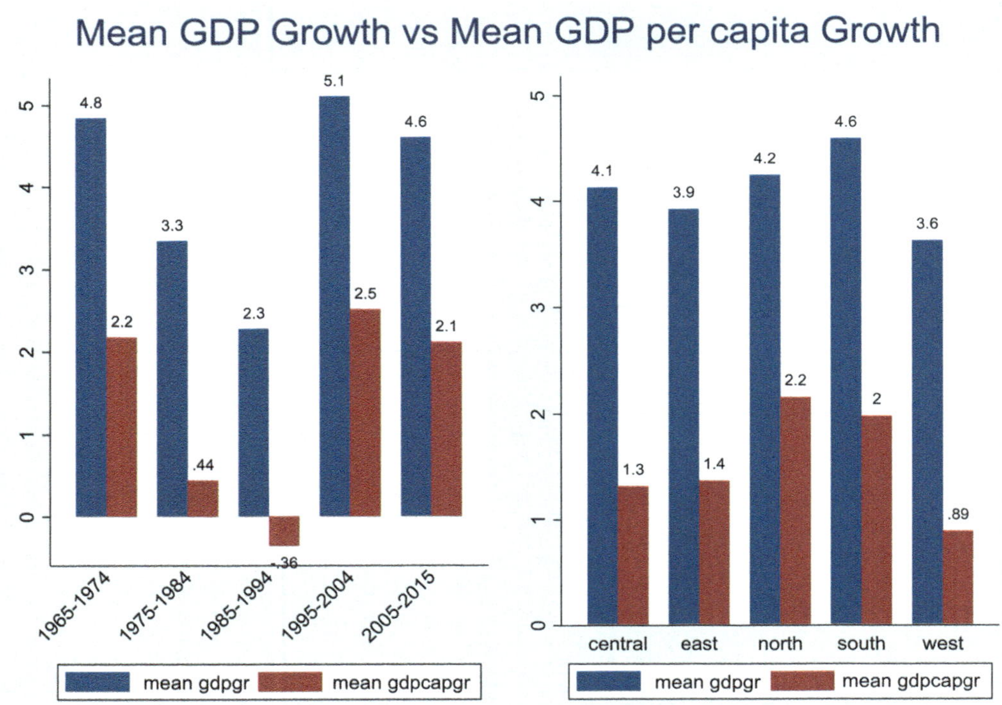

Fig. 7.3 GDP growth and Income per capita Growth
Notes: Variables are the annual percentage growth rate of GDP and the annual percentage growth rate of GDP per capita. (Source: World Development Indicators)

ing the growth for the overall period 1960–2015, recording an average of 4.6% real annual GDP growth. Interestingly, the rapid growth experienced during the 1960s was driven by economies in Southern Africa, while the economic boom between 1995 and 2004 largely came from Central Africa.

While economic growth on the continent recovered substantially in the 1990s and early 2000s, the improvements in per capita income over the same period seem to have been much less impressive. The average income per capita growth increased only moderately, suggesting that the effects of the rapid economic growth experienced in Africa failed to spill over to the broader population in the form of higher incomes and improvement in wealth. The overall income per capita growth for the full period 1960–2016 averaged 1.4% in comparison to the continent's average economic growth of 4%. The bar charts in Fig. 7.3 indicate that during the period of high growth in Africa, income per capita growth recovered at a relatively slower pace than the economic growth, averaging only 2.5%. The average growth in income per capita was driven by the average performance of countries in Northern and Southern Africa, most likely on the back of rising oil prices, but also due to structural reforms.

Despite the slowdown in economic growth after the financial crises, the growth performance on the continent still remains resilient and above the average levels of the 1970s and 1980s. The lack of spill over benefits on per capita income however, is an early indication that shows the deficiencies in the structure of the growth and the lack of policy measures to ensure that the wider population benefits.

Table 7.1 MDG progress in SSA, 1990–2015

MDG goals	1990	2000	2015
Goal 1: Eradicate extreme poverty			
% of people living in poverty	57	–	41
% of people living in extreme poverty	57		36
Goal 2: Achieve universal primary education			
% enrolment in primary education	52	60	80
Goal 3: Promote gender equality and empower women			
% of women in wage employment	14	17	21
Goal 4: Reduce child mortality			
Under-five mortality rate – number of deaths per 1000 live births	179	–	86
Goal 5: Improve maternal health			
Number of maternal deaths per 100,000 live births	990	830	510
Goal 7: Ensure environmental sustainability			
% access to an improved drinking source	48	–	68
% access to a sanitation source	24		30

Source: United Nations (2015)

7.3.2 Africa's Performance in the MDGs

The analysis of the African growth performance indicates that the poor growth performance on the continent turned around during the mid-1990s. However, at the end of the First Decade of Poverty, the persistence of poverty and conditions of extreme poverty had not significantly improved for the majority of poor people in the developing world. In 2000, the world leaders, in conjunction with the United Nations (UN), shaped a broad vision and entered into a commitment to "spare no effort to free our fellow men, women and children from abject and dehumanizing conditions of extreme poverty" (United Nations, 2015). The ambitious vision, termed the Millennium Development Goals (MDGs), consisted of eight goals and practical steps for the period 2000–2015 to lift more than one million people world-wide out of poverty.

At the end of the 15 years, the UN published the final report, summarising the successes and remaining challenges (United Nations, 2015). The report concludes that although significant progress has been made on many of the MDG targets since 1990, the progress has been unevenly spread around the developing regions and gaps still remain.

These stated goals influence the quality of life directly or indirectly. The performance of African countries on the MDGs varies substantially. Table 7.1 and Fig. 7.4 show the performance of Sub-Saharan Africa (SSA) on selected indicators.[2]

On Goal 1, the incidence of poverty has declined by 28% over the 25-year period, substantially lower than the 68% decline in poverty in the world over the same period. Forty-one percent of people still live in poverty and 36% of workers in Africa still live in extreme poverty. The portion of undernourished people also declined from 33% to 23%, but was still lower than the 13% for developing regions. The decline in the incidence of poverty also contributed to a decline in the hunger rate, as reflected in Fig. 7.4. However, it is disappointing that the number of under-nourished people has increased by 44 million since 1990, as a result of the high population growth (United Nations, 2015, p. 21).

SSA made the greatest progress in Goal 2, and especially in the access to primary education, in comparison with all developing regions – an improvement of 28 percentage points – to reach a primary enrolment rate of 80% in 2015. Despite the rapid population growth, the numbers of

[2]Only SSA is included in the discussion on the MDGs, since data gaps exist in the MDG data for Northern Africa.

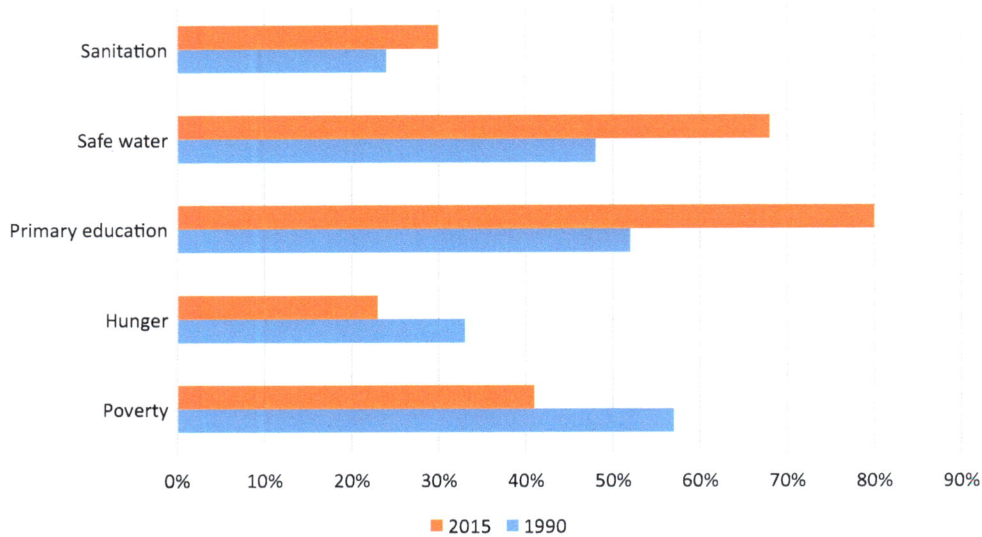

Fig. 7.4 Selected performance of MDG goals and sub-goals for sub-Saharan African countries, 1990 and 2015

Note: The analysis only covers Sub-Saharan Africa since the data on the performance of Northern African countries is lacking. (Source: United Nations, 2015)

enrolled children more than doubled from 62 million children to 149 million children (United Nations, 2015, p. 25).

With regard to the progress on gender equality (Goal 3), SSA achieved mixed results, with an underperformance in gender parity in primary education, reaching gender parity in secondary education and slipping back over the past 15 years in tertiary education. This is evident in the access to the labour force, where only 21% of African women are in wage employment, much lower than the 48% in all developing regions.

In contrast, impressive strides have been made to improve the under-five child mortality rate, where the deaths per 1000 live births declined since 1990 with an astonishing 52%, more or less in line with the decline in all developing regions (Goal 4).

Goal 5 represents the improvement in maternal health. The maternal mortality ratio in SSA has declined from 990 maternal deaths per 100,000 live births in 1990 to 510 in 2015. Despite the strong decline of 49% over the period, SSA is still way above the average of 230 for developing countries, and with Southern Asia, accounts for 86% of these deaths globally (United Nations, 2015, p. 39).

Although access to fresh drinking water has improved since 1990, SSA still falls below the set target. The same applies to access to sanitation, where the 30% in SSA is far short of the 62% in developing regions (Goal 7).

The performance of SSA in improving their quality of life as measured by their performance in the MDGs is mixed. Despite the substantive improvement in quality of life indicators such as primary enrolment and in the under-five child mortality rate, the continent still lags behind on the quality of life indicators in relation to other developing regions.

7.3.3 Relationship Between Economic Growth and the Quality of Life

The preceding overview indicates that African countries reversed their poor growth performance of the 1970s, 1980s and early 1990s, and have since the mid-1990s achieved significantly higher average growth rates, despite the impact of the global financial crises. However, we are also aware that the improvements in the growth performance since the mid-1990s did not necessar-

Table 7.2 Correlation matrix

	1960–2016 GDP growth	1960–1990 GDP growth	1991–2016 GDP growth
Child mortality	−0.1422	−0.4452*	0.0908
Life expectancy	0.1014	0.5149*	−0.0371
Primary education	−0.0695	0.2837	−0.0954
Secondary education	0.0102	−0.2272	0.0176
Fertility	−0.1530	−0.2509	0.1074

*Significant at 5%. Source: World Development Indicators

ily spill over to equal improvements in per capita incomes. Furthermore, though African countries achieved variable successes in their MDG performance since 1990, they still lag behind other developing regions today.

Quality of life captures the well-being of individuals through various aspects such as health, education, wealth, employment and security. We now analyse whether a correlation exists between economic growth in Africa and selected proxies for quality of life. The aim is to see whether the growth performance is associated with improved quality of life on the continent.

The selected proxies for the quality of life are:

- Under 5 child mortality rate per 1000 live births as proxy for access to health services;
- Life expectancy at birth as proxy for access to and quality of health services;
- Mean years in primary education as proxy for quality of education;
- Mean years in secondary education as proxy for quality of education;
- Total fertility rate (births per women) as proxy for both health and education;
- Sectoral growth in the economy to indicate access to employment opportunities;
- Measures for democracy and constraints on the executive of government accountability as proxies for the quality of institutions.

The data is obtained from the World Development Indicators and the Polity IV Project.

The correlation between the following variables and the mean GDP growth for African countries is conducted for the full period (1960–2016) and two sub-periods (1960–1990, 1991–2016). Table 7.2 reveals a concerning trend: the growth experienced during the 1960–1990 period appears to have had more of a significant effect on the quality of life than during the period of rapid economic growth in the late 1990s and early 2000s.

We observe the trends of child mortality and life expectancy as our measures for health. The correlations on child mortality in Fig. 7.5 highlight some interesting trends. The correlation for the entire period (1960–2016) is negative as expected. Child mortality is decreasing as economic growth increases. However, the two subperiods tell a different story. The correlation for the period 1960–1990 remained negative and significant, despite the poor growth performances during the 1970s and 1980s. The negative trend during the period 1960–1990 in child mortality may be a result of immunization campaigns, started in the 1970s, from international organizations such as the World Health Organisation (WHO) and the United Nations (Soares, 2007) to prevent child mortality in developing countries. The literature advances that declines in infant mortality rates were mostly driven by improvements in public health and better nutrition (Conley, McCord, & Sachs, 2007). In contrast, the correlation during the period 1991–2016, when a noticeable improvement in economic growth was evident, shows a positive but insignificant correlation.

The correlation between GDP per capita and life expectancy, the second health indicator, is also interesting (Table 7.2 and Fig. 7.6). The correlation for the full period (1960–2016) is again positive, indicating that improvements in economic growth contributed to improved levels of life expectancy. A stronger positive and significant correlation exists during the period 1960–1990, in contrast with the slight negative and insignificant correlation for the period 1991–2016, when improved growth was experienced. During the 1960–1990 period, improvements in medicines and technologies also contributed to better quality of life. However, this improved quality of life has reduced considerably over the

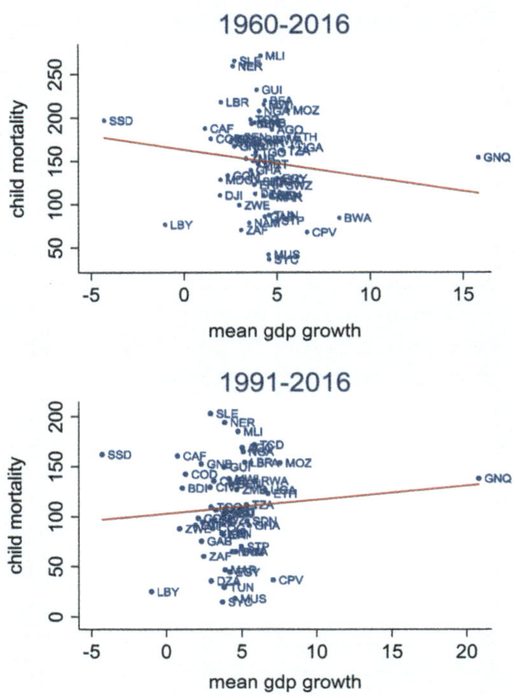

Fig. 7.5 Mean Under 5 Child Mortality Rate per 1000 live births and GDP Growth

Notes: Variable is the under 5 years of age mortality rate per thousand live births and the annual percentage growth rate of GDP. (Source: World Development Indicators)

course of the last 20 years for child mortality, less so for life expectancy, with the HIV and AIDS epidemic taking much of the blame.

While the slowdown in these health indicators may not have offset the overall declines in child mortality or increases in life expectancy, they are a worrying factor. Firstly, the slowdowns are taking place during the period that Africa was experiencing rapid growth and secondly, the slowdowns are taking place during the period that Africa should have been striving to meet the 2015 MDGs in order to reduce poverty and child mortality (Goals 1 and 4). If these current trends continue unchecked, they may pose serious delays in the improvements of Africans' standards of living and their efforts to meet the current Sustainable Development Goals (SDGs) for good health and well-being (Goal 3).

Another indicator of quality of life in the literature is education. We observe the trends in primary and secondary education in Figs. 7.7 and 7.8. We find that the effects of economic growth during the entire period had a minimal effect on primary education (contrary to the achievement of MDG Goal 3 for universal primary education), but appear to have a positive effect during the 1960–1990 period, again in contrast with the slower growth performance. Progress toward universal primary enrolment for children was steady in most of Africa in the 1960s and 1970s. However, this trend slowed down after the 1980s on the back of economic crises and debt restructuring, with the negative effects evident in the later period 1991–2016 (Lloyd & Blanc, 1996). The correlation coefficient for the period 1991–2016 is negative and insignificant, despite the positive growth performance over this period. This may be due to the underperformance in the gender parity in primary education (United Nations, 2015).

The correlation between GDP growth and mean years in secondary education over the full period is flat and the coefficient is insignificant.

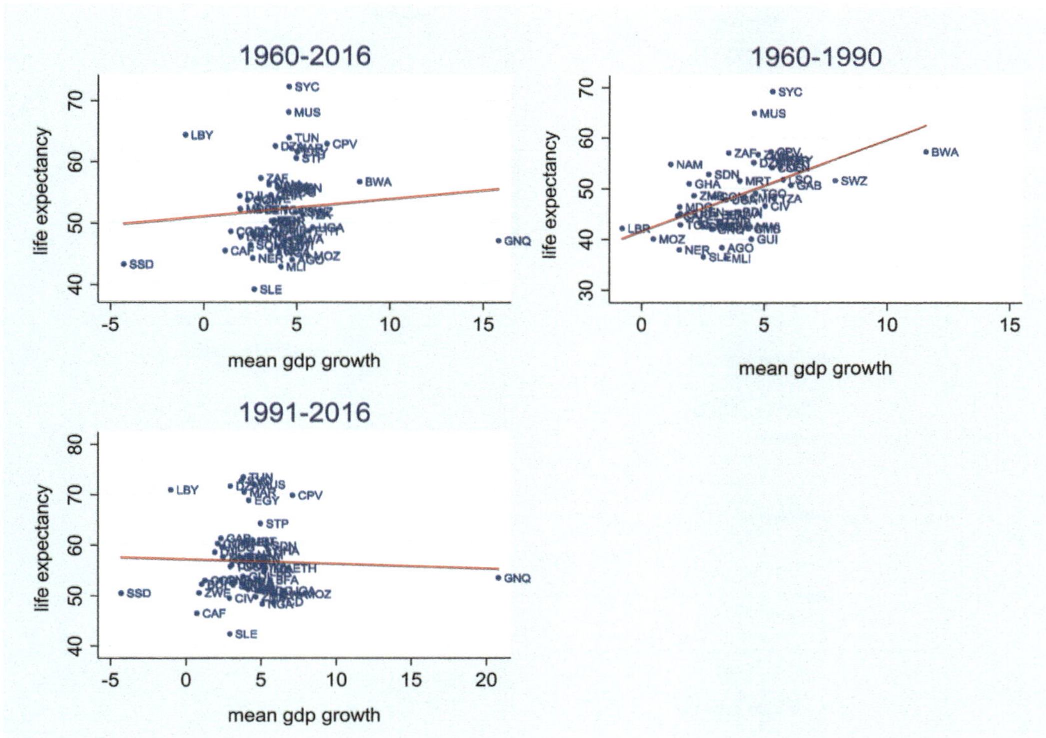

Fig. 7.6 Mean Years of Life Expectancy at birth and GDP Growth

Notes: Variable is the life expectancy at birth of the total population in years and the annual percentage growth rate of GDP. (Source: World Development Indicators)

The negative correlation during the 1960–1990 period may be reflective of the negative impact of the poor growth performance over this period on secondary education. This is not encouraging for Africa, as human capital accumulation feeds back into economic growth through increased labour productivity, increased innovative capacity and increased diffusion of knowledge (Benhabib & Spiegel, 1994; Mankiw, Romer, & Weil, 1992; Romer, 1990). One of the main factors contributing to Africa's sluggish total factor productivity growth is a lack of skilled labour. If the structure of growth in Africa fails to create the necessary incentives to encourage education, which seems to be the case given the weak correlations during 1991 and 2016 for primary and secondary education, the continent may well find itself in a never-ending cycle of poverty.

Lastly, the fertility rate could serve as proxy for both the quality and access to education, as well as the quality and access to health care services. Over the period 1960–2016, Africa recorded an average fertility rate of six children per woman, twice the rate in the rest of the world (Chisadza & Bittencourt, 2015). According to the literature, as incomes per capita continue to rise, countries begin to experience a demographic transition from high to low fertility rates (Becker, Murphy, & Tamura, 1990). Lower fertility rates allow families to invest in child education, bringing about a child quantity-quality trade-off as incomes continue to rise.

The evidence in Fig. 7.9 is in line with the literature for the period until 1990, showing a negative correlation between GDP growth and fertility rates: an increase in economic growth leads to a decline in fertility rates. Contrarily, in the latter period the correlation is positive, although insignificant, despite the fact that Africa was experiencing high growth.

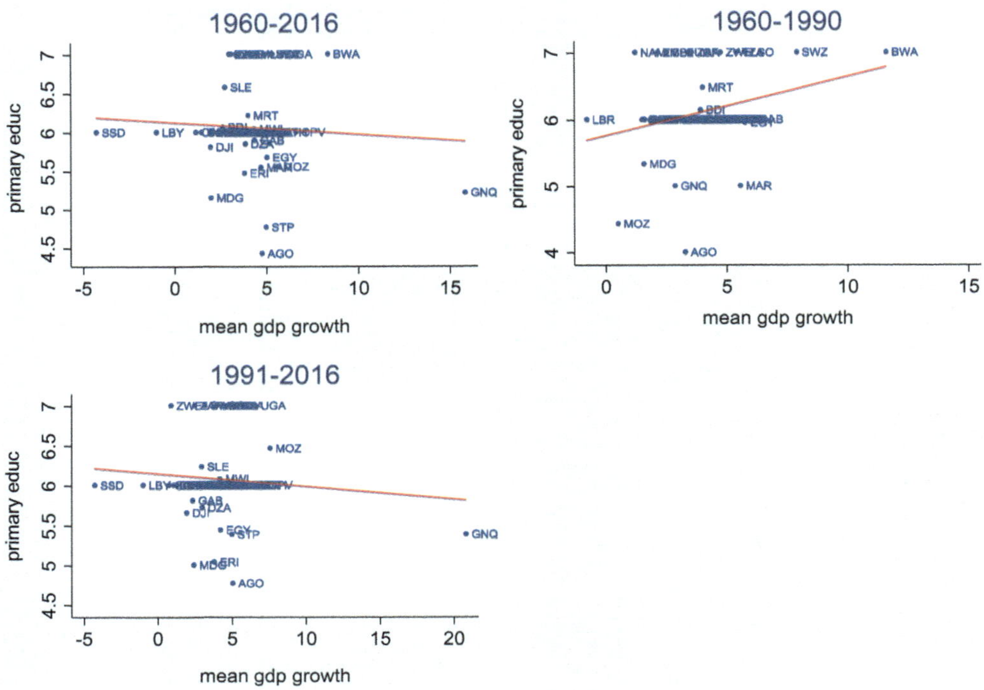

Fig. 7.7 Mean Years in Primary Education and GDP Growth

Notes: Variable is the number of years in primary education and the annual percentage growth rate of GDP. (Source: World Development Indicators)

The slowdown in fertility declines during 1991–2016 may be driven by several factors:

- The replacement effect for rising child mortality during the same period as illustrated in Fig. 7.5 (Conley et al., 2007),
- Low human capital stock delaying the child quantity-quality trade-off (Becker et al., 1990), also experienced in the same period (Figs. 7.7 and 7.8), or
- The gender differences in the desire for sex and the decision to use modern contraceptives (Strulik, 2016).

Furthermore, in low-income agricultural societies, children are more likely to be regarded as productive assets because they are a source of labour power and old-age security (Caldwell, Orubuloye, & Caldwell, 1992; Dreze & Murthi, 2001). Hence, developing countries in Africa are inclined to have more children with rising incomes.

The analysis to this point indicates that the effects from the rapid economic growth in the latter half have had limited impact on the quality of life measures. On the contrary, it appears that the growth effects from the 1960s and 1970s spilled over in improving the standard of living for Africans. A recent report by Smith (2016) places 15 African countries at the bottom end of the quality of life rankings. He highlights the irony of these countries being resource-rich, yet with so few of their citizens benefiting from it. Sadly, this is the reality for most Africans.

The quality of life of citizens of a country could be improved by access to employment opportunities. Figure 7.10 analyses the growth trends of three main sectors in Africa which con-

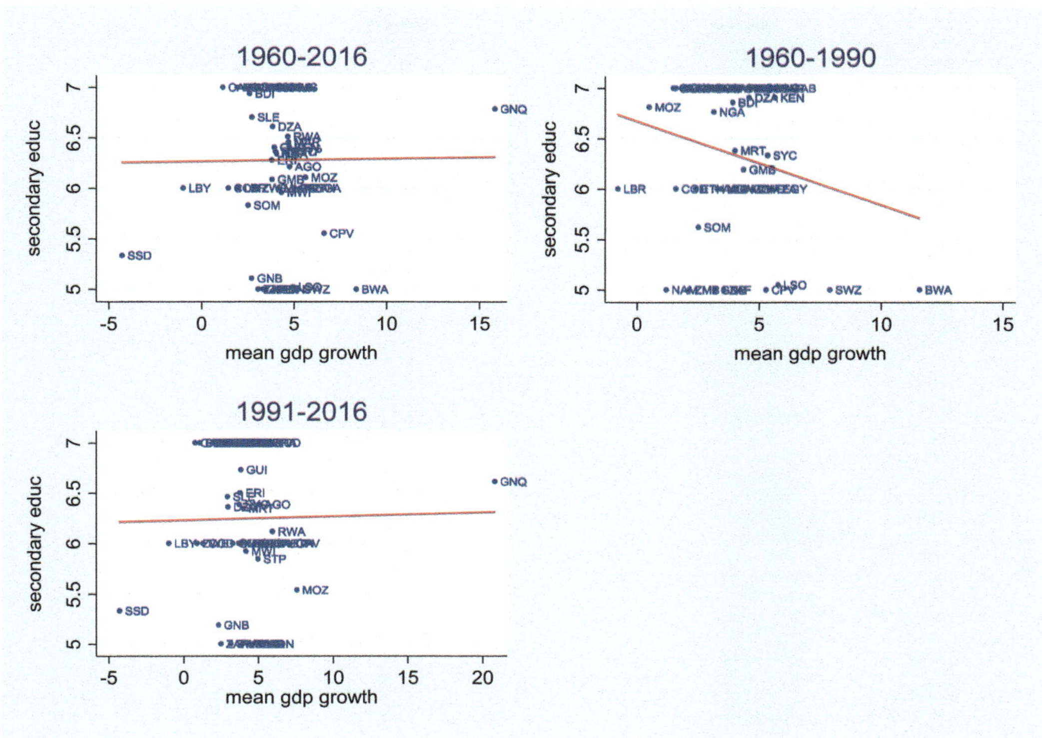

Fig. 7.8 Mean Years in Secondary Education and GDP Growth

Notes: Variable is the number of years in secondary education and the annual percentage growth rate of GDP. (Source: World Development Indicators)

tribute to job creation, skills development and innovation in technologies. Growth in Africa has been driven mainly by growth in the industry and services sectors. Unfortunately, the growth has not spilled over into the agricultural sector, which is Africa's primary productive sector for creating jobs for low-skilled workers. As such, it has been growth without jobs and therefore without reduction in poverty levels.

The quality of institutions also plays an important role in ensuring that policies to improve the quality of life are executed, in order to allow people the freedom to make choices about their lives and to allow for the general provision of services. Poor institutions can be detrimental to the functioning of an economic system. Figure 7.11 compares economic growth and institutions in Africa. While the economic growth in Africa seems to have increased the accountability of politicians, the democracy score is next to zero. The growth effects have had little impact on improving democracy in Africa. This is in line with evidence from several empirical essays that find a negative relationship between democracy and economic growth (Acemoglu, Johnson, Robinson, & Yared, 2008; Burke & Leigh, 2010; Chisadza & Bittencourt, 2018). Furthermore, this kind of negative relationship is typical of resource-rich countries (Fayad, Bates, & Hoeffler, 2012) and former colonies (Cervellati, Jung, Sunde, & Vischer, 2014).

7.3.4 Africa's Performance in the HDI

The human development index (HDI) is a composite index which includes wealth (gross

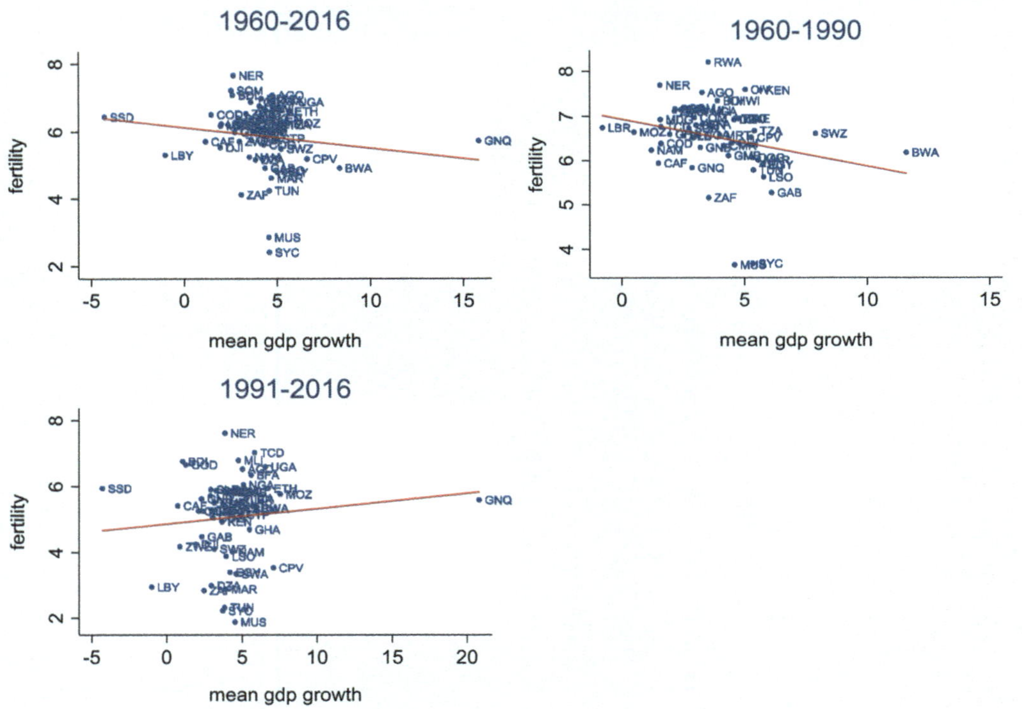

Fig. 7.9 Total Fertility Rate (births per women) and GDP Growth

Notes: Variable is the total fertility rate, number of births per woman and the annual percentage growth rate of GDP. (Source: World Development Indicators)

Table 7.3 HDI and GDP growth

HDI and GDP growth	1990–2000	2001–2015
HDI	0.43	0.49
GDP growth	3.7%	4.6%

Sources: World Development Indicators, United Nations Development Programme's Human Development Report
Variables are annual percentage growth rates of GDP and human development index

national income per capita, $PPP), health (life expectancy) and education (mean years of schooling). The index ranges from zero (low human development) to one (high human development). As was mentioned before, the HDI was developed to measure the progress made in development beyond the neo-classical per capita measure in isolation.

We find a similar story of delayed growth effects on the quality of life in Africa, when we compare the average HDI for Africa for two periods: 1990–2000 and 2001–2015. Table 7.3 shows that, despite the improved growth performance on the continent between the two periods, the HDI has improved only marginally for Africa, suggesting insignificant growth effects on improving standards of living. According to the classification of the HDI, Africa is still trapped in a low human development band.

7.4 Conclusion

This chapter discussed the growth performance in Africa and its potential impact on the quality of life in Africa. Three periods were included namely the period 1960–2016, as well as two sub-periods: 1960–1990 and 1991–2016. In general, the growth spill over effects were weak. In the first

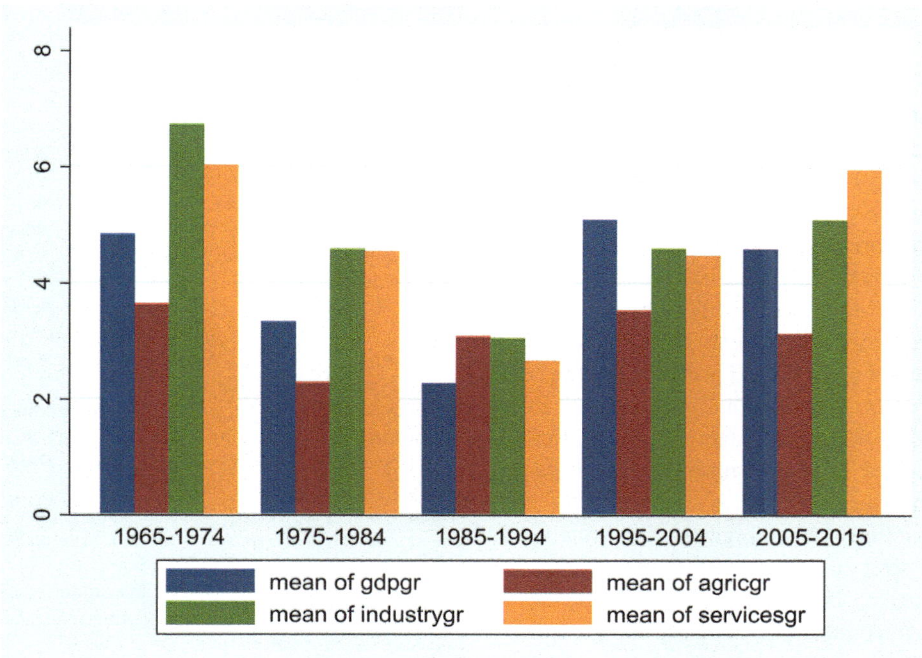

Fig. 7.10 Sectors and GDP Growth
Notes: Variables are the annual percentage growth of GDP, the annual percentage growth of the agriculture sector, the annual percentage growth of the industry sector and the annual percentage growth of the services sector. (Source: World Development Indicators)

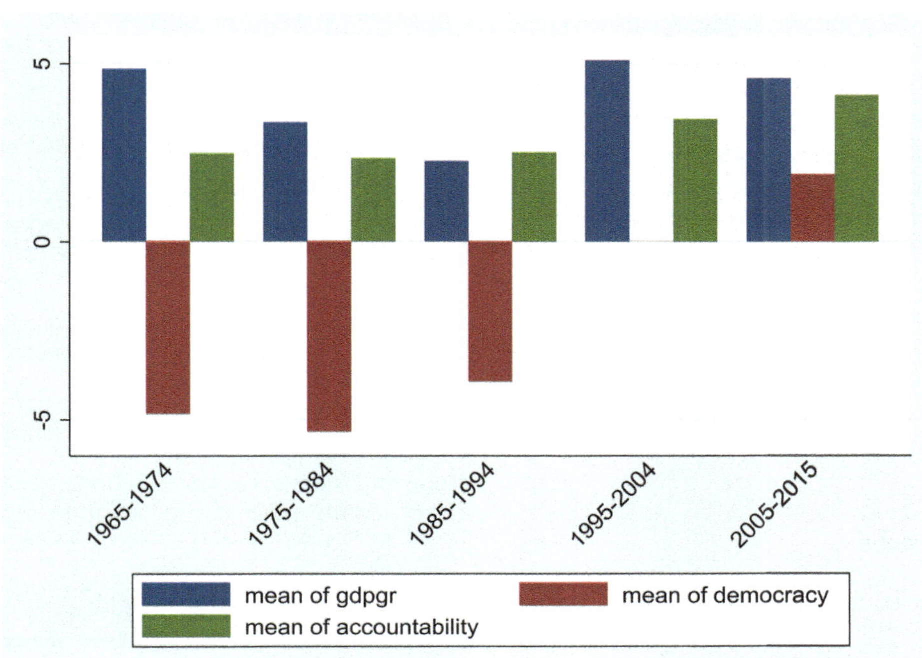

Fig. 7.11 Institutions and GDP Growth
Notes: Variables are the annual percentage growth rate of GDP, polity2 measure for democracy and constraints on the executive for government accountability. (Sources: World Development Indicators and Polity IV Project)

sub-period the correlation analysis shows more significant results on the impact of growth on the identified quality of life indicators than during the second sub-period, when the growth performance of the continent was not only on a higher level, but also on a more sustainable path. This is contrary to expectation that the rapid economic growth will translate into improved quality of life for the average citizen on the continent. This is also in contrast with the varied MDG performances over the past 25 years. The marginal improvement in the HDI since 1990 also substantiates that Africa has not benefitted from the improved growth performance over the two decades.

The picture is unambiguous: the growth pattern and structure on the continent in general is not inclusive. These preliminary findings raise some serious questions: why did the growth not have the desired effects on poverty reduction and improvements in the quality of lives? How can Africa generate sustained economic growth going forward? A possible answer is identifying the determinants which generate economic growth and ensuring that the policies in place facilitate the right incentives for enhancing these determinants. Such determinants include investment in physical capital and infrastructure, investment in education and skill accumulation, allowing for integration with global markets, and ensuring macroeconomic stability and institutions that encourage domestic investment.

The lack of inclusiveness of the growth pattern in Africa poses serious challenges to the continent. The participation in the early stages of the Sustainable Development Goals provides a renewed opportunity for Africa to change its policy and political environments, in order to ensure that the wider population receives the benefits of growth.

References

Acemoglu, D., Johnson, S., Robinson, J. A., & Yared, P. (2008). Income and democracy. *American Economic Review, 98*(3), 808–842.

Africa Population. (2017). Retrieved June 28, 2018, from http://worldpopulationreview.com/continents/africa-population/

Barro, R., & Lee, J. (1997). *Determinants of schooling quality*. Mimeo, Harvard and Korea Universities.

Barro, R., & Sala-i-Martin, X. (1995). *Economic growth*. New York, NY: McGraw-Hill.

Becker, G. S., Murphy, K. M., & Tamura, R. (1990). Human capital, fertility, and economic growth. *The Journal of Political Economy, 98*(5), 12–37.

Benhabib, J., & Spiegel, M. M. (1994). The role of human capital in economic development: Evidence from aggregate cross-country data. *Journal of Monetary Economics, 34*(2), 143–174.

Besley, T., & Cord, L. J. (2007). *Delivering on the promise of pro-poor growth: Insights and lessons from country experiences*. Washington, DC: World Bank and Palgrave Macmillan.

Bhanumurthy, H., & Mitra, H. (2004). Economic growth, poverty, and inequality in Indian states in the pre-reform and reform periods. *Asian Development Review, 21*(2., 2004), 79–99.

Boone, P. (1996, April). *Political and gender oppression as a cause of poverty*. Mimeo, London School of Economics.

Burke, P. J., & Leigh, A. (2010). Do output contractions trigger democratic change? *American Economic Journal: Macroeconomics, 2*(4), 124–157.

Caldwell, J. C., Orubuloye, I. O., & Caldwell, P. (1992). Fertility decline in Africa: A new type of transition? *Population and Development Review, 18*(2), 211–242.

Cervellati, M., Jung, F., Sunde, U., & Vischer, T. (2014). Income and democracy: Comment. *American Economic Review, 104*(2), 707–719.

Chisadza, C., & Bittencourt, M. (2018). Economic development and democracy: the modernisation hypothesis in sub-Saharan Africa. *The Social Science Journal,* in press (https://doi.org/10.1016/j.soscij.2018.10.007).

Chisadza, C., & Bittencourt, M. (2015). *The fertility transition: Panel evidence from sub-Saharan Africa* (Economic Research Southern Africa Working Paper Series 620).

Conley, D., McCord, G. C., & Sachs, J. D. (2007). *Africa's lagging demographic transition: Evidence from exogenous impacts of malaria ecology and agricultural technology* (National Bureau of Economic Research Working Paper 12892).

Dreze, J., & Murthi, M. (2001). Fertility, education, and development: Evidence from India. *Population and Development Review, 27*(1), 33–63.

Fayad, G., Bates, R. H., & Hoeffler, A. (2012). *Income and democracy: Lipset.s law inverted* (IMF Working Paper Series WP/12/295).

Fosu, A. (2013). Growth of African economies: Productivity, policy syndromes and the importance of institutions. *Journal of African Economies, 22*(4), 523–551.

Jerven, M. (2017). *Africa growing? Past, present and future* (Brief Issue 13). European Union Institute for Security Studies. https://www.iss.europa.eu/sites/default/files/EUISSFiles/Brief_13_African_economies.pdf

Leke, A., & Barton, D. (2016). *Africa, Lions on the move 2.0: The continuing progress of Africa's economies* (World Economic Forum on Africa

Series). https://www.weforum.org/agenda/2016/05/what-s-the-future-of-economic-growth-in-africa/
Lin, B. Q. (2003). Economic growth, income inequality, and poverty reduction in People's Republic of China. *Asian Development Review, 20*(2., 2003), 105–124.
Lloyd, C. B., & Blanc, A. K. (1996). Children's schooling in sub-Saharan Africa: The role of fathers, mothers, and others. *Population and Development Review, 22*(2), 265–298.
Mankiw, N. G., Romer, D., & Weil, D. (1992). A contribution to the empirics of economic growth. *Quarterly Journal of Economics, 107*(2), 407–437.
Olamosu, B., & Wynne, A. (2015). Africa rising? The economic history of sub-Saharan Africa. International Socialism, A quarterly review of socialist theory, Issue 146. http://isj.org.uk/africa-rising/
Pritchett, L., & Summers, L. H. (1993). *Wealthier is healthier* (Policy Research Working Paper Series 1150). Washington, DC: The World Bank.
Rodrik, D. (2007). *One economics, many recipes: Globalization, institutions and economic growth.* Princeton, NJ: Princeton University Press.
Rodrik, D. (2016). An African growth miracle? *Journal of African Economies* (Special Issue), 1–18.
Romer, P. (1990). Endogenous technological change. *Journal of Political Economy, 99*(5, pt. II), S71–S102.
Smith, M. N. (2016, July 1). The 17 countries with the worst quality of life in the world. In *Business Insider South Africa*.
Soares, R. R. (2007). On the determinants of mortality reductions in the developing world. *Population and Development Review, 33*(2), 247–287.
Strulik, H. (2016). *Desire and development* (Center for European Governance and Economic Development Research Discussion Paper No. 274).
United Nations. (2015). *The millennium development goals report 2015*. New York, NY: United Nations.
United Nations Development Programme (UNDP). (1990). *Human development report 1990. Conceptualisation and measurement of human development*. New York, NY: Oxford University Press.
World Bank. (1990). *World development report 1990: Poverty*. New York, NY: Oxford University Press.
World Bank. (1991). *World development report 1991: The challenge of development*. New York, NY: Oxford University Press.
World Development Indicators, The World Bank.
Young, A. (2012). The African growth miracle. *Journal of Political Economy, 120*(4), 696–739.

Improving Health Outcomes and *Quality of Life* for African Adolescents: The Role of Digital and Mobile Games

8

Tyra M. Pendergrass, Kimberly Hieftje, and Lynn E. Fiellin

Abstract

Quality of life has been defined as a multidimensional concept, that includes domains related to physical, mental, emotional, and social dimensions (Karimi & Brazier, Pharmacoeconomics, 2016). Along with other prominent factors such as labor market opportunities, education, and housing, health has been identified as a paramount and modifiable factor that can improve the quality of life for not only individuals, but for communities and nations as a whole (African Development Bank Group, Annual development effectiveness review 2017: transforming Africa, 2017). Though adolescents in Africa have experienced increases in access to education, more job opportunities, and longer lifespans when compared to previous generations, many inter-connected factors continue to adversely affect their quality of life. Furthermore, given that these adolescents are growing up in a different generation, novel approaches and interventions to impact and improve their health, well-being, and ultimately quality of life are sorely needed. This chapter will explore: (1) general definitions of well-being and its relation to factors associated with quality of life; (2) adolescents in Africa; (3) health burdens in Africa; (4) Serious Games; (5) Games for health on a global scale and (6) Games for health in Africa. In this chapter the term adolescent will refer to those individuals who are 10–19 years old and the term young people will include those who are 20–24 years old.

8.1 Well-Being

The term "subjective well-being" (SWB) emerged in the late 1950s as a result of researchers searching for useful indicators to reflect quality of life, to monitor social change, and improve social policy (Land, 1975). Andrews and Withey (1976) and Campbell, Converse, and Rodgers (1976) clarified that although people live in objectively defined environments, it is their subjectively defined worlds that they respond to, thus giving prominence to subjective well-being as a relevant index of people's life quality and their perception of it. There has been much discussion in the field of those who study well-being as to whether the terms happiness and life satisfaction can be used as synonyms for SWB (Ngamaba, Panagioti, & Armitage, 2017), or if they represent their own measurement of a person's view of their life. Happiness and well-being have often

T. M. Pendergrass (✉) · K. Hieftje · L. E. Fiellin
play2PREVENT Lab at the Yale Center for Health & Learning Games, Yale School of Medicine, New Haven, CT, USA
e-mail: tyra.pendergrass@yale.edu; kimberly.hieftje@yale.edu; lynn.fiellin@yale.edu

I. Eloff (ed.), *Handbook of Quality of Life in African Societies*, International Handbooks of Quality-of-Life, https://doi.org/10.1007/978-3-030-15367-0_8

had to be teased apart to get a more accurate picture of an individual's perspective as a whole. Happiness is most closely associated with emotions, feeling and moods (Diener, Suh, Lucas, & Smith, 1999). While SWB on the other hand is multifaceted; including both how happy individuals are at a point in time and how satisfied they are with their lives as a whole (Diener, 2006), this proxy for satisfaction could include evaluations about their work, personal relationships or perceptions of health status (Diener et al., 1999). In addition, different temporal frames differentiate SWB and happiness. SWB can be thought of as a judgmental, long-term assessment of one's life, whereas happiness is a reflection of pleasant and unpleasant affects in one's immediate experience (Keyes, Shmotkin, & Ryff, 2002). SWB has also routinely been defined as a person's mental and emotional evaluations of his or her life that incorporates both personal characteristics such as age, family experience, income, or health as well as external factors such as work satisfaction, government, values or religion (Reyes-García et al., 2016).

A more in-depth interpretation of SWB expands beyond just an individual and encompasses the perspectives and actual realities of communities. Michalos (2017) argues that the well-being of an individual or community can be thought of as a function of the actual condition of one's life and what an individual or community makes of those conditions. Michalos continues that well-being can be sorted into four categories that include components of both the perspective and reality of an individual or a community. What an individual or community makes of those conditions is in turn a function of how the conditions are perceived, what is thought and felt about those conditions, what is done, and finally which outcomes come from all of these inputs. Individuals' and communities' perceptions, thoughts, feelings and actions ultimately have an impact on their own and other's living conditions (i.e. their well-being) (Michalos, 2017). Regardless of how SWB is defined, there is a strong consensus that income, education, and health significantly influence one's well-being.

8.1.1 Income and Well-Being

Historically, there has been significant debate about the association and the strength of that association between income and well-being. In 1974 Richard Easterlin stated that increasing average income did not raise average well-being; this claim became known as the Easterlin Paradox (Stevenson & Wolfers, 2013). However, in more recent years many have highlighted that this claim is oversimplified and the nature of income's relation to well-being is multifaceted and often shows a positive correlation (Stevenson & Wolfers, 2013). Yet, others have pointed out that a hybrid of the two schools of thought is the actual representation of the relationship between income and well-being; the idea that there is a threshold after which basic needs are met and where income becomes unrelated to well-being, but before that threshold, income plays a bigger role in a person's well-being (Stevenson & Wolfers, 2013).

8.1.2 Education and Well-Being

Education is one of the strongest predictors of positive life outcomes in the areas of employment, income and social status, ultimately serving as a strong predictor of an individual's well-being. Research suggests that individuals with lower education levels have fewer prospects for higher level employment, and therefore lower levels of income, and a harder time developing a positive social identity (their understanding of themselves and their relationships with other people); negatively affecting their self-esteem and well-being (Economic and Social Research Council, 2014).

8.1.3 Health and Well-Being

The comprehensive definition of health, developed by the World Health Organization, highlights that health is complete physical, mental and social well-being and not merely the absence of disease or infirmity (WHO, 1948). This definition of health requires that in order to accurately measure one's overall health, the entire person must be the focal point. An inclusive representation of individual's over-all health should include the following components (Youth Health Education, 2018):

- *Physical health* can be described as what has, can and will affect your physical body such as genetics, diet exercise, illness, and disability.
- *Social health* can be defined as all forms of social interactions with two or more individuals including family, friends, colleagues, strangers; the potential of being influenced by other individuals or groups, either directly or indirectly such as media.
- *Cognitive health* has multiple factors which when combined, create an individual's intelligence. These factors are necessary to develop and/or maintain independence.
- *Emotional health* is not simply feeling happy all or most of the time but experiencing a large variety of emotions (positive and negative).
- *Cultural health* is a combination of social and physical health as it is influenced by our community laws, beliefs, attitudes, behaviors and values and has the potential to strongly influence emotional, social and physical health.
- *Spiritual health* is the most abstract and difficult to define; often including the belief of unity with a greater force, belief of a supreme being and/or a guiding sense of meaning and often includes higher values of hope, purpose, faith and peace.
- *Environmental health* focuses on the relationships between people and their environment (all the physical, chemical, and biological factors external to a person and all the related behaviors) (WHO, 2018).

All of these components of health shape an individual's SWB.

The Global Well-Being Index is often used in the global context to compare well-being between and across nations and encompasses many of the elements that have been associated with SWB (Gallup, 2017). It is organized into the five elements: purpose (liking what you do each day and being motivated to achieve your goals), social (having supportive relationships and love in your life), financial (your economic life to reduce stress and increase security); community (liking where you live, feeling safe and having pride in your community), physical (having good health and enough energy to get things done daily) (Gallup, 2017). These factors are important because they ultimately affect one's overall quality of life. The most recent report of the Global Well-Being Index, highlights the disparities that exist across nations, with regards to overall well-being and element of well-being (Standish & Witters, 2016) (Fig. 8.1).

8.2 Adolescents in Africa

In Africa in 2017, children and young people under the age of 25 accounted for 60% of the population (United Nations, 2017). More than half of the anticipated growth in global population between now and 2050 is expected to occur in Africa. Of the additional 2.2 billion people that are estimated to add to global population between 2017 and 2050, 1.3 billion will be born in Africa (United Nations, 2017). Beyond 2050, Africa will be the greatest contributor to the world's population growth. After 2050, it is anticipated that Africa will be the sole region in the world still experiencing substantial population growth (United Nations, 2017). As a result, Africa's share of the global population, which is projected to grow from roughly 17% in 2017 to around 26% in 2050, could reach 40% in 2100 (United Nations, 2017). In all plausible scenarios of future population trends, Africa will play a central role in shaping the size and distribution of the world's population over the next few decades by adding a multitude of adolescents. In fact, in some sub-Saharan African countries such as Niger, Uganda, Chad, and Burundi, their total populations are actually "youthening" rather than ageing, ultimately reflecting that the country's median age is declining (United Nations, 2017).

The United Nations highlights that recent shifts in the age structure towards younger populations present an unprecedented opportunity

ALL ELEMENTS OF WELL-BEING 10 LOWEST COUNTRIES AND AREAS

PURPOSE	% Thriving
Afghanistan	0.0
Tunisia	4.0
Bhutan	4.2
Palestinian Territories	6.0
Egypt	6.4
Hong Kong	6.6
Congo Kinshasa	6.6
Senegal	6.9
Morocco	7.2
Cameroon	7.7

SOCIAL	% Thriving
Afghanistan	0.0
Congo Kinshasa	6.5
Togo	6.9
Tunisia	7.4
Benin	7.9
Ghana	9.1
Haiti	10.0
Madagascar	10.0
Cameroon	10.2
Malawi	10.7

FINANCIAL	% Thriving
Afghanistan	2.7
Guinea	2.9
Benin	3.9
Togo	4.4
Burundi	4.5
Angola	4.8
Uganda	4.9
Rwanda	5.3
Madagascar	5.3
Niger	5.3

COMMUNITY	% Thriving
Bhutan	4.6
Angola	5.7
Burundi	6.9
Azerbaijan	8.3
Croatia	9.1
Montenegro	9.2
Congo Kinshasa	10.3
Gabon	10.9
Serbia	11.2
Armenia	11.4

PHYSICAL	% Thriving
Bhutan	6.4
Afghanistan	8.3
Tunisia	9.0
Ukraine	9.4
Cameroon	9.6
Hong Kong	10.0
Cambodia	10.9
South Korea	10.9
Singapore	11.0
Belarus	11.1

ALL ELEMENTS OF WELL-BEING 10 HIGHEST COUNTRIES AND AREAS

PURPOSE	% Thriving
Panama	60.5
Costa Rica	53.8
Puerto Rico	48.8
Chile	46.3
Guatemala	44.9
Denmark	42.7
Colombia	41.5
Belize	41.2
Mexico	40.5
Uruguay	39.2

SOCIAL	% Thriving
Puerto Rico	63.0
Panama	62.6
Costa Rica	59.3
Uruguay	57.8
Chile	54.5
El Salvador	49.4
Guatemala	49.3
Myanmar	48.4
Belize	48.2
Argentina	48.2

FINANCIAL	% Thriving
Norway	68.9
Sweden	67.9
Switzerland	66.1
Netherlands	60.8
Austria	59.5
Germany	57.4
Luxembourg	57.3
Denmark	55.0
Singapore	52.4
Finland	50.7

COMMUNITY	% Thriving
Sri Lanka	50.1
Panama	50.0
Belize	49.3
Denmark	48.8
Switzerland	48.7
Norway	47.8
Myanmar	47.7
Puerto Rico	47.7
United Arab Emirates	46.8
Costa Rica	46.1

PHYSICAL	% Thriving
Panama	52.2
Costa Rica	47.0
Belize	44.4
Puerto Rico	40.9
Uruguay	40.7
Guatemala	40.7
El Salvador	39.6
Colombia	39.4
Chile	39.2
Myanmar	38.8

Fig. 8.1 Ten highest and lowest country rankings, measured by elements of well-being. (Source: Gallup Healthways Well-Being Index. Based on surveys conducted in 145 countries and areas in 2014)

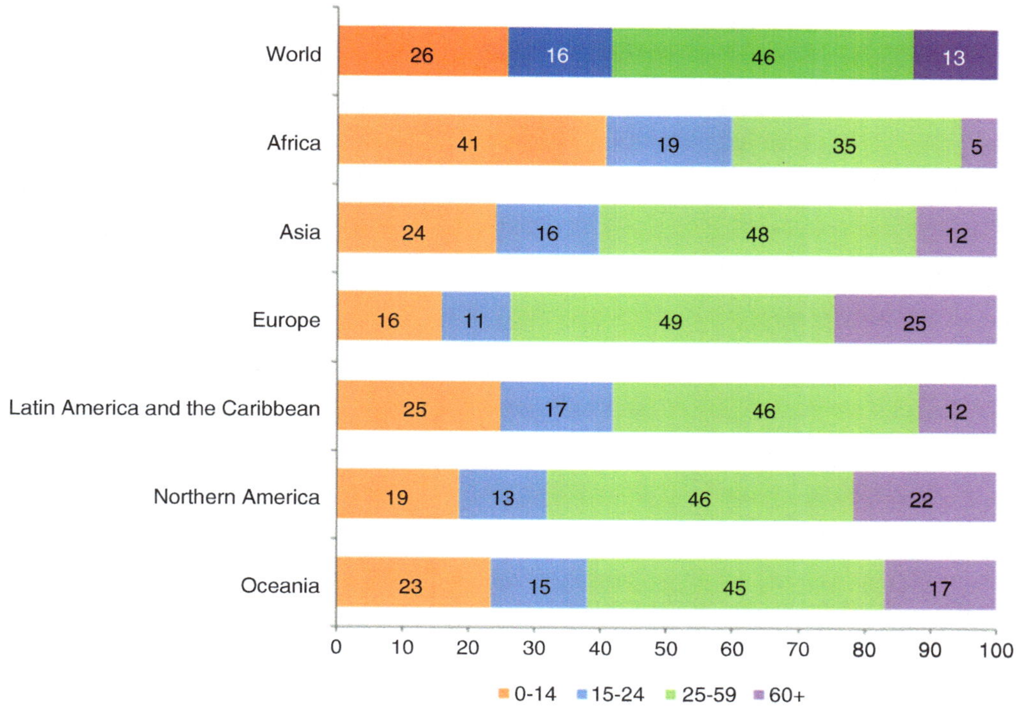

Fig. 8.2 Percentage of population in broad age groups for the world and by region, 2017. (Source: United Nations, Department of Economic and Social Affairs, Population Division, 2017)

to catapult developing countries forward through economic development (United Nations, 2015). For example, many East Asian economies experienced the "economic miracle" that saw a rapid growth in their economies in the late 1990s. With growing adolescent and young person populations, this same economic development could become a reality for many of today's economically developing countries, particularly in sub-Saharan Africa, if the well-being of adolescents is prioritized (United Nations, 2015) (Fig. 8.2).

8.3 Health Burdens in Africa

The immense continent of Africa comprises almost 17% of the world's population and is the home to almost 1.3 billion people. Africa has the burden of having to address a multitude of health issues, that have a significant effect on the well-being and quality of life of its citizens; both within country general populations as well as in sub-populations. The mammoth health issues of infectious diseases, non-communicable diseases, and malnutrition concurrently contribute to mortality, morbidity and decreased well-being in Africa (United Nations, 2016). Each of these health issues has distinct ramifications, but collectively they impact the health and well-being of Africans in a magnified fashion. In Africa, life expectancy increased from the 1950s until the early 1980s, where it was slowed by the HIV/AIDS epidemic in the late 1980s and through the 1990s (United Nations, 2016). More recently, the life expectancy at birth for the continent has reached almost 60 years; though it still lags significantly behind the rest of the world (United Nations, 2016) (Fig. 8.3).

The Sub-Saharan region of Africa encompasses 49 of the 54 countries that make up the African continent. Sub-Saharan Africa is home to 13% of the world's population yet represents 24% of the global disease burden (Agyepong

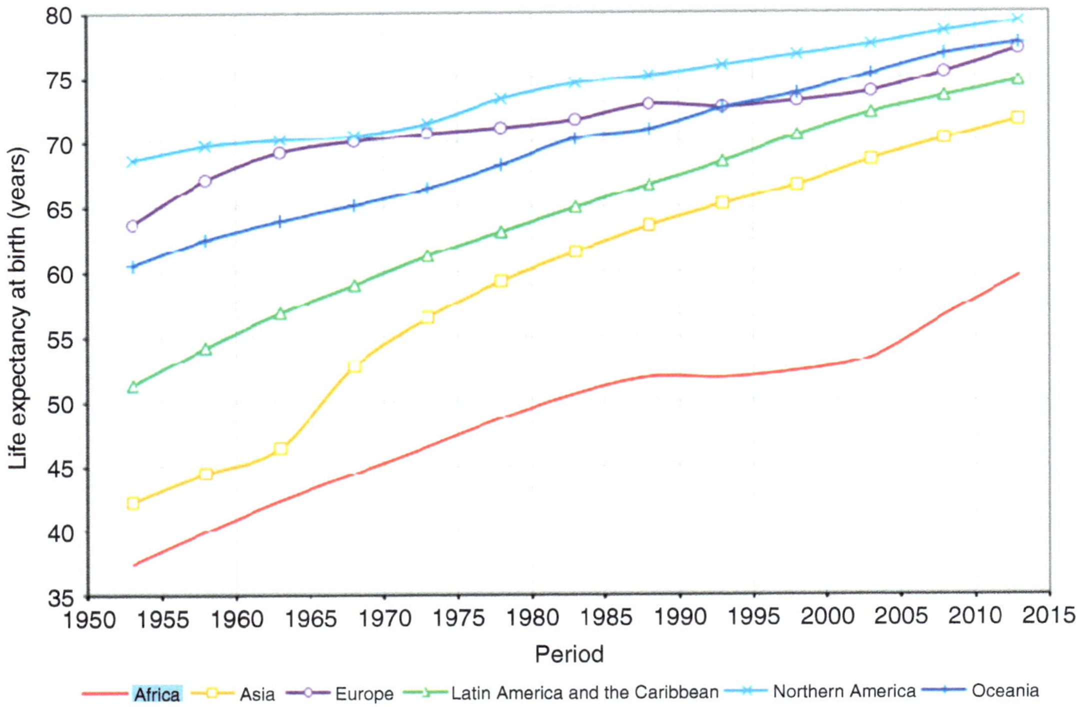

Fig. 8.3 Life expectancy at birth by major area, 1950–2015. (Source: United Nations Monitoring Report: Health, Morbidity, Mortality and Development, 2016)

et al., 2017). Sub-Saharan Africa's health challenges are unique in that, most sub-Saharan countries face a double burden of addressing conventional health challenges such as infectious diseases, malnutrition, and child and maternal mortality, and emergent challenges such as non-communicable conditions, mental health disorders, injuries, and health problems related to climate change and environmental degradation (Agyepong et al., 2017). Infectious diseases remain the leading causes of mortality and morbidity in Sub-Saharan Africa, with HIV/AIDS, lower respiratory infections, malaria, diarrheal diseases and tuberculosis ranking 1–5. Additionally, a combination of changing food habits, increased income and affluence, and increasing sedentary lifestyles has caused non-communicable diseases such as heart disease, stroke, diabetes, and pulmonary diseases to substantially increase their impact on health loss in the Sub-Saharan region (Agyepong et al., 2017). Africa is expected to experience the largest increase in non-communicable disease related mortality globally; about 46% of all mortality in Africa is expected to be attributed to non-communicable diseases by 2030 (Dalal et al., 2011; WHO, 2014).

Although adolescents in Africa are affected by the same health burdens as the general population, they also have their own health issues that disproportionately affect them in comparison to the general population. According to the World Health Organization, early pregnancy and childbirth, HIV, other infectious diseases, mental health, violence, malnutrition and obesity, and tobacco use are all health burdens that affect adolescents (WHO, 2018).

8.3.1 Early Pregnancy and Childbirth

Because the global population of adolescents continues to grow, projections indicate the number of adolescent pregnancies will increase globally by 2030, with the greatest proportional increases occurring in sub-Saharan Africa (United Nations Population Fund, 2013). The United Nations Population Fund asserts that adolescent pregnancies are of utmost importance, because they ultimately have irreparable consequences on adolescent health and well-being; compromising the individual's sexual and reproductive health and perpetuating the cycle of poverty.

8.3.2 HIV

HIV, or *Human Immunodeficiency Virus,* is spread through bodily fluids such as blood and semen and attacks the body's immune system. Over time, HIV can destroy many of the cells that the body depends on to stay healthy, eventually leading to the body not being able to fight off other infections and diseases. If not treated, HIV can develop into AIDS (*Acquired Immunodeficiency Syndrome*) at which point the body's immune system is severely damaged and the individual becomes ill with a number of infections called opportunistic infections. Although significant advances have been made in the areas of HIV/AIDS research, prevention, and treatment, the disease still has a significant impact on many countries in Africa. Notably, although HIV incidence rates have declined sharply in those countries that have the resources to invest in HIV prevention strategies, there are still almost 26 million people from the continent of Africa who are living with HIV/AIDS (WHO, 2018). Additionally, on a global level, almost two thirds of new HIV infections originate on the continent of Africa (WHO, 2018). HIV is the leading cause of death for adolescents in Africa, and the number of HIV deaths are continuing to rise in this age group (United Nations Population Fund, 2015). At a time when HIV-related deaths are declining rapidly in other age groups, HIV-related deaths among older adolescents aged 15–19 are not declining (United Nations Population Fund, 2015). In 2015, an estimated 29 adolescents acquired HIV every hour. Some of the factors that fuel the HIV epidemic in this population include poor uptake of HIV prevention strategies such as condom use and low rates of HIV testing (United Nations Population Fund, 2015).

8.3.3 Infectious Diseases

Although the burden of non-communicable diseases in African populations is expected to significantly rise, infectious diseases still have a greater impact on overall health, well-being, and mortality rates on the continent (Deaton & Tortora, 2015). Infectious diseases are caused by microorganisms (such as bacteria, viruses, parasites or fungi) that can be spread from person to person, either by direct contact (e.g., touching, intimate encounters) or indirect contact (e.g., coughing, sneezing, sharing infected objects). Africa is the only continent where deaths from infectious diseases still outnumber deaths from non-communicable diseases (Deaton & Tortora, 2015). Infectious disease can stunt children and adolescents' physical growth along with their cognitive development, ultimately having long-term consequences on their ability to learn and make a living (Alderman, Hoddinott, & Kinsey, 2006).

For example, tuberculosis is a disease that severely affect the lungs and is caused by bacteria. Tuberculosis is spread from one person to another through the air when an infected person coughs, sneezes or spits the tuberculosis germs into the air. Tuberculosis is the leading cause of death worldwide by an infectious disease, surpassing HIV (World Health Organization, 2017) and has had significant deleterious effects on the health and well-being of Africans. In 2016, 2.5 million people were affected by tuberculosis in Africa; accounting for a quarter of new cases worldwide (World Health Organization, 2017). Data has shown that the risk for tuberculosis increases dramatically during adolescence, due to challenges faced in case detection and effective

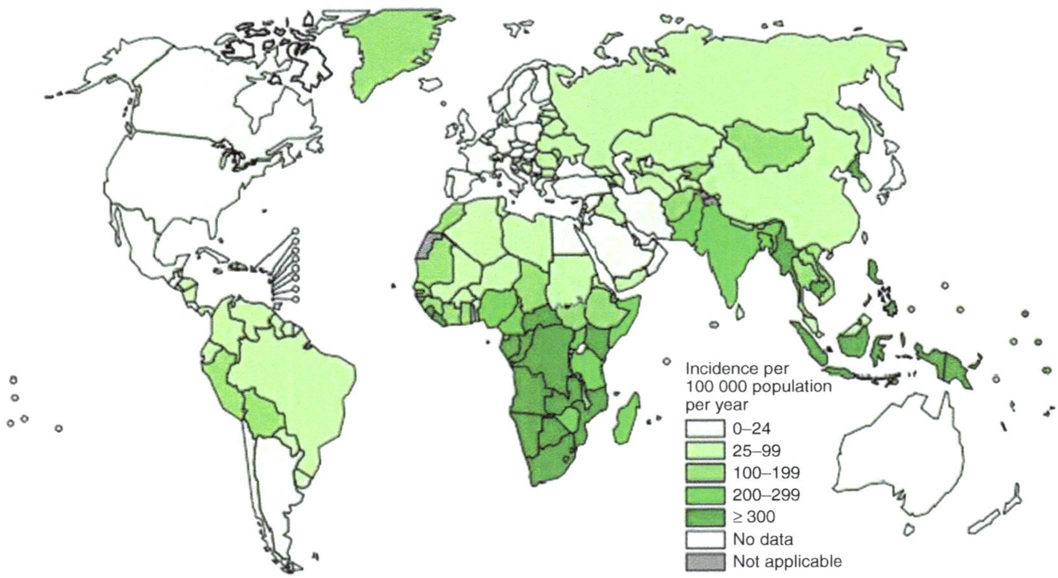

Fig. 8.4 Estimated tuberculosis incidence rates, 2016. (Source: World Health Organization's Global Tuberculosis Report, 2017)

treatment (Snow, Sismanidis, Denholm, Sawyer, & Graham, 2018). A recent study from Snow et al. estimates that approximately 1.78 million (uncertainty interval 1.23–3.00 million) adolescents and young adults developed tuberculosis each year (Fig. 8.4).

Malaria is another example of an infectious disease that significantly affects the health, well-being and quality of life for Africans. Malaria in humans is caused by five species of parasite. The majority of malaria incidence cases occur when a person is bitten by a mosquito that carries the disease. Even though the risk of acquiring malaria has been reduced by 37%, and the risk of dying from the disease has decreased by 60% since 2000, Africa still carries the greatest burden of the disease, leading in both number of cases and malaria-related deaths (WHO, 2016). The World Health Organization notes that the African countries continue to account for approximately 90% of malaria cases and deaths worldwide. Fifteen countries – all but one in sub-Saharan Africa – account for 80% of the global malaria burden (WHO, 2016). Most of the allocated resources to combat Malaria have gone to decreasing the incidence rates in children ages 5 and under; leaving adolescents as a vulnerable and understudied population (Fig. 8.5).

8.3.4 Mental Health

The growing awareness of the importance of mental health as a key component in adolescent development has begun to emerge in many African countries (Cortina, Sodha, Fazel, & Ramchandani, 2012). Although the majority of health resources in many countries are spent on HIV, tuberculosis, and malaria, the area of mental health is beginning to see increases in resources. The United Nations Millennium Development Goals specifically target mental health as a way to increase adolescents' overall well-being. Post-traumatic stress disorder is very common, given the history of many African countries in regards to conflict and war (Cortina et al., 2012). It has

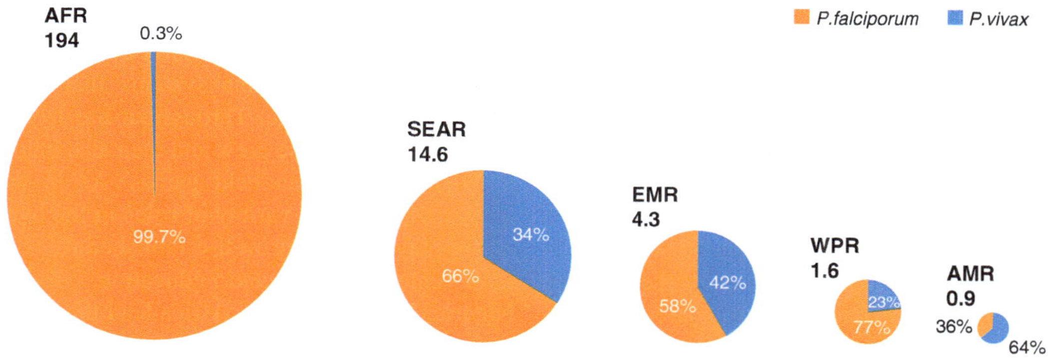

Fig. 8.5 Estimated malaria cases (millions) by mosquito species and World Health Organization region, 2016. The area of the circles is proportional to the estimated number of cases in each region. (Source: World Health Organization Global Malaria Report, 2016)

been estimated that 14% of adolescents have mental health problems and nearly 10% have diagnosable psychiatric disorders (Cortina et al., 2012), although it is argued that these numbers are not fully indicative of the region, given the limited number of resources and interventions that have specifically been dedicated to studying adolescent mental health in Africa.

8.3.5 Malnutrition

Malnutrition is defined as an impairment of health that is caused either from a deficiency, excess, or imbalance of nutrients. Malnutrition during childhood and adolescence has long term effects that extend into adulthood, affecting growth and development and increasing the likelihood of a premature death (Bain et al., 2013). According to the 2017 Global Nutrition report, Africa faces serious nutrition-related challenges. Over 60 million African children under age 5 are not growing properly, while at the other end of the spectrum it is estimated that at least 10 million children are overweight (Global Nutrition Report, 2017). This contributes to a high burden of allocating resources to combat these two, contrasting nutrition-related issues. Even with expanding economies, increased food production, and increased food waste (Dahir, 2017), many Africans still lack healthy amounts of food and nutrients needed to grow and develop; ultimately affecting their overall well-being. Because proper nutrition is essential for optimal brain development and function, as well as optimal physical function in adolescents, it has been estimated that the continent of Africa loses approximately 11% of its gross domestic product annually to malnutrition due to increased absenteeism, lost productivity, chronic illness and mortality (International Food Policy Research Institute, 2016).

8.4 Novel Interventions to Impact Health and Well-Being

Health interventions-whether they are behavioral, social, or environmental- have the potential to affect not only individuals, but communities, populations and nations as a whole. But in order for these interventions to have the desired and greatest impact, they must be: efficacious, contextually and culturally relevant, have high fidelity and be cost-effective. As interventions are designed to address current health concerns, there is a critical need for interventions that are adaptive to evolving priorities and populations and have the ability to not just mitigate health issues, but also prevent and/or eradicate these health burdens. Videogames are leading the way in this call for novel interventions, particularly among adolescent populations.

8.4.1 Videogames

The evolution of videogames can be traced back to the 1950s when scientists built the first videogames as instructional tools in academic settings (Desjardins, 2017). Following that, in the 1960s a group of students at the Massachusetts Institute of Technology (MIT) in the United States, were tasked with an assignment of using the school's new computer to create a demonstration program that (1) utilized as many of the computer's resources as possible, (2) remained interesting even after repeated viewings and (3) was interactive (Smithsonian, 2018). The result of the assignment was a dueling game between two spaceships, called *Spacewar* (Smithsonian, 2018). The development of this first game eventually led to the development of games that could be played on televisions in 1966. By the 1970s the pervasiveness of videogames had grown so much that prime time commercialization also began at this time and the first arcades were opened (Desjardins, 2017). Quickly following the arcades were the development of home gaming systems such as the Atari. In 1985, a Japanese company released the Nintendo Entertainment System (Smithsonian, 2018) which turned out to be widely popular and commercially successful; helping to solidify the videogame industry as a formidable industry in itself. Today, videogames in myriad forms (home entertainment games, computer games, mobile games, web-based games) are interwoven into the fabric of our society. In 2017, there were approximately 2.2 billion people world-wide that played some form of games (Research NGM, 2018). Additionally, it has been estimated that in 2017 almost $109 billion was spent on games.

8.4.2 Videogames in Africa

The first videogames in Africa were played in arcades. Some of the most popular videogames were PONG (1972), Space Invaders (1978), Asteroids (1979) and Pac-Man (1980) (Wolf & Iwatani, 2015). Similar to other places in the world, use of arcade games soon evolved into use of home-based game systems that were more easily accessible. Throughout the 1990s, home-based game use grew and then also incorporated portable handheld games. As in the past, games fulfill a variety of roles in the lives of the players; having well-established roles in both entertainment and education. Today, Nigeria, Egypt and South Africa lead the continent with the most videogame players and most money spent on videogames (Latzoo, 2016). However, within the last 20 years another role for games has emerged. This new use for games is neither solely for entertainment nor education, but an effective hybrid of both. This new genre of games is known as "serious games."

8.5 Serious Games

Serious games are officially defined as games that are created for a purpose other than solely just entertainment (Abt, 1970); these games can educate, train, and inform but still consist of enjoyable and entertaining components (Michael & Chen, 2005). Serious games can be utilized in an array of areas such as the military, government, educational, corporate, and healthcare (Susi, Johannesson, & Backlund, 2007). According to the Serious Game Classification System provided by Ludoscience (2014) and the serious game directory developed by the Serious Games Association (2014), serious games can be classified into different subcategories according to their goals. According to the classification system established by serious.gameclassification.com, these categories include:

- *Advergame*: a game used for marketing purposes
- A news game: a game broadcasting an informative message
- *Edugame*: a game broadcasting an educative message

- *Exergame*: a physical or cognitive training game
- *Edumarket*: a game broadcasting both a marketing or communication message and an informative or educative message (Ohannessian, Yaghobian, Verger, & Vanhems, 2016).

According to Corti (2006) serious games are "about leveraging the power of computer games to captivate and engage end-users for a specific purpose, such as to develop new knowledge and skills." The term "serious game" itself came into wide use with the emergence of the Serious Game Initiative in 2002. The initiative focused on uses for games in exploring management and leadership challenges facing the public sector (Susi et al., 2007).

When comparing serious games with traditional digital computer games, it has been argued that serious games have more than just story, art, and software. It is the addition of activities that educate or instruct, thereby imparting knowledge or skills, that sets serious games apart from other digital games (Zyda, 2005). Additionally, another element of serious games is that there is evidence that individuals who gain new knowledge and are able practice new behavioral skills in a virtual environment (through serious games) are more likely to use these new skills in real life settings (Bainbridge, 2007; Hubal, Kizakevich, & Furberg, 2007; Johnson & Beal, 2005; Schwebel, Gainesa, & Severson, 2008). Serious games also allow learners to experience situations that mimic the real world (Corti, 2006) and provide a novel approach to addressing sensitive behaviors, by allowing players to actively engage and process information within a private, virtual setting (Levin & Arafeh, 2002) and by stimulating and reinforcing learning by using multi-sensory, active, experiential, and problem-based learning (Oblinger, 2004). Serious game interventions have demonstrated effectiveness in affecting behaviors related to health promotion (Ferguson, 2012; Tarini, 2012) health prevention, emotional intelligence, environmental health and social good, and health and safety (Hieftje, Edelman, Camenga, & Fiellin, 2013). Serious games related to health and health care represent a significant portion of the serious games that have been developed.

8.6 Games for Health

Serious videogames for health ("games for health") are a special type of serious videogames that are specifically designed to change health or other behaviors while still being entertaining and engaging (Thompson et al., 2010). Health behaviors are often influenced by multiple competing factors, making them resistant to change (Baranowski, Lin, Wetter, Resnicow, & Hearn, 1997). Therefore, it is necessary for games for health to effectively target those factors to have the desired behavior outcome. To do this, in addition to including six essential components of effective game design (i.e. purpose, content and information, narrative, mechanics, graphics, and framing (Mitgutsch & Alvarado, 2012), games for health are often guided by psychology and health behavior models and theories (i.e. social cognitive theory, prospect theory, and the information motivation and behavior model). These theories and models are used in both the development and evaluation of the game for health. These theories and models address important factors that affect behavior such as: knowledge and information, attitudes, motivations, perceived susceptibility, perceived control, norms, benefits, penalties, barriers, and self-efficacy. By addressing these behavior mediators, games for health are able to address those multiple influences that would cause an individual to choose an unhealthy behavior over a healthy one, thereby affecting their overall health and well-being.

For example, social cognitive theory postulates that learning is a dynamic interplay between the person (personal and cognitive factors), the environment (social norms, influence by and on others), and behavior (skills, practice, self-efficacy) and that knowledge and skills provide the foundation for behavior change (Bandura, 1994). Therefore, basic knowledge of the health behavior and skills that enable the individual to act on this knowledge as well as elements that address environmental factors are critical

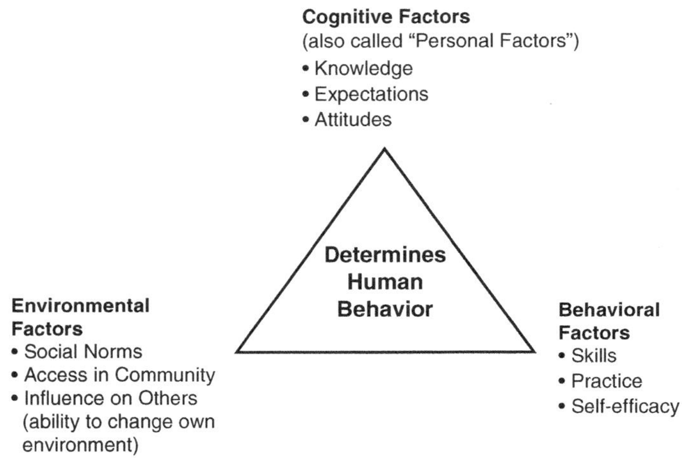

Fig. 8.6 Social cognitive theory

components for health behavior change and should be incorporated into a game for health. Additionally, social cognitive theory suggests that an important way to learn a new skill or behavior is to practice and perform the skill successfully yourself; games for health often provide the opportunity to practice this new skill in a virtual environment via repetition through different levels (Fig. 8.6).

Another example of a health behavior theory used in some games for health, is prospect theory. Prospect theory states that individuals avoid risks when they focus on the associated gains and are more willing to accept risks when they focus on the associated losses (Tversky & Kahneman, 1981). Prospect theory postulates that when gains are very relevant to the individual, people are averse to risks and that when losses are most important, individuals seek risk. By highlighting personal gains and losses associated with a specific health behavior, games for health are able to incorporate this theory into the game to relay trade-off costs to the player. Additionally, the Information, Motivation and Behavior Skills Model (IMB) has been used in games for health. The IMB model asserts that information is a prerequisite for changing behavior but is insufficient by itself to achieve this change; therefore, it is necessary for a game for health to identify and address motivations associated with the behavior and incorporate and teach familiar and uncomplicated behavioral skills to affect the desired behavior (Fisher & Fisher, 1992).

With the ubiquitous nature of and daily engagement with videogames globally among adolescents, games for health are increasingly being seen as a potential platform to teach knowledge and skills (Lenhart et al., 2008), and affect overall health and well-being of adolescents (Baranowski et al., 2008). Ultimately, games for health represent a novel intervention method to address health issues among adolescents. Because adolescents are constantly engaged with technology, games for health have the advantage of presenting information in a way that is relevant and relatable to them and on platforms with which they are familiar (i.e. smartphones, tablets, personal computers, the internet and game consoles).

8.7 Games for health Around the World

8.7.1 *The Baby Game*

An early example (1989) of a game for health, is *The Baby Game*. *The Baby Game* is a computer game designed with the purpose of increasing adolescents' desire and motivations to delay parenthood by having them engage in realistic simulations with caring for a baby; ultimately allowing them to evaluate their readiness for parenthood

(Paperny & Starn, 1989). *The Baby Game* aimed to teach adolescents about (1) their readiness to be a parent; (2) the amount of time needed to raise a child; (3) the costs of childbirth and raising a child in relation to the typical adolescents' finances; and (4) a more realistic understanding of the scope and responsibility of other demands of parenthood. Additionally, the game aimed to: increase adolescent's knowledge of the time and money needed for raising a baby, and foster attitudes favoring delayed parenthood and the use of contraception (Paperny & Starn, 1989).

The Baby Game is a 30-min color action game that was played on a standard personal computer. The effectiveness of the game was explored in secondary schools. Participants completed a pre- and post-test before and after playing the game, respectively. Participants in the control group were enrolled in only a health education class, while those participants in the experimental group played *The Baby Game.* Three hundred and fifty-one participants between the ages of 13 and 18 were enrolled in the study. In response to four assessment questions, all participants in the experimental group demonstrated significant learning; they exhibited increases in knowledge regarding: the financial costs of giving birth, the 1st year of life, and caring for a child to age 18, as well as the number of hour per day spent engaging in child care (Paperny & Starn, 1989).

8.7.2 *SPARX*

SPARX is a game for health comprised of a behavioral therapy intervention that aims to assist adolescents dealing with depression. The title *SPARX* is an acronym for: **S**mart, **P**ositive, **A**ctive, **R**ealistic, **X**-factor thoughts (Fleming et al., 2017). The intervention was initially designed for adolescents in New Zealand, but now other modified versions have been created to broaden the game's appeal to a wider range of adolescents. *SPARX* is an interactive fantasy game that incorporates both first person instruction and also a three-dimensional interactive game where the adolescent player chooses an avatar and navigates a series of challenges to restore the balance in a fantasy world dominated by GNATs (Gloomy Negative Automatic Thoughts) (Merry et al., 2012). In the game, the player travels through six provinces; each having their own theme such as (1) finding hope; (2) being active; (3) dealing with emotions; (4) overcoming problems (5) recognizing unhelpful thoughts, and (6) challenging unhelpful thoughts. At the beginning and end of each level, the player interacts with a "guide," who puts the game into context, provides education, gauges mood, and sets and monitors real-life challenges, equivalent to homework. *SPARX* is supplemented by a paper notebook with summaries of each level and with space for the participant to add comments about the challenges completed (Merry et al., 2012).

A randomized controlled trial to test the effectiveness of *SPARX* was completed, with the primary outcome being the change in score on the children's depression rating scale. Secondary outcomes were measured on a range of assessments examining depression, anxiety, quality of life (Merry et al., 2012). Participants were recruited from 24 sites across New Zealand, including 15 school-based counseling services, seven youth clinics, and two general practices. Outcome data were collected at baseline, post-intervention (approximately two months following baseline), and at follow-up five months following baseline. One hundred and eighty-seven participants were enrolled in the randomized controlled trial (Merry et al., 2012). At the two-month assessment, it was found that those participants who played *SPARX* had a higher average reduction in the raw scores on the children's depression rating-scale when compared to the control group (10.32 in *SPARX* and 7.59 in the control group; between group difference 2.73, 95% confidence interval −0.31–5.77; $p = 0.079$). Additionally, depression remission rates were significantly higher in the *SPARX* arm (n-31, 43.7%) than in the control group ($n = 19$, 26.4%) (difference 17.3%, 95% confidence interval 1.6–31.8%; $p = 0.030$). These improvements were maintained at the 5-month follow-up (Merry et al., 2012). All secondary measures supported the hypothesis that *SPARX*

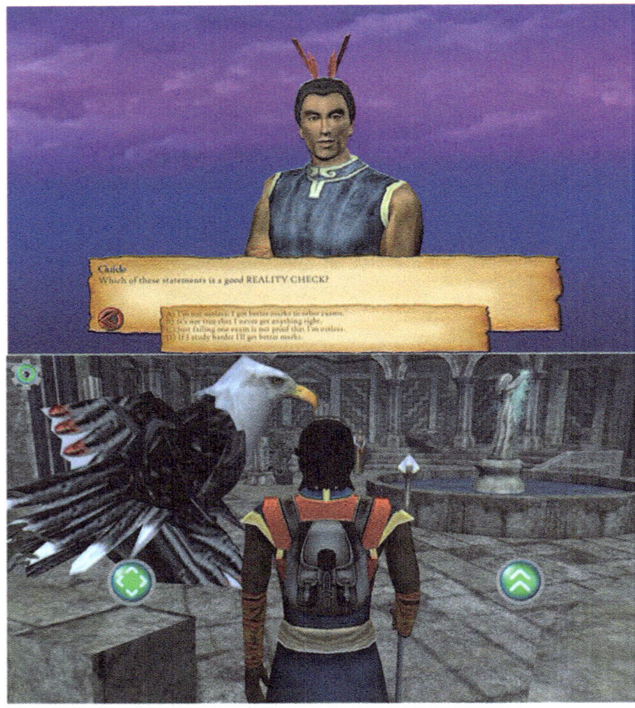

Fig. 8.7 Screenshots from the *SPARX* game

was not an inferior method of treatment to traditional treatments and practices and could be used as a novel intervention to impact adolescents' mental health (Fig. 8.7).

8.7.3 *PlayForward: Elm City Stories*

In 2009, the play2PREVENT Lab at the Yale University School of Medicine began the development of an original HIV prevention game that targeted risk behaviors in adolescents. The game intervention, *PlayForward Elm City Stories (PlayForward),* is a novel videogame intervention developed for adolescents aged 11–14 years old with the goal of reducing risk behaviors associated with HIV infection. *PlayForward* was developed with input from adolescents, researchers, educators, videogame designers/developers, and community organizations and incorporates social cognitive theory, prospect theory and message framing in its design (Camenga et al., 2014; Duncan, Hieftje, Culyba, & Fiellin, 2014; Hieftje, Duncan, & Fiellin, 2014; Hieftje, Rosenthal, Camenga, Edelman, & Fiellin, 2012). In *PlayForward* the adolescent player, using an *Aspirational Avatar* (Duncan et al., 2014; Fiellin, Hieftje, & Duncan, 2014) "travels" through life, encountering challenges related to sex, alcohol, drugs, and peer pressure and is required to make decisions in a range of situations. Through the game, the player is able to "fast-forward" to see how certain choices affect their lives, both in the present and in the future. The player is then able to go back in time in the game and make new choices to see how different actions affect their life in the game.

The game consists of 12 main storylines representing the player's avatar in the 7th–12th grades. Embedded within the main stories are five mini-games that help players build the skills to make healthy decisions when faced with difficult situations. The five skill-based mini-games are: *Me Power, Refusal Power, People Sense, Priority Sense, and Know Sense. Me Power* helps players think about who they are, what they care about, and what they want their future to look like and allows them to build their aspirations and values into the avatar. This mini-game encourages students to think beyond school to imagine what kind of future they would like for themselves, so they can better recognize how poor health decisions in the stories can impact that future. The *Know Sense* mini-game is designed to help players build their knowledge about health-related topics and model how they could convey such information to their peers in a relevant way. In *Refusal Power*, the player must identify how their friend is trying to pressure them, and then consider themes that would help them to say no. Within *People Sense,* the player has to decide which of their peers to keep close as a best friend or good friend and who they should avoid, given that one's circle of friends can heavily influence them and their decisions. The goal of *Priority Sense* is to teach players how to balance the consequences of different decisions on both the near and far future (Fiellin et al., 2016).

Following the development of *PlayForward*, a randomized controlled trial was conducted from 2013 to 2016 with 333 adolescents, aged 11–14, recruited and enrolled from their after-school, school, or summer-based program. The goal of the trial, was to evaluate the efficacy of the videogame intervention's impact on sex, alcohol and drug use behaviors and mediators of behaviors such as attitudes, knowledge, and intentions. Participants were randomized 1:1 to play up to 16 h of the experimental videogame (*PlayForward*) or control videogames over six weeks (Fiellin et al., 2017). Assessments were conducted at six weeks and at 3, 6, and 12 and 24 months. The primary outcome was delay of initiation of sexual intercourse. Secondary outcomes included sexual health attitudes, knowledge, intentions, as well as many other outcomes. Outcomes were examined by gender and age. In an analysis of specified outcomes at 12 months, the majority of participates in both the intervention and control groups (94.6% vs. 95.4%, respectively) had not yet started having sexual intercourse (relative risk = 0.99, 95% CI 0.94–1.05, $p = 0.77$); therefore, precluding the investigators from demonstrating a difference between the two groups at 12-month follow-up (Fiellin et al., 2017). However, the intervention group did demonstrate improved sexual health attitudes (least square means difference 0.37, 95% CI 0.01–0.72, $p = 0.04$). The intervention group also demonstrated increased sexual health knowledge over the 12-month follow-up (least square means difference 1.13, 95% CI 0.64–1.61, $p < 0.001$) (Fiellin et al., 2017) (Fig. 8.8).

Furthermore, the play2PREVENT Lab has also developed a spin-off game (*PlayTest!*) that is specifically geared toward increasing HIV testing and counseling in adolescents 14–18 years old. In addition to promoting HIV testing and counseling, *PlayTest!* also addresses personal health advocacy, communication in relationships around HIV testing and counseling, de-stigmatization of HIV and HIV testing, and utilizing

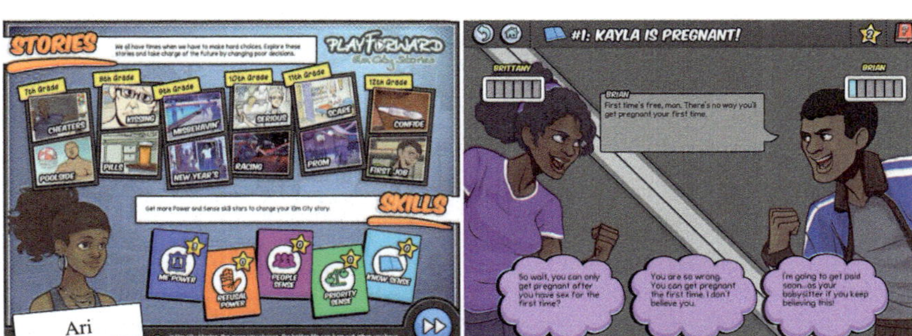

Fig. 8.8 Screenshots from *PlayForward: ElmCity Stories*

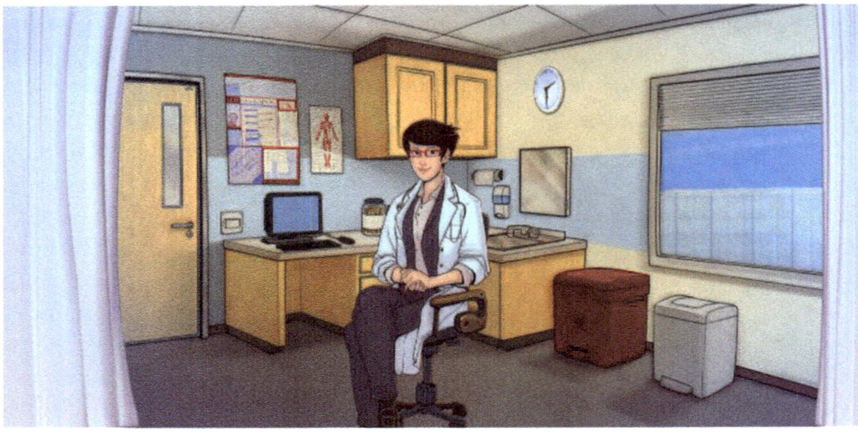

Fig. 8.9 Screenshot from *PlayTest!*

school-based health centers. The efficacy of *PlayTest!* on knowledge, attitudes, and behaviors surrounding HIV testing and counseling will be determined through a randomized controlled trial currently under way, that began in Fall 2018 (Fig. 8.9).

8.8 Games for health in Africa

Although the majority of serious games have been designed, developed and tested in middle and high income countries that often have the necessary resources, there is increasing potential to replicate these interventions in the African context. This section highlights several serious games that have been designed specifically in and for countries in Africa. These games have the goal of addressing a variety of issues that are relevant to the health and well-being of adolescents in African countries.

8.8.1 *SwaziYolo*

The Kingdom of eSwantini (formerly Swaziland) is a small, predominantly rural country in southern Africa that shares borders with South Africa and Mozambique (BBC Country Profile, 2018). The Kingdom of eSwantini is mostly homogenous in regards to language and cultural identity. Approximately 22% of the population are adolescents. Furthermore, the average life expectancy for citizens is 50 years for men and 48 years for women (BBC Country Profile, 2018). Unfortunately, the Kingdom of eSwantini has surpassed Botswana as the country with the world's highest known HIV/AIDS prevalence in the world (Central Intelligence Agency, 2018). It is estimated that approximately 210,000 of the 1.2 million citizens of Swaziland (18%) are living with HIV (BBC Country Profile, 2018). This fact has led to the need for strategies to combat this disease and increase the health, well-being and quality of life for its citizens, especially its adolescent population.

A unique game for health intervention that has been developed to address the high HIV/AIDS prevalence rate, is the game *SwaziYolo*. *SwaziYolo* was designed for mobile phones, making it highly accessible given that almost everyone in the country uses some form of smartphone. *Swaziyolo*'s creator, Bhekie Lukhele notes that with only $20, individuals can find a phone compatible to play *SwaziYolo* increasing its accessibility to a population that may be limited by technology (Lukhele, 2018).

The goal of *SwaziYolo* is to increase HIV risk perception, increase intention to reduce sexual partnerships, and increase the intention to know one's own and partner's HIV status. The target

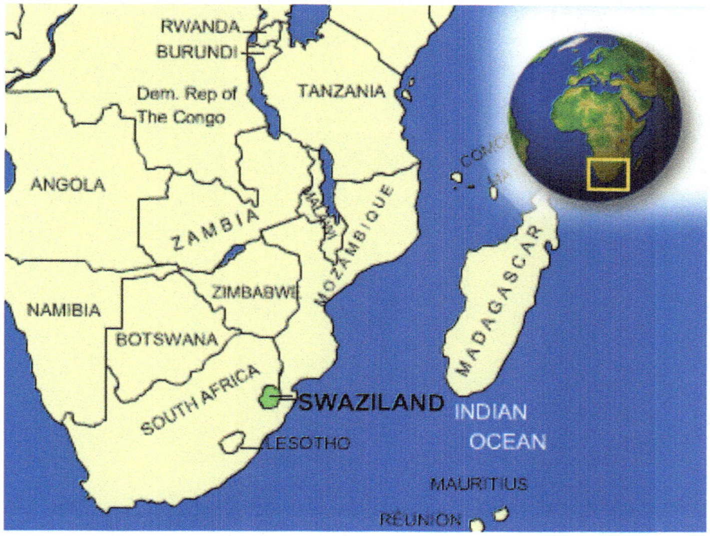

population for this game is Swazi males and females between the ages of 18 and 29 years old. The game targets this older adolescent age range because studies have shown that this age group is most vulnerable to HIV because of their low testing behavior (Lukhele et al., 2016). In the game, the player creates an avatar that is looking for love in the capital city of Mbabane. Throughout the game the player must make choices about relationships and their sexual health. A major component of the game includes the imaginary social network called *SwaziYolo* that is a combination of many of the popular social networking platforms that exist in the real world (i.e. Facebook, OKCupid and Whatsapp) (Lukhele et al., 2016). In the first part of the game the player creates a social profile that includes their interests and photos; in the second part of the game, the player can interact with computer generated characters at different locations around Mbabane, such as nightclubs and cafes. In both parts of the game, the player must choose between different storylines and interactions with their friends or love interest. The decisions they make influence the opinions and behaviors of the other characters and ultimately affect the player's health and safety (Lukhele et al., 2016).

The developers of *SwaziYolo* conducted a randomized controlled trial in 2016 with a target outcome being a change in risk perception in those that played the game. Those that participated in the study were exposed to the 4-week intervention (Lukhele, personal communication, 2018). A website was used to randomize participants to either the intervention or control group. Each participant was sent an SMS message that contained a code to enter into the system to take the pre- and post-game survey. Those in the intervention group immediately received the code to unlock the game after they completed their pre-game survey. Participants that were in the control group did not receive a code to play the game until after the randomized controlled trial concluded. The research team was able to use participants' cellphone numbers to track them; thereby creating a unique ID linked to their pre- and post-game surveys, as well as their gameplay. The results from the randomized controlled trial are currently being analyzed and are expected to be published later this year (Lukhele, personal communication, 2018).

In addition to the game itself, social media pages were used to increase game interest among adolescents. Lukhele notes that one of the challenges of the intervention was that most of the

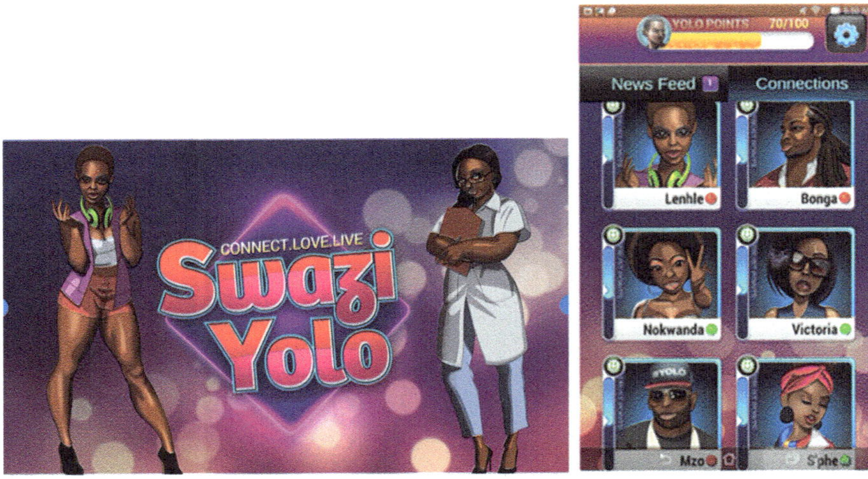

Fig. 8.10 Screenshots from *SwaziYolo*

users did not have a data package to access the internet. In order to access the game, they needed to buy air time to get data added to their cellphones. It was estimated that the game required approximately 64 MB to download to an individual's cellphone and therefore individuals needed approximately $6 to download the game (Lukhele, personal communication, 2018). Furthermore, moving forward, the developers intend to continue to develop the intervention package by making the game more interactive and developing more storylines that reflect some of the findings from the randomized controlled trial, and collaborating with universities in and outside of Africa (Fig. 8.10).

8.8.2 Pamoja Mtaani

The Republic of Kenya is located along the equator; surrounded by Ethiopia, South Sudan, Uganda, Somalia, and Tanzania. Kenya has experienced dramatic population growth since the mid-twentieth century as a result of its high birth rate and its declining mortality rate. Life expectancy in Kenya is 61.1 years for males and 65.8 years for females (Central Intelligence Agency World Fact Book, 2018). Approximately 20% of Kenya's population are adolescents. In 2015, it was reported that new HIV/AIDS infections among adolescents and young people increased by 17% even though the country as whole saw a decline of 19% in new HIV infection cases. In 2015, this finding translated to adolescents and young people contributing 51% of new HIV infection cases in 2015 (Kenyan Ministry of Health, 2016). This infection rate is equal to 97 adolescent and young people being infected on a daily basis (Kenyan Ministry of Health, 2016). To address the increased infection rates specifically in adolescents, Kenya developed a game to relay pertinent messages and address risky behaviors.

The online serious game entitled *Pamoja Mtaani* which is Swahili for "Together in the Hood," was created through a partnership between the U.S. president emergency plan for AIDS relief (PEPFAR) and Warner Bros. Studios (Fiorito, 2011) in attempts to address the HIV rates in the country. Warner Brothers selected the game development company, Virtual Heroes to develop the game.

The game was developed for 15 to 19-year olds, with the goal of educating them about HIV/AIDS. *Pamoja Mtaani* addresses the following five behaviors that can contribute to a reduction in HIV infection rates among adolescents: (1) delay in sexual initiation; (2) reduction in number of concurrent sexual partners; (3) increase in correct and consistent condom use; (4) increase in

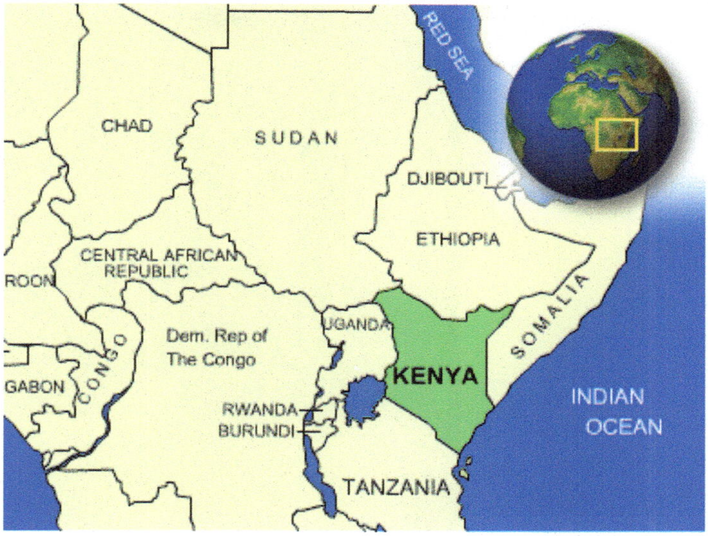

uptake of HIV testing and counseling services; and (5) increase in adoption of secondary abstinence (HIV Free Generation-Kenya, 2010). In the game, five strangers are brought together when they all have something stolen from them by a common character. The overarching game storyline, is that the players must work together to recover each of the stolen items and catch the thief. As the player progresses through the game, they encounter various neighborhoods that are based on real-life setting in the Kenyan capital of Nairobi (HIV Free Generation-Kenya, 2010). In these neighborhoods the players encounter barriers and facilitators to behavior change around HIV and must negotiate through different scenarios. There are also opportunities to play side missions and mini-games in addition to the main mission. The game uses a mix of English and Sheng, a local slang (HIV Free Generation-Kenya, 2010). The game can be played individually or in a group of up to five players. During the pilot phase, *Pamoja Mtaani* was implemented in three youth organization sites in Nairobi. In addition to being able to play the game, adolescents were also given access to health services such as: treatment for sexually transmitted infections, peer education sessions, and HIV testing and counseling. In addition, during this pilot phase, related activities that built skills and created economic opportunities for youth, were also implemented (HIV Free Generation-Kenya, 2010). A larger evaluation of the game was conducted from 2009 to 2011 and focused on risk perception and self-efficacy to perform the five previously mentioned HIV preventive behaviors. Over 4000 youth played the game, including 300 who participated in the evaluation (HIV Free Generation-Kenya, 2010) (Fig. 8.11).

Two levels of evaluation were conducted. Participants completed surveys at 30, 60, and 90-day intervals as well as shorter assessments that were embedded in the game after completing each level (HIV Free Generation-Kenya, 2010). The evaluation found a significant association between videogame exposure and overall change between baseline and post-baseline measures for both risk perception and self-efficacy related to the five behavioral objectives (HIV Free Generation-Kenya, 2010). Among males, exposure to the videogame increased their intention to initiate secondary abstinence, utilize services additional services, and reduce sex with older partners. Males also showed increased self-efficacy for condom use. Among females, expo-

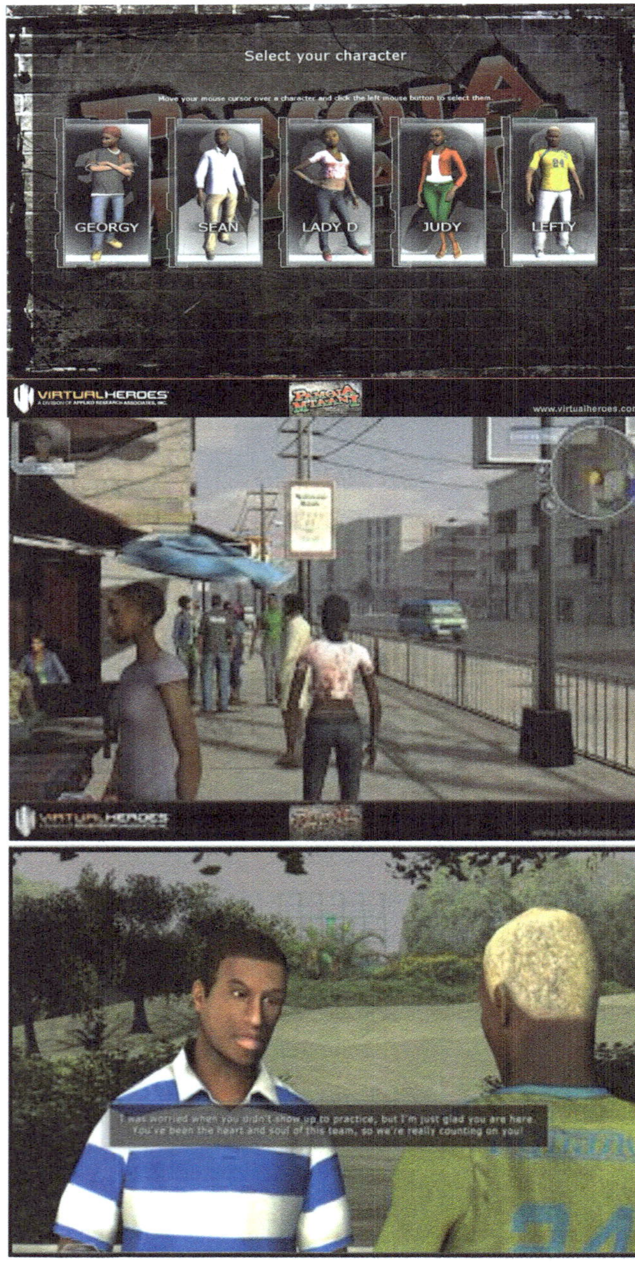

Fig. 8.11 Screenshots from Pamoja Mtaani. (Permission to use images obtained from Warner Brothers, Virtual Heroes and PEPFAR)

sure to the videogame increased their intention to delay sexual debut, self-efficacy for reducing concurrent sexual partners and for correct and consistent condom use (HIV Free Generation-Kenya, 2010).

8.8.3 *Cybersenga*

Uganda is located in East Africa and borders Kenya, Tanzania, South Sudan and Democratic Republic of the Congo. According to the BBC Country Profile, Uganda has transformed itself from a country with a troubled past to one of relative stability and prosperity. Uganda has one of the youngest and most rapidly growing populations in the world. Approximately 21% of the population are adolescents. Life expectancy in Uganda is 60.3 years for males and 64.3 years for

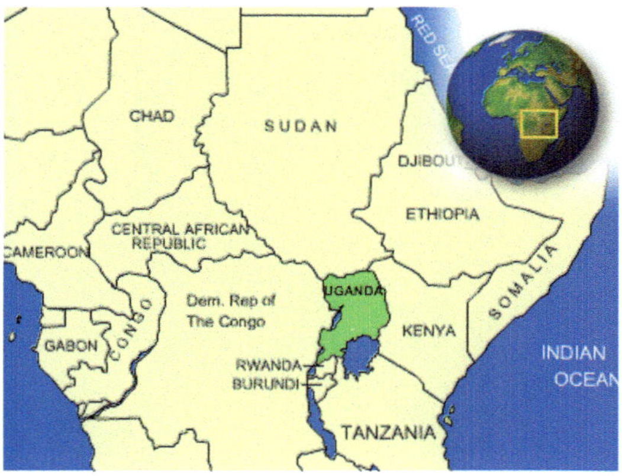

females (worldlifeexpectancy.com). Uganda is considered by UNAIDS (UNAIDS, 2004) to be one of the world's earliest and most compelling national success stories in combating the spread of HIV, with incidence rates plummeting from 16% in the 1990s to 6% were it remains today (Murphy, Greene, Mihailovic, & Olupot-Olupot, 2006). During the emergence of the HIV/AIDS epidemic in Africa during the 1990s, Uganda implemented a multi-pronged approach to address the epidemic that included: national messages about partner reduction and safe sex practices and significant increases in condom distribution to Ugandans (Kirby, 2008). Uganda has continued to experiment with novel methods and interventions to reduce HIV incidence rates, including the use of games for health.

Cybersenga is a school-based online game intervention that aims to help young people make healthy choices. The *Cybersenga* program provides information about HIV and illustrates relevant situations and useful ways for adolescence to problem-solve and communicate with others about their needs (Ybarra, Korchmaros, Prescott, & Birungi, 2015). Furthermore, *Cybersenga* uses culturally relevant aspects to connect with its adolescent audience. For example, *CyberSenga* uses the Ugandan concepts of Senga (father's sister; the auntie) and Koja (father's brother), both of whom are typically responsible for giving adolescents advice and guidance on issues related to sexual health (Ybarra et al., 2015). In the game, a virtual Senga or Kojja guides the player throughout the entirety of the game. The Senga introduces each topical area and then narrates the program for female participants, and the Kojja for male participants (Ybarra et al., 2015). *Cybersenga* focuses on: relaying facts about HIV (i.e. how HIV is and is not contracted, ways to reduce HIV risks, the prevalence rate of HIV in Uganda); problem-solving and communication skills; motivations to have sex or abstain from sex; condom use and negotiation skills; culturally specific issues related to HIV preventive behavior, and consensual relationships between adolescents (e.g., physical or emotional dating abuse) as well as romantic relationships with adults (e.g., sugar daddies and sugar mommies) (Ybarra et al., 2015).

A randomized controlled trial was conducted to test the acceptability and feasibility of the game. The study enrolled 366 sexually experienced and sexually inexperienced adolescents between the ages of 13 and 18 from across Uganda (Ybarra et al., 2015). The randomized controlled trial compared a control group that received sexual health education from their schools and an experimental group that played five one hour modules of the *CyberSenga* game, delivered in four tracks based on gender and sexual activity (Ybarra et al., 2015). Furthermore, half of the intervention group was randomized to receive a booster session after 3 months.

The study found significant improvement in the intervention groups (those groups that were assigned by gender and sexual experience) compared to the control in HIV prevention knowledge ($t\ (360) = 3.99$, $p < 0.001$, $B = 2.63$), motivation and attitudes for condom use. Attitudes toward condom use became more positive over time ($t\ (1057) = 5.13$, $p < 0.001$, $B = 0.28$). Subjective norms for condom use changed over time by becoming more positive over time ($t\ (1085) = 2.44$, $p = 0.015$, $B = 0.12$). Behavioral skills for condom use, and motivation

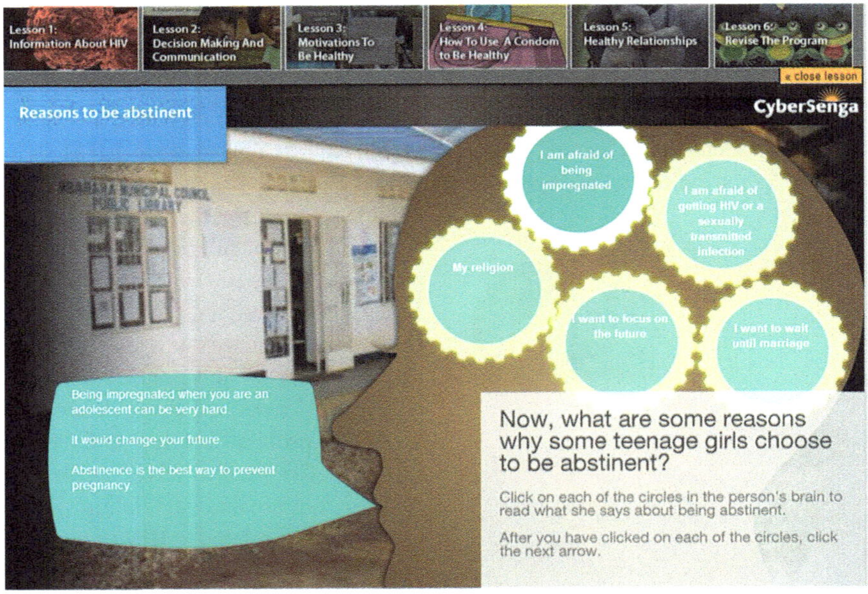

Fig. 8.12 Screenshots from *CyberSenga*

and behavioral skills for abstinence were statistically similar over time for both groups (Ybarra et al., 2015). Additionally, at the 3-month follow-up, 94% of intervention youth somewhat or strongly agreed that they had gains in learning, 76% said that the content addressed things they had experienced, and 93% reported they were very likely to recommend the program to their friends (Ybarra et al., 2015) (Fig. 8.12).

8.8.4 Easy-Care

Ethiopia is an inland country located in East Africa (the Horn of Africa) and is bordered by Somalia, Kenya, Sudan, Eritrea, and Djibouti. Ethiopia has a large adolescent and youth population. It is estimated that more than three out of five people in Ethiopia are under the age of 24; while about one in four people are between the ages of 10 and 19 (PMA 2020, 2017).

Low accessibility of educational information around nutrition and healthcare in the rural regions of Ethiopia has significantly contributed to Ethiopia having one of the highest maternal and child mortality rates in the world (Font, Hedvall, & Svensson, 2017), with a significant percentage of these mothers being adolescents.

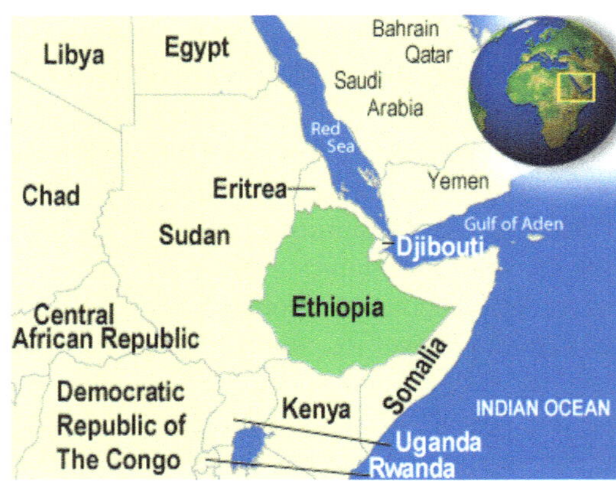

Based on many elements from the Tamagotchi game from the early 2000s (where users had to take care of an alien by feeding it, playing with it, and making sure it got enough rest for its survival), the game for health-*Easy-care*-was developed on the Android platform to help the player understand the importance of healthy nutrition during pregnancy. The player is given the task of taking care of a pregnant woman character living in an environment, that resembles rural Ethiopia.

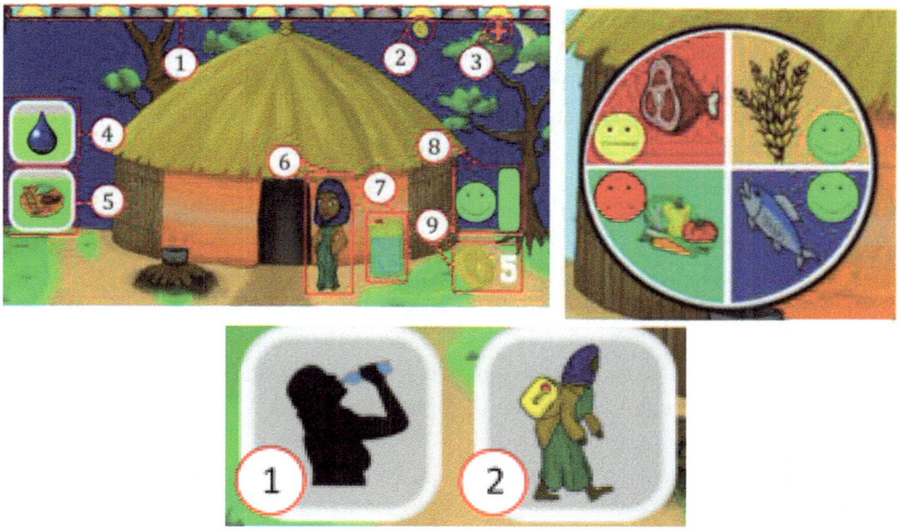

Fig. 8.13 Screenshots from *Easy-Care* Game

The main goal of the game is to keep the character healthy and nourished throughout her whole pregnancy by monitoring and controlling what she eats and drinks, the amount of healthcare she receives and ensuring that she maintains sufficient happiness levels (Font et al., 2017). A small field study with five women was conducted to test an early version of the game. The tests analyzed the usability of the user interface, the quality of the representation of the Ethiopian culture, and the general capability of *Easy-care* to teach maternal health concepts. It was found that the game succeeded in teaching the participants about principles about maternal healthcare and nutrition (Font et al., 2017). However, this small field study was only the first step in designing and developing a larger Game for Health that is not only culturally relevant but can also resonate with women who are mostly young, illiterate, living in rural areas and have almost no previous experience with digital games (Fig. 8.13).

8.9 Summary and Discussion

Africa is a uniquely diverse continent that has an array of concerns that need to be addressed in order to improve the overall health and well-being of its citizens. The growing number of adolescents across the continent has highlighted the need for special attention for the specific and unique heath needs and well-being of this population. Because the settings where adolescents live, work, and play are so influential to their health and well-being, prevention interventions to make these environments safe and conducive to optimal health and well-being are critical (Lansford & Banati, 2018). To be able to make choices that promote positive and healthy behaviors and decisions, adolescents need the support from many dimensions of their cultures and society as a whole. Large adolescent populations can have a profound effect on their respective countries and the world as a whole. Whether the effects are positive or negative depends on how well countries respond to their needs (United Nations Population Fund, 2015). Furthermore, because knowledge and behaviors learned in adolescence influence lifestyle choices during adulthood and ultimately have the ability to shape a society, investment in adolescents' health and well-being has increasingly emerged as an important area of focus in many countries.

The growing adolescent population has also emphasized the obligation that African countries have to develop novel ways to engage adolescents "where they are" in order to address these health issues with this new generation. The most powerful actions to address adolescent health and well-being are intersectional, multi-level and multi-component (Patton et al., 2016). The general challenge lies in the fact that many of the issues that burden African nations (i.e. poverty, access to jobs, education) and affect the overall quality of life for its citizens, often take precedence over interventions that promote positive behaviors in adolescents that could influence their heath and overall well-being in the long run.

Games for health have the potential to effectively address some of these health areas through platforms with which this young generation has the greatest familiarity. All of the serious games highlighted in the preceding section illustrate the potential that new technology-based interventions have to address issues that burden the overall health and well-being of adolescents (i.e. pregnancy, mental health, HIV, and nutrition). Although personal choices and behaviors are the prime focus of the serious game examples included in this chapter, serious games could also be used to address other health issues that are a strain on African citizens. For example, with an infectious disease such as TB or malaria, a serious game could be used to educate individuals on ways to reduce possible exposure through knowledge dissemination and role-playing.

However, it should also be noted that the limited available examples of how games for health are being used in the African context highlights the need for expansion in this area in terms of research, development, and evaluation. Often, both technology and available financial resources are the rate limiting factors to implementing these interventions among adolescent and youth populations. The interventions that were highlighted in the African context used mobile phones as a way to reach the greatest number of adolescents (as opposed to personal computers or iPads that were used in interventions in other countries); highlighting that this specific technology could be the most useful for effectively implementing these interventions. At the end of 2016, there were 420 million unique mobile subscribers in Sub-Saharan Africa. It has been estimated that more people in Africa have mobile phones than toilets (Hampshire et al., 2015); providing a unique platform and opportunity to address the technology shortcomings. The region is growing faster in terms of mobile phone use than any other region with an anticipated greater than half a billion unique mobile subscribers by 2020 (GSMC, 2017). Key factors that have supported the exponential growth of smartphone adoption in the region include the increasing affordability of new devices and the growing market for second-hand devices (GSMC, 2017).

Nevertheless, additional obstacles to using this type of technology exist not only in Africa, but in many middle and high income countries were serious game are most prevalent; one of these obstacles being the sustainability of the interventions. Even in high income countries, implementation, dissemination and sustainability remain large hurdles to the area of games for health. Because resources are often scarce, serious game development, efficacy testing, implementation, and dissemination, is almost always a challenge (Hightow-Weidman et al., 2015, 2017). Therefore, collaborations are sorely needed between universities and organizations who are developing these games and other governmental and non-governmental entities that can provide ample funding for the development of these game interventions for the benefit of Africa's adolescents.

Another limitation of this type of intervention, which is common to many behavioral interventions, is that it typically requires longitudinal engagement to demonstrate that the game is effective. Games for health must be able to show behavior change; it is not enough to solely change knowledge, perceptions, and attitudes to have a lasting impact and affect larger populations. The ultimate goal has to be behavior change, and that is where many interventions struggle, given the long temporal demands needed to observe and measure behavior change. But, adolescence is an opportune time to instill knowledge and skills in individuals to help positively shape their behavior into the future and as a result larger population, countries, and the continent as a whole.

The surging adolescent population in sub-Saharan Africa underscores the enormous potential for continent-wide development and advancement if adolescent health and well-being are made a priority. It is imperative to continue to address modifiable behaviors and circumstances that affect adolescents' health and well-being to ensure that this sub-population will thrive in the future. Games for health present themselves as novel ways to intervene with adolescents regarding their individual health and well-being by delivering information to them on familiar platforms and allowing them to practice behaviors and skills in virtual environments; ultimately having the potential to not just modify individual behaviors but affect the overall well-being of countries and the global community.

References

Abt, C. C. (1970). *Serious games: The art and science of games that simulate life*. New York, NY: Viking Compass Book.

African Development Bank Group. (2017). *Annual development effectiveness review 2017: Transforming Africa*.

Agyepong, I. A., Sewankambo, N., Binagwaho, A., Coll-Seck, A. M., Corrah, T., Ezeh, A., ... Mayosi, B. (2017). The path to longer and healthier lives for all Africans by 2030: The Lancet Commission on the future of health in sub-Saharan Africa. *The Lancet, 390*(10114), 2803–2859.

Alderman, H., Hoddinott, J., & Kinsey, B. (2006). Long term consequences of early childhood malnutrition. *Oxford Economic Papers, 58*(3), 450–474.

Andrew, F. M., & Withey, S. B. (1976). *Social indicators of Well-being* (Vol. 20, p. 31). New York and London: Plenum.

Bain, L. E., Awah, P. K., Geraldine, N., Kindong, N. P., Siga, Y., Bernard, N., & Tanjeko, A. T. (2013). Malnutrition in Sub–Saharan Africa: Burden, causes and prospects. *Pan African Medical Journal, 15*(1).

Bainbridge, W. (2007). The scientific research potential of virtual worlds. *Science, 317*, 472–476.

Bandura, A. (1994). Social cognitive theory and exercise of control over HIV infection. In *Preventing AIDS* (pp. 25–59). Boston, MA: Springer.

Baranowski, T., Buday, R., Thompson, D. I., & Baranowski, J. (2008). Playing for real: Video games and stories for health-related behavior change. *American Journal of Preventive Medicine, 34*(1), 74–82.

Baranowski, T., Lin, L. S., Wetter, D. W., Resnicow, K., & Hearn, M. D. (1997). Theory as mediating variables: Why aren't community interventions working as desired? *Annals of Epidemiology, 7*(7), S89–S95.

BBC Country Profile. (2018). eSwanti (Swaziland) Country Profile. https://www.bbc.com/news/world-africa-14095303. Accessed 14 April 2018.

Camenga, D. R., Hieftje, K. D., Fiellin, L. E., Edelman, E. J., Rosenthal, M. S., & Duncan, L. R. (2014). The use of message framing to promote sexual risk reduction in young adolescents: A pilot exploratory study. *Health Education Research, 29*(2), 360–366.

Campbell, A., Converse, P. E., & Rodgers, W. L. (1976). *The quality of American life: Perceptions, evaluations, and satisfactions*. New York, NY: Russell Sage Foundation.

Central Intelligence Agency World Fact Book. (2018).

Corti, K. (2006). *Games-based learning: A serious business application*. Coventry, UK: PIXELearning.

Cortina, M. A., Sodha, A., Fazel, M., & Ramchandani, P. G. (2012). Prevalence of child mental health problems in sub-Saharan Africa: A systematic review. *Archives of Pediatrics & Adolescent Medicine, 166*(3), 276–281.

Dahir, A. (2017). *Striking contrast: This is the only continent where children have both stunted growth and a rising obesity problem*. Quartz Africa.

Dalal, S., Beunza, J. J., Volmink, J., Adebamowo, C., Bajunirwe, F., Njelekela, M., ... Holmes, M. D. (2011). Non-communicable diseases in sub-Saharan Africa: What we know now. *International Journal of Epidemiology, 40*(4), 885–901.

Deaton, A. S., & Tortora, R. (2015). People in Sub-Saharan Africa rate their health and health care among the lowest in the world. *Health Affairs, 34*(3), 519–527.

Desjardins, J. (2017). *How video games became a $100 billion industry*. http://www.businessinsider.com/the-history-and-evolution-of-the-video-games-market-2017-1. Accessed 5 June 2018.

Diener, E. (2006). Guidelines for national indicators of subjective well-being and ill-being. *Journal of Happiness Studies, 7*(4), 397–404.

Diener, E., Suh, E. M., Lucas, R. E., & Smith, H. L. (1999). Subjective well-being: Three decades of progress. *Psychological Bulletin, 125*(2), 276.

Duncan, L. R., Hieftje, K. D., Culyba, S., & Fiellin, L. E. (2014). Game playbooks: Tools to guide multidisciplinary teams in developing videogame-based behavior change interventions. *Translational Behavioral Medicine, 4*(1), 108–116.

Economic and Social Research Council. (2014). *The well-being effect of education*. Accessed 5 May 2018.

Ferguson, W. (2012). The emergence of games for health. *Games for Health Journal, 1*(2), 1–2.

Fiellin, L. E., Hieftje, K. D., & Duncan, L. R. (2014). Videogames, here for good. *Pediatrics, 134*(5), 849–851.

Fiellin, L. E., Kyriakides, T. C., Hieftje, K. D., Pendergrass, T. M., Duncan, L. R., Dziura, J. D., … Fiellin, D. A. (2016). The design and implementation of a randomized controlled trial of a risk reduction and human immunodeficiency virus prevention videogame intervention in minority adolescents: PlayForward: Elm City Stories. *Clinical Trials, 13*(4), 400–408.

Fiellin, L. E., Hieftje, K. D., Pendergrass, T. M., Kyriakides, T. C., Duncan, L. R., Dziura, J. D., … Fiellin, D. A. (2017). Video game intervention for sexual risk reduction in minority adolescents: Randomized controlled trial. *Journal of Medical Internet Research, 19*(9), e314.

Fiorito, A. (2011). Gaming in sub-Saharan Africa. *The Four Peaks Review, 1*(1), 60–70.

Fisher, J. D., & Fisher, W. A. (1992). Changing AIDS-risk behavior. *Psychological Bulletin, 111*(3), 455–474.

Fleming, T. M., Bavin, L., Stasiak, K., Hermansson-Webb, E., Merry, S. N., Cheek, C., … Hetrick, S. (2017). Serious games and gamification for mental health: Current status and promising directions. *Frontiers in Psychiatry, 7*, 215.

Font, J. M., Hedvall, A., & Svensson, E. (2017). Towards teaching maternal healthcare and nutrition in rural Ethiopia through a serious game. In *Extended abstracts publication of the annual symposium on computer-human interaction in play* (pp. 187–193). ACM.

Gallup-Healthway Global Well-being Index (2014). Accessed 10 April 2018.

Gallup-Sharecare Well-being Index. (2017). Accessed 10 Apr 2018.

Global Nutrition Report 2017. (2017). *Nourishing the SDGs*. Bristol, UK: Development Initiatives.

Global System for Mobile Communications (GSMC). (2017). *The mobile economy: Sub-Saharan Africa 017*. London.

Hampshire, K., Porter, G., Owusu, S. A., Mariwah, S., Abane, A., Robson, E., … Milner, J. (2015). Informal m-health: How are young people using mobile phones to bridge healthcare gaps in Sub-Saharan Africa? *Social Science & Medicine, 142*, 90–99.

Hieftje, K., Duncan, L. R., & Fiellin, L. E. (2014). Novel methods to collect meaningful data from adolescents for the development of health interventions. *Health Promotion Practice, 15*(5), 714–722.

Hieftje, K., Edelman, E. J., Camenga, D. R., & Fiellin, L. E. (2013). Electronic media-based health interventions for behavior change in youth: A systematic review. *JAMA Pediatrics, 167*(6), 574–580.

Hieftje, K., Rosenthal, M. S., Camenga, D. R., Edelman, E. J., & Fiellin, L. E. (2012). A qualitative study to inform the development of a videogame for adolescent human immunodeficiency virus prevention. *GAMES FOR HEALTH: Research, Development, and Clinical Applications, 1*(4), 294–298.

Hightow-Weidman, L. B., Muessig, K. E., Bauermeister, J., Zhang, C., & LeGrand, S. (2015). Adolescence, technology, and HIV: Recent advances and future directions. *Current HIV/AIDS Reports, 12*(4), 500–515.

Hightow-Weidman, L. B., Muessig, K. E., Bauermeister, J. A., LeGrand, S., & Fiellin, L. E. (2017). The future of digital games for HIV prevention and care. *Current Opinion in HIV and AIDS, 12*(5), 501–507.

HIV Free Generation-Kenya. (2010). *Pamoja Mtaani fact sheet*. http://www.g-pange.com

Hubal, R., Kizakevich, P., & Furberg, R. (2007). Synthetic characters in health-related applications. In S. Vaidya & H. Yoshida (Eds.), *Advanced computational intelligence paradigms in healthcare 2*. Heidelberg, Germany: Springer.

Johnson, W. L., & Beal, C. (2005). *Iterative evaluation of an intelligent game for language learning*. Paper presented at: Proceedings of the international conference on Artificial Intelligence in Education. Amsterdam, The Netherlands.

Karimi, M., & Brazier, J. (2016). Health, health-related quality of life, and quality of life: What is the difference? *Pharmacoeconomics, 34*(7), 645–649.

Kenyan Ministry of Health. (2016). *Kenyan AIDS response progress report 2016*, Nairobi, Kenya.

Keyes, C. L., Shmotkin, D., & Ryff, C. D. (2002). Optimizing well-being: The empirical encounter of two traditions. *Journal of Personality and Social Psychology, 82*(6), 1007.

Kirby, D. (2008). Changes in sexual behaviour leading to the decline in the prevalence of HIV in Uganda: Confirmation from multiple sources of evidence. *Sexually Transmitted Infections, 84*, ii35–ii41.

Land, K. C. (1975). Social indicators models: An overview. In K. C. Land & S. Spilerman (Eds.), *Social indicator models* (pp. 5–36). New York, NY: Russell Sage Foundation.

Lansford, J. E., & Banati, P. (Eds.). (2018). *Handbook of adolescent development research and its impact on global policy*. Oxford, UK: Oxford University Press.

Latzoo, K. (2016). *12 facts demonstrating the RISE of a Video Game Industry in Africa*. https://medium.com/akoma-media/12-facts-demonstrating-the-rise-of-a-video-game-industry-in-africa-41a7e3ef8dbe. Accessed 4 June 2018.

Lenhart, A., Kahne, J., Middaugh, E., Macgill, A. R., Evans, C., & Vitak, J. (2008). Teens, video games, and civics: Teens' gaming experiences are diverse and include significant social interaction and civic engagement. Pew internet & American life project. Retrieved online from: http://www.pewinternet.org/2008/09/16/teens-video-games-and-civics/.

Levin, D., & Arafeh, S. (2002). *The digital disconnect: The widening gap between internet-savvy students and their schools*.

Ludoscience. (2014). *Game classification*. http://serious.gameclassification.com/. Accessed 25 Apr 2018.

Lukhele, B. W., Musumari, P., El-Saaidi, C., Techasrivichien, T., Suguimoto, S. P., Ono Kihara, M., & Kihara, M. (2016). Efficacy of mobile serious games in increasing HIV risk perception in Swaziland:

A randomized control trial (SGprev trial) research protocol. *JMIR Research Protocols, 5*(4), e224. https://doi.org/10.2196/resprot.6543

Merry, S. N., Stasiak, K., Shepherd, M., Frampton, C., Fleming, T., & Lucassen, M. F. (2012). The effectiveness of SPARX, a computerized self-help intervention for adolescents seeking help for depression: Randomized controlled non-inferiority trial. *BMJ, 344*, e2598.

Michael, D. R., & Chen, S. L. (2005). *Serious games: Games that educate, train, and inform*. Roseville, CA: Muska & Lipman/Premier-Trade.

Michalos, A. C. (2017). Education, happiness and well-being. In *Connecting the quality of life theory to health, well-being and education* (pp. 277–299). Cham, Switzerland: Springer.

Mitgutsch, K., & Alvarado, N. (2012). Purposeful by design? A serious game design assessment framework. In *Proceedings of the international conference on the foundations of digital games* (pp. 121–128). ACM.

Murphy, E. M., Greene, M. E., Mihailovic, A., & Olupot-Olupot, P. (2006). Was the "ABC" approach (abstinence, being faithful, using condoms) responsible for Uganda's decline in HIV? *PLoS Medicine, 3*(9), e379.

Ngamaba, K. H., Panagioti, M., & Armitage, C. J. (2017). How strongly related are health status and subjective well-being? Systematic review and meta-analysis. *The European Journal of Public Health, 27*(5), 879–885.

Oblinger, D. (2004). The next generation of educational engagement. *Journal of Interactive Media in Education, 2004*(1).

Ohannessian, R., Yaghobian, S., Verger, P., & Vanhems, P. (2016). A systematic review of serious video games used for vaccination. *Vaccine, 34*(38), 4478–4483.

Paperny, D. M., & Starn, J. R. (1989). Adolescent pregnancy prevention by health education computer games: Computer-assisted instruction of knowledge and attitudes. *Pediatrics, 83*(5), 742–752.

Patton, G. C., Sawyer, S. M., Santelli, J. S., Ross, D. A., Afifi, R., Allen, N. B., … Kakuma, R. (2016). Our future: A Lancet commission on adolescent health and well-being. *The Lancet, 387*(10036), 2423–2478.

Performance Monitoring and Accountability 2020-Ethiopia. (2017). *Adolescents and young women health brief.*

Research NGM. The games industry disrupted: 10 key moments towards 2017. http://www.newzoo.com/insights/games-industry-disrupted-10-key-moments-towards-2017/. Accessed 10 Apr 2018.

Reyes-García, V., Babigumira, R., Pyhälä, A., Wunder, S., Zorondo-Rodríguez, F., & Angelsen, A. (2016). Subjective well-being and income: Empirical patterns in the rural developing world. *Journal of Happiness Studies, 17*(2), 773–791.

Schwebel, D. C., Gainesa, J., & Severson, J. (2008). Validation of virtual reality as a tool to understand and prevent child pedestrian injury. *Accident Analysis & Prevention, 40*(4), 1394–1400.

Serious Game Association. (2014). *Serious games directory*. http://www.grandmetropolitan.com/. Accessed 25 Apr 2018.

Smithsonian National Museum of American History. (2018). *Video game history*. https://www.si.edu/spotlight/the-father-of-the-video-game-the-ralph-baer-prototypes-and-electronic-games/video-game-history. Accessed 5 May 2018.

Snow, K. J., Sismanidis, C., Denholm, J., Sawyer, S. M., & Graham, S. M. (2018). The incidence of tuberculosis among adolescents and young adults: A global estimate. *European Respiratory Journal, 51*(2), 1702352.

Standish, M., & Witters, D. (2016). *Americas lead highs, Sub-Saharan Africa lows in well-being*.

Stevenson, B., & Wolfers, J. (2013). Subjective well-being and income: Is there any evidence of satiation? *American Economic Review, 103*(3), 598–604.

Susi, T., Johannesson, M., & Backlund, P. (2007). *Serious games: An overview*.

Tarini, P. (2012). Curiosity, hope, and vision: The role of the Robert Wood Johnson Foundation's Pioneer Portfolio in funding early health game research. *Games for Health Journal, 1*(1), 7–8.

Thompson, D., Baranowski, T., Buday, R., Baranowski, J., Thompson, V., Jago, R., & Griffith, M. J. (2010). Serious video games for health: How behavioral science guided the development of a serious video game. *Simulation & Gaming, 41*(4), 587–606.

Tversky, A., & Kahneman, D. (1981). The framing of decisions and the psychology of choice. *Science, 211*(4481), 453–458.

UNAIDS/WHO. (2004). *Report on the global HIV/AIDS epidemic*. http://www.unaids.org/bangkok2004/report.html

International Food Policy Research Institute. (2016). *Global nutrition report: From promise to impact, ending malnutrition by 2030*. Washington, DC.

United Nations, Department of Economic and Social Affairs, Population Division. (2017). *World population prospects: The 2017 revision, key findings and advance tables* (Working Paper No. ESA/P/WP/248).

United Nations Monitoring Report Health, Morbidity, Mortality and Development. (2016).

United Nations Population Fund. (2013). *Adolescent pregnancy: A review of the evidence*. New York, NY: UNFPA.

United Nations Population Fund. (2015). *The power of 1.8 billion: Adolescents, youth and the transformation of the future*. New York, NY: UNFPA.

Wolf, M. J., & Iwatani, T. (2015). *Video games around the world*. Cambridge, MA: MIT Press.

World Health Organization. (1948). *Constitution of WHO*. Geneva, Switzerland.

World Health Organization. (2014). *Noncommunicable diseases country profiles 2014*. Geneva: WHO.

World Health Organization. (2016). *Global malaria report 2016*. Geneva, Switzerland.

World Health Organization. (2017). *Global tuberculosis report 2017*. Geneva, Switzerland.

World Health Organization. (2018). *Adolescents: Health risks and solutions*.

Ybarra, M. L., Korchmaros, J. D., Prescott, T. L., & Birungi, R. (2015). A randomized controlled trial to increase HIV preventive information, motivation, and behavioral skills in Ugandan adolescents. *Annals of Behavioral Medicine, 49*(3), 473–485.

Youth Health Education. (2018). http://www.youthhealtheducation.com.au/six-essential-components-of-health/. Accessed 1 May 2018.

Zyda, M. (2005). From visual simulation to virtual reality to games. *Computer, 38*(9), 25–32.

Part III

Health

9 Research, Innovation and Education Towards Malaria Elimination: Improving *Quality of Life* in Africa

Christiaan de Jager, Taneshka Kruger, and Cheryl Tosh

Abstract

Malaria is one of the African continent's major health challenges. According to the World Health Organization (WHO), 80% of the 216 million global malaria cases reported in 2016 occurred in sub-Saharan countries and India. Eighty percent of the 445,000 global fatalities occurred in these same countries. Eliminating malaria is intrinsically linked to the quality of life of communities affected by malaria. Communities need to perceive malaria as a significant health problem in order to make the behavioral changes required to successfully control vectors and parasites. Concurrently, governance and policies need to be in place to support health care and manage surveillance. We report on current initiatives in the Limpopo Province of South Africa that are connecting communities, researchers and policy makers. Novel materials are being developed to control mosquitoes in homes and various educational initiatives strive to teach school children about malaria control through music, dance and children's books. Mobile technology is being harnessed to spread information about malaria outbreaks and high risk areas. Researchers are focused on understanding the impact of invasive vector control strategies on local communities and are trying to understand the dynamics of insecticide and drug resistance. Eliminating malaria in African communities will reduce the burden of illness and mortality, releasing resources that can be channeled towards improving quality of life.

9.1 Background

9.1.1 What is Malaria?

Malaria is a serious, complex and often fatal vector-borne disease consisting of intermittent and remittent fever. The disease, malaria, is caused by single celled parasitic protozoans, *Plasmodium* (*P.*) *spp.* that are transmitted to humans when bitten by infected female mosqui-

C. de Jager (✉)
School of Health Systems and Public Health (SHSPH), University of Pretoria Institute for Sustainable Malaria Control (UP ISMC), Faculty of Health Sciences, University of Pretoria, Pretoria, South Africa
e-mail: tiaan.dejager@up.ac.za

T. Kruger
SHSPH, UP ISMC, Faculty of Health Sciences, University of Pretoria, Pretoria, South Africa
e-mail: taneshka.kruger@up.ac.za

C. Tosh
Faculty of Health Sciences, University of Pretoria, Pretoria, South Africa
e-mail: cheryl.tosh@up.ac.za

I. Eloff (ed.), *Handbook of Quality of Life in African Societies*, International Handbooks of Quality-of-Life, https://doi.org/10.1007/978-3-030-15367-0_9

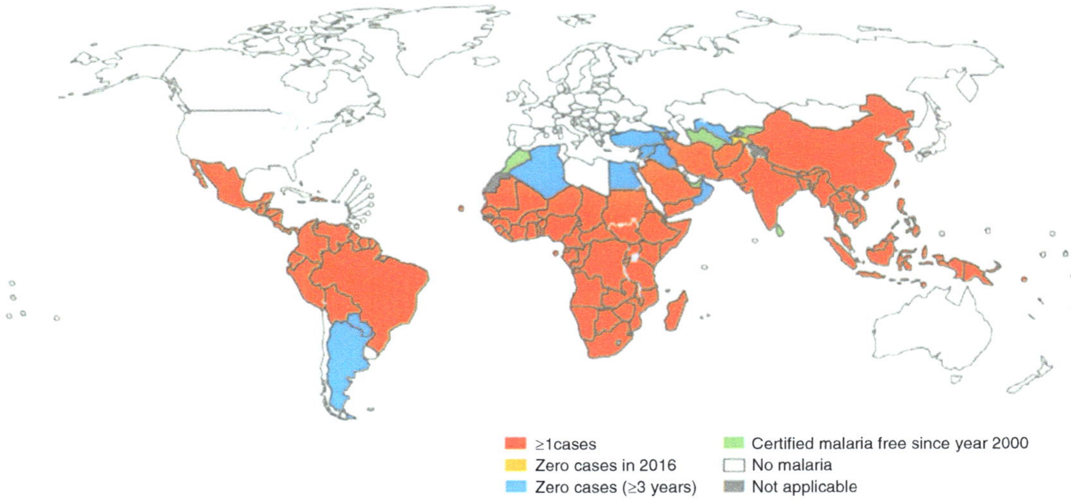

Fig. 9.1 The countries and territories with indigenous malaria cases in 2000 and their status by 2016 – Countries with zero indigenous cases over a minimum of three consecutive years are eligible to request malaria free status certification from the WHO (WHO, 2017)

toes belonging to the *Anopheles* (*An.*) genus (Birkholtz, Bornman, Focke, Mutero, & De Jager, 2012; Oyekale, 2015). Anopheline mosquitoes are infected with malaria parasites when taking a blood meal from a person with malaria. Female anopheline mosquitoes use the blood meal for egg production. When the infected mosquito feeds again, the parasites are injected with the mosquito's saliva into the person being bitten. Malaria parasites can also be transmitted from a mother to her unborn infant, prior to or during birth.

Malaria is an intricate mix of 3 biological systems namely human, mosquito vector (more than 30 *Anopheles spp.*) and parasite (5 *Plasmodium spp.*). Each of the vectors and parasites have their own complex lifecycle, habit, environment preference and patho-genesis (Birkholtz et al., 2012). Malaria transmission depends on the incidence and abundance of the mosquito vector, the susceptibility of the vector to the parasite, the host type being fed on and the survival, and subsequent ability of the mosquito to transmit the disease. Both vectors and parasites depend on high ambient humidity and relatively warm temperatures. Therefore, malaria is normally found in warmer tropical and sub-tropical countries. The disease is rife in large areas of Africa and South Asia, and parts of Central and South America, the Caribbean, the Middle East, Oceania and Southeast Asia (Fig. 9.1).

Malaria is preventable and treatable, but control, management and the prospect of eliminating the disease is impeded by the complexity of host-vector-parasite-environmental interactions. Over the past 70 years, controlling and eliminating malaria has been based on two strategies, namely, controlling the *Plasmodium* parasite and controlling *Anopheles* mosquitoes. Upscaling of control strategies over the past decade have resulted in significant reductions in the global malaria burden; however, despite control efforts, the disease remains a public health burden (Nixon, 2016). Malaria is recognized as a disease of poverty and a cause of poverty (WHO, 2011), affecting the poorest countries, which have to foot the bill for the high cost of prevention and treatment of the disease.

9.1.2 The Current Status of Malaria

Globally, the decrease in the incidence of malaria seen since 2010 has apparently stalled, with malaria incidence and mortality increasing in some regions. According to the World Health Organization (WHO), 216 million cases of malaria were reported from 91 countries in

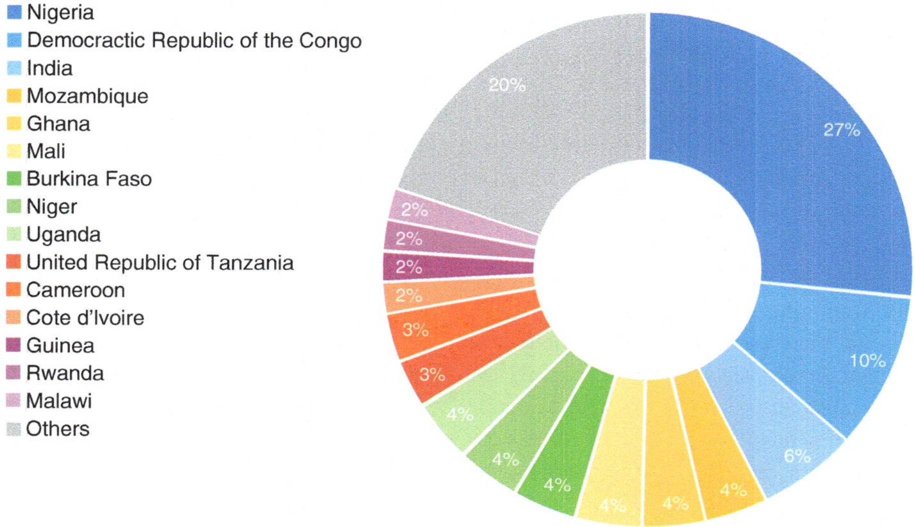

Fig. 9.2 The estimated country share of the 15 countries that together made up 80% of the global malaria cases for 2016 (WHO, 2017)

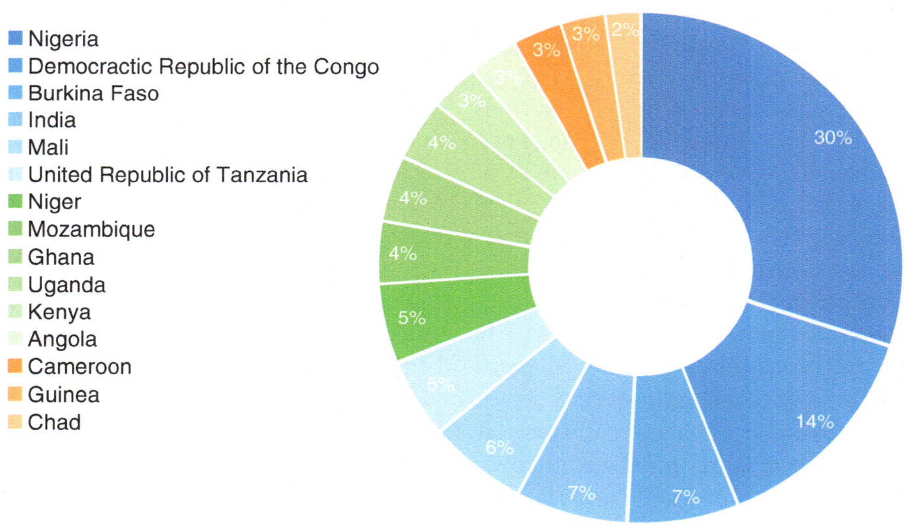

Fig. 9.3 Proportion of the estimated malaria deaths attributable to the 15 countries with nearly 80% of malaria deaths reported globally in 2016 (WHO, 2017)

2016, 5 million cases up from 2015. Eighty percent of the global malaria burden is carried by 15 countries, all but one (India) from sub-Saharan Africa (Fig. 9.2). Malaria mortality was estimated at less than half a million (~445,000 deaths) in both 2015 and 2016, where 80% of the fatalities – in 2016 (Fig. 9.3) – occurred in these same countries (WHO, 2017). At present, an estimated 3.3 billion people in 97 countries are at risk of contracting malaria, of these 1.2 billion are at high risk (Hemingway, Ranson, et al., 2016; Nixon, 2016).

In 2014, the WHO reported that 70% of malaria cases in Africa occurred in children under the age of 5 (WHO, 2015). The number of malaria-related deaths in children under the age of 5 years has decreased since 2000, but still contributes significantly towards morbidity in children from sub-Saharan Africa, with 10% of children under the age of 5 dying due to malaria – essentially one child dying of malaria every 2 min (Roberts & Matthews, 2016).

People who are heavily exposed to the bites of anopheline mosquitoes carrying *P. falciparum* are most at risk of dying from malaria. Young children, pregnant women or travelers from non-endemic areas tend to have little or no immunity against malaria and are more likely to become very sick and die. Poor people in rural areas who do not have quick or easy access to health care have a greater risk of contracting malaria and are most likely to die from the disease. Poor children living in rural areas, whose mothers have little or no education, are more likely to die from malaria due to an increase in susceptibility (Ingstad, Munthali, Braathen, & Grut, 2012). Whilst people living in poverty are known to be more susceptible to malaria (Stratton, O'Neill, Kruk, & Bell, 2008), other factors influence the spread of malaria, such as climate, geographic location, environmental conditions, human impact and the complexity of parasite-vector interactions.

Climate change has been linked to an increase in malaria transmission. In tropical countries, warm and wet climates create favorable breeding habitat for mosquitoes (Oyekale, 2015). In warm and wet conditions, mosquitoes breed faster and the disease in turn spreads faster. Malaria may also spread to areas that were previously unsuitable or be re-introduced to areas that were previously declared malaria free (Nkosi, 2017). Other vector species may also spread to new areas that become climatically suitable. Future increases in temperature may prompt an increase in malaria cases, especially in densely populated areas of Africa and South America that are at higher elevations (Siraj et al., 2014). In Ethiopia, researchers found that the 37 million people, living at an elevation between 5280 and 7920 ft, had an increased risk of malaria exposure during warmer climatic conditions (Siraj et al., 2014). A 1 °C increase in temperature could result in an extra three million cases of malaria annually in Ethiopian children under the age of 15 (Siraj et al., 2014). Newly exposed populations may be especially vulnerable due to a lack in protective immunity, eventually leading to severe malaria morbidity and mortality (Siraj et al., 2014).

In African communities, human factors play an important role in the occurrence of malaria. People living in African communities are known to have fluid movement patterns, often travelling across borders to work or to visit family, or because they have been displaced by war or natural disaster. People may become infected with malaria in malaria endemic areas and travel back to non-endemic areas providing a source for new malaria outbreaks. The settlement of people in large communities provides large populations as a blood source for mosquitoes. Human structures provide protection and shade for the mosquitoes. Land use practices and inadequate waste management can contribute to stagnant water bodies, which are ideal breeding habitat for mosquitoes. Water can accumulate in litter, including empty cans, vehicle tires, and packaging, in open channels, and in areas where there is poor sanitation. People living in low socio-economic areas such as rural communities or at the periphery of cities generally have poor-quality housing, unpaved roads, poor sanitation and reduced access to healthcare providing little protection against malaria (Mwangangi et al., 2012). It is predicted that sub-Saharan Africa's urban population will outnumber the rural population by the year 2035 (Parnell & Walawege, 2011). When screened at a health clinic, it was found that people living in the inner-city of Angola's capital, Luanda, were almost six times less likely to test positive for malaria than people living further than 15 km outside the capital (Thwing et al., 2009). The general agreement is that increasing urbanization will lead to a decrease in malaria transmission. Despite this expectation, De Silva and Marshall (2012) show that malaria transmission persists in African cities – in some cases, at even higher levels than in surrounding areas. The rapid urbanization of Africa has not been supported by the adequate development of infrastructure (Moller, Roberts, Tiliouine, & Loschky, 2017), resulting in high density, urban areas that are poor, with subsistence agricultural practices and poorly-monitored land use (Stoler, Weeks, Getis, & Hill, 2009).

9.2 Current Strategies in Malaria Control

The dramatic decline in malaria burden across the globe is largely due to the success of insecticide-based interventions (Thomas, 2018). The two principal methods of blocking malaria transmission are by using insecticide treated nets (ITNs) or long lasting insecticide treated bednets (LLINs), and by using long-lasting insecticides for indoor residual spraying (IRS) (Kruger, Sibanda, Focke, Bornman, & Jager, 2015; WHO, 2010). These two vector control methods aim to reduce vector capacity to below the threshold of continued infection (Birkholtz et al., 2012). A vector control method is usually selected based on epidemiological conditions and operational settings, including affordability, comparative efficacy and cost effectiveness (Djènontin et al., 2009; Guyatt, Corlett, Robinson, Ochola, & Snow, 2002; Kruger et al., 2015).

In sub-Saharan Africa, malaria control primarily consists of using ITNs/LLINs to prevent mosquitoes from biting humans whilst sleeping (WHO, 2017). While the use of bed nets has increased substantially since 2010 in sub-Saharan Africa, only 54% of people at risk were sleeping under an insecticide-treated mosquito net. The other important method used to control mosquito vectors is indoor residual spraying (IRS). The efficacy of IRS depends on adequate spatial and temporal coverage, which has dropped in African and other WHO regions since 2010 (WHO, 2017). The drop in IRS coverage may be attributed to a lack of resources and factors such as political instability, war and natural disasters. In Africa, the use of insecticide to control mosquitoes has also been associated with increasing resistance to various insecticides, prompting the development of alternative insecticides. Very few African countries have well developed resistance management plans, which are needed to maintain the efficacy of IRS. Insecticide resistance management strategies often include methods that are more expensive than existing interventions, which is problematic for control programs and donors working with fixed or declining budgets. Therefore, a balance is needed to maintain coverage levels whilst changing over to more costly insecticide classes to preserve insecticide susceptibility. The development and operational deployment of new insecticides is thus imperative (Hemingway, Ranson, et al., 2016).

Besides continuous and correctly administered vector control, malaria control programs today rely on the prompt diagnosis and effective treatment of malaria infection using rapid diagnostic tests (RDT) and artemisinin-based combination therapies (ACT), or intermittent preventive treatment for pregnant women (IPTp) (Hemingway, Ranson, et al., 2016). In Africa, most people seeking malaria treatment in the public health system receive the correct medication at the correct dose after a correct diagnosis had been made. Unfortunately, access to the public health system remains low in Africa, where only about a third or 34% of children with a fever are taken to a healthcare practitioner (WHO, 2017). The treatment of malaria is also complicated by increasing parasite resistance to existing anti-malarial drugs. The first case of resistance to the latest drug regimen was noted in Equatorial Guinea and cases have also been reported in Angola, Liberia and Uganda. This is concerning because drug resistance in Africa may result in similar transmission patterns as noted in South East Asia (Nkosi, 2017).

In 2010, the WHO stated that every person at risk of being infected with malaria must either have access to IRS or must own an ITN/LLIN by 2015 (WHO, 2010). Both vector control methods have seen a drastic upscaling in implementation since 2010 and have contributed to a significant reduction in malaria morbidity and mortality in a number of African countries over the last two decades (Birkholtz et al., 2012; Kruger et al., 2015). The success of vector control depends on continuous user cooperation, viable logistics behind implementation and the availability of appropriate delivery systems (Kruger et al., 2015; Messenger, Miller, Adeogun, Awolola, & Rowland, 2012). Regional malaria control programs are able to secure funds and capacity for implementation of vector control systems, but continuous user cooperation depends on individual compliance and awareness of the dangers of malaria. The success of malaria control programs depends on individual behavior and social organization (Carpenter, Pearson, Mitchell, & Oaks Jr, 1991). New malaria control programs thus need to factor in local communities during planning and inception. Within communities, education activities can create awareness and promote health. In communities that take ownership of their health, community representatives who are approached in the correct manner have participated in the planning and implementation of malaria prevention and control programs.

Between 2000 and 2009, interventions such as ACT, the increased use of bed nets and a drive to use IRS as a control method on the inner walls of dwellings have greatly contributed towards prohibiting malaria transmission (Ritha Njau, de Savigny, Gilson, Mwageni, & Mosha, 2009). To remain effective, a large percentage of the worldwide population must be reached (Ritha Njau et al., 2009). Widespread, free ITN/LLIN distribution has consistently been touted as the most feasible strategy to prevent malaria in people living in poor rural households (Joseph D Njau, Stephenson, Menon, Kachur, & McFarland, 2013). The distribution of free ITN/LLIN and medicine has certain pitfalls, such as not always reaching remote rural communities. In Zambia, women who attended antenatal clinics or had children under 5 years of age, were twice as likely to have bed nets in the household (Larsen et al., 2010). These women lived closer to healthcare facilities, and had the resources to attend antenatal clinics. In Malawi, people that lived far from health care facilities were less likely to have bed nets in their homes compared to people living closer to health facilities (Larson, Mathanga, Campbell, & Wilson, 2012).

9.3 Malaria and Quality of Life in Africa

Malaria poses one of Africa's greatest challenges. Bill Gates once said: "*For Africa to move forward, you've really got to get rid of malaria*". But why is malaria so common and such a burden in Africa or rather sub-Saharan Africa? Aside from the co-occurrence of major malaria mosquito vectors and parasites, sub-Saharan Africa is warm and wet, with large rural settlements that are characterized by poor sanitation, lack of health care and poor quality housing. Malaria impacts the quality of life in African communities by reducing community and household income, shortening the lives of children and adults, and through long term negative outcomes, such as anemia, neurological side effects and chronic kidney disease. These negative outcomes are exacerbated by poverty, malnutrition and inadequate access to healthcare, forming a vicious cycle that is difficult to break.

Birkholtz et al. (2012) stated that malaria is a major socio-economic, health and developmental challenge for many of the world's poorest countries. As a disease of poverty, malaria impacts adversely on the African continent's economic development. Malaria costs endemic countries about 1.3% of the gross domestic product (GDP) annually in lost productivity. This equates to an annual loss of US$12 billion of GDP for the whole African continent (Birkholtz et al., 2012; Gallup & Sachs, 2001). Currently, the drive towards controlling malaria in Africa can be compared to efforts made by WHO in the 1950s and 1960s by the Global Malaria Eradication Campaign. Originally, the campaign covered the entire globe, but excluded Africa. Realizing that global eradication efforts would be futile without controlling malaria in Africa, the WHO has shifted its target to Africa, including other malaria endemic regions (Coetzee et al., 2013). Funding toward malaria control has remained relatively stable since 2010, but inflation and high levels of population growth have resulted in inadequate investment required to reach a reduction of 40% in malaria incidence and mortality in 2016. An estimated US$ 6.5 billion is needed to achieve malaria control, whilst only US$ 2.7 billion was invested in global malaria control and elimination efforts in 2016 of which most of the funds (74%) funds were spent in the WHO African Region (WHO, 2017). Malaria imposes a heavy burden on the economics of individuals, households and endemic countries (Hailu et al., 2017) perpetuating the vicious cycle of poverty.

The economic burden of malaria is further exacerbated by the over-diagnosis of the disease. Over-diagnosis occurs when patients present with malaria symptoms, and self-diagnose, or when health care workers wrongly diagnose malaria based on clinical symptoms alone. Erroneous self-treatment can delay accurate diagnosis and lead to poor households spending money on the wrong medicine. Inaccurate diagnosis can lead to wasteful distribution of medicine in an already beleaguered health care system, as well as increase *Plasmodium* drug resistance (Hume et al., 2008). In Mozambique, between 30% and 70% of malaria cases are over-diagnosed, and led to more repeat visits to healthcare centres (Hume et al., 2008). Over-diagnosis of malaria in patients with severe febrile illness delays accurate treatment and can result in increased mortality (Reyburn et al., 2004). The problem of over-diagnosis has been reduced with the development of rapid diagnostic testing (RDTs) for malaria. Rapid diagnostic tests can detect specific malaria antigens from a blood smear, and may improve the targeting of anti-malarials and antibiotics in clinical settings where microscopy is not readily available (Ansah et al., 2010; Thiam et al., 2011). Rapid diagnostic testing also has the potential to improve the treatment of young children with febrile illness (Mtove et al., 2011).

The African childhood malaria burden is often underestimated (Murphy & Breman, 2001), with mortality often occurring due to secondary burden of disease. Women who contract malaria during pregnancy are more likely to have still births or give birth to low birth weight babies (Cottrell et al., 2015; Murphy & Breman, 2001). Alarmingly, infants who are exposed to placental malaria have a two times higher chance of contracting malaria in the first 30 months of life (Schwarz et al., 2008), increasing their chances of secondary outcomes such as cerebral palsy, blindness and other neurological outcomes (Ritha Njau et al., 2009). These neurological effects may affect the long term mental and physical development of children, increasing the demand for special education and additional educational support in poor, rural communities. Amongst school aged children, malaria is associated with increased absenteeism, especially during outbreaks (Nankabirwa et al., 2014), and malaria induced anemia can negatively affect cognitive ability. In Kenya, malaria was associated with increased absenteeism from primary school (King, Dewey, & Borish, 2015). These children fall behind in classes and may even drop out of school. Whilst children with malaria are unable to attend school, adults who have malaria are unable to work.

Malaria outbreaks are common in rural areas where most people rely on subsistence farming. During malaria outbreaks, many people can contract malaria at the same time, resulting in a large loss of work force, for days or weeks at a time. Loss of farm worker productivity leads to low harvests, resulting in food insecurity and eventual malnutrition in the community and weakened immune systems that are more susceptible to illness (Mayala et al., 2015). In Cameroon, women of very low socio-economic standing, the unemployed, people that were unable to afford modern housing facilities, and those living in very poor communities had an excessive malaria burden to handle (Oyekale, 2015). Health, agriculture, and food security are interdependent and, if one fails, then the others are negatively affected. Aside from reducing the number of days people are able to work, malaria can also incur significant healthcare costs, in terms of travelling to health centers and paying for medication (Hailu et al., 2017; Xu et al., 2003).

Social science research was considered to be anecdotal, unfocused on practical outcomes, and an overly academic approach to addressing malaria control; however, social sciences can reveal societal views and challenges associated with malaria, and how the experiences of communities are related to identifying the best malaria control methods (Carpenter et al., 1991). While current malaria control strategies focus on the mechanisms used over the past 70 years, malaria can only be eliminated if a holistic strategy involving multi- and trans-disciplinary efforts is used, which includes the participation and buy-in of affected communities.

9.4 Communities and Malaria

Community development is the process of empowering communities to improve their health and well-being, whilst the empowerment process enables people or whole communities to increase their power or control over events that influence their lives (Bang, 2010). In African communities, we need to understand how people perceive malaria and the barriers that prevent acceptance of prevention and control measures. Overcoming these barriers can ensure the success of control programs and target health promotion activities aimed at malaria (Carpenter et al., 1991). People need to perceive malaria as a serious problem or threat to change their behavior or their lifestyle to align with malaria control strategies or use self-protection methods to avoid malaria transmission (Carpenter et al., 1991). In rural communities that are affected by malaria, people often have dynamic cultural perceptions on health and disease (Tarimo, Lwihula, Minjas, & Bygbjerg, 2000) and a low level of literacy. Changing perceptions about malaria requires that people receive adequate information that is delivered in an appropriate manner (Bang, 2010).

Often communities see malaria as part of everyday life and the disease's symptoms are well known. Knowledge, Attitude and Practice (KAP) studies can determine community members' level of awareness of malaria. In rural, central Tanzania, most respondents had heard of malaria (97.5%) and acknowledged that mosquito bites cause malaria (Mayala et al., 2015). Almost all the participants (95.5%) indicated that ITNs/LLINs were the main method of vector control, with 78.7% believing that this was the most effective method (Mayala et al., 2015). In this community, few participants knew that environmental management was a possible way of reducing malaria, and that cleaning around dwellings (23.3%) and the clearing of grass and bushes around dwellings (12.5%) was important (Mayala et al., 2015). In the Republic of Guinea, a fifth of people understood how malaria was transmitted, but only 8.5% knew that mosquitoes bred in stagnant water (Ruberto, Camara, Banek, & Loua, 2014). Educating communities about the role of mosquitoes as a malaria vector is critical for prevention (Ruberto et al., 2014). Similarly, people living in Mozambique also knew much about malaria (Bingham et al., 2012). Almost all the participants suggested that malaria caused high death rates, severely affected attendance at school and work, with the overall loss of human resources in the workforce and in the fields negatively affecting the production of crops (Bingham et al., 2012).

The acceptance of malaria as a health issue is influenced by other aspects affecting quality of life. Grandmothers and unemployed mothers who were responsible for the daily care of children in the Vhembe District in Limpopo Province, South Africa, listed unemployment, poverty, crime and clean water as their main concerns towards survival (Bornman, Schlemmer, Van der Walt, Van Dyk, & Bouwman, 2012). Although malaria was not listed as an everyday concern, about half of women listed malaria as a concern when prompted (Bornman et al., 2012). People living in rural communities face daily challenges in food security, access to clean water and economic stability in the household, whilst malaria is seen as an important health challenge (Bornman et al., 2012; Dunkel, Hansen, Halvorson, & Bangert, 2016).

9.5 Socio-economic Disparities in Africa and Malaria

In Africa, poverty and lack of education are linked to low levels of awareness and low use of modern preventative methods against malaria (Clouston, Yukich, & Anglewicz, 2015; Omotayo & Oyekale, 2013). To understand the link between poverty and malaria in Africa, we need to consider the living conditions in rural communities, the attainment of education and level of household food insecurity in Africa. In sub-Saharan African almost 42% of the population are living below the poverty line of $1.90/day (World_Bank, 2018). Despite advances to increase educational levels, a third of children (~35 million from 33 low income countries across sub-Saharan Africa) who are of school going age, are still out of school (Majgaard & Mingat, 2012). Much of the socio-economic disparity observed in school attendance is either linked to poverty or living in a rural area.

People living in different socio-economic conditions are likely to respond differently to malaria prevention and treatment. In Madagascar, children's risk of contracting malaria was significantly higher if they lived in poor households and if their mothers had no primary education (Clouston et al., 2015). Women in Kenya, who had fewer than years of formal education, also had limited knowledge of how malaria is transmitted, which limits their understanding of malaria prevention strategies (Dunkel et al., 2016). In Zimbabwe, where 80% of respondents had either no or less than 7 years of formal schooling, the acceptability of IRS was linked to a lack of understanding about the intervention (Vundule & Mharakurwa, 1996). Assessing the impact of education on the perceptions about malaria and malaria control is complicated by the fact that such large proportions of vulnerable populations have no formal education (Diggle et al., 2014; Govere, Durrheim, la Grange, Mabuza, & Booman, 2000; Vundule & Mharakurwa, 1996).

In any society, there are people with little control due to their culturally and socially defined roles. The lack of control limits their ability to admit to illness, rally resources, access services, and make decisions. This lack of power and personal control leaves them socially vulnerable, which draws attention to factors that lead to inequality. Social vulnerability has a noteworthy impact on illness behaviors for example; women in some societies may appear weak if they admit to being ill, whilst men may be too proud to admit to being ill or they may be concerned about losing their jobs if they take time off from work. Social position also impacts on the use of resources, for example when someone is ill, money for treatment may be provided to the eldest son rather than an adopted child. Sociocultural considerations may impact on access to health care and services for example, in some societies women are unable to access health care due to cultural constraints (Jones & Williams, 2004).

9.6 Sustainable Malaria Control in Africa

The control of malaria in Africa is dictated by the rural lifestyles of people living in poor socioeconomic conditions, where education and food security remains a challenge. These communities are inherently more susceptible to contracting malaria due to having insufficient resources and lack of knowledge for implementing prevention strategies. Due to the vulnerable nature of these communities, controlling malaria will require collaborations between international, national, regional and local stakeholders that will combine safe, sustainable and innovative methods of malaria control. As previously mentioned, controlling malaria parasites and preventing mosquito bites remains the first line of defense, and is the focus of much research and most malaria control programs. With the rising resistance of mosquito vectors to insecticides and parasites to anti-malarial drugs (Thomas, 2018), these strategies are becoming outdated and ineffective. To eliminate malaria, the focus of malaria control needs to shift towards new innovative, sustainable methods.

Over the past decade, there has been a renewed worldwide effort in malaria control towards elimination, which has been accompanied by an increase in basic research. At present, it is unclear how these knowledge gains will translate into improved malaria control methods and strategies. While malaria has been eliminated in several, mostly developed countries, the worldwide call to eliminate malaria have been unsuccessful. To achieve elimination and, ultimately, eradication, the malaria community – scientists, control program managers, governments, funding agencies, and communities – need to approach malaria control with sustainability in mind (Birkholtz et al., 2012). Sustainable malaria control should incorporate methods and strategies that are safe to both humans and the environment. Once elimination has been achieved in an endemic area, continuous surveillance is key to ensuring that malaria is not re-introduced into that specific area. This is an important step towards worldwide elimination and is often not considered when annual malaria control program budgets are prepared.

Existing tools for malaria control are unlikely to lead to malaria elimination and eradication, if used singularly (Thomas, 2018). Lessons learnt from previous worldwide malaria-elimination attempts led to the conclusion that no single strategy can be effective, because unlike other infectious diseases such as smallpox, human immunodeficiency virus (HIV) and tuberculosis (TB), malaria is not caused by a single biological entity (Birkholtz et al., 2012). The eradication of malaria will only be achieved if a structured, multifaceted approach towards both malaria prevention and treatment, is implemented (Hemingway, Shretta, et al., 2016). It is highly unlikely that a drug campaign or future vaccine rollout, targeting only malaria parasites, will ever be effective on its own for sustainable malaria control. Vigilant coordination of the control strategies by reducing parasite numbers to prevent malaria transmission (Birkholtz et al., 2012), along with the inclusion of effective vector control strategies (Hemingway, Shretta, et al., 2016) are needed to eradicate malaria in Africa and across the globe.

Integrated Vector Management (IVM) combines diverse tools, tactics and resources to reduce malaria transmission (Thomas, 2018). According to the WHO, IVM is the "*rational decision-making process for the optimal use of resources for vector control*" (Mutero, Schlodder, Kabatereine, & Kramer, 2012; WHO, 2004). Integrated vector management uses a spectrum of control options that could better target the natural variation of vector populations (Birkholtz et al., 2012; Mutero et al., 2012). Aside from vector control, IVM encompasses five key aspects, namely evidence-based decision making; integrated approaches; collaboration with the health sector; advocacy; social mobilization and legislation; and capacity building (Beier et al., 2008). The WHO recommends a suitable combination of non-chemical and chemical methods of malaria vector control in an IVM framework suited to socio-economic, ecological and epidemiological settings (WHO, 2004). Despite the value of IVM, most countries have not adopted IVM strategies due to a lack of country-specific policies to guide development and implementation (Mutero et al., 2012). An essential component of implementation of IVM is the collaboration between the health sector and other public and private sectors, and engaging local communities and other stakeholders, because actions and policies outside of the health sector may affect malaria control (Birkholtz et al., 2012; Mutero et al., 2012).

9.7 The UNDP Sustainable Development Goals and Malaria

The United Nations Development Program (UNDP) has identified 17 sustainable development goals (SDGs) that imagines a future, by 2030, where there will be no poverty, no hunger and people will be safe from the worst effects of climate change (UNDP, 2018). The sustainable development goals aim to improve quality of life that can be sustained for future generations. Africa faces significant challenges in attaining these goals (Henao, Hui, & Shaw, 2017), which require significant infrastructure and investment. The fight against malaria can be seen as a microcosm of Africa's bid to achieve the SDGs by 2030, with malaria issues feeding into numerous goals. Attaining these goals will aid in the fight against malaria and vice versa.

The first SDG aims to eradicate poverty in all its forms (UNDP, 2018). Poverty is more than a lack of income or resources. People live in poverty if they lack basic services such as healthcare, security, and education. They also experience hunger, social discrimination, and exclusion from decision-making processes. In Africa, the fight against malaria will only succeed if communities perceive illness to be a major barrier to their desired quality of life. As long as extreme poverty persists, the fight against malaria will fall second to putting food on the table, which is linked to the SDG 2 or zero hunger (UNDP, 2018). Unfortunately, the costs associated with malaria will keep communities and countries in poverty and additional strategies are needed to tackle the problem.

The third SDG, aims to ensure health and well-being for all, including a commitment to end the epidemics of HIV/AIDS, tuberculosis, malaria and other communicable diseases (Henao et al., 2017). Malaria is the fourth most important cause of disability-adjusted life-years (DALYs) in Africa (Henao et al., 2017), and winning the fight against malaria will mean more men and women being able to work, parents able to care for their children, more children able to attend school, improved neonatal survival and a reduced secondary disease burden. The fight against malaria is not simply rooted in the provision of healthcare, vaccines, or treatment but links to other SDGs, such as quality education (SDG 4), clean water and sanitation (SDG 6), economic growth and decent work (SDG 8), and climate action (SDG 13). At the heart of attaining the SDGs lies the use of evidenced-based research to inform local, regional and national policies.

9.8 Malaria Research and Innovation in Africa

Despite malaria being a dominant disease in Africa, most malaria research is being conducted by researchers in developed countries where malaria does not necessarily occur. As a result, malaria research remains focused on traditional vector control and the development of new anti-malarial drugs, without considering the importance of community environment and identity. Researchers from countries with endemic malaria have a unique opportunity to develop new methods of malaria control, with the participation of affected communities. In Africa, researchers are often stymied by a lack of funding to develop proper and sustainable control methods despite having the knowledge skills and experience. Researchers from African countries also have the opportunity to collaborate to answer complex questions such as the importance of cross border control and influence of local climatic conditions on malaria.

Researchers from Africa, from malaria endemic countries, face inherent challenges in translating research to policy. In Malawi, malaria research was translated into policy when the government and the ministry of health revived the policy development unit and established the office for the director of research, the knowledge translation unit and, academic and non-academic research institutions (Mwendera et al., 2017). These institutions were supported by the national health research agenda, guidelines for policy development and analysis, and guidelines for evidence use in policy-making. In Malawi, barriers to the use of malaria research included researchers' inability to involve, collaborate and communicate their research findings to policy makers (Mwendera et al., 2017). Other barriers included lack of platforms for researcher-public engagement, politics, funder driven research, unknown WHO policy position, and a lack of a malaria research repository (Mwendera et al., 2017). Challenges to the implementation of malaria policies included inadequate resources, unavailability of trained staff, poor supervision and mentorship, politics, parallel implementation of policies, lack of a platform for engagement with communities, top-down approach in policy development, lack of understanding of socio-cultural factors affecting policy uptake by communities, and incomplete stakeholder analysis during policy development (Mwendera et al., 2017). Despite the barriers and challenges to the translation of malaria knowledge, the research activity on malaria in Africa is growing and gaining momentum.

In South Africa, the Vhembe district in northern Limpopo Province carries approximately 60% of South Africa's malaria burden (Raman et al., 2016) and forms a focal point for national elimination efforts. Researchers working in the Vhembe district are studying all aspects of malaria, including human and environmental health, parasite and vector control, with sustainability as a main focus. The research connects affected, rural communities, Malaria Control Program managers, policy makers and researchers, hoping to develop tailor-made malaria control strategies. Polymer mesh ITWLs were placed on the walls and tested in rural dwellings in communities in Thohoyandou, Limpopo. This mesh acted against indoor-resting mosquitoes and allowed for long-lasting residual efficacy of the insecticide and no insecticide dusting (Kruger et al., 2015). Dusting occurs when insecticide particles stick to dust particles during spraying, resulting in a loss of spray residue and thereby a decrease in insecticide effectiveness on surfaces and an increase in the human exposure potential. Researchers have reported that harmful levels of insecticide residues are still present in ambient air for up to 3 months after spraying (Van Dyk, Bouwman, Barnhoorn, & Bornman, 2010). The linings remained 100% effective after 5 years, based on laboratory efficacy tests. Community members that took part in the trial accepted the linings in their homes and were happy with the decrease in mosquito bites and the absence of other annoying insects. As with ITNs/LLINs, pyrethroids are currently the only insecticides approved by the WHO for use in insecticide treated wall linings (ITWLs). Due to vector pyrethroid resistance being a major concern, researchers are already investigating the use of new alternative insecticides in the ITWLs (Kruger et al., 2015).

Currently, communities from the Vhembe district municipality are also giving researchers an important opportunity to study the effects of existing mosquito control methods on human health. Indoor residual spraying with a range of insecticides including dichloro-diphenyl-trichloroethane (DDT), carbamates and pyrethoids are sprayed annually in rural villages that are severely affected by malaria. Over a 10 year period (2010–2015), almost two tons of DDT was sprayed in the area (Adebayo-Ojo et al., 2018, Unpublished). While the advantages of controlling malaria are undisputed, the cost of using large quantities of insecticides, with endocrine disrupting properties, on human health has to be considered.

In a large community experiment, the DDT levels in the plasma of young males was measured and related to various reproductive parameters (Aneck-Hahn, Schulenburg, Bornman, Farias, & Jager, 2007; Bornman et al., 2018; de Jager et al., 2009). Young men, who had a history of living in villages with high IRS coverage had high levels of DDT in their blood and plasma (Bornman et al., 2018). In the Limpopo Province, spray-workers exposed to DDT had higher estradiol (E_2) and total-testosterone levels (Dalvie et al., 2004). In young men living in IRS areas, DDT exposure was associated with impaired semen quality (Aneck-Hahn et al., 2007) and a high incidence of sperm with DNA breaks (de Jager et al., 2009). Results from a cohort study in the Vhembe district suggest that pre-natal exposure to pyrethroids may be associated with poorer language development by the time infants are 2 years old (Eskenazi et al., 2018). Evidence suggests that exposure to DDT during pregnancy may also be associated with hypertensive disorder during pregnancy (Murray et al., 2018). The negative effects of these chemicals on human health need to be quantified to inform malaria control programs in the 10 countries that are still using DDT.

Researchers have developed a new insect repellant formulation (Izadi et al., 2017) by mixing two existing repellent formulations. The resulting formulation has a longer lifespan and can knock down and kill mosquitoes at the same time (Izadi et al., 2017). Currently, researchers are also trying to identify the components of odor and chemical compounds that elicit a strong antennograph response from female mosquitoes, aimed at developing attractants (Rohwer, Naude, & Stoltz, 2017). Attractants can either lure mosquitoes to or away from a specific area or form part of a trap mechanism – toxic sugar baits, lethal ovitraps, mass trapping (Thomas, 2018) – where mosquitoes are killed by an insecticide in the trap or due to starvation. Attractants are considered safe for humans and the environment, are cheap to use, and are a very promising complimentary or alternative intervention (Birkholtz et al., 2012). Other novel developments include the use of nano-technologies as innovative, safer vector control methods. Researchers are using clay nano-technology, where clay particles are used as molecular reservoirs to stabilize insecticides. Nanomaterials can also be incorporated in fabrics, ceramics, paints, bracelets or other items that enable prolonged protection from mosquito vectors, such as socks and gloves (Nkosi, 2017; Sibanda et al., 2018).

Vector control is further complicated by the ability of mosquitoes to adapt to existing control methods by changing their behavior. For example, the biting behavior of mosquito vectors has shifted with the increased use of ITNs/LLINs and IRS (Gatton et al., 2013). Mosquitoes are now biting humans earlier in the evening and taking blood meals outdoors. Some mosquito vectors may avoid resting on insecticide treated surfaces inside houses after consuming a blood meal, leaving the home after feeding (Nkosi, 2017). To address the plasticity of mosquito vector behavior, we need to adopt a dynamic approach to vector control. For example, by protecting the lower limbs of people who are active outdoors at night, we may be able to decrease vector biting risk by wearing inexpensive repellent-impregnated anklets or sandals (Braack et al., 2015; Izadi et al., 2017). Similarly, people, especially children, sleeping at floor level – a common occurrence in poor rural communities – may be more exposed to mosquito bites while sleeping and treated bedding may protect children while sleeping at night (Braack et al., 2015).

When African rural houses are modified, mosquito entry can potentially be reduced by up to 80% (Nkosi, 2017). The windows of dwellings can be covered with mesh screens (Thomas, 2018) to prevent mosquitoes from entering dwellings. Another practice is to close up the eaves, the area where the roof meets the top of the wall, with mesh or other materials. Whilst closing up the eaves is very effective and cheap; it may cause indoor temperatures to rise. Whilst this method prevents biting, it does not reduce vector populations (Birkholtz et al., 2012).

The National Malaria Control Program in South Africa focuses on the use of IRS and limited larval source management through larvaciding, and does not promote the use of ITNs/LLINs. These control methods rely on chemical insecticides, which is a major concern due to known vector resistance; however, other biological control mechanisms or environmental management may also control adult and larval vectors (Birkholtz et al., 2012; Mutero et al., 2012). Biological control, such as fungal pathogens that infect mosquitoes, can be self-sustaining and self-spreading, cheap and novel delivery system, which is resilient to resistance, can target residual transmission, and can complement existing interventions, whilst allowing for community engagement and local production, enabling communities to take malaria prevention into their own hands (Thomas, 2018). Environmental management, or environmental sanitation (Mabaso, Sharp, & Lengeler, 2004) of potential mosquito breeding habitats is a very practical and easy way to control vector numbers, and complements other control measures (Birkholtz et al., 2012). People living in affected communities should clean up litter around their dwellings that allow water to pool and stagnate, and form breeding habitats for mosquito vectors. Environmental management and larval control should form part of malaria education and awareness campaigns.

9.9 Malaria Education, Health Promotion and Science Communication

Social scientists used to play a small part in the development or assessment of malaria control programs. At present, applied social science research and collaborations between basic and social scientists are informing malaria control programs and strategies in Africa. Societal perceptions influence how different communities accept control methods. Societal factors also drive local malaria epidemiology. These societal factors determine the choice of appropriate control methods for a specific community or region (Carpenter et al., 1991). Over the centuries, education has been a critical element of action to promote health and inhibit the spread of disease (Nutbeam, 2000; WHO, 1996). With education being a key factor in socio-economic development, school aged children should also be protected from malaria to prevent children from missing school for long periods (King et al., 2015)

Effective health education is adapted to the needs of learners that is specific to their epide-

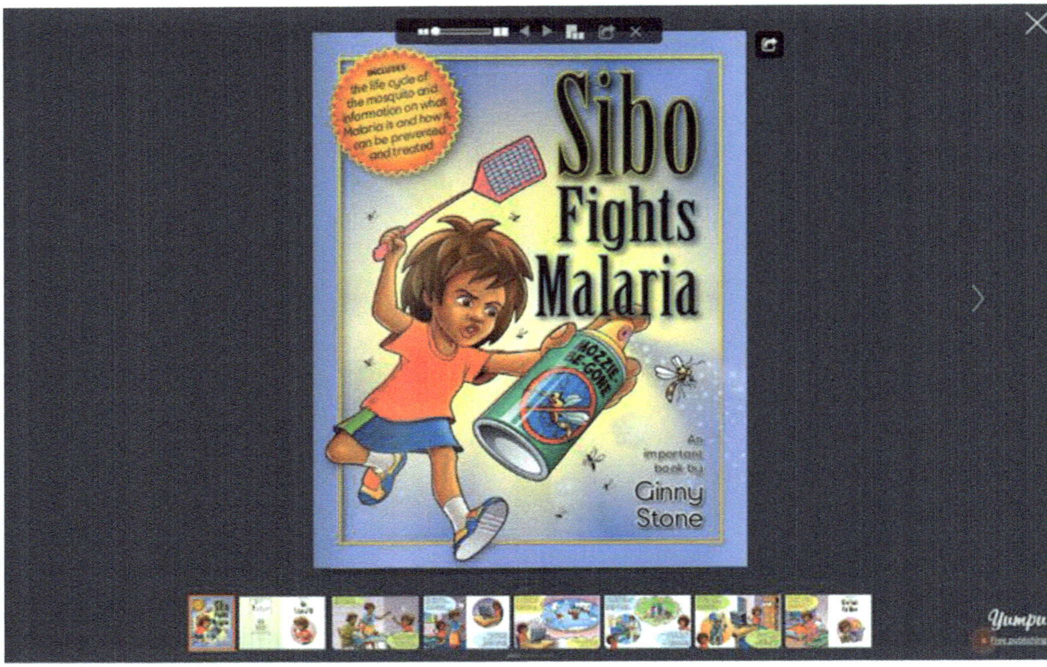

Fig. 9.4 The malaria educational children's book – 'Sibo Fights Malaria' – developed and written with the aim to inform children about malaria, its symptoms, how to prevent getting sick, and what to do if one is sick. The book is available to read on the internet (Stone, 2014)

miological, ecological, economic and social situation (Sachs & Malaney, 2002; WHO, 1996). For the promotion of health, schools are the most effective and easiest way to reach a large number of young children, families and community members (Ayi et al., 2010). In the Vhembe district of the Limpopo Province, researchers have integrated their research program with an extensive education and awareness campaign. Education researchers worked with children in primary schools in rural villages to assess the extent of malaria education in schools and found a need to develop an informative, educational resource that could be incorporated into the national curriculum. The group developed a colorful, easily accessible, children's book called 'Sibo Fights Malaria' (Fig. 9.4) (Stone, 2014). The book was used in malaria education projects in select primary schools as part of the formal curriculum, and for malaria awareness creation on World Malaria Day (Fig. 9.5a, b) – 25 April. The educational value of the book was expanded by drama performance and a song written for school children in TshiVenda. The culturally appropriate song was developed using participatory action research (PAR) where focus groups listened to and gave their input on how to make the song culturally and age appropriate for young children from a specific area (Anderson, McCrindle, Kruger, & McNeill, 2018). Researchers are using the song, along with other education techniques to develop a model for malaria education that could be followed in schools across Africa.

Music and song is known for its power of suggestion especially when used in the advertising business where songs known as "jingles" target a specific audience to purchase a specific product (Anderson et al., 2018). Music education is known to help teach good, educational and social habits to young children, who are able to follow the message in the song. Musical interventions have been used to prevent or manage disease by encouraging behaviour change in adolescents and adults (Anderson et al., 2018). Songs have been used to educate the public on how best to

a b
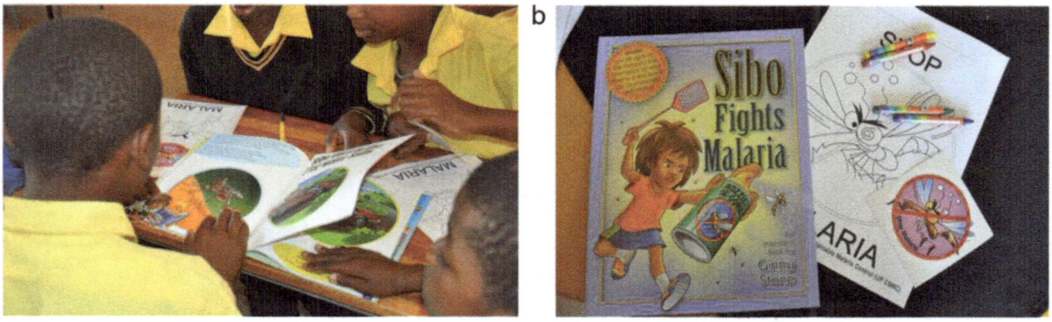

Fig. 9.5 (**a**) 'Sibo Fights Malaria' used by researchers in primary schools in malaria education projects, (**b**) 'Sibo Fights Malaria' used for awareness creation on World Malaria Day. (Photos by Ms. Ansa Heyl, University of Pretoria, 2015)

avoid getting Ebola and HIV/AIDS (Anderson et al., 2018). A song about the need to "Stomp out malaria" in Botswana was developed, and was sung by a well-known local artist along with a music video, in order to raise awareness about the disease (Anderson, 2014; Anderson et al., 2018).

Most importantly, education, awareness and health promotion work relies on a collaboration between researchers and community members. Educational projects rely on work conducted with young children in schools, who then become health messengers to inform others in their communities (Ayi et al., 2010; Midzi et al., 2011) and to promote lifestyle changes. Schools form important dissemination points for healthcare and health promotion. Awareness of malaria should enable rural, communities in endemic malaria areas to control their own vulnerability to malaria and contribute towards an integrated malaria management approach.

In the Vhembe district, community members have become lay health workers and project team members. Lay health workers, who were involved since the inception of the project play an important part in communicating with other community members. Local team members ensure that community members receive information in their local language and help to inform the greater community about the transmission of malaria. Researchers in the Vhembe district assessed the value of a Malaria Awareness Program (MAP) in improving malaria knowledge of households (Cox et al., 2018). Community health workers visited more than 1000 homes in the community to deliver information about malaria transmission and prevention. Community members who participated in the MAP had 3.3 times better scores about malaria transmission and 2.8 times better scores about malaria prevention than community members who did not participate in the MAP (Cox et al., 2018). Ideally, the MAP aims to change health seeking and prevention behavior of community members, and ultimately stop the transmission of malaria.

9.9.1 Social Media, Mobile Devices and Applications

Rural populations have limited access to technology and information, and encounter obstacles to obtain health information (Moonasar et al., 2012). This is especially true for the African continent but the tides may be changing. The Global Systems Mobile-Communication Association (GSMA) is a trade body that represents the interests of mobile network operators around the globe. In 2016, the GSMA reported that the number of smartphone connections in Africa had reached 226 million, and was on the rise. Growth in smartphone use was driven primarily by the massive uptake in the more technologically advanced mobile markets namely Egypt, Kenya, Nigeria, and South Africa. There were also some relatively new 3G markets, most notably Algeria, Cameroon and the Democratic Republic of Congo. It is estimated that the African region's smartphone connections will increase by a further 500 million by 2020 and will be driven mostly by the increase in available low-cost devices (Intelligent, 2016).

Information technologies, including smartphones, are transforming health promotion strategies. Effective communication is critical within any public health system. Social media are being used in numerous ways across the health sector to incorporate new ways to deliver care (Coiera, 2013). Social media are changing communication between individuals and organizations on a daily basis and also during disasters that threaten public health or to communicate health information (Merchant, Elmer, & Lurie, 2011). Health care programmes have started using social media to communicate important malaria related news to its researchers, stakeholders and the public. Health applications (apps) on smartphones are one of the most highly used apps covering a range of health topics including healthy lifestyles, fitness, disease management, and public health. Health apps support interventions for health behaviour changes (Kratzke & Cox, 2012). Public health services appear to use social media mainly for one way distribution of public messages (Thackeray, Neiger, Smith, & Van Wagenen, 2012), but social media could potentially reach a broader and more diverse audience (Thackeray et al., 2012). For example cancer patients use Twitter to offer emotional support and to discuss treatment (Sugawara et al., 2012). Online communities have helped people to quit smoking (van Mierlo, Voci, Lee, Fournier, & Selby, 2012). The mobile app, 'Malaria Buddy' is a health and travel app that was introduced with a very simple goal in mind. The app focuses on informing mainly tourists, about the disease, its symptoms, how to prevent getting malaria and what one should do if you suspected that you have the disease. The most recent version is more dynamic in its approach and includes the searchable locality function of clinics in South Africa and is slowly adding clinic information for the southern Africa region. A travel mode notifies the app user when entering or exiting malaria risk areas. The app uses Geographical Information System (GIS) technology and the phone's location to achieve this. The app also has a separate informative platform that allows health care professionals to advise patients on potential treatment. The ultimate end-goal is for the app to become a 'One-Stop' malaria information and prevention companion.

The emergence of 'mobile' as the platform of choice has been reported with regards to the "*creating, distributing and consuming of innovative digital solutions and services in Africa*". There is a growing interest from consumers in "*home-grown solutions that directly appeal to local interests and cultures*" that addresses the unique socio-economic challenges that are experienced by consumers in the African region. Some of these worldwide content providers, such as Facebook and Google, are tapping into Africa's increasingly technology-savvy consumer base by launching more localised services (GSMA, 2016). Thus far, no information technology, specifically social media platforms, have been used to inform and educate endemic rural communities about malaria. These technological marvels and social media platforms may not be accessible to the very remote and poor African rural communities yet, but may help to spread awareness and contribute towards malaria elimination in the not too distant future.

9.10 Eliminating Malaria Will Improve the Quality of Life Across Africa

With an increase in malaria awareness across the globe, many malaria researchers and policy makers have focused on the rapid expansion of effective malaria control programs without considering their sustainability. Worldwide malaria control programs received increased financial support to implement IRS at a large scale and distribute free ITN/LLIN across sub-Saharan Africa (Joseph D Njau et al., 2013). Over the last decade, malaria control programs have adopted a total policy overhaul regarding malaria case management; the use of more effective but expensive ACTs for malaria treatment; improved diagnosis of malaria using microscopy or RDTs; and increased support for IPTp for pregnant women, infants and school-age children.

9.10.1 A Case Study of Sustainable Integrated Malaria Management

According to the WHO, malaria elimination refers to zero local transmission, whilst eradication is the permanent zero, non-occurrence of malaria across the globe (Birkholtz et al., 2012; WHO, 2010). Very few examples of successful malaria control or local elimination have been reported from Africa. One example of elimination in a remote rural village was reported in Sanambele, Mali (Dunkel et al., 2013). Sanambele was chosen for the intervention based on focus groups with 11 villages. Only villagers from Sanambele identified malaria elimination as the highest priority for attaining their desired quality of life. Sanambele is 50 km south of Bamako, the capital city of Mali, and can be reached by a bus service that takes 8 h. The village has no electricity, municipal services or tarred roads.

The project started in 2005 and involved students from Montana State University (MSU, USA), scientists from Mali and an environmental engineer. Working with community leaders, Dunkel and co-workers (2013) identified sources or potential breeding sites for mosquitoes and focused their management efforts on managing larval breeding habitats. The students implemented larval control by living and working with the villagers to identify and manage larval breeding sites. During these homestay visits, outsiders were able to learn about the village situation. Living in the village, students were able to identify that most Sanambeleans did not use bed nets until three to 5 h after dusk, making them vulnerable to bites from *Anopheles* mosquitoes. The students educated and helped to build community capacity through storytelling and using adapted diagrams. Three MSU courses were transformed by eliminating lectures and holistically integrating traditional wisdom and participatory diagramming techniques. Traditional wisdom was integrated by mentors from the village who explained the importance of storytelling, the family and the tribal social systems to faculty and students from MSU. With this understanding, students from MSU were able to integrate and teach the villagers about malaria control using storytelling and song. Between 2005 and 2011, a handicraft enterprise was established to create cash flow, and was generating annual revenue of US$1464 by 2011, which improved financial security in the village. The revenue from this handicraft enterprise is used to buy ITNs/LLINs and medicines to treat malaria.

The interactions between villagers and MSU faculty and students led to villagers knowing more about malaria disease and malaria control. By the end of 2011, the women of Sanambele had improved their emergency plan for cerebral malaria, village leaders knew the life cycles of malaria protozoans and mosquitoes, and were able to communicate their knowledge through story telling. Village leaders and youth knew how to sample and identify mosquito larvae and were able to practice larval management using physical and botanical methods. Village school teachers and their students were able to use microscopes to diagnose malaria from blood smears. Village teachers were also able to impart protozoan and mosquito life cycle knowledge using the prescribed curriculum in Mali.

This community based program led to the elimination of malaria, 2 years after the start of the program. Following their successes, the Sanambelean villagers were able to extend their efforts to neighboring villages using storytelling. The villagers of Sanambele were able to eliminate malaria by reducing female *Anopheles* mosquito populations and were able to prevent mosquitoes from biting infected humans while they were in the fever state. The success of malaria control in Sanambele is linked to the environment, culture and attitudes of the villagers. The villagers were determined to eliminate malaria, and are thus also committed to maintaining larval control. The approach used in Sanambele, using a holistic process with transformed classrooms requires an informal approach that generates trust within the community. The elimination of malaria and the opportunity to generate revenue helped villagers to achieve their desired quality of life.

9.11 Conclusion

The intimate relationship between malaria and quality of life in Africa ties in with other aspects such as poverty (SDG 1), education (SDG 4) and food security (SDG 2). People living in remote, rural areas, who do not have access to healthcare (SDG 3) are often the most vulnerable. In many cases throughout Africa, malaria is seen as a perceived health threat but not an everyday concern. This perception needs to change if malaria is to be eliminated in Africa. Current methods used to control mosquito vectors are becoming less and less efficient. Insecticide treated bed nets are not always used correctly and indoor residual spraying is leading to increased insecticide resistance and evidence suggests that insecticides may have harmful endocrine disrupting effects, affecting human and environmental health. With these consequences in mind, malaria control programs need to reassess how they approach the problem and learn from experiences where countries have successfully eliminated malaria.

As long as the elimination of malaria is an international priority, externally funded control programs will remain the norm. These control programs will focus on the management of mosquito vectors and the development of new antimalarial drugs, which will have a limited impact without the understanding and trust of local communities. The history of malaria in Zanzibar (Smith et al., 2011) is a prime example. By 1969, Zanzibar had achieved malaria control and subsequently abandoned all intervention as there was not a perceived threat to health. Malaria quickly returned to levels seen before the control, and interventions were reintroduced in 2002. While malaria is almost negligible today, interventions need to be maintained to avoid resurgence (Smith et al., 2011). So how do we avoid this problem?

Researchers in Venda are researching more sustainable, natural methods of mosquito control. By interacting with the community, they are improving awareness and improving the quality of life in Vhembe villages, Limpopo, South Africa. The Sanambelean villagers provide a good example of the elimination of malaria coupled with achieving a desired quality of life, where eliminating malaria is a priority.

Africa is increasing its access to cell-phones, mobile data and ultimately information. Social media has created opportunities for the public to contact research entities, but without adequate healthcare resources in the public health sector, controlling and treating malaria will almost be impossible. Successful malaria elimination relies on partnerships between communities, healthcare providers, research entities and national policy makers.

References

Anderson, C. M. (2014). *Stomp it out*. https://www.youtube.com/watch?v=9r8deqdnKVs

Anderson, C. M., McCrindle, C. M., Kruger, T., & McNeill, F. (2018). Using participatory risk analysis to develop a song about malaria for young children in Limpopo Province, South Africa. *Malaria Journal, 17*(1), 181.

Aneck-Hahn, N. H., Schulenburg, G. W., Bornman, M. S., Farias, P., & Jager, C. (2007). Impaired semen quality associated with environmental DDT exposure in young men living in a malaria area in the Limpopo Province, South Africa. *Journal of Andrology, 28*(3), 423–434.

Ansah, E. K., Narh-Bana, S., Epokor, M., Akanpigbiam, S., Quartey, A. A., Gyapong, J., et al. (2010). Rapid testing for malaria in settings where microscopy is available and peripheral clinics where only presumptive treatment is available: A randomised controlled trial in Ghana. *BMJ, 340*, c930. https://doi.org/10.1136/bmj.c930. http://www.bmj.com/content/340/bmj.c930.abstract

Ayi, I., Nonaka, D., Adjovu, J. K., Hanafusa, S., Jimba, M., Bosompem, K. M., et al. (2010). School-based participatory health education for malaria control in Ghana: Engaging children as health messengers. *Malaria Journal, 9*(1), 98.

Bang, K. T. (2010). *Local community knowledge, perceptions, and experiences of malaria prevention in the Highlands of Papua New Guinea*. Unitec Institute of Technology.

Beier, J. C., Keating, J., Githure, J. I., Macdonald, M. B., Impoinvil, D. E., & Novak, R. J. (2008). Integrated vector management for malaria control. *Malaria Journal, 7*(Suppl 1), S4. https://doi.org/10.1186/1475-2875-7-S1-S4

Bingham, A., Gaspar, F., Lancaster, K., Conjera, J., Collymore, Y., & Ba-Nguz, A. (2012). Community perceptions of malaria and vaccines in two districts of Mozambique. *Malaria Journal, 11*(1), 394.

Birkholtz, L.-M., Bornman, R., Focke, W., Mutero, C., & De Jager, C. (2012). Sustainable malaria control: Transdisciplinary approaches for translational applications. *Malaria Journal, 11*(1), 431.

Bornman, M., Delport, R., Farías, P., Aneck-Hahn, N., Patrick, S., Millar, R. P., et al. (2018). Alterations in male reproductive hormones in relation to environmental DDT exposure. *Environment International, 113*, 281–289.

Bornman, M., Schlemmer, L., Van der Walt, T., Van Dyk, C., & Bouwman, H. (2012). Implications for health education and intervention strategies arising from children's caregivers concerns following successful malaria control. *Transactions of the Royal Society of Tropical Medicine and Hygiene, 106*(7), 408–414.

Braack, L., Hunt, R., Koekemoer, L. L., Gericke, A., Munhenga, G., Haddow, A. D., et al. (2015). Biting behaviour of African malaria vectors: 1. Where do the main vector species bite on the human body? *Parasites & Vectors, 8*(1), 76.

Carpenter, C. C., Pearson, G. W., Mitchell, V. S., & Oaks, S. C., Jr. (1991). *Malaria: Obstacles and opportunities*. Washington, DC: National Academies Press.

Clouston, S. A., Yukich, J., & Anglewicz, P. (2015). Social inequalities in malaria knowledge, prevention and prevalence among children under 5 years old and women aged 15–49 in Madagascar. *Malaria Journal, 13*(Suppl 1), 499. https://doi.org/10.1186/s12936-015-1010-y

Coetzee, M., Kruger, P., Hunt, R., Durrheim, D., Urbach, J., & Hansford, C. (2013). Malaria in South Africa: 110 years of learning to control the disease. *South African Medical Journal, 103*(10), 770–778.

Coiera, E. (2013). Social networks, social media, and social diseases. *British Medical Journal, 346*, f3007. https://doi.org/10.1136/bmj.f3007

Cottrell, G., Moussiliou, A., Luty, A. J., Cot, M., Fievet, N., Massougbodji, A., et al. (2015). Submicroscopic *Plasmodium falciparum* infections are associated with maternal anemia, premature births, and low birth weight. *Clinical Infectious Diseases, 60*(10), 1481–1488. https://doi.org/10.1093/cid/civ122

Cox, S. N., Guidera, K. E., Simon, M. J., Nonyane, B. A. S., Brieger, W., Bornman, M. S., et al. (2018). Interactive malaria education intervention and its effect on community participant knowledge: The malaria awareness program in Vhembe District, Limpopo, South Africa. *International Quarterly of Community Health Education, 38*(2), 147–158.

Dalvie, M. A., Myers, J. E., Thompson, M. L., Robins, T. G., Dyer, S., Riebow, J., et al. (2004). The long-term effects of DDT exposure on semen, fertility, and sexual function of malaria vector-control workers in Limpopo Province, South Africa. *Environmental Research, 96*(1), 1–8.

de Jager, C., Aneck-Hahn, N. H., Bornman, M., Farias, P., Leter, G., Eleuteri, P., et al. (2009). Sperm chromatin integrity in DDT-exposed young men living in a malaria area in the Limpopo Province, South Africa. *Human Reproduction, 24*(10), 2429–2438.

De Silva, P. M., & Marshall, J. M. (2012). Factors contributing to urban malaria transmission in sub-Saharan Africa: A systematic review. *Journal of Tropical Medicine, 2012*, 819563.

Diggle, E., Asgary, R., Gore-Langton, G., Nahashon, E., Mungai, J., Harrison, R., et al. (2014). Perceptions of malaria and acceptance of rapid diagnostic tests and related treatment practises among community members and health care providers in Greater Garissa, North Eastern Province, Kenya. *Malaria Journal, 13*, 502.

Djènontin, A., Chabi, J., Baldet, T., Irish, S., Pennetier, C., Hougard, J.-M., et al. (2009). Managing insecticide resistance in malaria vectors by combining carbamate-treated plastic wall sheeting and pyrethroid-treated bed nets. *Malaria Journal, 8*(1), 233.

Dunkel, F. V., Coulibaly, K., Montagne, C., Luong, K., Giusti, A., Coulibaly, H., et al. (2013). Sustainable integrated malaria management by villagers in collaboration with a transformed classroom using the holistic process: Sanambele, Mali, and Montana State University, USA. *American Entomologist, 59*(1), 45–55.

Dunkel, F. V., Hansen, L. M., Halvorson, S. J., & Bangert, A. (2016). Women's perceptions of health, quality of life, and malaria management in Kakamega County, Western Province, Kenya. *GeoJournal, 82*(4), 841–865. https://doi.org/10.1007/s10708-016-9701-7

Eskenazi, B., An, S., Rauch, S. A., Coker, E. S., Maphula, A., Obida, M., et al. (2018). Prenatal exposure to DDT and pyrethroids for malaria control and child neurodevelopment: The VHEMBE cohort, South Africa. *Environmental Health Perspectives, 126*(4), 047004. https://doi.org/10.1289/EHP2129

Gallup, J. L., & Sachs, J. D. (2001). The economic burden of malaria. *American Journal of Tropical Medicine and Hygiene, 64*(1_suppl), 85–96.

Gatton, M. L., Chitnis, N., Churcher, T., Donnelly, M. J., Ghani, A. C., Godfray, H. C., et al. (2013). The importance of mosquito behavioural adaptations to malaria control in Africa. *Evolution, 67*(4), 1218–1230. https://doi.org/10.1111/evo.12063

Govere, J., Durrheim, D., la Grange, K., Mabuza, A., & Booman, M. (2000). Community knowledge and perceptions about malaria and practices influencing malaria control in Mpumalanga Province, South Africa. *South African Medical Journal, 90*(6), 611–618.

GSMA. (2016). *The mobile economy Africa*.

Guyatt, H. L., Corlett, S. K., Robinson, T. P., Ochola, S. A., & Snow, R. W. (2002). Malaria prevention in highland Kenya: Indoor residual house-spraying vs. insecticide-treated bednets. *Tropical Medicine & International Health, 7*(4), 298–303.

Hailu, A., Lindtjørn, B., Deressa, W., Gari, T., Loha, E., & Robberstad, B. (2017). Economic burden of malaria and predictors of cost variability to rural households in south-central Ethiopia. *PLoS One, 12*(10), e0185315.

Hemingway, J., Ranson, H., Magill, A., Kolaczinski, J., Fornadel, C., Gimnig, J., et al. (2016). Averting a malaria disaster: Will insecticide resistance derail malaria control? *The Lancet, 387*(10029), 1785–1788.

Hemingway, J., Shretta, R., Wells, T. N., Bell, D., Djimdé, A. A., Achee, N., et al. (2016). Tools and strategies for malaria control and elimination: What do we need to achieve a grand convergence in malaria? *PLoS Biology, 14*(3), e1002380.

Henao, L., Hui, M., & Shaw, G. (2017). *Africa 2030: How Africa can achieve the sustainable development goals* (T. S. D. G. C. f. Africa). Tokyo, Japan: Japan International Cooperation Agency.

Hume, J. C., Barnish, G., Mangal, T., Armazio, L., Streat, E., & Bates, I. (2008). Household cost of malaria over-diagnosis in rural Mozambique. *Malaria Journal, 7*, 33. https://doi.org/10.1186/1475-2875-7-33

Ingstad, B., Munthali, A. C., Braathen, S. H., & Grut, L. (2012). The evil circle of poverty: A qualitative study of malaria and disability. *Malaria Journal, 11*(1), 15.

Intelligent, G. (2016). *The mobile economy Africa 2016.*

Izadi, H., Focke, W. W., Asaadi, E., Maharaj, R., Pretorius, J., & Loots, M. T. (2017). A promising azeotrope-like mosquito repellent blend. *Scientific Reports, 7*(1), 10273.

Jones, C. O., & Williams, H. A. (2004). The social burden of malaria: What are we measuring? *The American Journal of Tropical Medicine and Hygiene, 71*(2_suppl), 156–161.

King, N., Dewey, C., & Borish, D. (2015). Determinants of primary school non-enrollment and absenteeism: Results from a retrospective, convergent mixed methods, cohort study in rural Western Kenya. *PLoS One, 10*(9), e0138362.

Kratzke, C., & Cox, C. (2012). Smartphone technology and apps: Rapidly changing health promotion. *Global Journal of Health Education and Promotion, 15*(1), 72–82.

Kruger, T., Sibanda, M. M., Focke, W. W., Bornman, M. S., & Jager, C. (2015). Acceptability and effectiveness of a monofilament, polyethylene insecticide-treated wall lining for malaria control after six months in dwellings in Vhembe District, Limpopo Province, South Africa. *Malaria Journal, 14*(1), 485.

Larsen, D. A., Keating, J., Miller, J., Bennett, A., Changufu, C., Katebe, C., et al. (2010). Barriers to insecticide-treated mosquito net possession 2 years after a mass free distribution campaign in Luangwa District, Zambia. *PLoS One, 5*(11), e13129.

Larson, P. S., Mathanga, D. P., Campbell, C. H., & Wilson, M. L. (2012). Distance to health services influences insecticide-treated net possession and use among six to 59 month-old children in Malawi. *Malaria Journal, 11*(1), 18.

Mabaso, M. L., Sharp, B., & Lengeler, C. (2004). Historical review of malarial control in southern African with emphasis on the use of indoor residual house-spraying. *Tropical Medicine & International Health, 9*(8), 846–856.

Majgaard, K., & Mingat, A. (2012). *Education in sub-Saharan Africa: A comparative analysis*. Washington, DC: The World Bank.

Mayala, B. K., Fahey, C. A., Wei, D., Zinga, M. M., Bwana, V. M., Mlacha, T., et al. (2015). Knowledge, perception and practices about malaria, climate change, livelihoods and food security among rural communities of central Tanzania. *Infectious Diseases of Poverty, 4*(1), 21.

Merchant, R. M., Elmer, S., & Lurie, N. (2011). Integrating social media into emergency-preparedness efforts. *New England Journal of Medicine, 365*(4), 289–291.

Messenger, L. A., Miller, N. P., Adeogun, A. O., Awolola, T. S., & Rowland, M. (2012). The development of insecticide-treated durable wall lining for malaria control: Insights from rural and urban populations in Angola and Nigeria. *Malaria Journal, 11*(1), 332.

Midzi, N., Mtapuri-Zinyowera, S., Mapingure, M. P., Paul, N. H., Sangweme, D., Hlerema, G., et al. (2011). Knowledge attitudes and practices of grade three primary schoolchildren in relation to schistosomiasis, soil transmitted helminthiasis and malaria in Zimbabwe. *BMC Infectious Diseases, 11*(1), 169.

Moller, V., Roberts, B., Tiliouine, H., & Loschky, J. (2017). Waiting for happiness in Africa. In *World happiness report 2017*. New York, NY: Sustainable Development Solutions Network.

Moonasar, D., Nuthulaganti, T., Kruger, P. S., Mabuza, A., Rasiswi, E. S., Benson, F. G., et al. (2012). Malaria control in South Africa 2000–2010: Beyond MDG6. *Malaria Journal, 11*(1), 294.

Mtove, G., Hendriksen, I. C. E., Amos, B., Mrema, H., Mandia, V., Manjurano, A., et al. (2011). Treatment guided by rapid diagnostic tests for malaria in Tanzanian children: Safety and alternative bacterial diagnoses. *Malaria Journal, 10*(1), 290. https://doi.org/10.1186/1475-2875-10-290

Murphy, S. C., & Breman, J. G. (2001). Gaps in the childhood malaria burden in Africa: Cerebral malaria, neurological sequelae, anemia, respiratory distress, hypoglycemia, and complication of pregnancy. *American Journal of Tropical Medicine and Hygiene, 64*(1), 57–67.

Murray, J., Eskenazi, B., Bornman, R., Gaspar, F. W., Crause, M., Obida, M., et al. (2018). Exposure to DDT and hypertensive disorders of pregnancy among South African women from an indoor residual spraying region: The VHEMBE study. *Environmental Research, 162*, 49–54.

Mutero, C. M., Schlodder, D., Kabatereine, N., & Kramer, R. (2012). Integrated vector management for malaria control in Uganda: Knowledge, perceptions and policy development. *Malaria Journal, 11*(1), 21.

Mwangangi, J. M., Midega, J., Kahindi, S., Njoroge, L., Nzovu, J., Githure, J., et al. (2012). Mosquito species abundance and diversity in Malindi, Kenya and their potential implication in pathogen transmission. *Parasitology Research, 110*(1), 61–71.

Mwendera, C., de Jager, C., Longwe, H., Hongoro, C., Phiri, K., & Mutero, C. M. (2017). Development of a framework to improve the utilisation of malaria research for policy development in Malawi (journal article). *Health Research Policy and Systems, 15*(1), 97. https://doi.org/10.1186/s12961-017-0264-y

Nankabirwa, J., Brooker, S. J., Clarke, S. E., Fernando, D., Gitonga, C. W., Schellenberg, D., et al. (2014). Malaria in school-age children in Africa: An increasingly important challenge. *Tropical Medicine & International Health, 19*(11), 1294–1309.

Nixon, C. P. (2016). *Plasmodium falciparum* gametocyte transit through the cutaneous microvasculature: A new target for malaria transmission blocking vaccines? *Human Vaccines & Immunotherapeutics, 12*(12), 3189–3195.

Njau, J. D., Stephenson, R., Menon, M., Kachur, S. P., & McFarland, D. A. (2013). Exploring the impact of targeted distribution of free bed nets on households bed net ownership, socio-economic disparities and childhood malaria infection rates: Analysis of national malaria survey data from three sub-Saharan Africa countries. *Malaria Journal, 12*(1), 245.

Njau, R., de Savigny, D., Gilson, L., Mwageni, E., & Mosha, F. (2009). Implementation of an insecticide-treated net subsidy scheme under a public-private partnership for malaria control in Tanzania–challenges in implementation. *Malaria Journal, 8*(1), 201.

Nkosi, N. (2017). World Malaria Day: SA at forefront of fighting disease. *Pretoria News*.

Nutbeam, D. (2000). Health literacy as a public health goal: A challenge for contemporary health education and communication strategies into the 21st century. *Health Promotion International, 15*(3), 259–267.

Omotayo, A. O., & Oyekale, A. S. (2013). Effect of malaria on farming households' welfare in Ido Local Government Area of Oyo State, Nigeria. *Journal of Human Ecology, 44*(2), 189–194.

Oyekale, A. (2015). Do ownership of mosquito nets, dwelling characteristics and mothers' socio-economic status influence malaria morbidity among children under the age of 5 in Cameroon? *International Journal of Occupational Medicine and Environmental Health, 28*(3), 479–497. https://doi.org/10.13075/ijomeh.1896.00340

Parnell, S., & Walawege, R. (2011). Sub-Saharan African urbanisation and global environmental change. *Global Environmental Change, 21*, S12–S20.

Raman, J., Morris, N., Frean, J., Brooke, B., Blumberg, L., Kruger, P., et al. (2016). Reviewing South Africa's malaria elimination strategy (2012–2018): Progress, challenges and priorities. *Malaria Journal, 15*(1), 438. https://doi.org/10.1186/s12936-016-1497-x

Reyburn, H., Mbatia, R., Drakeley, C., Carneiro, I., Mwakasungula, E., Mwerinde, O., et al. (2004). Overdiagnosis of malaria in patients with severe febrile illness in Tanzania: A prospective study. *BMJ, 329*(7476), 1212. https://doi.org/10.1136/bmj.38251.658229.55

Roberts, D., & Matthews, G. (2016). Risk factors of malaria in children under the age of five years old in Uganda. *Malaria Journal, 15*(1), 246.

Rohwer, E. R., Naude, Y., & Stoltz, A. (2017). A new method for the collection and comparison of human skin volatile chemicals. In *MOMR 3rd Southern African malaria research conference*. Johhanesburg, South Africa.

Ruberto, I., Camara, S., Banek, K., & Loua, M. K. (2014). Knowledge, attitudes and practices of malaria control among communities from the health district of Forécariah in the Republic of Guinea, West Africa. *Journal of Vector Borne Diseases, 51*(2), 119.

Sachs, J., & Malaney, P. (2002). The economic and social burden of malaria. *Nature, 415*(6872), 680.

Schwarz, N. G., Adegnika, A. A., Breitling, L. P., Gabor, J., Agnandji, S. T., Newman, R. D., et al. (2008). Placental malaria increases malaria risk in the first 30 months of life. *Clinical Infectious Diseases, 47*(8), 1017–1025. https://doi.org/10.1086/591968

Sibanda, M., Focke, W., Braack, L., Leuteritz, A., Brünig, H., Tran, N. H. A., et al. (2018). Bicomponent fibres for controlled release of volatile mosquito repellents. *Materials Science and Engineering: C, 91*, 754–761. https://doi.org/10.1016/j.msec.2018.06.016

Siraj, A., Santos-Vega, M., Bouma, M., Yadeta, D., Carrascal, D. R., & Pascual, M. (2014). Altitudinal changes in malaria incidence in highlands of Ethiopia and Colombia. *Science, 343*(6175), 1154–1158.

Smith, D. L., Cohen, J. M., Moonen, B., Tatem, A. J., Sabot, O. J., Ali, A., et al. (2011). Infectious disease. Solving the Sisyphean problem of malaria in Zanzibar. *Science, 332*(6036), 1384–1385. https://doi.org/10.1126/science.1201398

Stoler, J., Weeks, J. R., Getis, A., & Hill, A. G. (2009). Distance threshold for the effect of urban agriculture on elevated self-reported malaria prevalence in Accra, Ghana. *The American Journal of Tropical Medicine and Hygiene, 80*(4), 547–554.

Stone, G. (2014). *Sibo fights malaria*. Pretoria, South Africa: Lets Look. Available at: https://www.yumpu.com/en/document/view/59165142/sibo-fights-malaria

Stratton, L., O'Neill, M. S., Kruk, M. E., & Bell, M. L. (2008). The persistent problem of malaria: Addressing the fundamental causes of a global killer. *Social Science & Medicine, 67*(5), 854–862. https://doi.org/10.1016/j.socscimed.2008.05.013

Sugawara, Y., Narimatsu, H., Hozawa, A., Shao, L., Otani, K., & Fukao, A. (2012). Cancer patients on Twitter: A novel patient community on social media. *BMC Research Notes, 5*(1), 699.

Tarimo, D. S., Lwihula, G. K., Minjas, J. N., & Bygbjerg, I. C. (2000). Mothers' perceptions and knowledge of childhood malaria in the holendemic Kibaha district, Tanzani: Implications for malaria control and the IMCI strategy. *Tropical Medicine & International Health, 5*(3), 179–184.

Thackeray, R., Neiger, B. L., Smith, A. K., & Van Wagenen, S. B. (2012). Adoption and use of social media among public health departments. *BMC Public Health, 12*(1), 242.

Thiam, S., Thior, M., Faye, B., Ndiop, M., Diouf, M. L., Diouf, M. B., et al. (2011). Major reduction in anti-malarial drug consumption in Senegal after nation-wide introduction of malaria rapid diagnostic tests. *PLoS One, 6*(4), e18419. https://doi.org/10.1371/journal.pone.0018419

Thomas, M. B. (2018). Biological control of human disease vectors: A perspective on challenges and opportunities. *BioControl*, 1–9.

Thwing, J. I., Mihigo, J., Fernandes, A. P., Saute, F., Ferreira, C., Fortes, F., et al. (2009). How much malaria occurs in urban Luanda, Angola? A health facility-based assessment. *The American Journal of Tropical Medicine and Hygiene, 80*(3), 487–491.

UNDP. (2018). *Sustainable development goals*. http://www.undp.org/content/undp/en/home/sustainable-development-goals.html. Accessed.

Van Dyk, J., Bouwman, H., Barnhoorn, I., & Bornman, M. (2010). DDT contamination from indoor residual spraying for malaria control. *Science of the Total Environment, 408*(13), 2745–2752.

van Mierlo, T., Voci, S., Lee, S., Fournier, R., & Selby, P. (2012). Superusers in social networks for smoking cessation: Analysis of demographic characteristics and posting behavior from the Canadian Cancer Society's smokers' helpline online and StopSmokingCenter.net. *Journal of Medical Internet Research, 14*(3), e66.

Vundule, C., & Mharakurwa, S. (1996). Knowledge, practices, and perceptions about malaria in rural communities of Zimbabwe: Relevance to malaria control. *Bulletin of the World Health Organization, 74*(1), 55–60.

WHO. (1996). *World malaria report*. Geneva, Switzerland: World Health Organization.

WHO. (2004). *Global strategic framework for integrated vector management*. Geneva, Switzerland: WHO.

WHO. (2010). *World malaria report*. Geneva, Switzerland: World Health Organization.

WHO. (2011). *Roll Back malaria: Economic costs of malaria*. Geneva, Switzerland: World Health Organization.

WHO. (2015). *World malaria report*.

WHO. (2017). *World malaria report*. Geneva, Switzerland: World Health Organization.

World_Bank. (2018). *Poverty and equity data portal*. Accessed.

Xu, K., Evans, D. B., Kawabata, K., Zeramdini, R., Klavus, J., & Murray, C. J. (2003). Household catastrophic health expenditure: A multicountry analysis. *The Lancet, 362*(9378), 111–117.

10 How Prioritised Policy Commitment Has Improved Food Security and Nutrition in Africa

Nokuthula Vilakazi and Sheryl L. Hendriks

Abstract

African governments have prioritised food security and nutrition over the past decade and a half. The benefits of this are starting to emerge. Food availability, access and nutrition have been improving and the proportion of people experiencing food insecurity and malnutrition has been declining. However, progress is not adequate to achieve the targets set by the international development goals or continental aspirations. So too, the gains are eroded by significant population growth that increased the absolute numbers of people still suffering. This chapter reviews the policy context of food security and nutrition in Africa and provides evidence of progress on reducing food insecurity and malnutrition – essential factors in ensuring a quality of life. However, more attention is needed to raise incomes and strengthen purchasing power to improve diets for all people in Africa. Overcoming food insecurity and malnutrition is fundamental to improving the quality of life of the current generation and breaking the inter-generational cycle of deprivation. African governments have shown that change and progress are possible. Scaling up the progress will take continued and sustained commitment and more concerted effort to ensure that economic growth drives positive changes in nutrition.

10.1 Introduction

Food insecurity is a state of deprivation that manifests in malnutrition, and at its most severe form, as hunger and famine. Malnutrition manifests as undernourishment, micronutrient deficiencies and also as overweight and obesity (imbalances in food intake). Being food secure means that all members of a household enjoy adequate, diverse diets of safe and nourishing food that meets their individual requirements for living an active and health life. Being food insecure robs children of their potential for optimal growth and development and denies people the opportunity to productively engage in livelihoods, enterprises and employment. Such deprivation creates a cycle of poverty and perpetuates inequality within society, transmitting this to future generations. Improving the quality of life for all means addressing the fundamental human right to be free from hunger and worry about future food insecurity.

Malnutrition is both a consequence of and contributor to underdevelopment. As a constraint to development, it is, concentrated among the

N. Vilakazi · S. L. Hendriks (✉)
Institute for Food, Nutrition and Well-Being and the Department of Agricultural Economics, Extension and Rural Development, University of Pretoria, Pretoria, South Africa
e-mail: Sheryl.hendriks@up.ac.za

I. Eloff (ed.), *Handbook of Quality of Life in African Societies*, International Handbooks of Quality-of-Life, https://doi.org/10.1007/978-3-030-15367-0_10

poor who do not have the means to purchase enough nutritious food. Increasing incomes is an essential remedy to both development and improving food security. Raising incomes raises the demand for more nutritious foods, leading to more diversified diets and better nutrition. More demand for food and non-food goods and services in turn drives employment growth and further development. Development programs should include interventions that address many direct and underlying determinants of malnutrition which include increasing income; food availability and access; micronutrient adequacy; gender equity; nutrition, health, as well as hygiene knowledge and practices (Ruel, Quisumbing, & Balagamwala, 2018).

In Africa, priority policy areas include striving for inclusive economic growth that reduces inequality and ensures sustainable agriculture, food self-sufficiency, and nutrition security for all which commits to use agricultural growth for eradicating undernutrition instead of leaving achievement of this goal solely to the health sector as in the past (AU, 2015a, 2015b). Policy makers have realised that improving agricultural production can make staple foods more accessible, bring prices down, making food more affordable to meet the nutritional needs (Hendriks, 2018; Pinstrup-Andersen, 2000). But achieving food security requires more than just providing the staples, agriculture also needs to include food diversification, to provide a varied diet. Focusing only on producing or making available low-cost, energy dense staple foods is not the answer to the problem of malnutrition (AfDB, forthcoming).

Eradicating extreme hunger and poverty were targets of Millennium Development Goal 1 (MDG1 for the period 2000–2015), while eliminating hunger, reducing food insecurity and improving nutrition are the aim of Sustainable Development Goal 2 (SDG2 for the period 2016–2030). Both MDG1 and now SDG2 are prioritised in the policy frameworks of the African Union. These commitments are embodied in a number of declarations, commitments and programmes in Africa and reflected in many national policies, strategies and priority development and investment programmes.

Overtime, there has been an improvement in the food security and nutrition of populations, raising prospects for improvements in the quality of life for the current and future generations. While direct attribution of these improvements to policy changes is difficult, there is overall agreement in development circles that much of the progress can be attributed to prioritising agriculture, food security and nutrition in development agendas in Africa through, in particular, the Comprehensive Africa Agriculture Development Programme (CAADP). While the numbers and scale of food insecurity and malnutrition are still considerable, African governments and their partners have made considerable strides to improve the situation. Population growth will remain a challenge in Africa in the near future, negating the improvements made in the overall proportions of destitute people but increasing the absolute numbers of those in need. This chapter explores the policy priorities related to food security and nutrition in Africa over the period MDG period and relates these to improvements in various food security and nutrition indicators that are indicative of an improved quality of life.

The chapter begins with an overview of the food security and nutrition policy commitments in Africa that have been made during the Millennium Development Goal era (2000–2015) and more recent start of the Sustainable Development Goal (2016–2030) period. This section will set out the context of the African development agenda with regard to these important elements essential to the quality of life. The chapter then turns to a review of progress made towards the commitments made to improving the quality of life in terms of food security and nutrition.

10.1.1 Understanding Food Security and Nutrition

At the centre of Africa's development agenda are food security and nutrition which calls for multi-sectoral and evidence-based decision making processes to end hunger, achieve food security and advance optimal nutrition (FAO, 2017).

Within the African food security policy landscape, there is a need for activities that have direct links to nutrition and stabilize food availability and prices contributing to food availability, diversification of diets and improved consumption of nutritious food (Lokosang, Osei, & Covic, 2016). Delivering on these commitments requires multisectoral action in implementing both nutrition-specific (direct provision of food and nutrients to address nutritional deficiencies) and nutrition-sensitive (indirect pathways to addressing nutrition) interventions across sectors (Lokosang et al. 2016).

The Food and Agriculture Organization defines food security as a situation when all people, at all times, have physical, social and economic access to sufficient, safe, and nutritious food that meets their dietary needs and food preferences for an active and healthy life (FAO, 2003). This ensures a measure of a quality of life where a population, household or individual must have access to adequate food at all times without any impending risk of losing access to food as a consequence of sudden shocks or cyclical events (FAO, 2017).

Food security has four essential elements – namely the availability of food (and safe drinking water), access by households to food, nutrition and the resilience of food systems and livelihoods. Nutrition requires not only adequate consumption of enough nutritious food to meet the specific requirements of an individual but also includes access to care and sanitation. At the heart of food security is adequate food supply. In Africa this is a major concern.

10.1.2 Food Security and Nutrition Policy Context in Africa

Africa has aligned its food security and nutrition policy frameworks with the global context set by the Sustainable Development Goals (SDGs) that seeks sustainable solutions to end hunger in all its forms by 2030, achieve food security and improve nutrition. To align with the SDGs, African leaders set their sights on striving for inclusive economic growth that reduces inequality and ensures sustainable agriculture, food self-sufficiency, and nutrition security for all (AU, 2015a). This has led to increased political will to nutrition actions, leading to even greater commitment among all stakeholders to tackle the nutrition problems on the continent (Lokosang et al. 2016).

However, despite this growing commitment over the past two decades, malnutrition remains a key challenge to good health and strong economies in Africa. Increasingly, governments in Africa have sought to create an enabling environment for achieving food security and improving nutrition. The Malabo Montpellier Panel (2017) investigated the success factors driving the progress in reducing the levels of child malnutrition (as determined by the Global Hunger Index) between 2000 and 2016 in seven African countries (Senegal, Ghana, Rwanda, Angola, Cameroon, Ethiopia and Togo respectively) that have shown the greatest progress. The Panel reported that in each country, success was driven by multi-sectoral nutrition actions and high-level accountability at every sphere of public policy and action.

Numerous statements, decisions and declarations commit Africa's leaders to realizing the continent's aspiration for equitable growth and socio-economic development through improving food security and human nutrition. These demonstrate the strong political commitment to food security and nutrition. The key elements of this are discussed below.

10.1.2.1 The African Union Agenda 2063 and the Maputo and Malabo Commitments

The African Union's Agenda 2063 (AU, 2015a) is the policy framework for the Continent's development over the next 50 years (2014–2063). Agenda 2063 prioritises healthy and well-nourished African citizens as an overarching goal for realizing a "prosperous Africa that is based on inclusive growth and sustainable development" (AU, 2015a). The priority areas include striving for, "inclusive economic growth that reduces inequality and ensures sustainable agriculture, food self-sufficiency and nutrition security for all" (AU, 2015a).

Based on the realization of the positive contribution that agriculture has on the economic transformation on the Africa continent, African Union (AU) leaders in the AU's Second Ordinary Assembly held in July of 2003 in Maputo, Mozambique endorsed the Comprehensive Africa Agriculture Development Programme (CAADP) (NEPAD, 2003). As part of the New Partnership for Africa Development (NEPAD), CAADP was endorsed as Africa's policy framework for agriculture and agriculture-led development meant to create ambitious institutional and policy transformation in the agriculture sector (NEPAD, 2003). CAADP's aim is to eliminate hunger and reduce poverty through agriculture. CAADP provides an overarching policy framework for attaining food security, nutrition and sustainable development through agriculture-led investment at a national and regional level within Africa (UN, 2015). CAADP has been particularly successful in raising the profile of agriculture and reclaiming African ownership and leadership of the strategic agenda in the agricultural sector through national investment planning (Badiane, Benin, & Makombe, 2016). CAADP initiated a transition to evidence-based planning and implementation and thereby increased the technical credibility of the agenda itself at the global level and national agricultural strategies and programs at country level (Badiane, Odjo, & Ulimwengu, 2011).

The African Union Commission (AUC) and the NEPAD Planning and Coordinating Agency (NPCA) developed the CAADP Implementation Strategy and Roadmap, Program of Work, Results Framework, and refined second generation national agriculture and food security investment plans (NAIPs) to make sure that the commitments set in CAADP framework for agricultural sector transformation are implementable (Badiane et al., 2016). Post-Malabo, the Implementation Strategy and Roadmap recognises that agriculture-based activities have the potential to achieving nutrition targets, particularly through stabilization of food availability and prices and diversification of available nutritious foods for local consumption for improving the diversity of diets (Lokosang et al. 2016). CAADP has demonstrated that Africa has well-crafted, home-grown framework guiding policies, strategies and actions for agricultural development and transformation suitable for its people.

As the flagship programme of the AU for agriculture and food security under the Maputo Declaration on agriculture and food security in Africa, CAADP called for the allocation of at least 10% of public expenditure to the agricultural sector and a 6% agricultural growth rate at the national level to reach the MDG targets (NEPAD, 2003). Ten years later, in June 2014 in Malabo, Equatorial Guinea the AU adopted the Malabo Declaration on Accelerated Agricultural Growth and Transformation was endorsed (AU, 2018). The Malabo Declaration acknowledged the progress as defined in the National and Regional Agricultural and Food Security Investment Plans developed through the CAADP process and they recommitted to the principles and values set. The Malabo commitments take on board the developments around nutrition that occurred in the global development agenda, especially the Rome Declaration on Nutrition (2014) and the World Health Assembly targets for nutrition (Fig. 10.2) (2011).

The Malabo Declaration sets the Africa 2025 Vision for agriculture which is implemented within the framework of CAADP as a vehicle to implement and achieve the First Ten Year Implementation Plan of Africa's Agenda 2063 (AU, 2014). The Malabo commitments highlight the importance of nutrition in Africa's economic and development agenda as put in AU's Agenda 2063 (AU, 2015a). The seven Malabo Commitments translated into seven (7) thematic areas of performance which are: (i) re-committing to the principles and values of the CAADP process; (ii) enhancing investment finance in agriculture; (iii) ending hunger in Africa by 2025; (iv) reducing poverty by half, by 2025, through inclusive agricultural growth and transformation; (v) boosting intra-African trade in agricultural commodities and services; (vi) enhancing resilience of livelihoods and production systems to climate variability and other related risks; and (vii) strengthening mutual accountability to

Declaration on Nutrition Security through Inclusive Economic Growth and Sustainable Development in Africa

1. Ending hunger by 2025 through strengthening development policies
2. Ending child hunger and bringing down stunting to 10 percent and underweight to five percent by 2025, including:
    a. Focusing on the first 1000 days of a child's life
    b. Prioritizing this goal in national development plans and strategies
    c. Establishing long-term targets that give all children an equal chance for success
3. Continuing the dialogue and strengthening advocacy in support of improved nutrition

Declaration on Ending Preventable Child and Maternal Deaths in Africa

1. Ending preventable child and maternal deaths by 2035 in line with the Post 2015 Sustainable Development Framework
2. Developing and implementing country-led roadmaps to accelerate ending preventable deaths among children and mothers

Declaration on Accelerated Agricultural Growth and Transformation for Shared Prosperity and Improved Livelihoods

1. Ending hunger by 2025
2. Improving nutritional status and eliminating child undernourishment by bringing down stunting to 10 percent and underweight to 5 percent by 2025

Fig. 10.1 The Malabo declaration commitments to nutrition (AU, 2014)

actions and results. The three Malabo Declarations nutrition commitments are presented in Fig. 10.1 (AU, 2014).

Most countries have internalised or domesticated the CAADP/Malabo policies, institutions, targets and principles. However, more work still needs to be done to fully domesticate the Malabo Declaration into their national policy and programme frameworks (AU, 2018). Table 10.1 sets out the progress made by Member States in implementing the Malabo declaration's seven thematic. The Table shows that only 20 countries are on-track for achieving the commitments by 2025; with Rwanda having the highest score in terms of progress on agricultural transformation in Africa (AU, 2018).

Twenty-six countries have increased the yields of key national food commodities (AU, 2018). Countries that are on-track are expected to increase Agricultural Research Spending to at least 1% of the Agricultural GDP by 2025. These countries are: Botswana (2.7%), Burundi (2.7%), Ghana (11.9%), Kenya (2.5%), Mauritius (3.0%), Mozambique (2.9%), Namibia (3.2%), Seychelles (6.3%), and South Africa (1.6%). Twenty-five countries have achieved a 6% increase in agricultural GDP in 2016.

Only nine countries are on track for bringing down undernourishment to 5% or less, by the year 2025 (AU, 2018). These countries are Egypt, Ghana, Lesotho, Mali, Mauritania, Morocco, Niger, Senegal and Togo. Egypt (4.5%), Ghana (5%), Mali (5%), Mauritania (3.9%), Morocco (0.1%), and Niger (1.1%) have the lowest prevalence in undernourishment (≤5%).

10.1.2.2 Africa Regional Nutrition Strategy (ARNS)

CAADP has been instrumental in bringing about increased food production on the continent.

Table 10.1 Country progress in implementing the Malabo Declaration on agriculture transformation in Africa (AU, 2018)

Country	Re-committing to CAADP process	Enhancing investment finance in agriculture	Ending hunger by 2025	Halving poverty through agriculture by 2025	Boosting intra-african trade in agriculture commodities	Enhancing resilience to climate variability	Mutual accountability for actions and results
Algeria	[grey]	[grey]	[grey]	[grey]	[grey]	[grey]	[grey]
Angola	[green]	[red]	[red]	[red]	[red]	[red]	[red]
Benin	[green]	[red]	[red]	[red]	[green]	[red]	[green]
Botswana	[green]	[red]	[red]	[green]	[green]	[red]	[green]
Burkina Faso	[green]	[red]	[red]	[green]	[green]	[red]	[green]
Burundi	[green]	[red]	[red]	[green]	[green]	[green]	[green]
Cameroon	[green]	[red]	[red]	[green]	[red]	[red]	[red]
Cape Verde	[green]	[red]	[red]	[green]	[green]	[green]	[green]
Central African Republic	[red]	[red]	[red]	[green]	[red]	[red]	[red]
Chad	[green]	[red]	[red]	[red]	[green]	[red]	[red]
Comoros	[grey]	[grey]	[grey]	[grey]	[grey]	[grey]	[grey]
Congo (Republic of the)	[green]	[red]	[red]	[red]	[green]	[red]	[red]
Cote d'Ivoire	[green]	[red]	[red]	[red]	[red]	[red]	[green]
Democratic Republic of the Congo	[green]	[red]	[red]	[red]	[red]	[red]	[red]
Djibouti	[green]	[red]	[red]	[green]	[green]	[red]	[green]
Egypt	[red]	[green]	[red]	[green]	[green]	[red]	[red]
Equatorial Guinea	[green]	[red]	[red]	[red]	[green]	[green]	[red]
Eritrea	[grey]	[grey]	[grey]	[grey]	[grey]	[grey]	[grey]
Ethiopia	[green]	[red]	[red]	[green]	[green]	[red]	[green]
Gabon	[green]	[red]	[red]	[green]	[red]	[red]	[red]
Gambia	[green]	[red]	[red]	[green]	[green]	[red]	[green]
Ghana	[green]	[red]	[red]	[green]	[green]	[red]	[green]
Guinea	[green]	[red]	[red]	[red]	[green]	[red]	[green]
Guinea-Bissau	[grey]	[grey]	[grey]	[grey]	[grey]	[grey]	[grey]

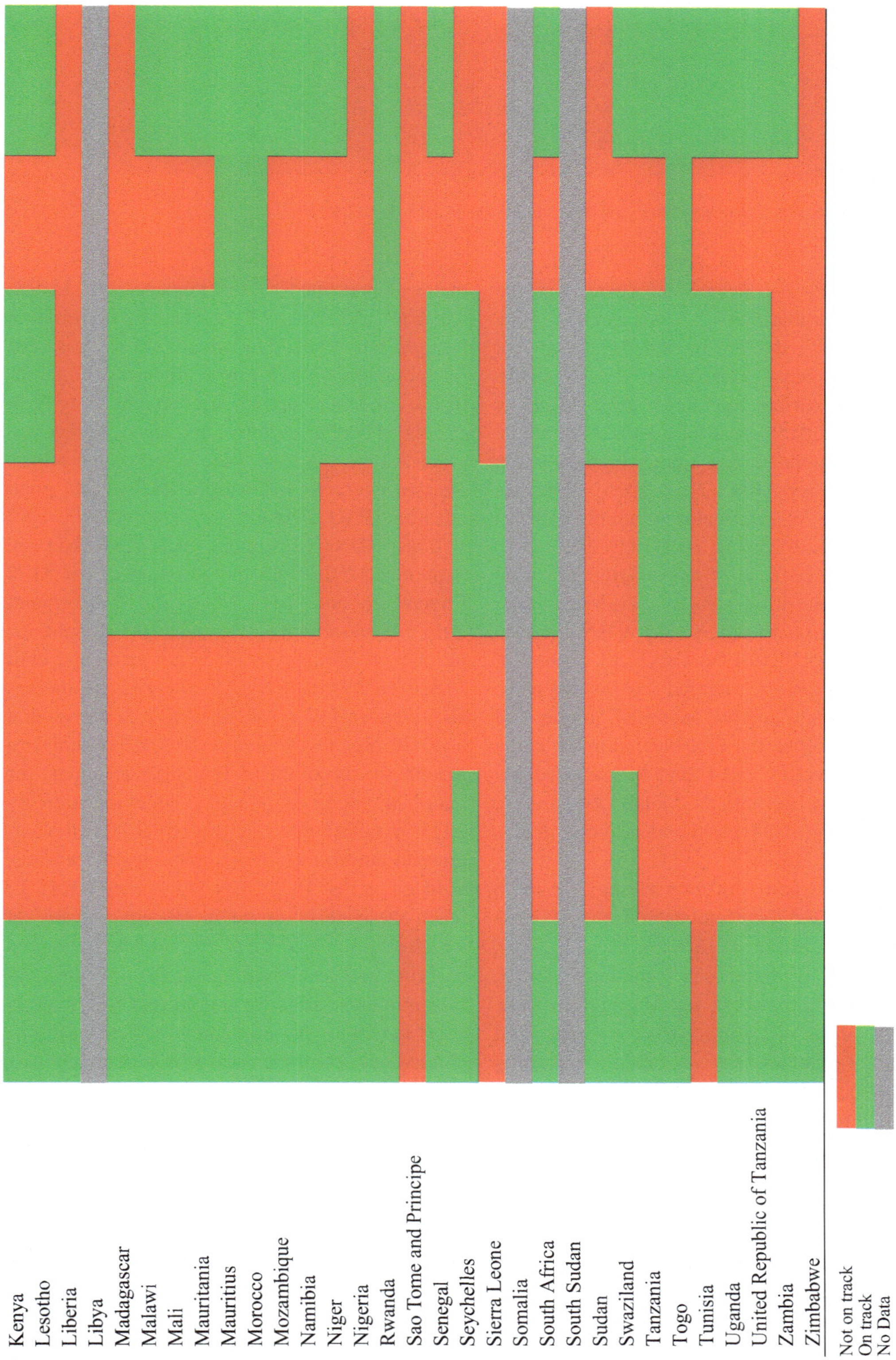
Kenya
Lesotho
Liberia
Libya
Madagascar
Malawi
Mali
Mauritania
Mauritius
Morocco
Mozambique
Namibia
Niger
Nigeria
Rwanda
Sao Tome and Principe
Senegal
Seychelles
Sierra Leone
Somalia
South Africa
South Sudan
Sudan
Swaziland
Tanzania
Togo
Tunisia
Uganda
United Republic of Tanzania
Zambia
Zimbabwe
Not on track
On track
No Data

1. Achieve a 40% reduction in the number of children under-5 who are stunted
2. Achieve a 50% reduction of anaemia in women of reproductive age
3. Achieve a 30% reduction in low birth weight
4. Ensure that there is no increase in childhood overweight
5. Increase the rate of exclusive breastfeeding in the first 6 months up to at least 50%
6. Reduce and maintain childhood wasting to less than 5%

Fig. 10.2 The World Health Assembly global nutrition targets 2025 (WHO, 2014)

However, it is also widely accepted that the increased food production has not resulted in the same levels of reduction in under-nutrition that would be expected (Lokosang et al., 2016). Therefore, the African Regional Nutrition Strategy (ARNS) (AU, 2015b), was formulated to reinforce the nutrition policies and frameworks targeting nutrition. The six ARNS 2015–2025 targets are aligned to the World Health Assembly (WHA) nutrition targets 2025 (Fig. 10.2) (AU, 2015b).

The ARNS 2016–2025 has concrete nutrition specific and nutrition sensitive evidence-based interventions to help achieve the WHA nutrition targets 2025 (AU, 2014). These are consistent with the globally agreed Comprehensive Implementation Plan for Maternal, Infant and Young Child Nutrition that was adopted at the 2012 WHA (WHO, 2014) and by the 23rd AU ordinary session through the Malabo Declaration on ending preventable child and maternal deaths in Africa (AU, 2014).

The ARNS spells out four strategic areas to guide the AU and the Member States in the governance of nutrition (Lokosang et al. 2016). These include: (i) definition of standards, norms, policies, and frameworks for AU member state adoption and ratification, (ii) convening and facilitation of consensus on matters regarding nutrition security in Africa, (iii) nutrition security policy and program advocacy and (iv) promotion and establishment of decision-making architecture for the implementation of the strategy (Lokosang et al. 2016)

10.1.2.3 The Scaling Up Nutrition (SUN) Movement

The Scaling Up Nutrition (SUN) Movement is an intergovernmental formation initiated in 2008 to address the recent gap in the nutrition situation that was presented by the January 2008 Lancet series (World Bank, 2011). The new information brought much needed evidence showing a need for more action to eliminate all forms of malnutrition and its largely irreversible long-term effects on health, cognitive and physical development. All these actions were based on the principle that everyone has a right to food and good nutrition (FAO, 2016).

The SUN Movement was launched in September 2010 with the adoption of the SUN Framework and Road Map (SUN Movement, 2011). It was endorsed by over 100 global entities which brought together governments, civil society, the United Nations, donors, businesses and scientists (World Bank, 2011). Countries that had indicated their intention to scale up nutrition agreed to reach the WHA global targets for maternal, infant, and young child nutrition by 2025, in addition to relevant targets for preventing and controlling non-communicable diseases as listed on Fig. 10.2 (SUN Movement, 2014). To reach these goals, strategic objectives were set which are (Table 10.2): (i) expand and sustain an enabling political environment (ii) prioritise and institutionalise effective actions that contribute to good nutrition (iii) implement effective actions aligned with common results (iv) effectively use, and significantly increase, financial resources for nutrition (SUN, Undated).

To realise the SUN Movement's strategic objectives, in-country capabilities are encouraged aligning the Movement's vision with national nutrition priorities. The roadmap therefore builds on what already exists in the countries and it encourages stakeholders to 'learn by doing' (SUN, Undated). The SUN Movement is founded on the principle of country ownership and continuous improvement towards implementation

Table 10.2 Progress in prioritising and institutionalising effective actions that contribute to good nutrition (SUN Movement, 2017)

Effective actions that have been prioritised and institutionalised that contribute to good nutrition	Countries that have taken action	Actions taken
1. Expand and sustain an enabling political environment	Somalia, Côte d'Ivoire, Senegal, Malawi	Development of advocacy and communication strategies
		Integrate nutrition into sector-specific plans (in agriculture, gender equality and climate change) to alignment with the SDGs
	Benin, Burkina Faso, Côte d'Ivoire, Madagascar, Niger and Tanzania	Auditing their coordinating structures to identify capacity strengths and gaps of individuals, and of the overall structure
	Madagascar, Guinea, Chad, Burkina Faso and Cameroon, Côte d'Ivoire, Niger and	Forming new networks with Academia, the media, champions, parliamentarians in their multi-stakeholder platform (MSP)
	Benin, Burundi, Chad, Côte d'Ivoire, Mali, Malawi and Madagascar	Decentralising MSP's to high-burden areas at national, district and community levels
2. Prioritise and institutionalise effective actions that contribute to good nutrition	Niger, Zimbabwe, Central African Republic, Côte d'Ivoire, Democratic Republic of the Congo, Ethiopia, Guinea, Kenya, Madagascar, Malawi, Mali, Senegal, Togo and Tanzania	Constitutions explicitly implicitly putting the right to adequate food
	Burkina Faso, Cameroon, Kenya, Sierra Leone, Somalia	Putting in place regulations on the marketing of breastmilk substitutes
	Burkina Faso,	
	Cameroon, Central African Republic, Chad, Comoros, Congo, Gabon, Madagascar, Mauritania and Togo	Provide for up to 10 days' paternity leave
	Kenya	Providing for 14 days' paid leave for fathers
	Senegal and Zambia	To bring parliamentarians together to make nutrition priority
3. Implement effective actions aligned with common results	Madagascar	Finalising its third multi-sectoral plan for the Common Results Frameworks (CRF)
	Burkina Faso, Cambodia, Chad and Tanzania	Developing and assessing their CRFs
	Mali, Congo, and Senegal	Involved members of parliament in the process of strategy and action plan development
	Democratic Republic of the Congo	In-country capacity used to organise and implement priority actions at local and national levels
4. Effectively use, and significantly increase, financial resources for nutrition	Chad, Comoros, Ghana, Liberia, Madagascar, Democratic Republic of the Congo, Guinea-Bissau, Lesotho, and Zambia	Increases in spending on nutrition-specific programmes
	Sudan, Ethiopia	Actively investigating shortfalls in the capital needed to fund nutrition

and ensuring that malnutrition in all its forms comes to an end leaving no one behind (SUN Movement, 2017).

SUN Movement countries are making progress in ensuring that actions contributing to good nutrition are prioritised and institutionalised effectively. Table 10.2 gives an overview of progress that has been made by some of the countries taking specific actions to prioritise and institutionalise actions that contribute to good nutrition

(SUN Movement, 2017). To date 59 countries are Scaling Up Nutrition, 40 of them from African (SUN Movement, 2017). Thirteen SUN "Early Risers" from Africa have been eager to do more to scale up nutrition with governments active involvement in scaling up nutrition (WHO, 2011).

There is strong evidence that countries that have been part of the SUN Movement for longer have been able to establish evidence-based nutrition policies and legislation that support lasting human impact (SUN Movement, 2017). Progress toward achieving the strategic objectives has been shown by countries that joined between 2010 and 2013 which include Congo, Kenya, Lesotho, Madagascar, Malawi, Somalia, South Sudan, Togo, Uganda, United Republic of Tanzania, Zambia and Zimbabwe (Table 10.3). Notably, Uganda's progress in bringing people into a shared space for action (objective 1) reached a 100% in 2017. Uganda is one of the first countries to align its national and subnational development plans and budget with the SDGs with multi-stakeholder participation (United Nations Development Group, 2016).

SUN Movement countries are working hard at making sure that multi-stakeholder platforms (MSP), involving more sectors and stakeholders are formalized to work together with high level government officials for maximum impact (SUN Movement, 2017). Countries that are working on formalizing MSP's include Congo, where the MSP is hosted by the Committee for the Fight against Malnutrition and Guinea-Bissau where they are hosted by the Presidential Commission for the Reduction of Chronic Malnutrition (Table 10.3). Other countries include Namibia which has developed the Ministry of Poverty Eradication and Social Welfare. Benin, Burundi and Madagascar have brought in new sectors such as the water and sanitation sector, the Ministry of Decentralisation, and ministries of environment, finance and social protection (SUN Movement, 2017).

Countries that have formed networks with non-governmental stakeholders in the MSP include Madagascar including academia and the media, Chad is using the media and champions and Côte d'Ivoire, Niger and Cameroon networking with the media (Table 10.2) (SUN Movement, 2017). Benin, Burundi, Chad, Côte d'Ivoire, Mali, Malawi and Madagascar have decentralised their MSP to high-burden areas at national, district and community levels and are taking matters further to do organisational, or institutional, audits to help identify capacity strengths and gaps of individuals, and of the overall structure (SUN Movement, 2017).

10.1.3 Agricultural Progress in Africa

It is estimated that 70% of the African population depends on agriculture for food, income and employment (World Economic Forum, 2016). Even though the percentage of the population dependant on agriculture in Africa is said to have dropped, by 2012, the proportion of agricultural population in the total population in Central, Eastern, North, Southern and Western Africa was approximately 55%, 70%, 28%, 50%, 45% and 30% respectively (FAO, 2014). Agriculture is said to contribute between 4% and 27% of Gross Domestic Product (GDP) in many countries in the region (SADC, 2011a, 2011b).

African governments have made progress towards achieving the CAADP goals since 2010. Since 2003, many African countries have increased the volume of public agriculture expenditure from an average of $128.55 million in 1995–2003 to $219.62 million in 2008–2014 (Badiane et al., 2016). Even though they could not make the CAADP target of 10%, low-income countries were reported to be allocating the highest share of 5.1–7.5% of public expenditures to the agricultural sector in 2008–2014. In 1999–2003, the agriculture expenditure as a share of total expenditure (%) in only five countries managed to meet or exceed the 10% target (Badiane et al., 2016). These are Burkina Faso, Ethiopia, Madagascar, Malawi and Zimbabwe (Fig. 10.3).

The share of agriculture expenditure in total expenditure increased by 1.8% on average per year for the countries that signed CAADP compact in 2007–2009. These countries include Benin, Burundi, Cape Verde, Ethiopia, Gambia, Ghana, Liberia, Mali, Niger, Nigeria, Rwanda, Sierra Leone and Togo (Badiane et al., 2016).

Table 10.3 Country progress towards the SUN movement strategic objectives (SUN Movement, 2017)

Country	Year of joining SUN Movement	Objective 1 Bringing people into a shared space for action (% change between 2014 and 2017)	Objective 2 Ensuring a coherent policy and legal framework (% change between 2014 and 2017)	Objective 3 Aligning actions around a common results framework (% change between 2014 and 2017)	Objective 4 Financial tracking and resource mobilization (% change between 2014 and 2017)
Benin	2011	54–64 (10)	46–75 (29)	73–63 (−10)	50–30 (−20)
Botswana	2015				
Burkina Faso	2011	59–69 (−10)	56–63 (7)	30–58 (28)	52–54 (2)
Burundi	2013	35–69 (34)	28–58 (30)	52–54 (2)	5–38 (33)
Cameroon	2013	23–33 (10)	36–40 (4)	0–39 (39)	4–26 (22)
Central African Republic	2017				
Chad	2013	85–82 (−3)	72–69 (−3)	42–52 (10)	39–23 (−16)
Comoros	2013	0–21 (21)	0–22 (22)	0–3 (3)	0–2 (2)
Congo (Republic of the)	2013	46–81 (35)	42–75 (33)	8–78 (70)	0–54 (54)
Cote d'Ivoire	2013	70–97 (27)	62–79 (17)	43–88 (45)	51–84 (33)
Democratic Republic of the Congo	2013	47–42 (−5)	46–42 (−4)	37–38 (1)	25–29 (4)
Ethiopia	2010				
Gabon	2016				
Gambia	2011	80–79 (−1)	54–96 (42)	29–40 (11)	40–54 (14)
Ghana	2011	63–69 (6)	38–63 (25)	20–65 (45)	0–51 (51)
Guinea	2013	38–63 (25)	32–75 (43)	29–74 (45)	29–50 (21)
Guinea-Bissau	2014	34–57 (23)	48–22 (−26)	29–4 (-25)	0–38 (38)
Kenya	2012	35–58 (23)	44–69 (25)	39–54 (15)	44–56 (12)
Lesotho	2014	4–28 (24)	8–34 (26)	8–26 (18)	0–4 (4)
Liberia	2014	0–8 (8)	0–4 (8)	0–4 (4)	0
Madagascar	2012	62–76 (14)	56–73 (17)	54–75 (21)	54–63 (9)
Malawi	2011	75–85 (10)	74–79 (5)	61–75 (14)	69–69 (0)
Mali	2011	59–12 (−47)	46–9 (37)	50–38 (12)	40–12 (28)
Mauritania	2011	44–69 (25)	42–54 (12)	34–50 (16)	40–37 (−3)
Mozambique	2011	43–78 (35)	34–69 (35)	43–57 (14)	39–39 (0)
Namibia	2011	54–79 (25)	34–71 (37)	43–76 (33)	41–76 (35)
Niger	2011	51–54 (3)	46–52 (6)	21–35 (14)	37–44 (7)
Nigeria	2011	50–69 (19)	46–90 (44)	29–39 (10)	25–46 (21)
Rwanda	2011				
Senegal	2011	64–68 (4)	62–75 (13)	55–71 (16)	62–61 (−1)
Sierra Leone	2012	75–64 (−11)	58–65 (7)	53–58 (5)	44–48 (4)
Somalia	2014	29–48 (19)	12–8 (−4)	21–0 (−21)	22–0 (−22)
South Sudan	2013	11–30 (19)	0–16 (16)	0–36 (36)	0–4 (4)
Sudan	2015				
Swaziland	2013				
Togo	2014	8–15 (7)	26–36 (10)	23–0 (−23)	19–9 (−10)
Uganda	2011	37–100 (63)	34–88 (54)	41–84 (43)	43–75 (32)
United Republic of Tanzania	2011	52–74 (22)	54–79 (25)	42–47 (5)	40–69 (29)
Zambia	2010	53–83 (30)	66–44 (22)	63–81 (18)	44–62 (18)
Zimbabwe	2011	33–86 (53)	58–66 (8)	21–75 (54)	40–52 (12)

Negative progress	
Positive progress	
No Data	

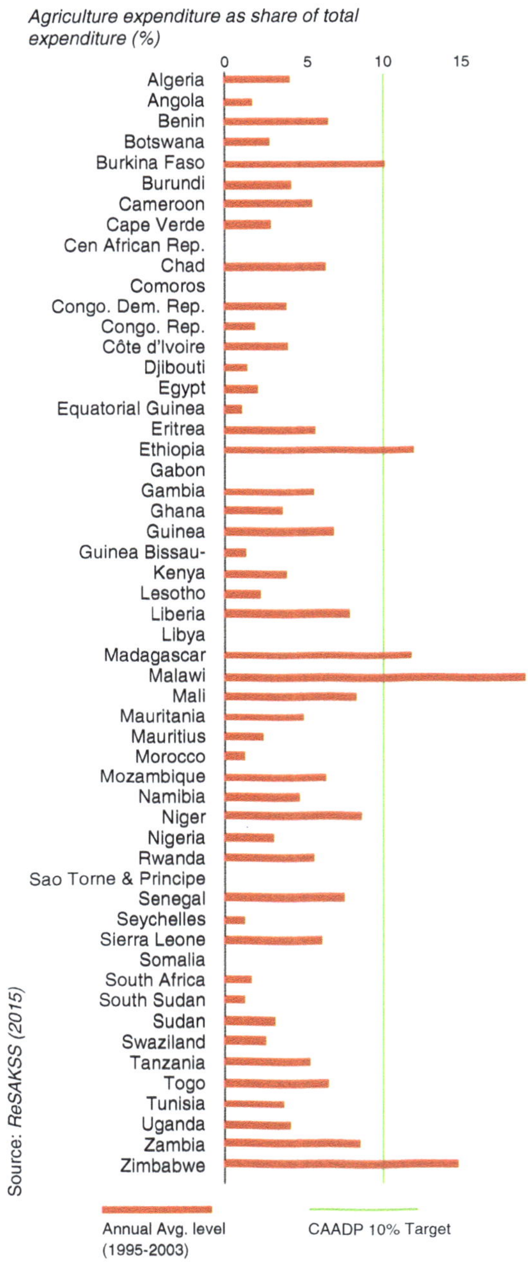

Fig. 10.3 Progress in meeting CAADP 10% target (Badiane et al., 2016)

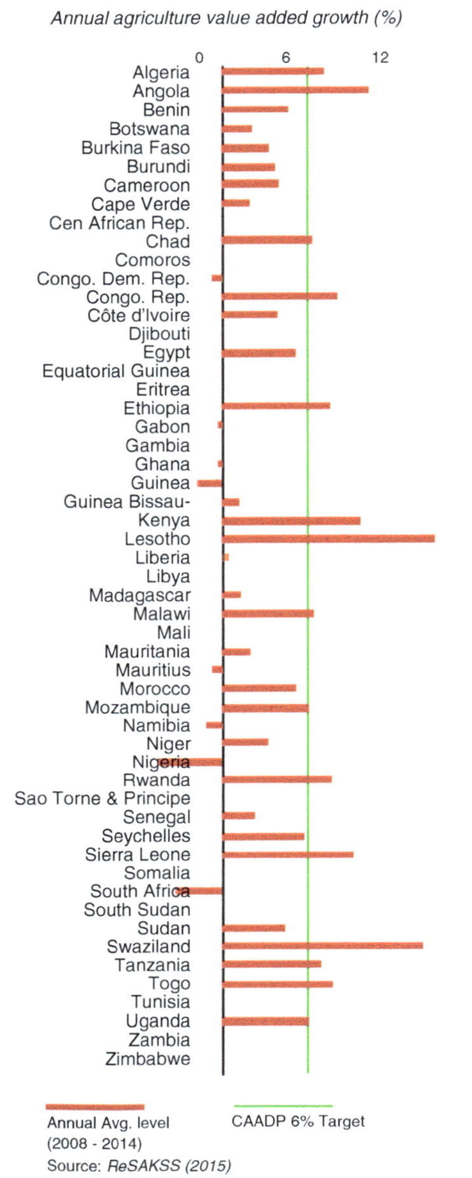

Fig. 10.4 Progress in meeting CAADP 6% target (Badiane et al., 2016)

Countries that signed in the period 2010–2012 (Burkina Faso, Central African Republic, Congo, Côte d'Ivoire, Djibouti, Guinea, Guinea Bissau, Kenya, Malawi, Mauritania, Mozambique, Senegal, Swaziland, Tanzania, Uganda and Zambia) had an increase of 2.4% while the countries that signed last (2013–2014) had a negative increase −2.6%. These are Angola, Cameroon, Chad, Congo, Lesotho, Madagascar, Sudan and Zimbabwe (Badiane et al., 2016).

In as far as meeting the 6% agricultural growth rate target of CAADP, 15 countries met or surpassed the 6% target during the periods 2008–2014 (Fig. 10.4) (Badiane et al., 2016). As a whole, the income (GDP per capita), increased

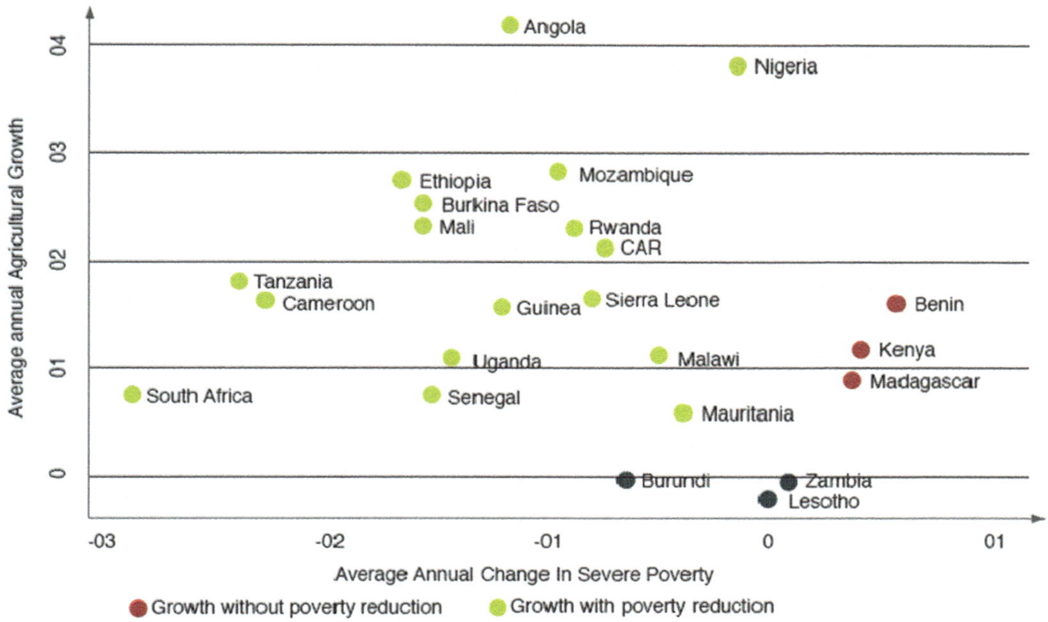

Fig. 10.5 Changes in annual agricultural productivity per agricultural person and annual changes in poverty rates, 2000–2013, in 23 African countries (Badiane et al., 2016)

from an annual average of US$987 in 1995–2003 to $1289 in 2008–2014. However, during 2008–2016, GDP growth slowed to less than 1% per year notably due to the impact of the fuel and financial crisis of 2007 and 2008. During the 2008–2016 period, consistent with GDP growth, household consumption expenditure also increased substantially from an average of US$1014 in 1995–2003 to US$1296 in 2008–2016, being at the highest during the 2003–2008 period (Makombe, Tefera, Matchaya, & Benin, 2016).

Agriculture production has had a positive impact on reducing poverty which declined from 25.0% in 1995–2003 to 17.1% in 2008–2016 (Makombe et al., 2016). The incidence of poverty was lowest in the middle-income group at 29.8% and highest in the mineral-rich group at 55.9% in the period 2008–2014 (Badiane et al., 2016). Growth in agricultural productivity over the 2000–2012 period helped to reduce poverty in countries where the workforce is still engaged in agriculture (Fig. 10.5).

10.1.4 Progress on Nutrition and Health Outcomes

Malnutrition is manifested through, among other indicators, child stunting, wasting, vitamin A deficiency, iodine nutrition and anaemia. Stunting (being short for height) and wasting (being underweight for age) are used as indicators of growth faltering and deprivation (WHO, 2010). These measures are used to determine children's development potential and are indicators of the quality of life.

Stunting arises because of prolonged periods of nutritional deprivation from a poor diets or recurrent infections and illness (WHO, 2010). Stunting is defined as shortness for age. Wasting on the other hand comes as a result of having insufficient food intake or a high incidence of infectious diseases. It is defined as low weight for height (WHO, 2010).

Anaemia, vitamin A deficiency and iodine deficiency are micronutrient deficiencies often resulting from insufficient intake. Micronutrient deficiencies affect many physiological and psychological functions. Even though anaemia can come about as a result of a wide variety of causes, the most common and most concerning is iron deficiency anaemia (WHO, 2008). Iron deficiency affects cognitive and physical development in children and work productivity in adults. Vitamin A deficiency can lead to high rates of infection diarrhoea and measles in young children and women of reproductive age (WHO, 2009). This deficiency is of major concern because it can lead to night blindness, poor outcomes of pregnancy, slow growth and maternal mortality. Iodine-deficiency on the other hand can cause stillbirth, spontaneous abortion and congenital abnormalities and serious mental damage in children (WHO, 2004).

10.1.4.1 Reducing Malnutrition

The Hunger and Nutrition Commitment Index (HANCI) Africa revealed how countries had varying levels of commitment in their efforts to tackle hunger and undernutrition. South Africa was ranked 4th, making it the leading African country committed to end hunger and malnutrition and Malawi is the second highest African country ranking 7th (HANCI, 2018). Both countries constitutions have shown commitments to protect the right to food and provide good social safety nets (IDS & NEPAD, 2017). They have also made significant investments towards improving availability and access to health services. Other countries that have done well include Tanzania and Sudan whose governments have made good efforts to address hunger which has improved their standing on the HANCI ranking to 10th and 36th place respectively (HANCI, 2018).

A review of the most recent Demographic and Health Surveys (2006–2016) of 32 countries in sub-Saharan Africa grouped by sub-region revealed that the prevalence of malnutrition was highest within countries in East Africa and West Africa compared to the WHO Millennium development goals target for 2015 (Akombi, Agho, Merom, Renzaho, & Hall, 2017). By the end of the Millennium Development Goals (MDGs) era in 2015, Africa had made good to fair progress to meet the target of reducing extreme poverty and hunger by half (UN, 2015). Even though there are fears that the world might not meet the global nutrition targets adopted by the World Health Assembly, some African countries have made significant progress towards meeting the 40% reduction in the number of children younger than five who are stunted (WHO, 2016).

Measures of hunger and food and nutrition security (undernourishment, underweight, stunting, and wasting) have generally improved across Africa (Badiane et al., 2016). The latest data from the Global Nutrition Report (Development Initiatives, 2017) lists and ranks countries according and the nutrition indicators (Table 10.4). In Table 10.4, the countries are ranked according to whether they are on or off course on the World Health Assembly stunting target. Of the 54 African countries, 48 have sufficient data with nine on course to meet the target and 34 off course with some progress and only 6 making no progress.

Wasting affects an estimated 52 million children under the age of 5 years globally while an estimated 17 million is reported to be severely wasted (UNICEF, WHO, World Bank Group, 2017). However, despite these statistics that reflect what is going on the region, individual country commitments to reducing the prevalence in their nations have been impressive. The data shows that 18 countries are on course while 22 countries are making good progress (Table 10.4).

Between 1993 and 2005 anaemia was reported to have affected an estimated 24.8% of the world's population, a majority of which were women and children (WHO, 2008). Anaemia affects an estimated 47.4% of the world's child under 5 year's population which is almost half of the children globally. In 2011, the prevalence went down to 42.6%, but was still very high in children under 5 years (WHO, 2015). The data shows that most countries (24) are making slow progress in reducing the prevalence of anaemia in women of reproductive age (15–49 years old) (Development Initiatives, 2017). Despite the overall slow progress, supplementation and fortification programs are being successfully implemented. On average, countries managed to reach

Table 10.4 Country progress to reach the World Health Assembly global nutrition targets 2025 (Development Initiatives, 2017)

Country	Stunting (%)	Progress	Wasting (%)	Progress	Anaemia prevalence in women of reproductive age (%)	Progress	Vitamin A prevalence (%)	Iodine nutrition	HANCI (%)
Algeria	11.7		4		36		11		
Angola	29.2		5		48		45		38
Benin	34		5		47		53		30
Botswana	31.4		7		30		36		
Burkina Faso	32.9		8		50		52		14
Burundi	57.5		6		27		46		29
Cameroon	32.6		5		41		45		30
Cape Verde	No data		No data		33		42		
Central African Republic	40.7		7		46		60		
Chad	38.7		13		48		47		
Comoros	32.1		11		29		46		
Congo (Republic of the)	32.1		8		52		49		33
Cote d'Ivoire	29.6		No data		53		52		24
Democratic Republic of the Congo	42.6		8		41		64		
Djibouti	33.5		22		33		58		
Egypt	22.3		10		29		8		
Equatorial Guinea	26.2		3		44		24		
Eritrea	50.3		15		38		56		
Ethiopia	40.4		10		23		50		32
Gabon	17.5		3		59		40		
Gambia	24.5		11		58		54		19
Ghana	18.8		5		46		50		22
Guinea	31.3		10		51		51		
Guinea-Bissau	27.6		6		44		No data		44

Table 10.4 (continued)

Kenya	26	4	27	49	12
Lesotho	33.2	3	27	44	41
Liberia	32.1	6	35	60	45
Libya	21	7	33	8	
Madagascar	49.2	15	37	52	8
Malawi	42.4	4	34	47	7
Mali	38.5	15	51	66	15
Mauritania	22	15	37	56	27
Mauritius	13.6	No data	25	29	
Morocco	14.9	2	37	15	
Mozambique	43.1	6	51	55	34
Namibia	23.1	7	23	39	
Niger	43	19	49	56	19
Nigeria	32.9	7	50	42	38
Rwanda	37.9	2	22	39	12
Sao Tome and Principe	31.6	4	46	48	
Senegal	19.4	8	50	40	17
Seychelles	7.9	4	22	25	
Sierra Leone	37.9	9	48	53	34
Somalia	25.9	15	44	60	
South Africa	23.9	5	26	45	4
South Sudan	31.1	22	34	No data	
Sudan	38.2	16	31	44	36
Swaziland	25.5	2	27	31	
Togo	27.5	7	49	53	40
Tunisia	10.1	3	31	6	
Uganda	34.2	4	29	39	25
United Republic of Tanzania	34.7	5	37	43	9
Zambia	40	6	34	49	27
Zimbabwe	27.6	3	29	57	

Stunting
Insufficient data to make assessment
On course, good progress
Off course, good progress
Off course, no progress
No Data

Wasting
No progress or worsening
On course
Some progress
No Data

Iodine
Optimal iodine nutrition
Mild iodine deficiency
Moderate iodine deficiency
Risk of iodine-induced hyperthyroidism
No Data

a 79% coverage among children aged 6–59 months who received two doses of the vitamin A supplement leading to countries such as Uganda dropping the vitamin A deficiency prevalence to almost 6% (Development Initiatives, 2017).

While the majority of the African countries have done well in addressing iodine deficiencies, nine countries have been reported to show excessive iodine intakes (Development Initiatives, 2017). This a major health risk for a type of autoimmune condition where the thyroid gland produces an excess amount of the thyroid hormone, causing the thyroid to grow producing more thyroid hormone than the body needs (Franco, Amaya-Amaya, & Anaya, 2013). Actions need to be taken by these countries to bring the excess iodine intake levels down to an acceptable level.

10.2 Conclusions

The progress that Africa has seen on food security and nutrition has been as a result of effective implementation and delivery of policies and investment plans aligned with the SDG's, AU Agenda 2063, CAADP-Malabo Declarations, SUN Movement and the ARNS 2015–2025. The policies have contributed significantly to raising agricultural productivity leading to positive impact promoting agriculture growth (through African agricultural transformation), reduce poverty, improve food security, eliminating hunger and reduce poverty in sub-Saharan Africa.

While the direct attribution of these policies and programmes to reducing food insecurity and malnutrition cannot be established, it is clear that African governments have prioritised food security and nutrition over the past decade and a half. The benefits of this are starting to emerge. Food availability, access and nutrition have been improving and the proportion of people experiencing food insecurity and malnutrition has been declining. However, progress is not adequate to achieve the targets set by the international development goals or continental aspirations. So too, the gains are eroded by significant population growth that increased the absolute numbers of people still suffering.

To significantly change the situation, more attention is needed to increasing incomes, reducing inequality and generating inclusive and employment-generating growth. This is necessary to raise incomes, improve purchasing power to improve diets for all people in Africa. Overcoming food insecurity and malnutrition is fundamental to improving the quality of life of the current generation and breaking the intergenerational cycle of deprivation. African governments have shown that change and progress are possible. Scaling up the progress will take continued and sustained commitment and more concerted effort to ensure that economic growth drives positive changes in nutrition.

References

Adesina, A. A. (2016). *Inaugural address of the eighth elected president of the African Development Bank Group on the 1st of September 2015*. Available via DIALOG. https://www.afdb.org/en/news-and-events/inaugural-speech-akinwumi-a-adesina-phd-president-african-development-bank-group-september-1-2015-abidjan-cote-divoire-14629/. Accessed 5 June 2018.

AfDB (African Development Bank). (Forthcoming). *Investing in nutrition: Harnessing 'grey matter infrastructure' to unlock the human and economic potential of Africa, 2017–2021 multisector nutrition action plan for the operations of the African Development Bank*. Abidjan, Côte d'Ivoire: AFDB.

AfDB Food Cuisine. (2017). *The high 5 for transforming Africa*. http://www.afdbfoodcuisine.com/afdbs-high-5s/#1487684277718-5979396f-7ae7. Accessed 8 June 2018.

AU (African Union). (2015a). *Agenda 2063: The Africa we want*. Addis Ababa. http://archive.au.int/assets/images/agenda2063.pdf. Accessed July 10 2016.

AU (African Union). (2015b). *Africa regional nutrition strategy 2015–2025*. Addis Ababa, Ethiopia: AU. http://sa.au.int/en/sites/default/files/Africa%20Regional%20Nutrition%20Strategy%202015-2025%2013.3.2015%20-%20English_0.pdf. Accessed 16 Jan 2017

AU (African Union). (2015c). *Agenda 2063 first ten-year implementation plan 2014–2023*. Agenda_2063_First_Ten_Year_Implementation_Plan_2014_2023_EN.pdf. Accessed 7 June 2018.

Agenda 2063. (Undated). *Progress report of the commission on the Africa 2063 Agenda*. https://au.int/sites/default/files/newsevents/workingdocuments/12582-wd-agenda_2063_e_0.pdf. Accessed 2 June 2018.

Akombi, B. J., Agho, K. E., Merom, D., Renzaho, A. M., & Hall, J. J. (2017). Child malnutrition in sub-Saharan Africa: A meta-analysis of demographic and health surveys (2006–2016). *PLoS One, 12*(5), 1–11. e0177338. https://doi.org/10.1371/journal.pone.0177338

AU (African Union). (2014). *Decisions, declarations and resolution*. Assembly of the African Union, twenty-third ordinary session, June 26–27, 2014, Malabo, Equatorial Guinea. Assembly/AU/ /Dec.517–545(XXIII); Assembly/ AU/ /Decl.1-4(XXIII); Assembly/AU/ /Res.1 (XXIII). http://au.int/en/sites/default/files/decisions/9661-assembly_au_dec_517_-_545_xxiii_e.pdf. Accessed 12 May 2018.

AU (African Union). (2018). *The 2017 progress report to the assembly. Highlights on intra-African trade for agriculture commodities and services: Risks and opportunities*. file:///C:/Users/u25354192/Downloads/2017%20Full%20Report.pdf. Accessed 3 June 2018.

Badiane, O., Benin, S., & Makombe, T. (2016). Chapter 2: Strengthening the continental agricultural agenda and accountability framework – The road from Maputo to Malabo. In *Africa Agriculture status report 2016: Progress towards agriculture transformation in Sub-Saharan Africa* (pp. 24–47). Washington, DC: International Food Policy Research Institute. https://reliefweb.int/sites/reliefweb.int/files/resources/assr.pdf. Accessed 2 June 2018.

Badiane, O., Odjo, S., & Ulimwengu, J. (2011). *Emerging policies and partnerships under CAADP implications for long-term growth, food security, and poverty reduction* (IFPRI Discussion Paper 1145). Washington, DC: International Food Policy Research Institute.

Development Initiatives. (2017). *Global nutrition report 2017: Nourishing the SDGs*. Bristol, UK: Development Initiatives.

FAO. (1996). *World food summit 1996 report of the world food summit*, 13–17 November 1996. Food and Agriculture Organization of the United Nations. www.fao.org/docrep/003/w3548e/w3548e00.htm. Accessed 13 May, 2018.

FAO. (2003). *Trade reform and food security. Conceptualizing the linkages*. ROME: Food and Agriculture Organization of the United Nations.

FAO. (2014). *FAO statistical yearbook 2014 Africa, food and agriculture*. Accra, Ghana: Food and Agriculture Organization of the United Nations Regional Office for Africa.

FAO. (2016). *Compendium of indicators for nutrition-sensitive agriculture*. ROME: Food and Agriculture Organization of the United Nations.

FAO (Food and Agriculture Organization). (2017). *Regional overview of food security and nutrition in Africa 2017*. The food security and nutrition–conflict nexus: Building resilience for food security, nutrition and peace. Accra, Ghana.

Franco, J.S., Amaya-Amaya, J., Anaya, J.M. (2013). Chapter 30: Thyroid disease and autoimmune diseases. J-M. Anaya, Y. Shoenfeld, A. Rojas-Villarraga, R.A. Levy, R. Cervera, . Autoimmunity. From bench to bedside. Bogota, Colombia, El Rosario University Press. https://www.ncbi.nlm.nih.gov/books/NBK459466/. Accessed 7 June 2018

HANCI (Hunger and Nutrition Commitment Index). (2018). *Hunger and nutrition commitment index Africa*. http://www.hancindex.org/countries/angola/#.WxlOpVUzaJA. Accessed 6 June 2018.

Hendriks, S.L. (2018). *Food policy and nutrition economics in the SDG era*. Tomlinson commemorative lecture, 22 February, University of Pretoria. http://www.up.ac.za/media/shared/238/food-policy-and-nutrition-economics-in-the-sdg-era-24-feb-2018-speech-publication-version.edited.zp144306.pdf. Accessed 5 Mar 2018.

Institute of Development Studies & African Union's New Partnership for Africa's Development (IDS & NEPAD). (2017). *South Africa tops new hunger and nutrition commitment index – Africa*. http://www.ids.ac.uk/news/south-africa-tops-new-hunger-and-nutrition-commitment-index-africa?utm_source=feedburner&utm_medium=feed&utm_campaign=Feed%3A+IDS_Newsfeed+%28IDS+News+Feed%29. Accessed 5 June 2018.

Lokosang, L., Osei, O., & Covic, N. (2016). The African Union policy environment toward enabling action for nutrition action in Africa. In N. Covic & S. Hendriks (Eds.),. 2016 *Achieving a nutrition revolution for Africa: The road to healthier diets and optimal nutrition* (ReSAKSS Annual Trends and Outlook Report 2016) (pp. 5–11). Washington, DC: IFPRI.

Makombe, T., Tefera, W., Matchaya, G., Benin, S. (2016). Chapter 11: Tracking CAADP indicators and processes. A. De Pinto, J.M. Ulimwengu. A thriving agricultural sector in a changing climate: Meeting Malabo Declaration goals through climate-smart agriculture. ReSAKSS Annual Trends and Outlook Report 2016. 146–157. International Food Policy Research Institute. Washington, DC. http://www.resakss.org/sites/default/files/Ch11%20ReSAKSS_AW_ATOR_2016_Final.pdf. Accessed 2 June 2018.

NEPAD (New Partnership for Africa's Development). (2003). *Introducing the Comprehensive Africa Agriculture Development Programme (CAADP)*. Johannesburg, South Africa: New Partnership for Africa's Development (NEPAD).

Pinstrup-Andersen, P. (2000). Improving human nutrition through agricultural research: Overview and objectives. *Food and Nutrition Bulletin, 21*(4), 352–355.

Ruel, M. T., Quisumbing, A. R., & Balagamwala, M. (2018). Nutrition-sensitive agriculture: What have we learned so far? *Global Food Security*. First published online on February 1, 2018. https://doi.org/10.1016/j.gfs.2018.01.002. Accessed 2 June 2018.

SADC. (2011a). *Regional agricultural policy (RAP) country summary agricultural policy review reports*. Gaborone: Food, Agriculture and Natural Resources (FANR) Directorate.

SADC. (2011b). *Southern African Development Community Regional Agricultural Policy*. Gaborone: Food, Agriculture and Natural Resources (FANR) Directorate.

Scaling Up Nutrition (SUN). (Undated). *Sun movement: Strategy and roadmap (2016–2020)*. http://sun-csn-assets.s3.amazonaws.com/resources/files/000/000/005/original/SUNRoadmap.pd. Accessed 27 May 2018.

Scaling Up Nutrition (SUN) Movement. (2014). *An introduction to the scaling up nutrition movement*. http://scalingupnutrition.org/wp-content/uploads/2015/06/Orange_Internal_InOutline_ENG_20140415_web.pdf. Accessed 29 May 2018.

Scaling Up Nutrition (SUN) Movement. (2017). *Annual progress report 2017*. Geneva, Switzerland.

UN (United Nations). (2015). *The millennium development goals report*. United Nations Department of Economic and Social Affairs (DESA). http://www.un.org/millenniumgoals/pdf/MDG%20Report%202010%20En%20r15%20-low%20res%2020100615%20-.pdf. Accessed 19 Apr 2018.

UNICEF, WHO, World Bank Group. (2017). *Joint malnutrition estimates. Stunting prevalence 1990–2016*. https://data.unicef.org/topic/nutrition/malnutrition/. Accessed 24 Apr 2018.

United Nations Development Group. (2016). *The sustainable development goals are coming to life: Stories of country implementation and UN support*. New York, NY: United Nations Development Group.

WHO. (2004). *Iodine status worldwide. WHO Global database on iodine deficiency*. Geneva, Switzerland: World Health Organization.

WHO. (2008). *Worldwide prevalence of anaemia 1993–2005 WHO global database on anaemia*. Geneva, Switzerland: World Health Organization.

WHO. (2009). *Global prevalence of vitamin A deficiency in populations at risk 1995–2005. WHO global database on vitamin A deficiency*. Geneva, Switzerland: World Health Organization.

WHO. (2010). *Nutrition landscape information system (NLIS) country profile indicators: Interpretation guide*. Geneva: World Health Organization.

WHO. (2011). *Scaling up nutrition in the African region. A consultation in response to the WHA resolution* (WHA 63.23). http://www.who.int/nutrition/Harare_regionalconsultation_May2011.pdf. Accessed 2 June 2018.

WHO. (2014). *Global nutrition targets 2025: Policy brief series (WHO/NMH/NHD/14.2)*. Geneva, Switzerland: World Health Organization.

WHO. (2015). *National health account tracking, 2015*. http://apps.who.int/nha/database/Country Profile/Index/en. Accessed 2 June 2018.

WHO. (2016). *Global targets 2025: Poster*. www.who.int/nutrition/topics/nutrition_globaltargets2025/en/. Accessed 2 June 2018.

World Bank. (2011). Scaling up nutrition: A framework for action (English). Washington, DC; World Bank. http://documents.worldbank.org/curated/en/920621468326172212/Scaling-up-nutrition-a-framework-for-action. Accessed 29 May 2018.

World Economic Forum. (2016). *70% of Africans make a living through agriculture, and technology could transform their world*. https://www.weforum.org/agenda/2016/05/70-of-africans-make-a-living-through-agriculture-and-technology-could-transform-their-world/. Accessed 11 June 2018.

Changing Trends in the Provision of Psychosocial and Health Resources for Quality Childhood Development in Cameroon

11

Therese Mungah Shalo Tchombe

Abstract

The chapter sets out to examine the changing trends in the provision of psychosocial and health resources for quality childhood development in Cameroon. Providing appropriate psychosocial and health resources is vitally important from birth to 11 years, as childhood ages are filled with developmental mile stones which, if not well managed, would lead to inappropriate developmental trajectories with long term negative effects through youth and adulthood. Despite the progress made under the Millennium Development Goals (MDGs), much work remains to move the new global agenda, the Sustainable Development Goals (SDGs), forward for children. Inequities in opportunities for children, ranging from education to health prevent them from reaching their developmental potential (World Bank. GINI index). (World Bank estimate, 2017). https://data.worldbank.org/indicator/SI.POV.GINI?locations=ZA-MA-TN-DZ-EG-NG-KE-LR-SO). Based on the above literature the main objectives of the chapter was aimed at examining (a) access to Quality and Equity Education (b) acquisition of social and personality skills by children (c) enabling psychosocial environment and (d) access to health. A cross sectional survey research design was employed. The survey method was used to collect descriptive data on parents and children's opinions in four regions of Cameroon out of ten regions. Two Anglophone (North West and South West) and two Francophone (West and Littoral) regions were chosen for the study. Two hundred (200) parents and children were used as participants in the study. On the whole 64.15% indicated that there was improvement in the provision of psychosocial and health resources for children in Cameroon. The implication of these findings is that despite the fact that some progress has been made, Cameroon still falls below excellent standards hence, need for more improvement on the provision of services. The current progress can be leveraged to ensure that even more progress is made in the years to come. Amongst other factors, it was specifically recommended that early childhood is the most effective and cost efficient time to ensure that all children develop their full potential. The returns on investment in early child development are substantial.

11.1 Introduction

Cameroon like the rest of world is dynamic with determination on improving the wellbeing of children during childhood years as they are the

T. M. S. Tchombe (✉)
University of Buea, Buea, Cameroon

I. Eloff (ed.), *Handbook of Quality of Life in African Societies*, International Handbooks of Quality-of-Life, https://doi.org/10.1007/978-3-030-15367-0_11

youths, adults and above all workers and leaders of tomorrow, on whom social and economic growth depend. Providing appropriate support is vitally important as the period from birth to 11 years is pregnated with many developmental mile stones which, if not well managed, would lead to inappropriate developmental trajectories with long term negative effects. Accordingly, the need for changing the trends that affect the well-being of children and the livelihood conditions of the family and society draws from an increasing awareness for the need for a change in the mind-set on the value of enabling an enriched and healthy environment for development. Changing trends in the provision of psychosocial resources is the realisation that these resources play a major role in the development of children during their childhood years. The quality of resources and support provided during these significant years of physical, personality, social and cognitive development are crucial in today's world. Therefore, psychosocial resources are individual differences and social relationships that have beneficial effects on mental and physical health outcomes, as well as playing an important role in the quality development of human beings throughout the lifespan (Taylor & Broffman, 2011). Kern, Friedman, Martin, Reynolds, and Luong (2009), also provide additional examples of psychosocial resources such as self-esteem, close attachments, health, optimism, mastery/perceived control, self-related resources, social support, financial support and other factors that are linked to beneficial mental and physical health outcomes The examples of the resources given above illustrate two groups of resources; psychological and social, which are somewhat inter correlated, but are also sufficiently independent to warrant independent consideration. Psychosocial resources have also been divided between those that are distal and proximal to the self, internal and external, and biological and cultural. Psychosocial resources include only those constructs that are held as resources for a wide range of people who share a set of cultural traditions (Kim, Sherman, & Taylor, 2009).

Social relationships experienced within social support structures, are the best established psychosocial resources for protecting mental and physical health, because these create the basis for psychological balance for individuals. Social support, a major Africentric philosophy is defined as the perception or experience that one is loved and cared for by others, esteemed and valued, and part of a social network of mutual assistance and obligations (Wills, 1984). Early research on social support classified support into several explicit forms. Informational support occurs when one person helps another to understand a stressful event better and determine what resources and coping strategies may be needed to deal with it. Instrumental support involves the provision of tangible assistance, such as financial aid, food, housing, education or transportation. Emotional support involves providing warmth and nurturance to another person, and reassuring that person that he or she is a valuable person for whom others care. This commonly employed taxonomy implies that the benefits of social contact are achieved primarily during or following the enactment of social support. All of these are crucial for the growing child (Kim et al., 2009).

However, many of the benefits of social support accompany the perception that social support is always available if needed. Today in Cameroon, there are many schools and health centers and hospitals found in all of the country's 58 sub-divisions. Families, children and youths have to, however, show interest to access the resources. These resources offer both implicit and explicit support though most often explicit support from others may also undermine self-esteem, through marginalisation and communicating a sense of one being inefficacious (Bolger & Amarel, 2007). Psychosocial resources, therefore, play an important role in the quality development of individuals throughout the entire lifespan. In this light, this review sets out to explore the changing trends in the provision of psychosocial and health resources for quality development of children from birth to 11 years old in Cameroon.

11.1.1 Background

Children are at the centre of the concern for sustainable development. Developmental sciences through the theories inform clearly on the importance of childhood as a whole for the human development. Childhood is a sensitive period for cognitive development (Piaget, Vygotsky), social development (Erikson) personality (Freud) and moral development (Kohlberg). Evidently from literature and theories these are critical years for health and intellectual development (Erikson, 1982; Freud, 1921; Kohlberg, 1984; Piaget, 1962; Vygotsky, 1978). Realisation of these issues necessitates the need for people to change their attitudes towards life. Children more than ever are entitled to a healthy and productive life in harmony with nature. The goals of sustainable development cannot be achieved when there is a high prevalence of debilitating illnesses. Population health cannot be maintained without ecologically sustainable development. Despite undoubted health advances, poor health among children and youth in Cameroon continues to be a constraint on sustainable development efforts (Davis, 2000). In some cases, the process of development itself is creating conditions wherein the health of children suffers as a result of economic, political and social upheaval, environmental degradation, rapid urbanisation and uneven development or increasing inequalities in access to psychosocial resources (Davis, 2000). The World Health Organisation (WHO) according to its 1948 constitution defines health as a state of complete physical, mental and social well-being of an individual and not merely the absence of disease or infirmity (WHO, 2011). Access to education and health are important determinants and indicators of psychosocial development among children as these play an important role in the development of children's self-esteem, cognitive skills and socio-cultural well-being.

The Sustainable Development Goals (SDGs) offer a more holistic vision of child and youth development than in previous agendas. Developmental science has been influential in shaping the SDGs in relation to early childhood development (Britto et al., 2017; Engle et al., 2011; Walker, Chang, Powell, Simonoff, & Grantham-McGregor, 2007) and in highlighting the importance of health and well-being in children and adolescence (World Health Organization, 2014). For example, SDG 4 on learning and education is more comprehensive than the education goal in the Millennium Development Goals (MDGs) (see Table 11.1). It covers "lifelong learning" and thus emphasises the developmental outcome of education, rather than simply access to education itself. It also covers human development from early childhood (Target 4.2) through primary and secondary schooling (Target 4.1), technical and vocational education and university (Target 4.3), and certain other aspects of adolescence and young adulthood, including acquisition of skills and knowledge to promote sustainable development (Target 4.7), and prepa-

Table 11.1 Access to quality and equity in education

Indicator	Sample quotation
Access	*There is some degree of increase in access to education though the country has not achieved 100% access rate. The educational policy in Cameroon ensures the accessibility of all children of school going age. Primary education is free in the public sector and secondary and tertiary education is affordable with a few registration cost. In the private sector, fees are paid but the government subsidizes cost by granting subventions to ensure access to all. There is also the creation of many public schools in all communities. The missionary movements have also done a lot to bring education closer to the people*
Equity	*There have been improvements in terms of inclusion of girls, persons with disabilities and vulnerable people due to renovations in school environments, school curricula, didactic materials and learner centred approaches. These need further improvements. Today there are 68 experimental basic education schools for inclusive education created by government*
Quality	*There is a new shift from content based curriculum to competency based approach which has led to increase in quality. But the educational system still faces problems like large class sizes, diversity, infrastructure, assessment, teacher training etc. in the full realization of competency based approach*

ration of youth for employment and entrepreneurship (Target 4.4).

Mental health is also included explicitly in the SDGs under Goal 3, which includes language on prevention and promotion of mental health and well-being. However, few other specific references to outcomes related to socio-emotional development occur in the SDGs, although understanding of the importance of social and emotional development in learning is growing (Learning Metrics Task Force, 2013), which highlights the recent and rapid acceptance of holistic-development concepts. The SDGs maintain emphasis on the unfinished agenda of the MDGs in poverty reduction, nutrition, health, clean water, and sanitation (SDGs 1, 2, 3, and 6, respectively) exacerbated today by immigration and urbanisation creating overcrowded unhealthy environments. A strong gender-equity lens is added in the call for ending discrimination against girls and an equitable distribution of psychosocial and health resources among children of both sexes (SDG 5). The SDGs also recognize the many influences on children's development that go beyond access to basic services, such as promotion of peace (Goal 16) and the reduction of violence against children and of their trafficking, torture, and exploitation (Goal 16.2). The larger prominence of child and youth development in the SDGs relative to the MDGs acknowledges that without a next generation that achieves its human potential in growth, learning, and development, none of the goals of the ambitious agenda to achieve a sustainable planet will be realized. In addition, children are the most affected by the degree of progress in all areas of the SDGs. The impact of climate change will fall heavily on children and youth (Broome, 2008; Currie & Deschenes, 2016; Sheffield & Landrigan, 2011), affecting both physiological and psychological well-being and threatening to reverse progress made in recent years on mortality and morbidity (Phalkey, Aranda-Jan, Marx, Hofle, & Sauderborn, 2015). Especially dire implications for health and well-being among children in low-resource settings are predicted—for example, among urban children in low- and middle income countries (Bartlett, 2008), migrant and refugee populations, and children residing in all parts of the Global South (Hanna & Oliva, 2016). Developmental sciences thus can figure prominently to help make the voices of these children heard.

Despite the progress made under the MDGs, much work remains to move the global agenda forward for children. Gross inequities in opportunities for children—from lack of access to clean water, lack of literacy materials in homes, recurrent poor health, and pervasive and persistent poverty—prevent them from reaching their developmental potential (Armah-Attoh, Selormey, & Houessou, 2016; World Bank, 2017). Developmental science is needed to promote action in three areas: (1) generating locally and globally relevant information on the nature of human development in diverse contexts, including experimental studies, primary and secondary data analyses, programme evaluations, and longitudinal studies to inform policy development; (2) ensuring reliable measurement and monitoring; and (3) building capacity for SDG- and policy-relevant developmental science across and within all countries (Abbie, Hirokazu, Iheoma, & Pia, 2017).

First, the generation of knowledge on normative and at-risk development in diverse contexts should accompany the implementation of the SDGs. This could include outlining similarities and differences in child and youth development across environmental contexts, cultures, and in the wake of climate change, conflict, and migration; studying the impact of various interventions on children's development; and documenting the experiences of all children in longitudinal and panel studies that include children in emergency situations, children who are not in school, and other groups who are hard to reach and not typically included in research or measurement. The substantial body of literature outlining the interactions between biology and environment on development has changed how human development is understood, helping policy makers and practitioners conceptualise the sensitivity and responsiveness of human beings to their environments. These ideas now need to be expanded and applied to more diverse contexts so that the mechanisms that promote healthy development in all places can be better identified and understood—and eventually addressed as needed (Abbie et al., 2017).

Second, developing new approaches to measurement and monitoring to generate data and indicators to accurately track progress towards policy implementation and improved outcomes for children and youth is urgently needed. Drawing attention to children, especially those most at risk, is achieved in part by accurately measuring and reporting on children's development. This is especially critical for the millions of children who live on the margins, due to lack of birth registration and migration that create "invisible" populations of children who face severe risks in reaching their developmental potential. Today in Cameroon there are legislation insisting on the registration of births and marriages to enable the government to determine the scope of psychosocial provisions such as financing, establishing infrastructure and other supports, including human resources.

Finally, partnerships and capacity building are required to build research and measurement infrastructures in each country. Most immediately, effort is needed to train and support students in developmental science from a range of countries and backgrounds. Partnerships between research institutions and implementation agencies are also needed to create research studies that address novel and timely approaches to developmental science that will inform policy on the direction of change. Funding for research on normative development and partnerships can effectively lead to new theories and approaches for developmental science (Requejo et al., 2015).

11.1.2 Situational Analysis of Psychosocial/Health Resources for Children in Cameroon

If education, learning and skills are to be seen as both enablers and drivers of inclusive and sustainable development, it is important to review the experience of education within the framework of the international development agenda. The more comprehensive international education agenda is that of the six 'Education for All' (EFA) goals adopted in the 2000 Dakar Framework for Action. The annual EFA Global Monitoring Report (GMR) has been monitoring progress towards these goals since 2002/2003. What do these trends tell us that can help define future perspectives? While there has been rapid progress made in expanding access to formal basic education worldwide, significant inequalities between countries persist, and national averages in many countries continue to mask striking inequalities in levels of educational attainment and outcomes (The Africa-America Institute, 2015; World Bank, 2012). Traditional factors of marginalization in education such as gender and urban/rural residence continue to combine with income, language, minority status, HIV and AIDS, age (particularly in the case of young adolescent girls), and disability, to create "mutually reinforcing disadvantages", particularly so in low-income and conflict-affected countries (UNESCO, 2011).

11.1.2.1 Access to Education

Cameroon has a pre-primary population of 1,402,610 pupils, primary population of 3,806,736 pupils, secondary population of 3,722,513 students and a tertiary population of 2,231,240 students (UNESCO, 2016). Although youth in the age group of 15–24, may still be in school and working towards their educational goals, it is notable that approximately 10% of youth have no formal education and 20% of youth have attained at most incomplete primary education, meaning that in total 30% of 15–24 year olds have not completed primary education in Cameroon (UNESCO, 2016). In Cameroon, 17% of children of official primary school age (6 years old) are out of school. For example, approximately 15% of boys of primary school age are out of school compared to 19% of girls of the same age. Nearly 33% of females of secondary school age (12 years old) are out of school compared to 22% of males of the same age. For youth of primary and secondary school age, the biggest disparity can be seen between the poorest and the richest youth (UNESCO, 2016).

Many factors contribute to this low enrolment rate such as financial crunch, especially at the secondary level, shortage of classrooms and teachers, lack of educational technologies, and quality of teachers particularly in more remote areas. For girls, the rate of enrolment is further affected by socio-cultural biases, early marriage, sexual harassment, unwanted pregnancy, and domestic responsibilities (International Children's Awareness, 2011).

According to the Child, Youth & Family Development (CYFD) Annual Report of 2004 & 2005, most children in Sub-Saharan Africa, especially those living in the rural areas still lack access to formal education. Poverty (which is SDG 1) is a burden on families rendering them incapable to send children to schools. The provision of primary education was actually revealed to be one of the least important problems of villages surveyed in Southwest Region in Cameroon with children walking to schools in neighbouring villages for a distance of more than 4 km (Davis, 2000). School fees in Cameroon were also withdrawn in the year 2000, hence financial access to education in rural areas is no longer deemed problematic with the exception of uniforms, exercise books and other educational needs (Davis, 2000).

On a positive note, according to UNESCO (2016) access to primary school in Cameroon rose to 95% in 2015, partly due to the government's decision to eliminate public school fees. School completion rate has remained low (65.75%), indicating that only one out of two children entering primary school manages to successfully complete the cycle because of high rates of repetition (12.17%) and dropout. Also, 67.9% of pupils who complete primary school make a successful transition to secondary education. However, weak completion and retention rates are indicative of underlying structural problems which have considerable social and economic costs involved because of rapid population growth and urbanisation which government is addressing. Children's access to education in Adamawa region of Cameroon was subjected to a gender split with many girls being excluded from schools teaching the national curriculum, but rather being encouraged to attend Islamic schools to learn Arabic and teachings of the Koran (Amin & Dubois, 1999). Today this is changing (Tchombe, 2014a, 2014b) as the gap in gender split is being reduced through much sensitisation and removal of barriers and creations of avenues for providing other specific teachings and cultural values, including reducing the incidence of repetition.

11.1.2.2 Acquisition of Social and Personality Skills

Social and Personality skills form important aspects of psycho-social development of children between 0 and 11 years of age as evident in the Erikson psychosocial theory (1969). This period is important for developing a strong personality with support from the society. Positive personality is built very early and based on positive experiences. Apart from formal education, children acquire these skills through social interaction and through parental engagements of children's indigenous knowledge systems.

Social Interaction

The family is the most basic of all institutions of socialisation. According to Nsamenang (2005), this primary agent of socialization makes the deepest impression on the child's intellectual development because it provides the first cultural experiences and training in cultural learning. Thus, through parents, the family is the place where the foundation of learning in later life is laid. Children learn from their parents in three principal ways. This is done by observation, imitation and co-participation in parent's activities (Nsamenang, 2005; Tchombe, 2011). Other important factors include parental narratives with children through proverbs and folktales that are rich in African philosophy and which constitute important teaching principles. Today, more than ever, parents are listening to their children by encouraging them to ask questions and share their worries and fears. There is more follow up of their school activities. Partnerships between home, schools and university is often technology driven. This is facilitating collaboration and cooperation to ensure good practices in terms of relevance, inclusion and quality. Schools are becoming more accountable and ensuring good governance. The principle of decentralisation is being respected as more schools are opened in different catchment areas to ensure access. Children's voices are heard in parliament. These and many more such best practices are driving home changes in a mind-set for a positive move to ensure sustainable development.

Indigenous Games

The importance of play in the development of intellectual abilities has been emphasized in developmental psychology. Play is more than what children do to pass time. Instead, play serves an important purpose, helping children to develop socially, cognitively and physically (Power, 2000). According to Piaget (1962) play is derived from the child's working out of two fundamental characteristics of his mode of experience and development. The pioneering social constructivist developmental psychologist Lev Vygotsky (1978) thought that, in the preschool years, play is the leading source of development. Through play children learn and practice many basic social skills. They develop a sense of self; learn to interact with other children, how to make friends, how to lie and how to role-play. Bronfenbrenner's (1979) ecological model provides an important framework for considering play as part of a child's development in the midst of various social systems, with the family occupying a central role.

Participation in social games and play have many important implications for development and learning. Discussions on the above issues of social interactions, indigenous games and folklore and proverbs reminds us of two major perspectives that are; (1) the value of the neglected African epistemologies and (2) its pedagogic principles. This paper considers the above as embedded in psychosocial concerns that make demands on socio-cognitive processes that relate to culture. The dominant western form of education eroded these content and pedagogic practices. Parents, because of many societal and economic pressures, reduce their efforts to continue to employ these strategies to enhance developmental processes. Today efforts are being made to focus on these indigenous practices in the formal school system (Tchombe, 2016) and also at community levels. Parents have come to realise the importance of play as a function of childhood and so planned and organised play grounds are now available in schools and most communities. Current curriculum reform in nursery and primary schools are addressing these cultural assets and the pedagogical implications making education more child-centred, inclusive and relevant.

11.1.2.3 Healthy Psycho-social Environment

Children interact with their environment. Keeping a healthy environment is therefore vital for their social and personality development. Some environmental problems faced by both rural and urban areas in Cameroon include inadequate water and sanitation, lack of rubbish disposal and industrial pollution. The health implications of these environmental problems include respiratory infections and other infectious and parasitic diseases. The majority of peri-urban residents lived in poorly drained and poorly serviced areas. The water supply and sewage sector is particularly affected by the deterioration of public services. Consequently, health indicators are seriously hampered. Because of this poor environment children are exposed to social vices like drug addiction, substance abuse, smoking, alcoholism, promiscuous social activities, poor sexual behaviours, antisocial games, thieves and vandals. Today, government has put in place strategies for rubbish disposal in the entire town. There are public water points in key points in most towns and drainage systems are being cleared. This effort increases peoples' awareness of having a clean and healthy environment.

11.1.2.4 Access to Health

Health intervention coverage in Cameroon stands at 55%, which is relatively low (WHO, 2016). More so, children mortality rate stands at 51 deaths/1000 live births (Cameroon Demographics Profile, 2018), which is also relatively high. As with many rural communities throughout Sub-Saharan Africa, formal health care is often sought only in emergencies, when the cost of service provision and transport to the nearest hospital can be justified. The same is true of rural Cameroon where the most common frequency of travel to health clinics is by pregnant women and those in labour. In some rural areas in the Southwest region, patients are transported in push trucks or on the back of relatives for some 5–20 km to the nearest Rural Health Centre (RHC). If fortunate, they can catch a lift with a transporter, but often settle for giving birth at home in the absence of passing vehicles (Davis, 2000). A particular complaint of participants was that after travelling up to 20 km to the nearest RHC and paying between 200 and 600 FCFA for a consultation, they receive prescriptions only, therefore requiring them to travel to the nearest town to obtain drugs. Sassa Mbersi in Adamawa region of Cameroon is a case in point; the RHC is 50 km from the nearest town at Mbe and only has facilities to treat malaria and typhoid (Davis, 2000).

This scenario is now changing. Health centres are now spread out in the rural and urban towns and some of them are equipped with a pharmacy where certain regular drugs are sold. There are also outreach programmes and community health workers who operate between one and six times a year providing child vaccinations and primary treatments.

In recent years, UNICEF and its partners, including United Nations High Commission for Refugees (UNHCR) and the Ministry of Health have been working to reach vulnerable Cameroonian children and youth in some of the most isolated areas of the Eastern and North regions (Barón & Melton, 2010).

High incidence of malnutrition has negative developmental outcomes among children. According to WHO (2009), vitamin and mineral deficiencies impact well-being, and are highly prevalent in Cameroon. Preschool aged children (39%) and pregnant women (18%) are deficient in vitamin A and a supplementation with dietary diversification can eliminate this deficiency. Half of the households in Cameroon do not consume iodized salt, leaving children in those households unprotected from iodine deficiency disorders. Current rates of anaemia among preschool aged children and pregnant women are 68% and 51%, respectively (WHO, 2009).

Today much effort is now being made to support the knowledge and outreach capacity of rural health centres in order to better educate and engage caregivers and communities in basic child care in order to enhance sustainable psycho-social development of children (Barón & Melton, 2010).

With the growing recognition of the challenges of "reaching the unreached, the expansion in access to basic formal education has resulted in a shift from a quantitative focus on access and participation in formal education to a concern with qualitative aspects and the results of learning and their social distribution. The expansion of access to primary education has also resulted in the recognition of a growing demand for secondary and tertiary education and increasing concern for vocational skills development, particularly in a context of growing youth unemployment. Indeed, too many young people and adults are currently unable to develop the skills, knowledge and attitudes they need for today's rapidly changing technologies and world of work. This inadequate access to higher levels of learning is resulting in a knowledge divide that includes the 'e-literacy' gap (UNESCO, 2011).

The 'e-literacy' gap which was pronounced between genders, where girls generally have a lower literacy rate is also experiencing a changing trend. The gender gap is gradually closing up with girls having greater opportunities to access ICT knowledge given its implication for employment opportunities. The President of Cameroon in many of his speeches to the youth emphasised computer literacy. Recently, all university students of good academic standing received a laptop.

11.2 Emerging Trends in the Provision of Psychosocial and Health Resources

The Cameroonian society is confronted with the challenge of promoting the emotional, social and intellectual development of all children, while facing the odds of inappropriate structures and specific programmes for vulnerable children due to poor governance. There is a growing awareness of the pressures being placed on public financing of education. This has resulted in the need to seek more efficient use of these limited resources, to ensure greater accountability in the investment of public resources for education, and ways in which to supplement these public resources through greater fiscal capacity, new partnerships with non-public actors, as well as through advocacy for increased official development assistance. Notwithstanding these adverse conditions, the Cameroonian child possesses psychosocial resources that could act as protective factors. These include family and community solidarity, age group membership and participation in collective action (Asangha, 2015). With respect to solidarity, in typical Cameroonian societies, an individual receives social support from members of the immediate family, the extended family and the members of the community, which aids him or her to cope with the vicissitudes of life. As to age group membership, it provides the child with peer support and prevents social isolation. Lastly, participating in community activities such as collective farming allows the child to develop, at an early age, an appreciation for working in a group. These elements of social capital in African cultures could be related to the concept of resilience and thus helps young people in gaining skills and realise the significance of investing in the sustainable development of their communities (Asangha, 2015).

According to Tchombe (2011), socialization for adult roles begins early for children. Children of the Bamiléké ethnic group in Cameroon engage very early in various forms of interaction with persons in the social milieu and with available, rich, physical and material resources. These experiences are meaningful, sustainable and transferable. The adolescent is already the owner of a farm or a petty business and a member of "thrift and loan" or Njangi group, which is an avenue to raise capital through loans to start or sustain an existing business. The activities and abilities to participate are fostered by the inculcation of the values of endurance, patience, persistence, honesty, respect and hard work, which are indelible characteristics of the Bamiléké people. Perseverance, according to the people is a key to success. As they develop, deprived children participate in these economic activities depending on the nature and difficulty level of such tasks as selling and participating in the bargaining and negotiation of the prices of commercial wares.

In the same light, according to Fomba (2011), such a human development strategy that young people benefit from, is common through sustainable livelihood activities such as farming, carpentry, mechanics, craft, fishing, animal rearing, blacksmithing and small businesses. Investment in life skills through traditional preparation strategies has been drawn from the firm belief that young people through peer cultures are agents of change with the potential of taking a leading role in the socio-economic development of their communities as they transit from childhood to the world of work. Such life skills acquired by these young people as highlighted in SDG 4.7, is highly important with regard to achieving sustainable development. This is also in line with SDG 4.4 which advocates for a substantial increase in the number of youth and adults who have relevant skills, including technical and vocational skills, for employment, decent jobs and entrepreneurship.

According to the National AIDS Control Committee (2010), providing social support for orphaned and vulnerable children, especially those affected by HIV-AIDS poses a great challenge for both families and the society. Many disadvantaged children live out of the family support and hence they are marginalized, stigmatized and

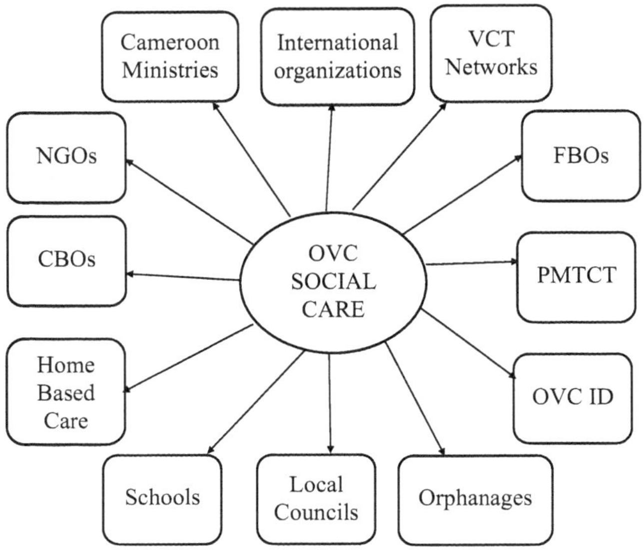

Fig. 11.1 Sources for Identifying and Providing Care to OVC in Cameroon
Source: Adapted from Nsagha, Ngowe, Nguedia, and Longdoh (2014)

Key: NGO = Non-governmental organization, FBO = Faith-based organization, CBO = Community-based organization, PMTCT = Prevention of Mother-To Child Transmission of HIV, VCT networks = Voluntary Counselling and Testing, OVC ID = Orphans and vulnerable children identification

exposed to vulnerable conditions such as lack of schooling, begging, paedophilia, juvenile delinquency, prostitution, and transmission of STIs. In 2006, when the Cameroon Government integrated Orphans and vulnerable children (OVC) into its health and education policies, key services such as education, birth registration, health, nutrition, water and sanitation, judicial protection and placement services were identified as crucial for children and youth without family care (UNICEF, UNAIDS and the Future Group, 2006). Nonetheless, the country possesses a good number of social support institutions that cater for the needs of orphaned and vulnerable children. Figure 11.1 above illustrates these support systems.

In 2006, taking into consideration all categories of orphaned and vulnerable children, there were 183, 523 identified for assistance by the national AIDS Control Committee, of which assistance was provided to 25,643 (14%). In 2007, assistance was given to 43,505 of them, an increase by 69.6%. However, when AIDS orphans were examined, 12,776 and 28,319 (121.7% rise) were respectively catered for in 2006 and 2007 (Mbanya, Sama, & Tchounwou, 2008). Cameroon therefore has been able to put in place support services that can cater for the health and education needs of disadvantaged children.

For any meaningful sustainable development to take place, children and youth themselves must be active participants in the developmental process. Today's children are those to herald sustainability by, assuming an active role in the educative process that empowers them. The human person is not strictly shepherded by external events or other persons because children and youth have cognitive power to influence their own actions in order for them to produce certain results. It is important to reiterate that the socio-cognitive challenges experienced by children and even youths such as poverty and hunger (SDG 1&2) most often are well managed through personal decision making as they occur. Children, like other individuals, do have their personal mind theory illustrated through socio-cognitive processes as they express their feelings, thoughts about persons, self and events base on their perceptions. It is worth noting that children encounter a myriad of personal, social, and environmental barriers which they address through their personal efforts using socio-cognitive processes to change, adapt and adjust in the circumstances without external assistance. Most often this decision is made independent of those around them. So children do have the capacity to exercise control over their own thought processes, actions and those of others, motivating and affecting their actions which operate through their personal agency. On this account the mediated mutual reciprocity theory can be presented here as a valuable tool to explain how the children's personal role in changing can be appreciated.

Mediated mutual reciprocity (MMR) is characterised by action that is need-interest-driven, based on learning initiated and sustained by the learner (Tchombe, 2004, 2011). Children's personal initiated involvements offer new directions for understanding their involvement. The theory (MMR) postulates equal responsibility to all with varying degrees of accountability. Children have the ability to monitor and control their own cognitive resources which are frequently lost sight of when explaining their participatory roles in relation to others. Tchombe (2009), Tchombe et al. (2012) argues that the MMR explains learner's inputs as they assume responsibility and determine the direction of their learning activities in solving problems through reflecting, questioning, encouraging, negotiating and being creative. In finding out how children and youth cope with everyday challenges, this holistic theoretical framework, the MMR (Tchombe et al. 2012) is action oriented leading to the use of different competences and techniques such as:

- Sharing of behaviour based on the mutual need for collaboration and cooperation in any learning task or decision making.
- Assuming a transforming role by redirecting processes through initiating, negotiating and modulating to suit an individual's rhythm, and modifying the learning behaviours of others.
- Monitoring a task in order to adjust one's behaviour appropriately is an unconditional give and take process with no hierarchy.

Mediated Mutual Reciprocity is a new paradigm shift theorizing the view that development is from the child rather than from the adult's perspective. On this account the child demonstrates how he/she learns through influencing and effecting change initiated by their inputs. So in the learning context they are not being dictated to, but rather being an important and equal partner in the learning process. Deprived children and youth can participate fully in different cultural activities of interests that match their needs. MMR sees the child and adult as co-constructors of knowledge, whereby both are active participants, but the child is the focal point. This is so because the ability to transform knowledge into ideas for transferability is to be creative, analytic and to solve problems with the child as the learner. Teachers, parents and other significant others neglect the fact that for learning to be effective there must be mutual reciprocity. The learning act is a symmetrical action that is a process that is two way and interactive with no one having a dominant position on the basis of them being co-constructors in the knowledge creation process. MMR therefore enables us to understand that children are very active in the learning process and are not passive recipients of knowledge in the teaching learning transactional process. Thus, we cannot talk of quality health and education for deprived children and youth without identifying their roles. Mediated mutual reciprocity can explain the important role of learners to help facilitate health and education through their participation in controlling, negotiating, discussing issues concerning drug abuse, alcoholism, malaria, teenage pregnancy and sexually transmitted infections like HIV-AIDS that are key concerns of Cameroonian youth today (Tchombe, 2011; Tchombe et al. 2012).

The MMR provides a broad theoretical framework with potentials that can explain the interactions between cultural amplifiers or assets and the processes of development and learning in social-cultural contexts. These amplifiers generate different actions, cognitive and social skills and knowledge contents which create rich opportunities for children's development and learning through observation, participation and recognition. Some of these cultural amplifiers are hunting, fishing, weaving, farming, trading, and pottery, compound cleaning, singing, dancing and doing household chores. Worthy to note is the fact that the norms of the African empirical world enable the enhancement of competencies such as spatial linguistic, perceptual, temporal, interpersonal, cognitive and mathematical competencies. Appropriate explanations for such indigenous actions and processes in development pose challenges for mainstream psychological theories, research methods, teaching and assessment (Tchombe, 2014a, 2014b).

Learning in Africa is a cultural construct whereby individuals continuously interact and share ideas and knowledge with each other reciprocally. Mutual Reciprocity encourages recognition and the values of give and take, acting as an intrinsic motivational factor with respect for one another in the transaction game (Tchombe, 2014a, 2014b). MMR addresses shared knowledge of the perspectives of others. This suggests mutual influences or reciprocal effects. So in the context of socialisation, parents are aware of the tacit norms as they appraise children's performance, assess their progress and understand their actions and verbal behaviours. Parents also discern their children's motives, emotions and are able to encourage, correct and sanction when and where necessary.

The study sought to answer four specific research objectives, namely, to examine the perception of parents on changing trends in relation to:

(a) Access to Quality and Equity Education
(b) Acquisition of Social and Personality Skills by Children
(c) An Enabling Psycho-social Environment
(d) Access to health

11.3 Methodology and Design

A descriptive research design sought to describe the current situation of changing trends to illustrate change. It did this through a survey of parents' perceptions using both qualitative and quantitative paradigms in relation to the objectives of the study.

11.4 Area of Study

The study was carried out in four regions out of the ten regions of Cameroon through purposive sampling technique. Two Anglophone (North West and South West) and two Francophone (West and Littoral) regions were chosen for the study.

11.5 Sample and Sampling Technique

A purposive sampling technique was used to choose participants of the study based on defined criteria. All participants ought to be of at least 45 years of age and have children within the defined age bracket for the study. The reason for this was because the items in the questionnaire as well as the focus group discussion required an appraisal of the provision of education and health in Cameroon for the past 17 years that is from 2000 to 2017, marking the advent of MDGs, EFA goals and the SDGs. Fifty (50) parents were chosen from each of the four regions to make a sample of 200 participants. The study employed both qualitative (focus group discussions) and quantitative (questionnaire) methods for data collection.

11.6 Instrumentation

The four point scale (Agreed, Strongly Agreed, Disagreed and Strongly Disagreed) questionnaire had four parts based on each objective set for the study, including the section for demographic information not to be considered in the analyses. Objective one examined three indicators concerned with Access to Quality and Equity in formal Education. Objective two examined the acquisition of social and personality skills by children using two indicators, namely, indigenous knowledge systems and social interaction via mediated mutual reciprocity. Objective three addressed the enabling psycho-social environment using multiple indicators including environments that expose children's vices like drug addiction, substance abuse, smoking, alcoholism, promiscuous social activities, sexual behaviours, antisocial games, thieves and vandals. Objective four questioned access to health using three indicators, namely, nutrition, and sanitation and health facilities.

Focus group discussions were conducted with four groups of ten each from each of the regions studied, raising questions on issues from the questionnaire for in-depth discussions.

11.7 Data Analysis

Descriptive statistics and a systematic process of thematic analysis were used to analyse both quantitative and qualitative data respectively.

11.8 Presentation of Findings and Discussion

The findings of the study are represented in terms of the four stated objectives for the study.

11.8.1 Objective One: Access to Quality and Equity Education

This objective was examined using three indicators, namely, access, equity and quality in education. According to the findings, 60% of the participants perceived an improvement in access to education. Furthermore, 62.8% thought that there was equity in education and 74.2% accepted that the quality of education has improved. Hence a total of 65.7% of the participants perceived improvements in access to quality and equity education. Their views from focus group discussion are qualitatively summarised in the table below.

11.8.2 Objective Two: Acquisition of Social and Personality Skills by Children

This objective was examined using two indicators, namely, indigenous knowledge systems and social interaction via mediated mutual reciprocity. According to the findings 67.2% of the participants perceived that children acquire social and personality skills more effectively from indigenous knowledge systems, while 53.3% acknowledge social interaction as explained by the theory of mediated mutual reciprocity. Hence a total of 60.2% of the participants perceived that children acquired social and personality skills via social interactions where there is respect and autonomy. Their views are qualitatively summarised in the table below (Table 11.2).

11.8.3 Objective Three: Enabling Psycho-social Environment

This objective was examined using multiple indicators including environments that expose children's vices like drug addiction, substance abuse, smoking, alcoholism, promiscuous social activities and sexual behaviours, antisocial games, thieves and vandals. According to the findings

Table 11.2 Acquisition of social and personality skills by children

Indicator	Sample quotation
Indigenous knowledge systems	*Cameroon is blessed with a rich cultural diversity that enables the learning process. There is a program for cultural manifestations during the youth week where students show case the different cultural aspects that they learn in school or from home. Arts and crafts are another aspect that brings out the psycho-social development of Cameroonian youths. These indigenous ways of knowing (like proverbs, riddles, folktales, idioms, dances, songs and games) are however facing stiff competition and neglect due to advance of modern technologies like gadgets and internet*
Social interaction via mediated mutual reciprocity	*Children normally cultivate talents and skills by working at home as a way of training. Most children assist their parents in the various trades in which the parents are found. In the Tiko neighbourhood for instance where most parents are traders, children assist their parents in the market and end up creating their own personal businesses. But this phenomenon of children helping parents is now being confused as child labour. This has made some parents to be reluctant in giving their children task for fear of being accused of child labour. There is need to educate the population on the difference between the two scenarios*

57.5% of the participants perceived the environments to be enabling to children. Qualitatively, the participants stated that:

> There are some environments like in "new lay outs" that are very conducive and free from the above vices. But in other localities, there are slums that have met with little or no improvements and keep on breeding the above vices.

11.8.4 Objective Four: Access to Health

This objective was examined using three indicators, namely, nutrition, sanitation and health facilities. Accordingly, 68.9% of the participants believed there has been improvement in food quantity and quality. In addition, 66.7% believed in improved sanitary situations and 84% stated that children are more exposed to better health facilities. Hence, a total of 73.2% of participants perceived improved access to health. Their views are qualitatively summarised in the table below (Table 11.3).

11.9 Implications of the Study

The summary of the findings of the present study reveal that generally 64.15% (as opposed to 35.85%) of the participants agreed that Cameroon had made progress in improving the provision of psychosocial and health resources for quality development of children 0–11 years old. Cameroon, however, still falls below international standards in these domains, hence, a need for more improvement on the provision of services still exists. The positive perceptions, and the subjective indications of progress, may however, serve as a solid foundation to accelerate the betterment of access to quality and equity education, the acquisition of social and personality skills by children, the creation of enabling psycho-social environments and access to health, for the younger section of the population.

11.10 Conclusion

Cameroon is a lower-middle income country with an estimated population of 22.8 million, with a GDP of 5.5 and 5.9% between 2013 and 2015. The country is endowed with natural resources. Nonetheless there is a slow pace of socio economic growth, leaving about 40% of the population below the poverty line. The provision of psychosocial and health resources for quality development of children (0–11 years old) in Cameroon remains an issue that poses serious challenges for sustainable development. The government has some policies on the improvement of health and education, but these have met with little or no success at the implementation level. Cameroon faces serious problems of government accountability and decentralization of services to

Table 11.3 Access to health

Indicator	Sample quotation
Nutrition	*Our environment is very rich as far as nutritional value of food types is concerned. There is the availability of a wide range of food types like protein, starch, carbohydrates etc. we have a lot of vegetables, plantains, beans, fish and meat. etc. we can boost of good foods; the community only needs more education and sensitization on how to make a balance diet from these types of foods*
Sanitation	*Apart from slums and some localities that have poor sanitary conditions, there have been moves in helping to keep the environment clean. The local council has set aside 1 day per month that is used for keeping the town clean. The presence of waste disposal company (HYSACAM) has equally helped. What is most important of all is the education of the public on the proper management of waste especially stopping dirt litter that is found almost everywhere. The drainage system of some roads needs further maintenance and construction*
Access to health facilities	*There has been remarkable improvement on this sector though there are still a good number of challenges. There are periodic immunization campaigns (vaccination) which the government administers to children from 0 to 11 years. There is also the distribution of mosquito nets to families, especially pregnant women to help prevent malaria. There has been increase in access and availability of hospitals and health centres to improve on the condition of children. There is need for continuous equipment of these health centres as well as increase in medical personnel*

meet the demands of the civil society. Meaningful sustainability can only be achieved, if the children and youth themselves are engaged in the process of development. This review has highlighted key issues with regards to changing trends in the provision of psychosocial and health resources for quality development of children 0–11 years old in. The review has proposed the mediated mutual reciprocity theory as an important theoretical perspective whereby all children and youths' engagements in achieving the sustainable development goals can be explained. In this light as developmental scientists, it is imperative to pay attention to our children and their spaces which are quite agentive and to see how we can involve them in decision making so as to enhance sustainable development and to facilitate the implementation of sustainable development goals.

The following recommendations may assist in this regard:

- Investing in parenting interventions that promote parent–child interactions to improve responsiveness in feeding infants and young children; increase attachment; and encourage learning, book reading, play activities, positive discipline, and problem-solving related to children's development, care, and feeding. Parenting education and support are often delivered through home visits, community groups, regular clinic visits, and media or in combination with other components, and should be expanded. Parenting interventions and centre-based programmes can improve children's cognitive and social–emotional development and school readiness.
- The returns on investment in early child development are substantial.
- Investment inearly childhood is regarded as the most effective and cost efficient time to ensure that all children develop their full potential. Reducing inequalities through integrated interventions early in life that target the many risks to which vulnerable children are exposed.

Unless governments allocate more resources to quality early child development programmes for the poorest people in the population, economic disparities will continue and widen. Scientists will, in the meantime, continue to provide empirical evidence that can serve as directives for strategic planning in sustainable development.

References

Abbie, R., Hirokazu, Y., Iheoma I., & Pia, R. B. (2017). Social policy report. *Children, Youth and Developmental Science in the 2015–2030 Global Sustainable Development Goals.* Volume 30, Number 3.

Amin, A., & Dubois, J. L. (1999). *A 1999 update of the Cameroon poverty profile*. Washington, DC: World Bank.

Armah-Attoh, D., Selormey, E., & Houessou, R. (2016). *Despite gains, barriers keep health care high on Africa's priority list* (Afrobarometer Policy Paper No. 31).

Asangha, M. N. (2015). Peer group activities and resilient identity among mid adolescents (15–17years old): Case of Mbengwi sub division. *The African Journal of Special Education, 3*(1), 157–164.

Barón, E. V., & Melton, R. J. (2010). *Health promotion and early childhood development: Some emerging global research issues*. Geneva, Switzerland: World Health Organization.

Bartlett, S. (2008). Climate change and urban children: Impacts and implications for adaptation in low- and middle-income countries. *Environment & Urbanization, 20*, 501–519. https://doi.org/10.1177/0956247808096125

Bolger, N., & Amarel, D. (2007). Effects of social support visibility on adjustment to stress: Experimental evidence. *Journal of Personality and Social Psychology, 92*, 458–475.

Britto, P. R., Lye, S., Proulx, K., Yousafzai, A., Perez-Escamilla, R., Rao, N., & Bhutta, Z. (2017). Nurturing care: Promoting early childhood development. *The Lancet, 389*, 91–102. https://doi.org/10.1016/s0140-6736(16)31390-3

Bronfenbrenner, U. (1979). *The ecology of human development*. Cambridge, MA: Harvard University Press.

Broome, J. (2008). The ethics of climate change. *Scientific American, 298*, 96–102. https://doi.org/10.1038/scientificamerican0608-96

Cameroon Demographics Profile (2018). https://www.indexmundi.com/Cameroon/demographics_profile.html.

Child, Youth & Family Development (CYFD). *Annual Report (2004 & 2005)*. Retrieved on 11th of March, 2011 at 4:55pm from http://www.hsrc.ac.za/Annual_Report-18.phtml

Currie, J., & Deschenes, O. (2016). Children and climate change: Introducing the issue. *The Future of Children, 26*, 3–9. https://doi.org/10.1353/foc.2016.0000

Davis, A. (2000). *Transport versus service provision: A sustainable livelihoods profile of Cameroon*. Retrieved 16 March, 2011 at 5:30pm from http://www.google.com

Engle, P. L., Fernald, L. C., Alderman, H., Behrman, J., O'Gara, C., Yousafzai, A., & Iltus, S. (2011). Strategies for reducing inequalities and improving developmental outcomes for young children in low-income and middle-income countries. *The Lancet, 378*(9799), 1339–1353. https://doi.org/10.1016/s0140-6736(11)60889-1

Erikson, E. H. (1982). *The life cycle completed: A review*. New York, NY: Norton.

Freud, S. (1921). *Group psychology and the analysis of the ego. The standard edition of the complete psychological. Works of Sigmund Freud*, Volume XVIII (1920–1922): Beyond the Pleasure Principle, Group Psychology and Other Works, 65–144.

Hanna, R., & Oliva, P. (2016). Implications of climate change for children in developing countries. *The Future of Children, 26*, 115–132.

International Children's Awareness (ICA 2011). *Schooling in Cameroon*. http://icacanada.org/projects/schooling-in-cameroon.

Kern, M. L., Friedman, H. S., Martin, L. R., Reynolds, C. A., & Luong, G. (2009). Conscientiousness, career success, and longevity: A lifespan analysis. *Annals of Behavioural Medicine, 37*, 154–163.

Kim, H. S., Sherman, D. K., & Taylor, S. E. (2009). Culture and social support. *The American Psychologist, 63*, 518–526.

Kohlberg, L. (1984). *The psychology of moral development: The nature and validity of moral stages* (Essays on Moral Development, Volume 2). Harper & Row.

Mbanya, D., Sama, M., & Tchounwou, P. (2008). Current status of HIV/AIDS in Cameroon: How effective are control strategies? *International Journal of Environmental Research and Public Health, 5*, 378–383. https://doi.org/10.3390/ijerph5050378

National AIDS Control Committee (2010). *The impact of HIV and AIDS in Cameroon through 2020*, 1–40.

Nsagha, D. S., Ngowe, N. M., Nguedia, J. C. A., & Longdoh, N. A. (2014). A public health model and framework to mitigate the impact of orphans and vulnerable children due to HIV/AIDS in Cameroon. *World Journal of AIDS, 4*, 27–37.

Nsamenang, A. B. (2005). *Developmental psychology: Search for diversity paradigm*. Bamenda, Cameroon: Anoh's Printing Services.

Phalkey, R. K., Aranda-Jan, C., Marx, S., Höfle, B., & Sauerborn, R., (2015). Systematic review of current efforts to quantify the impacts of climate change on undernutrition. Proceedings of the National Academy of Sciences, 112(33)

Piaget, J. (1962). *Play, dreams, and imitation in childhood*. New York, NY: W. W. Norton & Company.

Power, T. G. (2000). *Play and exploration in children and animals*. Mahwah, NJ: Erlbaum.

Requejo, J. H., Bryce, J., Barros, A. J., Berman, P., Bhutta, Z., Chopra, M., & Victora, C. G. (2015). Countdown to 2015 and beyond: Fulfi lling the health agenda for women and children. *The Lancet, 385*, 466–476. https://doi.org/10.1016/s0140-6736(14)60925-9

Sheffield, P., & Landrigan, P. (2011). Global climate change and children's health: Threats and strategies for prevention. *Environmental Health Perspectives, 119*(3), 291. https://doi.org/10.1289/ehp.1002233

Taylor, S. E., & Broffman, J. I. (2011). Psychosocial resources: Functions, origins, and links to mental and physical health. In J. M. Olson & M. P. Zanna (Eds.), *Advances in experimental social psychology* (pp. 1–57). New York, NY: Academic.

Tchombe, T. M. (2009). *Entrepreneurship, education and National Development*. Jos: University of Jos press.

Tchombe, M. S. T. (2011). Cultural strategies for cognitive enrichment in learning among Bamilike of west region of Cameroon. In Nsamenang & Tchombe (Eds.), *Handbook of African educational theories and practices; a generative teacher education curriculum*. Yaounde, Cameroon: Presses Universitaires d'Afrique.

Tchombe, M. S. T. (2014a). *Gender in secondary school classroom practices in Cameroon*. London, UK: Commonwealth Secretariat.

Tchombe, M. S. T. (2014b). *Mediated mutual reciprocity for enhancement of cognitive and ecological impact in developing cognitive competences in arithmetic.* Paper presented at the inaugural conference of the South African Psychological Association in Durban, September 2014.

Tchombe, M. S. T. (2016). Shifting the paradigm from misconceptions about Africa's nonproductivty to new narratives on its achievements and contributions: Implications for research. *Journal of Educational Research in Africa (JERA), 8*, 13–29.

Tchombe, T. M. S., Shumba, A., Lo-Oh, J. L., Gakuba, T.-O., Zinkeng, M., & Teku, T. T. (2012). Psychological undertones of family poverty in rural communities in Cameroon: Resilience and coping strategies. *South Africa Journal of Psychology, 42*(2), 232–242. https://doi.org/10.1177/008124631204200210

Teaching Metrics Task Force (LMTF). (2013). *Toward universal learning: Recommendations from the learning metrics taskforce*. Montreal, Canada/Washington, DC: UNESCO Institute for Statistics/Brookings Institution. http://www.brookings.edu/research/reports/2013/09/learning-metrics-task-force-universal-learning

The Africa-America Institute (2015). "State of Education in Africa Report," http://www.aaionline.org/wpcontent/uploads/2015/09/ AAI-SOE-report-2015-final.pdf

UNESCO. (2011). *EFA global monitoring report 2010*. UNESCO-UIS (2005) Children Out of School: Measuring Exclusion from Primary Education.

UNESCO. (2016). Cameroon I UNESCO UIS - UNESCO Institute for Statistics. uis.unesco.org/country/CM.

UNICEF, UNAIDS and the Future Group. (2006). National responses to orphans and other children in sub-Saharan Africa—*The OVC Programme Effort Index* 2004, September; and Demographic and Health Surveys.

United Nations Educational, Scientific and Cultural Organization. (2011) *EFA global monitoring report.* Paris: 2011.

United Nations Educational, Scientific and Cultural Organization (2012). *Education and skills for inclusive and sustainable development beyond2015.* Retrieved from http://www.un.org/milleniumgoals/pdf/Think%20pieces/4_education.pdf.

Vygotsky, L. S. (1978). *Mind and society: The development of higher mental processes*. Cambridge, MA: Harvard University Press.

Walker, S. P., Chang, S. M., Powell, C. A., Simonoff, E., & Grantham-McGregor, S. M. (2007). Early childhood stunting is associated with poor psychological functioning in late adolescence and effects are reduced by psychosocial stimulation. *The Journal of Nutrition, 137*, 2464–2469.

WHO. (2009). *Global prevalence of vitamin A deficiency in populations at risk 1995–2005. WHO Global Database on Vitamin A Deficiency.*

WHO. (2011) *Global response: Epidemic update and health sector progress towards Universal Access* 2011.

WHO. (2016). *Public financing for health in Africa: From Abuja to the SDGs* (p. 27). Geneva, Switzerland: WHO Press. 20 Avenue Appia, 1211.

Wills, T. A. (1984). Supportive functions of interpersonal relationships. In S. Cohen & L. Syme (Eds.), *Social support and health* (pp. 61–82). New York, NY: Academic.

World Bank. (2012). *Assessing progress in Africa toward the millennium development goals.* http://www1.uneca.org/Portals/mdgreports/2012/Goal02.pdf

World Bank. (2017). *GINI index (World Bank estimate).* https://data.worldbank.org/indicator/SI.POV.GINI?locations=ZA-MA-TN-DZ-EG-NG-KE-LR-SO

World Health Organization. (2014). *Health for the world's adolescents: A second chance in the second decade: summary*. Retrieved from: http://www.who.int/maternal_child_adolescent/documents/second-decade/en/

Humanising Silence: The Representation of HIV & AIDS in South African Narratives

12

Vasu Reddy

Abstract
This chapter focuses on an analysis of HIV & AIDS and its representation in South African autobiographical narratives produced in the post-apartheid context. The chapter will zoom in on a selection of texts (largely memoirs, journals and general life writing) that provide perspectives on representations of living with and through the HI virus and AIDS to show resistances to silence and denial. The chapter centres on a descriptive reading of selected texts as representations of a social world in the way authors engage disclosure, sexuality, and identity in relation to how these narratives bear witness to the complexities of disease and its' modalities.

12.1 Introduction

The pioneering anthology titled *Nobody Ever Said Aids* (Rasebotsa, Samuelson, & Thomas, 2004) comprises 20 short stories and 22 poems by both established and new writers that show the human side of HIV that manifest life and experience in an African context. The texts manifest experiences of people living with and dying of HIV with the vast majority of authors being South African (a third of the contributions emanate from Zimbabwe, Botswana, Malawi, Zambia and Lesotho). At its core, the volume features texts that engage processes of mourning, feelings of despair and an awareness of tragedy (notably the injustices towards women in prostitution, childbearing, marriage and divorce) centred on the context of HIV and AIDS. The collection also directs attention to the consequences of silence and denial and points fingers at the evasions and untruths espoused by some African politicians about HIV. *Nobody Ever Said AIDS* concludes with a poem by Mthuthuzeli Isaac Skosana's poem "When I rise":

I shall defeat HIV
I shall defeat AIDS
I shall defeat anger
When I rise
Yes when I rise I shall smile
Oh, when I rise

However, most striking is the title of the volume, drawn from Eddie Maluleke's (Rasebotsa et al., 2004: 20) poem of the same name, as he writes in the final stanza in his poem:

We all died
Coughed and died
We died of TB
That was us
Whispering it at funerals
Because nobody ever said AIDS.

V. Reddy (✉)
University of Pretoria, Pretoria, South Africa
e-mail: vasu.reddy@up.ac.za

I. Eloff (ed.), *Handbook of Quality of Life in African Societies*, International Handbooks of Quality-of-Life, https://doi.org/10.1007/978-3-030-15367-0_12

An arresting chord is struck with the collective "we" that comments on the illness, death and disgust associated with HIV as experienced by Africans. These words register a direct alignment with AIDS as a disease that is embodied and lived, and more that this is a disease that expresses notable silences; even more, it is exceptionalised instead of normalised (see Cameron, 2007). The words are not empty nor abstract musings but rather reflective, as they call into question contemporary struggles about the silences surrounding AIDS that circumscribe lived realities in African contexts that compromise the quality of life experiences. An underlying feature of Maluleke's words is a rejection of a romantic or sentimental attitude for the sake of the struggle for survival. Not only does Maluleke make a plea for perseverance in the fight against the disease, but also the lines in the text provide a lamentation about the loss of human life that call into question the centrality of the human cost. The human cost of silence is a central refrain in writing about HIV and AIDS, and is less about disease, and indeed more about directing us to the cost and consequences of silence. The text responds to some extent to large-scale denials, misconceptions and political neglect and discomfort that characterise the discourse surrounding the epidemic in many contexts that marginalise people living with HIV in African locations.

Taking the cure from the above examples relating to the discourses of suffering, blame, shame and stigma associated with HIV, this chapter focuses on a descriptive interpretation of a selection of narratives (some novels, and life writing informed by autobiographical and biographical accounts) from South Africa (I shall explain the uses of (auto)biography later). Along the lines of Plummer (1995: 168) I approach these stories (including the narratives in poems) as modes of life writing – as acts as well as texts, sociological as well as aesthetic phenomena in which "story tellings may come very close to the life as experienced". Plummer takes up the 'narrative turn' from cultural studies within sociology and suggests that a sociology of stories asks different questions about the meaning of navigating disease and direct us to the role of the social and political (see also Plummer, 2001). In addition the social processes through which lives are constructed and consumed also speak back to earlier theoretical encounters with autobiography (explained briefly in a later section) that have returned to the "paradox of the referential aesthetic" (see Eakin, 1992). By 'referential aesthetic', I mean locating the speaking voice in a real world.

The chapter provides a brief explanation of a location of the texts aligned in relation to a developing critical analytical literature in the field. Thereafter it turns to an overview of some key texts focused on the representation of central meanings shaped by authors. The chapter also builds on the insight by Brophy (2004: 4) that "personal testimonies written in response to HIV and AIDS attempt to intervene in cultural memory by rewriting the story of the body and its locations, thus significantly altering how readers receive and respond to these imaginings and re-imaginings." "AIDS," wrote Susan Sontag (1989: 122), "reinstates something like a premodern experience of illness," a throwback to an era when sickness was, by its nature, immutable, mysterious, and fatal. However, it also marked a major shift, as motivated from viewing purely the medicalised language of suffering and the relationship to death but rather more a preoccupation with life and living as espoused by the texts.

12.2 Location and Context

The texts chosen represent a growing body of cultural perspectives of HIV and the AIDS diagnosis that build on the formidable writing as a canon of established Northern accounts of HIV and a growing body of creative and documentary writing in African contexts.[1] With the former, I

[1]There is a growing body of writing in the African context. This chapter does not provide a comprehensive representation of the texts but references these in abbreviation in this note. See for example, Attree (2010), Coovadia (2009), Dow and Essex (2011), Greene (2005), Koch (2002), Moele (2009), Morgan and the Bambanani Women's Group (2003), Mpe (2001), Nolen (2008), Odhiambo (2017), and Steinberg (2008)

am reminded by established classics such as Paul Monette's *Borrowed Time* (1988), and the Dutch writer Frans Kellendonk's *Mystiek lichaam: een geschiedenis* (1990) amongst others that mediate and depict looming death in the face of the AIDS diagnosis. These texts were published at a time when the HIV diagnosis was in its infancy. These accounts characterise first the shaping of lives of infected gay men in a context where stigma and prejudice were rife, and second, where the knowledge base was fairly thin compared to the body of knowledge that we have today (see for example, Caron, 2001; Herdt & Lindenbaum, 1992; Murphy & Poirier, 1993; Ranger & Slack, 1992). Notwithstanding the advances in biomedical and scientific knowledge, including medical technologies to combat HIV and the AIDS diagnosis, stigma, shame and pathologisation are still prevalent (see Dilger & Luig, 2010; Rödlach, 2006). Central to the pathologisation and the founding metaphors of sexual pollution associated with HIV and the AIDS diagnosis is the connection between illness (HIV) and a group of people (gay men). Jeffrey Weeks (1985: 46) prophetically articulated over three decades ago an observation that still has merit today inspite of the massive developments we have seen in our understanding, interpretation and responses to HIV:

> AIDS is a metaphor that "has come to symbolize … the identity between contagion and a kind of desire." In the fear and loathing that AIDS evokes there is a resulting conflation between two plausible, if unproven theories – that there is an elective affinity between disease and certain sexual practices, and that certain sexual practices cause disease – and a third, that certain types of sex are diseases. In the climate produced by such assumptions, rational thought is very near impossible.

The above view also direct us to the crude historically ascribed categorisations of people affected by HIV, as Crimp (1988) noted between *innocent victims* (haemophiliacs, women, and children) versus the *guilty perpetrators* (promiscuous men, intravenous drug users, homosexuals, sex workers, pimps). The ideas emphasise an important perspective that the chapter takes as a cue, namely that sexual practices, sexuality and identity opens up debate that respond to how we can see HIV and the AIDS diagnosis as a "liberating force that enables us to break the borders and controls, and to create a new social and sexual understanding" (Reddy, 2011: 12). These views also build on what Treichler (1999: 11) memorably articulated as a plague of images as an "epidemic of signification". In other words the idea of the AIDS epidemic as a transmissible lethal disease is also simultaneously an epidemic that amplify meanings at a symbolic level of interpretation as loss, as tragedy, as social history, as sexual politics, as racism, as a practical problem (see Aggleton, 1989 for a more detailed discussion of the symbolic meanings associated with these issues).

The founding perspectives by Aggleton (1989) remain not only relevant but also central to how we understand the shape, architecture and patterns of HIV and the AIDS diagnosis beyond the statistics and the biomedical identity of a patient with HIV to how we understand lived, material realities of the person living with HIV in relation to the quality of life. This is in part the response by Nyanzi (in Tamale 2011: 47) when she claimed that "preventative interventions against HIV/AIDS reignited the overt medicalisation of sexuality, such that the sexual self became restricted by intricate ties to the body, to bodily functions of coitus and reproduction, to illness and death … sexual health programmes focused on disease, pregnancy and death". The idea that biomedicine maintains hegemony over what knowledge is valued (Cáceres, in Parker, 2001: 241) can therefore be countered by alternative forms of knowledge that prioritise the social and the cultural. This chapter locates the cultural in the context of narrative accounts (life stories, auto/biographies, fiction) as one possible data source of information.

In other words, another nodal entry point to making sense of HIV is the way culture, sexuality, sexual practices and mediations of HIV and the AIDS diagnosis have been articulated, shaped by narrative accounts of HIV that provide what I have termed humanising effects to counteract silence and through these writings, a wider conception of culture is evoked. I view AIDS writing as political and personal acts as far as the texts direct readers' attention to providing a sense of self in relation to location, culture, context and indeed the qualities of life shaped by disease and illness. The chapter motivates that narrative accounts of HIV lifts the veil of silence by providing more nuanced, textured and humanising effects of the self. If silence is perceived as an omission in communication interactions, Picard (1988: 15–16) also reminds us that "[s]ilence is an autonomous phenomenon. It is therefore not identical with the suspension of language … Language and silence belong together: language has knowledge of silence as silence has knowledge of language". More importantly, silence is not just linked with some active human performance; it is an active human performance (Dauenhauer, 1980: 4). The humanising effects that this chapter speaks to is a view that the texts provide an antidote to dehumanisation, alienation and instrumentalism, by placing a premium on the value of knowledge, culture, and life experiences. Issues that inform the analysis section of the chapter address the discourses generated by the texts in so far as the silences and constructions they address. Taken up briefly in the conclusions are the kind of stories that are being told about HIV and the AIDS diagnosis and the possible implications for thinking about HIV and the AIDS diagnosis in cultural terms and their prospects for enhancing the quality of life. The latter encapsulates in broad terms the needs and expectations of what may be considered the goals, hopes and aspirations that entail a good life where life domains and needs are met along physical and health status, psychological status, well-being, social interactions and economic status) (see for example, Anderson, 2014; Michalos, 2017; Møller, 1997, 2007; Sirgy, 2012). Central it seems is the fact that the interrelationship between these domains are meaningful when all aspects of human suffering decline in the engagement of life. With respect to HIV and AIDS, health outcomes and life quality is weakened when there is an absence of treatment, stigma and exclusion.

12.3 The Political Context of AIDS

The texts featured in this chapter are shaped in some ways in South African AIDS discourse when HIV became a deeply divisive and politicised issue in a context where poverty, inequality, unemployment and disease were rife. The latter, namely poverty, inequality, unemployment and health more broadly minimise life opportunities, reduce and ultimately weaken the quality of life experience (see Møller & Dickow, 2002; Møller, 2013). The presence of HIV, including misunderstanding and stereotypes about the virus have been notably shaped by socio-cultural and political crises over leadership and management of the disease represented by former President Mbeki's AIDS denialism (see Geffen, 2010; Kalichman, 2009; Lawson, 2007; Mbali, 2013; Nattrass, 2007). AIDS denialism produced much confusion about the biomedical 'truth' of HIV and AIDS and restricted antiretroviral medications in public state hospitals and centred on the belief, contradicted by conclusive medical and scientific evidence that HIV does not cause AIDS during the period 1999–2008. Where politicians such as Mbeki sowed doubt about the existence of the virus, he sought out scientists (the so-called aids dissidents) to support his view. Public health researchers have attributed 330,000–340,000 AIDS-related deaths, along with 171,000 other HIV infections and 35,000 infant HIV infections, to the South African government's former embrace of HIV/AIDS denialism (see Chigwedere et al., 2008; Nattrass, 2008). Upon becoming president in 2008, Mbeki's successor, Kgalema Motlanthe, appointed Barbara Hogan as health minister to replace Tshabalala-Msimang on the 1st day of his presidency. Hogan told *The New York Times*, "The era of denialism is over completely in South Africa" (Dugger, 2008). The period of significant change that closed the chapter on AIDS Denialism was sustained into the Jacob Zuma Presidency (2009–2018).[2]

[2]It should be noted that the Zuma presidency was riddled, beyond the accusations of corruption related to state entities and resources, by much controversy, in part related to HIV and AIDS. In the preceding 2 years leading to his appointment as president of the African National Congress, he was charged with rape in the Johannesburg High Court on 6 December 2005. On 8 May 2006, the Court dismissed the charges, agreeing that the sexual act in question was consensual. During the rape trial in 2006 Zuma told the court during cross-examination (he was accused of raping Fezekile Ntsukela Kuzwayo (known in court proceedings 'Khwezi'), an HIV positive woman that

Prevention and treatment therefore remain the two core challenges for the South African government in responses that entail improvements to the quality of life of citizens with respect to HIV. These challenges abound in South African society and inspite of the availability of antiretroviral therapy and many awareness campaigns that promote treatment literacy and awareness, deep-seated stigmatisation remains. These are shaped in part by struggles over gendered and patriarchal attitudes towards transfer modes (modes of transmission) and infection modes (modes of infections) which the person with HIV draws as a victim. In this tension, it appears that the human catastrophe and the human stories remain forgotten as Ndebele (2004: 9) notes that "the intimate ways in which people across all communities are being affected with HIV/AIDS are all too often lost" (2004: 9). Stories about HIV infection and AIDS especially in the media is concentrated on the anxiety or the so-called 'moral panic' within society. However, statistical data alone is not sufficient to represent the actual experiences of those whose existence are affected by HIV. Therefore, the questions arise as to how human experiences are shaped in relation to the virus, as well as experiences regarding living with the virus, and further, what the narrative reveals about the construction of self.

12.4 Positioning Genre

As a term which may be traced to the beginning of the eighteenth century, autobiography as a word is shaped by three Greek root terms *autos* (self) + *bios* (life) + *graphe* (to write), translating into *self-life-writing*, which as Olney (1980: 6) argues existed as literary phenomenon as memoirs and confessions. Memoirs demonstrate some affiliation to autobiography, except that members of an elite grouping (such as generals and eminent judges) often write it and earned the label of being an aristocratic genre. In autobiography, *personality* is primary, *history* is secondary and there is a privileging of the *autos* and *bios* of the autobiographical act over the *graphe.* In earlier studies, Pascal (1960) analyses autobiography as a narrative deployment of symbolic personality, which is based on truth as a central design. Olney (1972) maintains that autobiography is a structured "ideal act" (20) that gives rise to "symbolic man" (318). For Bruss (1976) autobiography is a performative act that works with speech acts. For Weintraub (1978: 4) the concept of individuality is a distinctive quality to create a modern self-image. For Egan (1984) autobiography shows mythic correspondences to childhood, youth and maturity with an emphasis on the evolutionary pattern of the autobiographical self. For Stone (1982: 4) autobiography is a creative act of "re-inventing a plausible and satisfying history" of the self. For Easkin (1985) autobiography is a mode of self-invention with the self being a fictive structure at the centre of the narrative. For Jongeneel (1989) autobiography assesses the historical and the generic in relation to fiction, history and society. Moreover, for Kerby (1991) autobiography is about language and persons, and the various ways in which narration gives meaning to the self. Central in these studies is the premium placed on the self. Biography on the other is the interpretation of another's life story (Broughton, 2006; Chansky & Hipchen, 2016).

Kruger (1996) formulates two types of narratives about AIDS in which perspectives are taken about the disease: one is what he calls 'microcosmic narrative', in which the individual's life story is depicted; the other he calls 'macroscosmic' which according to him is an epidemiological or population narrative which allow the focus to fall on the historical course of the epidemic. I focus on the microcosmic narrative where the 'autos' (self) and "bios" (life) provide not only an accounting of the self or a meticulous self-

he showered rather than worn a condom to ward off the risk of HIV. The statement revealed that Zuma had been taking regular HIV tests, and for him showering entailed a form of hygiene, keeping clean that held the prospect of risk reduction which goes against the grain of scientific evidence. Inspite of his views Zuma supported disclosure and launched several scaled-up counselling and testing campaigns to stem the spread of the epidemic during his presidency. See also Motsei (2007), Reddy and Potgieter (2006), and Suttner (2009).

directed attitude, but also the 'events' that shape the construction of the self are described in terms of a special history of the self. Underlining autobiographical narrative is a form of protest against AIDS, which must apply to a degree of discomfort. By this I mean that the aids narrative (again, the *autos* and the *bios*) who are painted against the background of events about the self, are activated as a form of resistance to so-called dominant discourses such as cultural traditions, nation, race, family structure, friendship, gender, biomedical discourses and so on.

A striking aspect of writing about AIDS, particularly texts that offer a perspective from the viewpoint of the HIV-positive subject is that the narrative not only constitutes the matter of AIDS as a public matter of ideology and representation, but also how the disease as an internalised personal event of the subject, supports the narrative. This idea is not new, and can also be traced back to narratives about other diseases such as cancer, also the investigation of the social role of disease (in fact, there is an extensive literature on disease as literature; see Brody, 2003; Gerhardt, 1989; Herzlich & Pierret, 1988; Lupton, 1994; O'Leary, 2002; Sontag, 1988). Disease is traditionally interpreted as a form of punishment (for example in the work of Sontag (1989) and Sander Gillman, 1988). Sontag (1989: 93) ascribes the 'metaphoric trappings' of AIDS to its status as a not-yet-understood disease, as according to her "[e]ven the disease most fraught with meaning can just become an illness".

Often this narrative underscores blame. Moreover, in the AIDS narrative, just as in the broader illness narrative, there is a point where illness stimulates the sick subject to construct disease as it is experienced and stands in stark contrast to the clinical medical illness report which Arthur Frank (1991) described as 'the voice of medicine' versus the 'voice of life' (see also Frank, 1995). In the case of narratives about AIDS, the disease is often framed as the foundation of guilt, while the AIDS patient is the accused. In the case of a person with AIDS, it is often the case that HIV infection is aligned to the idea that the contamination is the result of unsafe sex emanating from cultures of prejudice and stigma. The association is further connected to misconceptions about sexual practice deriving from perceptions about excess, promiscuity and decadent behaviour leading to infection. In the case of gay men, the pathologisation is the strongest, shaped in part by moral judgements located in homophobic and patriarchal understanding about the AIDS diagnosis.

The project of memory, and to remember, is central to discourses about AIDS. Constructions of the self in narrative accounts indicate that knowledge about the self navigates the need for correctives and counter perspectives about life and living with HIV that are shaped by memory and grief. The texts offer complex rhetorical and ethical questions about living with HIV and work against dominant discourses such as homophobia, racism and sexism that shape the representation of AIDS. Writing about AIDS in cultural accounts challenge so-called master narratives as singular truths. In her discussion of AIDS losses, social identity, and grief in *The Psychic Life of Power*, Butler sketches how feelings of grief, fear and ambivalence simultaneously produces the desire for victory (triumph). Butler (1997: 29) asks: "How might we begin to imagine the contingency of that organisation (or social life), and performatively reconfigure the contours of the incorporate life? ". What is relevant for Butler is the question about how people negotiate the social conditions of identity against the background of social norms. These narratives comment on issues such as belonging, and work deliberately and against strategies of eradication and exclusion, and forgetting that may come with the possibility of stigma, prejudice and ultimately erasure. In this sense, the texts work toward countering dehumanisation and silence. I turn to selected texts in the following section.

12.5 The Texts in This Analysis

In February 2000, the South African Ministry of Health published a collection of stories titled *Living Openly: HIV positive South Africans tell their stories* (Department of Health). The publication features 32 stories that feature the disclosures of HIV positive people across race, class and gender lines. The cover shows a collage of black and white close-ups of people (together with their photos) whose stories and images represent what can be termed autofiction. Each photo carries the suggestion of an intimate (perhaps a leisured and relaxed image) of people who would otherwise be known to be healthy and unencumbered by disease if the narratives that accompany them do not disclose the information. We are also informed by the editors of this collection that this publication "is about the experiences of people who have publically declared their HIV status" (Department of Health, 2000: 1). The key word is *experience* as it is this that is to be recovered. These published stories place HIV and the AIDS diagnosis as central to individuation, where each person's existential sense of belonging is enacted in the act of disclosure. Disclosure helps to navigate a pathway to improve the quality of life. In some respects the type of disclosure framed in this collection is similar to confession (a form of self-examination centralised around some form of truth about the self), a known mode of writing as a precursor to what today is designated as autobiography. This is especially true when one considers Foucault (1990) who illuminates the link between confession and autobiography. There is some relevance to the claim by Foucault (1990: 59–60) that confession represents an individual who attempts to extract "from the depths of oneself", "in the self-examination", the "truth" of the "basic certainties of consciousness". In this sense the "obligation to confess" in this publication of HIV positive stories represents an act of countering silence by disclosing a secret truth that has to be surfaced.

In this collection focusing on living positively with HIV we are dealing with a type of autobiographical AIDS narrative where people resist death and dying. There is a clear desire to live, for presence, for hope. *Living Openly: HIV positive South Africans tell their stories* invokes classical forms and traditions of autobiography as narratives of revelation and conversion. Reworking a history of forced confession, coming out has expressed the political and historical moment of early gay liberation. I preface four extracts from the life stories that speak to the importance of the healing effects of countering silence in the context of disclosure.

Brett Anderson-Terry (Department of Health, 2000: 7) was diagnosed in March 1999 and disclosed a week after his diagnosis:

> For me, talking about my status was my saving grace. I'm expecting the day that some ignorant idiot will say something rude to me, but I think South Africa is finally waking up to the disease. As much as I don't believe in notification, I do believe that South Africans do need to get ready for people to start talking. The only way that that is going to happen is for people to realize that disclosure is a healing process. To come out and take control of the disease rather than letting the disease take control of you. Your life doesn't necessarily have to change and you just wait to die. I'm not planning on dying for a long time.

Martin Vosloo (Department of Health, 2000: 29) was diagnosed in 1990 and disclosed in 1997:

> The more that I speak about it, the less I worry about it. If you keep this to yourself, I think it contributes to you dying sooner. From that time that I started speaking openly about it, I really experienced an improvement in my health. I'm not sick. I'm never sick, yet I'm HIV positive.

Valencia Mofokeng (Department of Health, 2000: 53) was diagnosed in 1998 and disclosed in September 1998:

> When I was diagnosed with HIV I was angry, and for the first time in my life I thought of suicide. I thought maybe if I died, things would be better for my son. After a few weeks, I realized I was making a big mistake because my two older daughters also needed me. So I decided it was better to live and teach people how to live with AIDS.

Portia Yalezo (Department of Health, 2000: 57) was diagnosed in 1992 and disclosed in 1997:

> In 1997 I started going out and telling people that I was HIV positive because people don't know that a person with HIV can live for a long time. I thought if I came out as a young person, they will change too and they will learn to tell their parents. They will learn to accept that HIV is not a death sentence.

The above passages highlight a preoccupation with the experiences of public declarations about HIV status associated with openness, courage and meanings about infection that were hidden markers of embodiment. The language of the disclosure direct the readers' attention to the urgency to prioritise openness over silence. These attributes, namely openness over silence; voice over silence, are navigational markers that help mediate and moderate a more meaningful life.

Suffering in Silence by Xoliswa Busakwe (2004) is a short life story about a 30 year old South African domestic worker living in Cape Town. Through no fault of her own she contracts AIDS. The title of the text discloses the ambiguities of living with HIV centred mainly on cultures of secrecy and shame; and hence the title is in large measure ironic. By speaking about the life, the story disrupts the silences around AIDS. The text is structured in six chapters, each offering a specific perspective on people in Xoliswa's life, such as her mother, sister, her friends, her doctor, and her boss, Mary. The story assigns sharp criticism about culture, by debunking stigmatising stereotypes that describe the AIDS patient, the refusal to discuss any sexuality in the black culture, and gendered issues in a strong patriarchal environment. In the opening chapter Xoliswa describes her feelings when she receives her results for her AIDS test: "He gently breaks the news, and the bottom line is that I have AIDS [...] I reach home and I am angry, I want to kill my boyfriend; He is the only man in my life" (2004: 14–15).

The passage illustrates the emotional and psychological effect of the initial response to an HIV test diagnosis, followed by the accompanying anger over the realisation of her partner's infidelity towards her. The gendered implication of the diagnosis suggests that black women especially are often framed as the dangerous AIDS carriers. Black women are perceived as the source of diseases, and which further implies that women are viewed as the cause of contamination. Xoliswa's words, 'he was the only man in my life' is a further illustration that she was not the source of disease, echoing Crimp's (1988) earlier formulation that women are a group of innocent victims, except in this instance, in Africanised settings, women are also perceived as guilty perpetrators and carriers of disease.

In the subsequent chapter of her life story, she speaks out about her fear of death and the possibility of estrangement from her family and friends: "I am alone, the fear of dying alone is killing me. If I had cancer, I would be able to tell the whole world. I don't want to lose my friends and family [...]" (2004: 15). Her thoughts highlight why there is such a strong culture of silence around AIDS, since the disclosure of her status leads to alienation and discrimination.

Beyond the above publication, other texts have also shed light on aspects of living with HIV in varying contexts in the South African landscape. The biography titled *Khabzela: The Life and Times of a South African* (McGregor, 2005) provides a compelling account of Fana Khaba (affectionately known as Khabzela), a black Johannesburg-based disc jockey at Yfm radio. Soon after learning about his HIV status, around May 2003, he publicly announced on his show telling listeners that he was HIV positive and that he needed time to heal and recover. He disclosed his HIV status in a recorded message aired as an insert on the station's breakfast programme in April 2003 after he had been off air for a while:

> Guys, I'm sick, very sick. I've taken some bit of rest. And I went to see a doctor to see why I'm always tired. I thought it might be stress-related because I'm working all the time. The doctor told me that I'm HIV positive. I took that bad because I always preach protection every Sunday at PYT. Well, mistakes like those happen in life. I'm asking for your support, guys. Thank you to Greg. Thank you to Dirk. Thank you to Dre. Thank you to Mama. Thank you to Sibongile for taking care of me. Support all the time. If you can see me, I've gained some weight. Thanks for the support, guys. I will be back on the show. This is my show. All I need is support.

At this point Khaba was very ill and rejected ART on the ground that he believed antiretrovirals were dangerous and likely to kill him despite the fact that he was middle class and had access to private medical care. His employer even purchased the first supply of ART that he took for several weeks and then stopped. Instead, he undertook his own journey for alternative healing technologies, largely 'traditional' medicines from traditional healers and quack remedies. One of the key people who treated him was a woman called Tine van der Maas, who was sent personally by the Minister of Health at the time and treated him with a diet programme made up of amongst others, lemon juice and olive oil while his CD4 count was only 2 and while he was living with full-blown AIDS. He was severely ill at the time, and McGregor (2005: 7) describes the condition of his death and dying:

> Fana Khaba died a horrible death. The HI virus had destroyed his brain, leaving him demented and hallucinatory. He could no longer move his arms or legs. He could neither defecate nor urinate. The colostomy bag attached to his bowel to drain his waste was leaking blood. Pus seeped from the wound left by the operation to remove his intestines. A vast bedsore had eaten away his right buttock. More bedsores festered on his back, hips, ankles and elbows. It must have been a relief to him when, at 12.10 on January 14, 2004, he finally stopped breathing.

Khaba's story also reflects the context of the political moment during which the South African government was agonising over acceding to the pressure of civil society to provide life-prolonging medication to people living with AIDS in the public health sector. Khabzela's life story is located in the heart of the AIDS Denialist period and is in several ways an account that reflects what we could label as treatment failure, silence and denial. His story provides some marked contrasts to the life narratives of other South Africans to which we turn.

In *AIDSAFARI: A Memoir of my Journey with AIDS*, Levin (2005), a white gay man chronicles his struggle to survive with the daily trials of living with AIDS. Diagnosed HIV positive in July 2003 Levin engages his promiscuity, denial and terrors of mortality. He writes about castigating himself for thinking in the past that somehow he would be immune to the virus even while engaging in unsafe sex. The text details the progression of the disease and reflects the experiences and emotions about how his health deteriorated into full-blown AIDS and the opportunistic battles encountered with various ailments, not the least of which were debilitating neuropathy, losing his teeth, cancer, and tuberculosis. Levin (2005: 205) expresses the physical and psychological pain experienced:

> I'll tell you something, mate, it's one damn pain in the tummy, the neck, the feet and the ass, this thing they call AIDS. ... When I wonder if it's really worth all the drama ... then I remember the other possibility: Not living with it. Not living at all.

Levin (a journalist and cultural critic) explains that he coined the title of this memoir based on his journeys through Africa doing research for an earlier book on African art: "I realized that the hardest, most frightening safari of all had been ... the journey in my head and through every aching nerve in my body. The journey inside" (2005: xii). In other words, the journey within about life and love forms a neat backdrop to the physical toll on the body. Levin (2005: x) also explains that when he first became ill, he looked for books that might help him but found none, and he hopes that his memoir "helps to chip away at a single brick of that immense wall of silence". Deep into the text, Levin (2005: 226) indicates, "It doesn't matter if you are HIV-positive or negative" because "the world has AIDS. And if you give a shit about the world, you have it too."

Levin explains as a white homosexual the response he received by his family members and friends, how he was rejected by his illness, about his loneliness and his suffering, and with the use of antiretroviral drugs antitrust laws how he reconstructed his life.

Positively Alive by Alan Brand (2005) is a memoir written to be an inspirational text. Brand lives openly with his HIV status and uses his personal life story to break the silence and change the mind-set of those who he meets. Brand is a middle-aged and divorced man with two adult daughters who has been living as a gay man for many years. He learned of his HIV status in 1997 (leaving his doctor's room in shock) and shortly thereafter he met his life partner, Johan. He worked as a district manager for a national catering company, and was later appointed group national HIV/AIDS manager for the same company. His memoir contains information and advice about adopting a holistic approach to the disease combined with experiences both before and after his diagnosis. The second half of the text is dedicated to diary entries from June 2004 to June 2005 derived from an online AIDS diary project in which he participated (Brand, 2005: 21):

> I decided to remain silent about my status until I was ready to deal with it. I knew I needed information but didn't know where to find it. Information about HIV/AIDS was mostly about prevention and was based on frightening people into using condoms. I already knew I should have practiced safe sex. I was well informed about the risk of HIV and that I would die of AIDS. This information was useless at this point of my life. But every poster and pamphlet seems intent on propagating this type of fear-based information. Information about living with HIV was difficult to attain. I felt that if I asked for help, people would suspect that I had HIV.

In an interview over 10 years later, Brand (2016) had the following to say on reflecting about breaking his silence and disclosure of his status:

> Today there is still a taboo about the subject of HIV and AIDS, but back in 1997 the subject was even more "in the dark". Most of the information that was available was aimed at scaring people into using condoms and preventing the transmission of the infection, rather than being useful on what to do if you have it. If I had asked for information, that would have signalled to others (and to myself) that I had HIV – and I wasn't ready for that. So I kept quiet, which I think is what many people still do, but that has dire consequences.

The text is equally designed as a motivational humanising response to living with HIV by examining the way we treat others and ourselves and expresses the need for a united, compassionate response to those living with HIV.

Perhaps one of the most striking life stories about HIV is *Witness to Aids* (Cameron, 2005). The text charts the life of Edwin Cameron, a human rights lawyer and former South African judge in the appeal court (he now is a Judge in the Constitutional Court) and a well-known advocate for gay rights. In a profound engagement with the meanings of AIDS, Cameron (2005: 42) unknowingly also engages Treichler's "epidemic of signification". He draws attention to the rich array of meanings that cluster around the social, physical, moral and representational; directing the reader to the reality that in the end, AIDS is, as natural as, "the ocean and the moon" and nothing other than "a disease":

> AIDS is a disease. It is an infection, a syndrome, an illness, a disorder, a condition threatening to human life. It is an epidemic – a social crisis, an economic catastrophe, a political challenge, a human disaster. AIDS is known. It has been analysed assessed assayed tested measured surveyed considered reflected documented depicted exhaustively described. Its virus is primal particular subcellular mutant enveloped nitrogenous. Our knowledge of it is clear and precise. But the disease is also unknown. It is guessed, estimated, projected, approximated, sketched, debated, disputed, controverted, hidden, obscured. Still, it is mere fact: an event, a circumstance, a happening, a reality as present as the ocean or the moon. AIDS is mouth and tongue, and scar and nerve and eye and brain and skin and tum and gut. AIDS is smell and feel – of sweat and grime and snot and breath and bowel and secretion, discharge, pus, putrescence, disintegration, excrement, waste. Human waste. AIDS is feeling – painful sharp tingling burning heavy dull weakening wasting enervating diminishing destroying bereaving. AIDS is fear. It is breathless and nameless. AIDS is stigma, disgrace, discrimination, hatred, hardship, abandonment, isolation, exclusion, prohibition, persecution, poverty, privation. AIDS is metaphor. It is a threat a tragedy a blight a blot a scar a stain a plague a scourge a pestilence a demon killer rampant rampaging murderer. It is made moral. It is condemnation, deterrence, retribution, punishment, a sin a lesson a curse rebuke judgment. It is a disease.

The narrative is designed along the lines of overcoming a deep, personal and embedded sense of self-stigmatisation in a journey involving disclosure of his HIV status before going onto ART. His account is informed by poignant personal, social, medical, cultural and legal understanding of living with HIV. For Cameron the ambiguities of life necessitate a concomitant ethical duty, to be a witness to AIDS and an advocate for ART. The connections between treatment for AIDS and inequality remain a central metatext of his writing. He was one of the very few people who in 1997 underwent ART, and he reflects on his privileged middle class position that enabled this possibility.

The high cost of the stigma and denial that plague AIDS both in South Africa and Africa receive prominent attention, and he feels a strong moral obligation to speak out. "To survive AIDS," he says, "is to feel the joy of escape, and the elation of continued life. It is also to bear the duty to speak, and the responsibility to bear witness" (Cameron, 2005: 122). To bear witness, it will seem, is to take responsibility for the truth: to speak, explicitly within the legal pledge and the juridical imperative of the witness's oath (Felman & Laub, 1992: 204). Cameron (2005: 45) reminds the reader about this possibility for writing as the *raison d'etre* earlier in the text, namely to confront "shame, the humiliation or distress that arises from self-knowledge of dishonour or offence or impropriety or indecency". In other words to survive AIDS is to enter into an act of naming a set of conditions by confronting death and silence and to remain faithful to the urgency to develop a form of knowledge and truth about the self.

More than a life story, the text also provides a powerful historical reading of patent protection, stigma and the problem of AIDS denialism (a particular African form rooted in race and sexual shame). In response to the "agony of denialism" that enveloped South Africa in the context of the Mbeki administration, Cameron (2005: 155) says:

> I felt called to speak, and to speak out, and to challenge untruth and obfuscation in the debate about AIDS and its causes and to speak the truth about the proper treatment for AIDS. I did not feel I could or should remain silent.

Primo Levi prefaces the idea of silence earlier in the motto: "For these survivors, remembering is a duty. They do not want to forget, and take all they do not want the world to forget, because they understand that their experiences were not meaningless". In an interview Cameron (in Anthony, 2005: 17) said:

> I very carefully calculated my own voice [...] In this epidemic or so many millions, there are so few voices. In affluent North America and Western Europe, you have these loud, expressive voices. In Africa it's different. Poverty, stigma and discrimination, the linked or have muted the response. But I deliberately set out to speak at a very personal level, to find the hearts or a wide range of people.

The conclusion provides a poetic summary of his life with AIDS:

> I carry in me now, a memory like blood, the shock of my own diagnosis, the long years of muteness and secrecy, the fear of fleshly failure, the allies I harboured and therefore just that I refuse to forget. It's that I cannot. Remembering is in me, like blood. (Cameron, 2005: 214)

Inherent in this passage is an idea that a life with AIDS is a life presumed polluted by the virus. Infection it seems induces in some ways a further stimulant for identity, derived from visceral foundations, namely the physical and psychological changes that are caused by his disease, giving rise to a new form of identity. HIV and AIDS are therefore represented as a process where the health of the person living with HIV is measured in terms of seropositivity, in terms of physical signs and symptoms rather than anything else. This idea is initiated in the opening paragraph of the narrative: "I knew I had AIDS when I could no longer climb the stairs from the judge's common room [...] My energy seemed to have drained from my legs. I was perspiring grey exhaustion. My lungs felt waterlogged. My mouth rough and dry. No pain. Just overwhelming weariness" (Cameron, 2005: 9).

We note in this passage the debilitating effects of the virus and an estrangement and alienation experienced between the struggle to live while confronting simultaneously the debilitating symptoms of physical degradation and violation of the body. In Cameron's (2005: 17) case the physical damage in the earlier stages of his illness was connected to the fear to disclose HIV status:

> Each illness in turn weakens the body [...] All this I knew. [...] That I had reached the diagnostic point where I was not 'just' living with HIV – but that I actually had AIDS. And that without immediate, expert intervention I faced near-certain death.

Only the symptoms and physical signs of AIDS-related diseases are at stake here. The physical signs that refer to the dismantling of the body, focus the reader's attention on the scarring physical aspects of AIDS, on the person living with HIV's changed attitude towards the body and its relationship to society. In this reconstruction of the self there is simultaneously the rejection of death for the sake of the necessity to live: "To stop work would be to admit defeat. And admitting defeat meant death" (Cameron, 2005: 24).

Beyond the side effects of medication, the desire to live in the wake of physical limitations combines with Cameron's (2005: 38–39) recognition of the benefits of treatment in restoring the immune system, thereby giving him back the opportunity to renew life and living:

> But all this was quite trivial besides the growing realisation that something quite unmistakably dramatic was taking place within my body. My tiredness was lessening. It was disappearing. In its place, I could feel a daily access of miraculous new energy. Life forces were coursing through my body. Illness was yielding to a nearly novel feeling – renewed and joyful wellbeing.... I not only regained my appetite – despite the nausea the protease inhibitors induced when I took them, I became ravenously and continuously hungry. For the first time in months, my stomach was digesting food properly. And my gaunt body avidly claimed every morsel of it to make up for the twelve kilograms (twenty five pounds) in weight I had lost.
> There was only one word for it. It was glorious. The drugs were working. I could feel that I was getting healthy again. I knew that I would be well again. That, in tum, spurred my inner confidence. Physiological wellbeing had a pronounced psychic effect. If the drugs were working – and it was utterly clear they were – it meant that for the first time since my infection more than twelve years before, the virus was no longer multiplying within me. It was no longer progressively taking over my body, taking over my life. It was being beaten back to some deeply secluded (although latently dangerous) viral reservoirs. But outside these recesses, the rest of my body was free of it. And my immune system was, for the first time in all these years, free of its burdens.
> The feeling was exhilarating. For the first time in more than a decade I was no longer – no longer felt – contaminated. From the world I had little to hide, and less to fear.

Cameron's efforts through his writing and public appearances have made a significant contribution to advancing the case for ART in ways that advance the case for normalising HIV and AIDS rather than exceptionalising it (see Cameron, 2007). He reflects: "We have responded to the epidemic with silence; and our doing so has rendered it and those who suffer under it unspeakable. We have too often placed those suffering the effects of the virus beyond the reach of our embrace, beyond word and comfort and help and remedy (Cameron, 2005: 213).

12.6 Conclusions

'Humanising Silence' is perhaps a misnomer. Inherent in the phrase is the conjunction of two interrelated meanings: the idea of *being human* and the attributes of *being human*. Therefore to be human opens up the reality of being able to speak, to activate voice and articulate ideas and experiences of the self. Recourse to the social realities of living with HIV in African contexts indicate that there are other ways of countering social silences. The texts assembled in this chapter suggest that there are in fact nuanced ways of interpreting the meaning of disease and illness. HIV and AIDS are not just simply biomedical realities, but rather also embodied human life stories. The construction of self (and consequently the construction and declaration of identity through disclosure about HIV status) is formed in tandem with destigmatising metaphors. While varying and multiple in respect of the issues they represent the texts featured in this chapter mobilise the reconstruction of life beyond being a patient. Here we find resistance against the stigma in relation to various cultural, social and ethical codes. Life writing about HIV and AIDS provide perspectives on resisting silence when the virus infects. In this way, the idea is revealed, through processes of reflection and discovery of the self that the virus is not a punishment for moral offense, but rather that HIV is instead a stage in the disease process where certain silences are unmasked. These thoughts are presented as externalised memories of self-discovery to render identity as compatible with and integral to living with disease.

It seems plausible to conclude that in the broader context of the quality of life trends in South Africa, notably the subjective components (such as well-being, life satisfaction and happiness), that living standards, and by extension, quality of life has improved (Møller & Dickow, 2002) in the post-apartheid context. Møller (2013: 934) provides the following important evidence: "Between 2001 and 2010 the proportion of black South Africans with the highest living standard according to the Living Standards Measure increased from 3 to 19% [...] Some

52% of all South Africans were satisfied with life, 65% were happy and 51% felt life was getting better."

The fact that HIV is now generally controllable, and HIV management is centred more on the quality of life rather than simple survival, requires ongoing efforts to nevertheless curb stigma and discrimination. For people living with HIV this also entails controlling the impact of disease on their psychological, social and physical aspects of daily life. The power of the narratives featured in this chapter provide an entry point to suggest that there seems to be a healing effect in their acts of disclosure that has curative properties that enable coping with life, but also their ability to enable normalisation that leads to a fulfilling existence.

What is additionally striking about the representation of AIDS is the emphasis on the restoration of identity as a human being by focusing on hope, love, compassion and a new sense in (and about) life. Efforts to humanise silence are achieved by uncovering ways of speaking that resist human suffering, as well as countering perceptions of disease as punishment for a prior life. AIDS therefore in some ways – via the texts – rewrites the politics of life by directing readers to the relationship to biosecurity, self, sociality, integration, inclusion and belonging. Inspite of the taboos and realities that persist, writing AIDS authorises identities that defy silence, exclusion and invisibility. In this way, discourses of shame, suffering and perversion that normally cloud HIV are challenged and made audible.

References

Aggleton, P. (1989). *AIDS: Social representations, social practices*. Lewes, UK: Falmer Press.

Anderson, R. E. (2014). *Human suffering and quality of life: Conceptualizing stories and statistics*. New York, NY/London, UK: Springer.

Anthony, L. (2005). Force of the truth. *Sunday Times Lifestyle*, 1 May 17.

Attree, L. (Ed.). (2010). *Blood on the page: Interviews with African authors writing about HIV/AIDS*. Newcastle-upon-Tyne, UK: Cambridge Scholars Press.

Brand, A. (2005). *Positively alive, by Alan Brand*. Johannesburg, South Africa: Jacana Media.

Brand, A. (2016). *Alan Brand – living a life that is "positively Alive"*. https://www.cipla.co.za/medi-hub/cipla-people/alan-brand-living-life-positively-alive/. Accessed 4 Apr 2018.

Brody, H. (2003). *Stories of sickness* (2nd ed.). Oxford, UK: Oxford University Press.

Brophy, S. (2004). *Witnessing AIDS: Writing, testimony, and the work of mourning*. Toronto, Canada: University of Toronto Press.

Broughton, T. L. (Ed.). (2006). *Autobiography: Critical concepts in literary and cultural studies* (Vol. 4). London, UK: Routledge. 2006.

Bruss, E. (1976). *Autobiographical acts: The changing situation of a literary genre*. Baltimore, MD: John Hopkins University Press.

Busakwe, X. (2004). *Suffering in silence*. Durban, South Africa: New Generation Publishers.

Butler, J. (1997). *The psychic life of power: Theories in subjection*. Stanford, CA: Stanford University Press.

Cáceres, C. (2000). The production of knowledge on sexuality in the AIDS era: Some issues, opportunities, and challenges. In R. Parker, R. M. Barbosa, & P. Aggleton (Eds.), *Framing the sexual subject: The politics of gender, sexuality and power*. Berkeley, CA/Los Angeles, CA: University of California Press.

Cameron, E. (2005). *Witness to AIDS*. New York, NY: Palgrave Macmillan.

Cameron, E. (2007). Normalizing testing – Normalizing AIDS. *Theoria: A Journal of Social and Political Theory, 112*, 99–108.

Caron, D. (2001). *AIDS in French culture: Social ills, literary cures*. Madison, WI: The University of Wisconsin Press.

Chansky, R. A., & Hipchen, E. (Eds.). (2016). *The Routledge Auto|Biography Studies Reader* (Routledge Literature Readers). London, UK/New York, NY: Routledge. 2016.

Chigwedere, P., Seage, G. R., et al. (2008). Estimating the lost benefits of antiretroviral drug use in South Africa. *Journal of Acquired Immune Deficiency Syndromes, 49*(4), 410–415.

Coovadia, I. (2009). *High low in-between*. Cape Town, South Africa: Umuzi.

Crimp, D. (1988). *AIDS: Cultural analysis, cultural activism*. Cambridge, MA: MIT Press.

Dauenhauer, B. P. (1980). *Silence: The phenomenon and its ontological significance*. Bloomington, IN: Indiana University Press.

Department of Health. (2000). *Living openly: HIV positive South Africans tell their stories*. Pretoria, South Africa: Department of Health.

Dilger, H., & Luig, U. (Eds.). (2010). *Morality, hope and grief: Anthropologies of AIDS in Africa*. New York, NY: Berghahn.

Dow, U., & Essex, M. (2011). *Saturday is for funerals*. Cambridge, MA: Harvard University Press.

Dugger, C. W. (2008). Study cites toll of AIDS policy in South Africa. *The New York Times*, 25 November.

Eakin, J. P. (1992). *Touching the world: Reference in autobiography*. Princeton, NJ: Princeton University Press.

Easkin, J. P. (1985). *Fictions in autobiography: Studies in the art of self-invention*. Princeton, NJ: Princeton University Press.
Egan, S. (1984). *Patterns of experience in autobiography*. Chapel Hill: University of North Carolina Press.
Felman, S., & Laub, D. (1992). *Testimony: Crises of witnessing in literature, psychoanalysis, and history*. New York, NY: Routledge.
Foucault, M. (1990). *A history of sexuality: An introduction* (R. Hurley, Trans.). Harmondsworth, UK: Penguin.
Frank, A. W. (1991). *At the will of the body: Reflections on illness*. Boston, MA: Houghton Miffin.
Frank, A. W. (1995). *The wounded storyteller: Body, illness, and ethics*. Chicago, IL: University of Chicago Press.
Geffen, N. (2010). *Debunking delusions: The inside story of the treatment action campaign*. Johannesburg, South Africa: Jacana.
Gerhardt, U. (1989). *Ideas about illness: An intellectual and political history of medical sociology*. London: Macmillan.
Gillman, S. (1988). *Disease and representation: Images of illness from madness to AIDS*. Ithaca, NY: Cornell University Press.
Greene, M. F. (2005). *There is no me without you: One woman's odyssey to rescue Africa's children*. New York, NY: Bloomsbury.
Herdt, G. H., & Lindenbaum, S. (1992). *The time of AIDS: Social analysis, theory, and method*. Newbury Park, CA: Sage.
Herzlich, C., & Pierret, J. (1988). *Illness and self in society* (E. Forster, Trans.). Baltimore, MD: The John Hopkins University Press.
Jongeneel, E. (Ed.). (1989). *Over de Autobiografie*. Utrecht, The Netherlands: HES uitgevers.
Kalichman, S. (2009). *Denying AIDS: Conspiracy theories, pseudoscience, and human tragedy*. New York, NY: Copernicus Books.
Kellendonk, F. (1990). *Mystiek lichaam: een geschiedenis*. Amsterdam, The Netherlands: Meulenhof.
Kerby, A. P. (1991). *Narrative and self*. Bloomington, IN: Indiana University Press.
Koch, B. (2002). *In, around, through and out: An actor's life*. New York, NY: Spearhead Press.
Kruger, S. (1996). *AIDS narratives: Gender and sexuality, fiction and science*. New York, NY: Garland Press.
Lawson, L. (2007). *Side effects: The story of AIDS in South Africa*. Cape Town, South Africa: Double Storey.
Levin, A. (2005). *AIDSAFARI: A memoir of my journey with AIDS*. Cape Town, South Africa: Zebra Press.
Lupton, D. (1994). *Medicine as culture: Illness, disease and the body in Western societies*. London, UK: Sage.
Mbali, M. (2013). *South African AIDS activism and global health policies*. New York, NY: Palgrave Macmillan.
McGregor, L. (2005). *Khabzela: The life and times of a south African*. Auckland Park, South Africa: Jacarna Media.
Michalos, A. C. (2017). *Development of quality of life theory and it's instruments: The selected works of Alex C. Michalos*. New York, NY/London, UK: Springer.
Moele, K. (2009). *The book of the dead*. Cape Town, South Africa: Kwela Books.
Møller, V. (Ed.). (1997). *Quality of life in South Africa*. Dordrecht, The Netherlands: Kluwer.
Møller, V. (2007). Researching quality of life in a developing country: Lessons from the South African case. In I. Gough & J. A. McGregor (Eds.), *Wellbeing in developing countries: From theory to research* (pp. 242–258). Cambridge, UK: Cambridge University Press.
Møller, V. (2013). South African quality of life trends over three decades, 1980 – 2010. *Social Indicators Research, 113*(3), 915–940.
Møller, V., & Dickow, H. (2002). The role of quality of life surveys in managing change in democratic transitions: The South African case. *Social Indicators Research, 58*(1), 267–292.
Monette, P. (1988). *Borrowed time: An AIDS memoir*. San Diego, CA: Harcourt Brace Jovanovich.
Morgan, J., & the Bambanani Women's Group. (2003). *Long life: Positive HIV stories*. Cape Town, South Africa: ABC Press.
Motsei, M. (2007). *The kanga and the kangaroo court. Reflections on the rape trial of Jacob Zuma*. Auckland Park, South Africa: Jacana.
Mpe, P. (2001). *Welcome to our Hillbrow*. Pietermaritzburg, South Africa: University of Natal Press.
Murphy, T., & Poirier, S. (Eds.). (1993). *Writing AIDS: Gay literature, language, and analysis*. New York, NY: Columbia University Press.
Nattrass, N. (2007). *Mortal combat: AIDS denialism and the struggle for Antiretrovirals in South Africa*. Scottsville, VA: University of KwaZulu-Natal Press.
Nattrass, N. (2008). AIDS and the scientific governance of medicine in post-apartheid South Africa. *African Affairs, 107*(427), 157–176.
Ndbele, N. (2004). Preface. In N. Rasebotsa, M. Samuelson, & K. Thomas (Eds.), *Nobody ever said AIDS*. Cape Town, South Africa: Kwela Books.
Nolen, S. (2008). *Stories of AIDS in Africa*. New York, NY: Walker.
O'Leary, P. (2002). *Gnostic contagion: Robert Duncan and the poetry of illness*. Middletown, CT: Wesleyan University Press.
Odhiambo, E. A. (2017). *Auma's long run*. Minneapolis, MN: Carolrhoda Books.
Olney, J. (1972). *Metaphors of self: The meaning of autobiography*. Princeton, NJ: Princeton University Press.
Olney, J. (1980). *Autobiography: Essays theoretical and critical*. Princeton, NJ: Princeton University Press.
Parker, R. (2001). Sexuality, culture and power in HIV/AIDS research. *Annual Review of Anthropology, 20*, 163–179.
Pascal, R. (1960). *Design and truth in autobiography*. Cambridge, MA: Harvard University Press.

Picard, M. (1988). *The world of silence*. Washington, DC: Regnery Gateway.

Plummer, K. (1995). *Telling sexual stories: Power, intimacy and social worlds*. London: Routledge.

Plummer, K. (2001). *Documents of life 2: An invitation to a critical humanism* (2nd ed.). London, UK: Sage.

Ranger, T., & Slack, P. (Eds.). (1992). *Epidemics and ideas: Essays in the historical perception of pestilence*. Cambridge, UK: Cambridge University Press.

Rasebotsa, N., Samuelson, M., & Thomas, K. (Eds.). (2004). *Nobody ever said AIDS*. Cape Town, South Africa: Kwela Books.

Reddy, V. (2011). *AIDS review*. Pretoria, South Africa: Centre for the Study of AIDS, Sexuality & Gender.

Reddy, V., & Potgieter, C. (2006). 'Real men stand up for the truth': Discursive meanings in the Jacob Zuma rape trial. *Southern African Linguistics and Applied Language Studies, 24*(4), 511–521.

Rödlach, A. (2006). *Witches, Westerners, and HIV: AIDS and cultures of blame in Africa*. Walnut Creek, CA: Left Coast Press.

Sirgy, M. J. (2012). *The psychology of quality of life: Hedonic well-being, life satisfaction, and Eudaimonia* (2nd ed.). New York, NY/London, UK: Springer.

Sontag, S. (1988). *Illness as a metaphor*. New York, NY: Farrar, Straus and Giroux.

Sontag, S. (1989). *AIDS and its metaphors*. New York, NY: Farrar, Straus and Giroux.

Steinberg, J. (2008). *Sizwe's test: A young man's journey through Africa's AIDS epidemic*. New York, NY/London, UK/Toronto, Canada: Simon & Schuster.

Stone, A. E. (1982). *Autobiographical occasions and original acts: Versions of American identity from Henry Adams to Nate Shaw*. Philadelphia, PA: University of Pennsylvania Press.

Suttner, R. (2009). The Jacob Zuma rape trial: Power and African National Congress (ANC) masculinities. *NORA—Nordic Journal of Feminist and Gender Research, 17*(3), 222–236.

Tamale, S. (Ed.). (2011). *African sexualities: A reader*. Dakar, Senegal/Nairobi, Kenya/Oxford, UK: Pambazuka Press.

Treichler, P. A. (1999). *How to have a theory in an epidemic: Cultural chronicles of AIDS*. Durham, BC: Duke University Press.

Weeks, J. (1985). *Sexuality and its discontents: Meanings, myths and modern sexualities*. London, UK: Routledge and Kegan Paul.

Weintraub, K. J. (1978). *The value of the individual: Self and circumstance in autobiography*. Chicago, IL/London, UK: University of Chicago Press.

The Use of Support Groups to Facilitate Resilience and *Quality of Life* in Families Affected by HIV

13

Michelle Finestone

Abstract
HIV has a potentially detrimental effect on South African families. Families exposed to HIV are overwhelmingly single-parent families living in extreme poverty and exposed to high levels of violence. Caregivers do not only have to cope with being HIV positive and the stigma related to HIV, but they also have to manage as parents of vulnerable children. Children exposed to maternal HIV are vulnerable to develop long-term emotional and psychological difficulties. There is thus a definite need for meticulously researched, theory-based intervention programmes that recognize the importance of psychosocial needs and resilience of young children in order to enhance the quality of family life in South Africa. It is essential that families exposed to maternal HIV receive adequate support. The Kgolo Mmogo intervention support group programme was grounded in a systematic review of accrued evidence of compelling vulnerability and protective processes that tend to reduce the negative effects of parental HIV-infection. This intervention programme is resultant of the first African based randomised control trial for HIV affected caregivers and their young children attending support group sessions. The intervention provides empirical data from which community workers, researchers, and practitioners can tailor-make group sessions for the South African population and promote resilience in young children.

13.1 Introduction

Evidence from various studies indicate that HIV affected children have a higher propensity to display internalising and externalising problems, lower cognitive scores, developmental delays, attention deficit, increased sexual risk-taking behaviour and more exposed to abuse than non-affected peers (Arikawa, Rollins, Newell, & Becquet, 2016; Roux, Abrams, Nguyen, & Myer, 2016). Support to HIV positive parents and subsequent positive parenting may reduce these difficulties. There is, therefore, an increased need for culturally adapted interventions focussing on HIV-positive parenting (Goldberg & Short, 2016; Rochat, Netsi, Redinger, & Stein, 2017).

Knowledge of the psychosocial impact of maternal HIV on African children is limited and therefore also little is known of the traumatic effect of HIV on the psychological well-being of young children. Advanced life-saving medical treatment has the positive effect that parents live

M. Finestone (✉)
Department of Educational Psychology, Faculty of Education, University of Pretoria, Pretoria, South Africa
e-mail: michelle.finestone@up.ac.za

I. Eloff (ed.), *Handbook of Quality of Life in African Societies*, International Handbooks of Quality-of-Life, https://doi.org/10.1007/978-3-030-15367-0_13

longer than in the early days of HIV treatment and it is of vital importance that countries and researchers plan for psychological interventions to support children affected by parental HIV/AIDS. Literature places emphasis on rigorous research of maternal-child psychosocial interventions and interventions targeting positive parenting which can be implemented by careworkers in the community. The interventions need rigorous evaluation and have to be sustainable. Evaluations using a randomised control-group study design are scarce not only in Africa but also globally (Betancourt, Meyers-Okhi, Charrow, & Hansen, 2012; Boeving-Allen et al., 2014; Skerfving, Johansson, & Tobias, 2014).

13.2 Background

HIV and AIDS are not unique to South Africa, but it demands special attention as sub-Saharan Africa is the most affected region in the world by this pandemic. According to the 2013 UNAIDS report, the global infection rate for new HIV infections is approximately 2.3 million and 80% of these infections occur in sub-Saharan Africa (UNAIDS, 2012, 2013, 2016). In 2005 a North-South collaboration between researchers from Yale University and the University of Pretoria applied for an NIH grant to develop an intervention to promote resilience in young children affected by maternal HIV and AIDS. A randomised control trial followed with pre- and post-measures of the theory-based support intervention. This was the first study in South Africa that endeavoured to provide empirical evidence of the impact of a caregiver and child group intervention for children affected by maternal HIV (Eloff et al., 2014) The participants were selected from a group of women who were enrolled in an earlier HIV-focused study[1] of children aged three and HIV-infected caregivers with children in the age range of 6–10 years and who were referred to hospitals and clinics in the resource-poor communities in Pretoria, South Africa. The participants enrolled for the study included 32 caregivers with children aged 3 years old and 429 caregivers with children aged 6–10 years.

The caregivers and their children were randomly assigned to the treatment group or interview-only group. A comparison group of 118 age- and gender-matched children (3 years and 6–10 years old) of non-HIV infected caregivers were identified from the same sites in the same communities. In 2007 a pilot study of two caregiver and children groups preceded the main intervention study (Forsyth, 2005).

The primary objectives of this study were specified as: "indicate the psychosocial effects of parental HIV disease on young children in South Africa (3-year-old and 6 to 10-year-old children); to assess the effectiveness of a theory-based support intervention for caregivers and their children; and to identify maternal, medical and psychological factors and child-related mediating variables that contributed to adaptive functioning of children with HIV-infected caregivers" (Forsyth, 2005).

The hypotheses of the Promoting Resilience in Young Children Study were stated as:

> Hypothesis 1: Children of HIV-infected women have significantly decreased adaptive functioning when compared to children of mothers who are not HIV-infected.
> Hypothesis 2: A structured support intervention for HIV-infected mothers that includes support groups, home visiting for those who are ill, and parenting education that focuses on promoting resilience, results in improved adaptive functioning among children in both age groups.
> Hypothesis 3: Strengths of HIV-infected women, such as increased self-esteem and positive coping, promote more positive adaptive functioning among their children and this positive effect is most evident among pre-school-aged children. Furthermore, as a woman's medical condition improves following the initiation of antiretroviral therapy, the adaptive functioning of her child also improves (Forsyth, 2005, p. 7)

[1] Serithi project. It refers to a previous NIH-funded study concerning prevention of mother to child HIV transfer (PMTC).

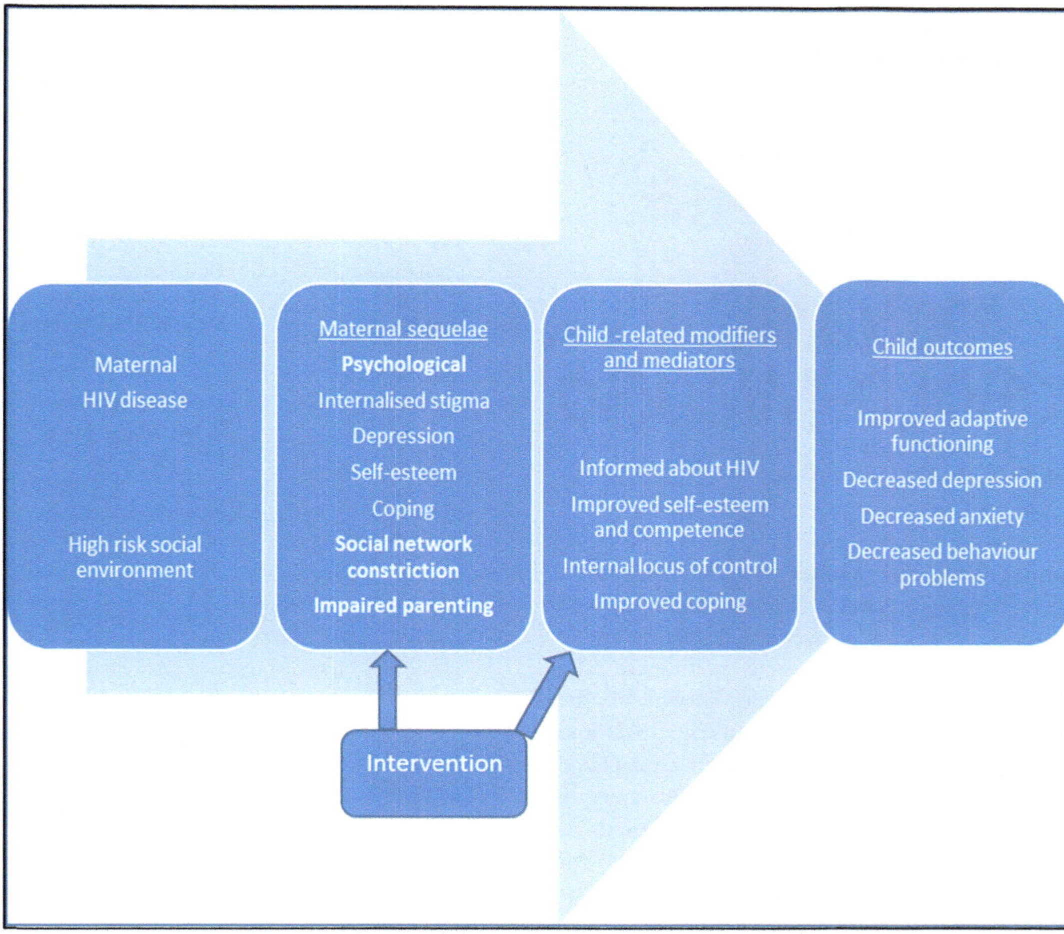

Fig. 13.1 The conceptual model underlying the support group intervention study. (Forsyth, 2005. Promoting resilience in young children of HIV-infected mothers in South Africa. Research Proposal submitted to the National Institutes of Health, April 2005)

The conceptual model for the intervention was modelled on resilience theories[2] and included elements of culturally appropriate interventions previously used in other African communities.

Van Breda and Theron (2018) advocate the importance for enhancing the resilience of young children in order to buffer them against the negative effects of adversity. The focus on resilience becomes especially important in the South African context with its high levels of structural disadvantage. The theory-based conceptual model (refer to Fig. 13.1), as architected by Forsyth (2005), regards maternal HIV/AIDS and insecure social milieus as risk indicators for negative child behaviour outcomes. The intervention focused on the provision of support to caregivers regarding the psychological effects of the disease, identified as diminished social support due to the accompanying stigma, increased the occurrence of depression, poor self-esteem and avoidant coping. It also focussed on the enhancement of the caregiver's ability to

[2] The Promoting Resilience in Young Children Intervention was based on the resilience and coping theories of Baldwin.

Fig. 13.2 The Kgolo Mmogo logo

communicate and interact with her child in an age-appropriate manner. This action was aimed at ultimately improving the child's adaptive functioning and to promote resilience. The intervention sessions became known as the *Kgolo Mmogo* sessions (refer to Fig. 13.2) and referred to as such by the group participants and careworkers. *Kgolo Mmogo* is translated in English from the African language Sepedi as 'We grow together'. A logo was developed for the sessions and used to guide participants to the session sites. Participants were more willing to attend a group session referring to resilience and growth. This reference also protected the caregivers' HIV positive status and therefore enhanced group participation.

13.3 Intervention Manual

A 6-month intervention was developed where HIV-positive women and their children engaged in a structured support group intervention that concentrated on the enhancement of child resilience. The intervention was presented in a group support format (Forsyth, 2005). In total, 12 groups of caregivers and their children partook in the intervention support sessions. There were on average eight participants in each wave who attended the support groups (Table 13.1).

Table 13.1 A summary of the Kgolo Mmogo intervention manual for mothers and children (6 to 10-year-olds)

Separate sessions (sessions 1–14)			
Caregiver intervention sessions		**Child intervention sessions (6–10 years)**	
1.	Introduction, orientation, and relationships of trust	1.	Introduction, orientation, and relationships of trust
2.	Living positively "How do I look after myself?" (Basic HIV and Aids info)	2.	Developing relationships within the group "Let's get to know each other"
3.	Disclosure	3.	Describe self and self in the family "Let's get to know each other"
4.	HIV and relationships	4.	Describe self and family within the community "My community"
5.	The emotional experience of having HIV "how do I feel?"	5.	Identify strengths within self "What do I look like? I have. I am. I can!"
6.		6.	Identify coping that is linked to strengths identified "What can I do/what am I good at?"
7.	Coping, problem-solving and stress management	7.	Problem-solving "How can I do it?"
8.	HIV in the household, human rights, and stigma	8	Protecting self and identifying boundaries "Protecting myself"
9.	Knowing and understanding myself as a parent (parenting skills)	9.	Social skills "Socialising with peers"
10.		10.	Identifying emotions (focus on self) "How do I feel?"
11.	Knowing and understanding my child (development of children)	11.	Identifying emotions (focus on others and communication) "How do others feel?"
12.		12.	Survival skills "Look and learn"
13.	My child and HIV	13.	Survival skills "Let's practice our skills"
14.	Life planning and goal setting	14.	Identifying meaning, purpose and future orientation "Let's live life"

(continued)

Table 13.1 (continued)

Joint sessions (sessions 15–24)			
15.	Caregiver and child getting to know each other		
16.	"Knowing me, knowing you"		
17.			
18.	Creating a legacy "Let's make a family memory"		
19.			
20.	The interaction between mother and child "Let's		
21.	have fun"		
22.	Caregiver sessions revised "Where are we at know"	22	Child sessions revised "Where are we at know"
23.	Planning for the future "Let's dream together"		
24.	Family celebration "Let's celebrate life"		

The complete Kgolo Mmogo manual is available at https://www.up.ac.za/en/faculty-of-education/article/1971976/upyale-project

13.4 Design and Content of the Support Group Intervention

The intervention was initially developed for the HIV positive caregivers and their 6 to 10-year-old child who was randomly selected for the intervention study. The intervention was tailor-made for latent phase children. The initial intervention design proposed a childminder to take care of the younger children during the support sessions. In the pilot phase, it became clear that this was not a feasible design. Caregivers were unable to leave their children at a guardian and there were safety risks involved for leaving their children in other's care. Therefore it was common practice during the support sessions for caregivers to bring all their children along for the sessions. The intervention had to adapt to the larger number of attending children to ensure the safety of attendees and positive experiences for all. The researchers subsequently developed an additional intervention programme for the 3 to 5-year-old children attending the groups with their mothers as it was felt that this opened up an opportunity for intervention.

13.4.1 Culturally Relevant and Accepted Manual Content by the Community

The intervention sessions were planned to be culturally relevant for the specific community in which it was implemented. In the pilot phase some of the activities had to be amended or replaced for this particular reason. A board game for children was initially incorporated in the sessions. It depicted among other objects pictures of fairies and magicians. These characters caused anxiety as they are equated with witchcraft in the community. They were replaced by more appropriate figures. Some of the stories the children could not relate to and they had to be changed to be culturally more relevant. The reference to animals in the stories made it more acceptable to the intended audience. Children showed difficulty in understanding some of the more abstract constructs that were not part of their frame of reference such as future orientated exercises. These exercises were made more relevant by placing them in the children's context such as referring to a situation where the children imagined a 'future taxi'.

As many of the caregivers did not disclose their HIV status to their children, all reference to HIV or AIDS were removed from the group session content. The memory box exercise where caregivers leave tangible objects or memories for their children, left some of the caregivers distressed. The activity was then renamed as 'a family legacy' exercise and both the caregiver and child contributed to the contents of the memory box.

Two culturally played games were included in the intervention namely *morabaraba* and *masekitlana. Morabaraba* was a game used during the joint sessions where the caregivers and their children could engage with each other by playing a board game. *Masekitlana* is a traditional game played with stones and chosen as projection method during the children's intervention sessions. The game is also known as the

Table 13.2 A summary of the manual for the 3 to 5-year-old child intervention sessions

Separate child intervention sessions (3 to 5-year-olds)	
1.	The cognitive domain "This is the way I think"
2.	The emotional domain "This is the way I feel"
3.	The social domain "This is the way I play"
4.	The physical domain "This is the way I move"
5.	The spiritual domain "This is the way I believe"
6.	The conative domain "This is the way I want"
Joint sessions	
15–24	Join caregiver and older child groups for joint sessions

'talking stones game'. Each stone gets a role and name of a family member. The child then acts out roles in their real-life family and life experiences while knocking the stones together.

13.4.2 Intervention Sessions for the 3–5 Year Child Groups

The intervention sessions for the 3 to 5-year-old children (see Table 13.2) were initially not indicated in the original planning of the intervention study, but the need for young child care necessitated the design of a separate manual to engage constructively with them. The goals for the sessions were to assess and support young children's resilience. The basic coping skills of the 3 to 5-year-olds were explored in order to determine their level of resilience. Individual assets and skills of each individual child were identified in order to conceptualise their resilience. Potential areas that could be stimulated in order to enhance their resilience was subsequently identified. An additional aim for the sessions was to provide support and knowledge to caregivers to assist their children to cope with adversity. The manual guided the separate sessions and each session stretched over more than 1 day to accommodate individual developmental differences. Time for free play was also indicated in the manual. The younger children joined their mothers and siblings in the joint sessions. The children who were younger than 3 years old were either accommodated in the young children group or they attended with their mothers in the group.

13.4.3 Intervention Sessions for the 6–10 Year Child Groups

The intervention sessions for the 6 to 10-year-old children (see Table 13.1) incorporated content that was purposefully selected to enhance the children's resilience and subsequent adaptive behaviour.

Each session was designed to incorporate the following themes:

1. Coping
   (a) Coping with stress
   (b) Coping with life challenges
   (c) Engaging with stress in an adaptive manner
2. Optimism
   (a) To reinforce children's positive behaviour
   (b) Encourage optimistic and hopeful statements and behaviours
   (c) Encourage positive future perspectives
3. Emotional Intelligence
   (a) Naming and identifying emotions
   (b) Appropriate expression of own emotions
   (c) Appropriate responses to other's emotions
4. Social Skills
   (a) Reinforce appropriate social skills demonstrated in sessions
      (i) Sharing
      (ii) Communication
      (iii) Support of peers/group members
5. Identifying meaning and purpose (Finestone, 2013).

Every session had furthermore a repetitive order where it started with a 'feeling thermometer' and 'climbing up and down the tree' exercise to indicate the beginning and end of each session. The 'feeling thermometer' exercise was particularly important for the careworkers to gauge the emotional level of the group members before each session. Homework related to the topic of the group session was indicated after each session and the caregivers and children were encouraged to work together to complete the tasks.

The children groups were designed to complement the caregiver sessions and to empower them to cope with their caregiver's illness. Although caregivers generally did not disclose their HIV positive status to their children before the intervention, many of the children indicated that they experience anxiety or know their caregivers are ill. The group had to first learn to trust one another and to get to know each other before self-discovery could occur. They then had an opportunity to explore their roles and strengths in their families. Problem-solving skills and self-protection awareness were taught in the groups. Emphasis was additionally placed on the development of emotional intelligence with reference to the identification of feelings, expression of feelings and socialisation. Practical skills were taught to the children to support them for the possibility of parental illness and their role in the household. The children's separate sessions concluded with an exercise to help them to set goals for their future.

The group activities were carefully chosen for the children sessions to be developmentally appropriate and engaging. Role-play was used in the form of puppet play and real-life scenario interaction. Arts and crafts were useful activities and helped them to construct a 'feel-good quilt' and doing body mapping exercises. Board games were well accepted by the group members and they played 'don't talk to strangers'-, 'emotions'- and '*morabaraba*' board games. Physical activities were encouraged in the sessions such as 'blind snake'-, and 'falling trust'- games. After each session and time allowed for it the children could play outside under supervision. Bibliotherapy activities included many culturally relevant stories and also a session where they could watch a DVD.

Projective methods were incorporated to support the development of the children's emotional intelligence and included '*masekitlana*' and 'future train' exercises.

13.4.4 Caregiver Intervention Groups

The caregiver intervention sessions were drafted on a previous community HIV project, the Serithi project and adapted to the outcomes as envisaged by the Kgolo Mmogo intervention (Mundell, Visser, Makin, Forsyth, & Sikkema, 2012). The caregiver sessions had the requirements to:

- Empower women living with HIV to have the knowledge to make better choices for them and their children
- Empower women with knowledge and skills to enable them to assist their children to become more resilient
- Empower caregivers to improve their relationships with their children and partners
- Reduce stigma
- Advocate the right of people living with HIV
- Provide support and a referral system for caregivers
- Provide parenting skills and support
- Support caregivers to disclose their status in a responsible manner

The caregiver and child sessions were constructed to overlap and for caregivers to learn new skills and knowledge to support their children. The intervention for the caregivers acknowledged that they first had to come to terms with their own HIV status and relating emotions before they could be expected to support their children. Open conversation, relevant HIV/AIDS information, disclosure exercises, and group support helped them to cope with their diagnosis. The second part the intervention included information and exercises that focussed on child development and positive parenting. This was done in preparation of the joint session with their children.

13.4.5 Joint Intervention Phase

The main objective of the Kgolo Mmogo intervention was to increase the adaptive behaviour of young children by strengthening the caregiver-child relationship. The joint sessions for the caregivers and children were designed to enhance communication and interaction between them. The ten joint sessions were purposefully planned to slowly introduce the caregivers and children to the interactive phase of the intervention. Fun activities were incorporated to engage the participants and help them to get to know each other. The caregivers were not used to partake in play activities with their children.

The first session involved a picnic where caregiver and child pairs had the opportunity to prepare food together and to play games with other caregiver and child pairs. The Marschak Interaction Method (M.I.M) was used as orientation in session 16 where the emphasis was placed on structuring, engaging, nurturing and challenging activities. These activities were chosen to strengthen the caregiver and child bond.

Session 17 involved activities to enhance interaction between the caregiver and child, to express verbal and non-verbal communication skills and to support planning as a pair. A body map and puppet socks were created by the pairs. With the puppet sock activity, the pairs had the opportunity to switch roles. In sessions 18 and 19, the caregiver and child pairs worked together to create a family legacy and memories. Photos of each family unit were taken for the memory box they created. Sessions 20 and 21 incorporated craft activities and the culturally played *morabaraba* board game to increase communication and planning strategies of the caregiver and child pairs. Session 22 was a separate session for the caregiver and child pairs where revision of the sessions took place. In session 23 the pairs were encouraged to plan for the future by constructing a collage together and to discuss their future dreams.

In the final session, the participants were surprised by a farewell party and they received a certificate of attendance to indicate their commitment to reach the goals they set for themselves during the intervention sessions.

13.5 Planning and Preparation for the Support Group Intervention

The initial planning and preparation phases of an intervention require particular consideration in the South African context. The choice of the intervention site, the support group size, the duration of the support group sessions and the training and responsibilities of the group facilitators are important to support group design aspects. Optimal circumstances and preparation for an intervention are crucial to predicting the success of a support group.

13.5.1 Intervention Sites

The site of an intervention requires careful planning and selection. Transport and safety are two issues in the South African context that necessitates special consideration. The location of the two intervention sites was carefully chosen to ensure that it was in reach for most of the participants. The sites had to be on a bus or taxi route and it had to be secure for both the participants and careworkers. Other prerequisites were that it had to be big enough for the different groups, consist of at least three rooms to accommodate the caregivers, 6 to 10-year-old children, and 3 to 5-year-old children (refer to Fig. 13.3), a kitchen area to prepare the lunch and a play area for the children. The children rooms were decorated to be child-friendly and toys for the younger children were made available.

13.5.2 Proposed Group Sizes

The participants were randomly selected for the group sessions. A decision was made by the research team to select 15 caregivers and their children for each of the 6-month intervention groups. The group size was chosen to ensure max-

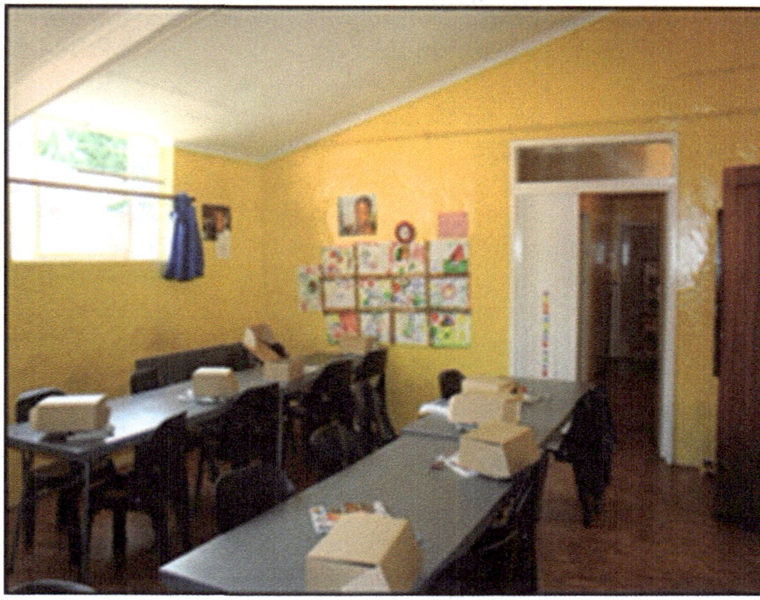

Fig. 13.3 Intervention site

imum attendance. The projection was that some of the caregivers might receive medical treatment, obtain employment or withdraw from the sessions during the 6-month intervention period. The careworkers reported in their concluding evaluation that they experienced the group sizes to be optimal if more than two and less than 12 members attended a session. The activities of the support group intervention were designed for high-level group interactivity and if the groups were too big or too small the sessions were not deemed ideal to reach the proposed outcomes.

The groups had both a facilitator and co-facilitator which supported the group processes. During the joint sessions both the separate child- and caregiver groups combine and this factor, in particular, make the choice of group size important.

13.5.3 Duration of Group Support Sessions

A 6-month or 24 weeks intervention was designed to ensure optimum support to the group members. The caregivers and their children attended weekly support groups and although uncontrollable external factors as for instance transport problems, school holidays and maternal illness did influence the continuity of the sessions this effect was countered by repeating sessions or home visits. The research team was initially concerned that the 6-month period of the sessions might be too long but the caregiver, child, and careworker post-intervention evaluation indicated that they experienced the group sessions as acceptable and in many instances, they suggested more sessions. The support group sessions were developed with a definite structure and the activities arranged accordingly. The themes built on each other and they had a direct correlation with the parallel caregiver sessions. The sessions were planned for an hour and a half each. An extra half hour was added for lunch which totaled up to 2 h. The careworkers did have leeway to allow the children to do organised outside play activities if the session ended earlier for them, but this rarely occurred. The duration of the sessions was planned to ensure attention and maximum participant cooperation. One aspect that needs special consideration when planning for an intervention with school-aged children is that the session schedule has to be flexible enough to accommodate them if they have extra-mural school activities or if they experience transport problems from school.

13.5.4 Group Facilitator Training and Implementation Process

The researchers intended for the intervention to be replicable, affordable and sustainable. Therefore it was necessary that the careworkers were volunteers and recruited from the identified community in which the intervention was to take place. Eight female volunteers from surrounding communities indicated their interest and availability to be trained as careworkers (group facilitators) for the intervention study. Some of the volunteers were HIV positive themselves, but it was not a prerequisite. The most important requirement was that the careworkers were proficient in both English and one or more of the languages in their community. None of them had any previous experience as group facilitators or a background in counselling and nor was it required.

Training and monitoring were important aspects of the intervention to ensure fidelity and replicability of the sessions. To ensure that the sessions were exactly executed as indicated in the manual a quality assurance questionnaire had to be completed after every group session and a social worker attended the sessions. Every session had a facilitator and co-facilitator. This ensured that there was a careworker available at all times and leave or sickness did not impact on the delivery of the session.

Training focussed on basic communication skills, counselling skills, group facilitation skills, identification of problematic behaviour and emotional difficulties, identification of social problems, referral skills, and HIV and Aids information. Each of the sessions in the manual was practiced during the pilot phase and also practiced among each other under the guidance of a psychologist.

Weekly group discussions with the careworkers ensured that problems, referrals, and other observations were dealt with. Many socio-economic problems were experienced by the group members. These observed problems and difficult personal circumstances of the careworkers made it essential for the researchers to include debriefing sessions for the careworkers.

13.5.5 Responsibilities of the Careworkers

The careworkers were paid a small stipend and worked flexible hours depending on how many group sessions were arranged per week. There were approximately two intervention sessions planned per week in both of the identified communities. The careworkers had to be available for practice sessions, preparation for group sessions and reflection sessions. The preparation for the support sessions did extent to phoning or texting the caregivers before each session to remind them of attending. Most of the children who attended the sessions did so directly after returning from school and it necessitated that lunch was provided to the groups. The lunch had to be nutritious and affordable. Churches and supermarkets were approached by the social workers for food donations. The careworkers in conjunction with the social worker had to plan and prepare for the lunches according to the weekly donations as received from the community organisations. The lunches were mostly cooked meals and for many of the participants the only warm meal for the day. The careworkers also had to ensure that each group member received an envelope with the correct travelling stipends. After the sessions, they completed a quality assurance questionnaire.

In situations where the caregivers were ill and unable to attend a specific support session, the careworkers visited the caregiver and her child at their house. This measure increased group attendance and retention as the caregiver and child did not miss out on any of the group content.

13.6 Instruments Used to Measure the Effectiveness of the Intervention Groups

The quantitative instruments selected to measure the effectiveness of the intervention groups were translated to the participants' home languages. The instruments were translated with the permission of the instrument distributors to isiZulu, Sesotho, Sepedi, and Setswana and back-translated into English. The questionnaires were culturally adapted by inviting community members to conversation groups with the research team to ensure the items were culturally accepted and understood. A follow-up pilot phase tested the items' reliability and validity. Research assistants received training to administer the assessment battery. All questions were read aloud to the participants to ensure that any uncertainty from the interviewees is addressed.

The translated instruments produced its own set of challenges as the languages the instruments were translated into having a restricted emotive vocabulary matched to the larger emotion vocabulary of English. The instruments chosen for the intervention study was thus ultimately a limited selection of instruments available for measuring the resilience of young children in South Africa.

13.6.1 Child Results

The instrument battery used for the child participants (refer to Table 13.3) were selected with the aim of measuring resilient and adaptive behaviour. Depression, anxiety, emotional intelligence, coping skills and self-concept were indicated as the intervention's intended resilience outcomes.

Table 13.3 Child participant instrument battery

Instrument	Intended resilience outcome/s measured
Child Depression Inventory (CDI)	Depression
Kidcope	Cognitive and behavioural coping strategies
Revised Children Manifest Anxiety Scale (RCMAS)	Anxiety
Child Spiritual Coping Scale (CSCS)	Religious and existential coping methods
BarOn EQ-i: Youth Version	Self-consciousness and expression
	Social awareness and interpersonal relationships
	Coping with change
	Emotional coping and regulation
Self-Description Questionnaire (SDQ)	Self-concept

The researchers of this randomised control study reported that the primary quantitative outcomes of the group intervention study indicated that the children displayed a decrease of externalising behaviour problems and an increase of adaptive behaviour, in particular, the areas of communication and daily living skills. An important finding was that this effect persisted for at least 12 months after the group intervention sessions took place and thus indicated a long-lasting effect on the children's resilience (Eloff et al., 2014).

The child participants completed a group evaluation questionnaire after attending the 6-month intervention sessions. A large percentage of the children indicated that they felt comfortable and accepted in the group (85%). The participants felt that they made new friends (78%) who cared about them (80%) and they cared about their new friends (83%), they learned new skills in the group (85%) that will help them outside of the group (78%) and understood what they were supposed to do during each group session (80%) (Finestone, 2013). The support groups were a positive experience for the children.

13.6.2 Caregiver Results

A premise of the intervention study was that when a caregiver's self-esteem and positive coping skills increase, it will promote enhanced parenting skills resulting in the more positive adaptive functioning of their children. The instruments used to measure caregiver participant outcomes (refer to Table 13.4) were selected to measure their coping skills and depression. The second part of the instrument battery focussed on the caregiver's experience of parental stress and they reported on their children's behaviour and emotions.

There were no significant changes indicated on the caregivers' psychological or parental measurements but the quantitative data did show that caregivers who attended the sessions regularly

Table 13.4 Caregiver instrument battery

Instrument (caregiver focused)	**Intended outcome/s measured**
Socio-demographic questionnaire	Socio-demographic information of caregiver and child
Center for Epidemiological Studies Depression (CES-D)	Screening for depression
Brief Cope Questionnaire	Coping skills
Positive Religious Coping Scale	Religious coping skills
Instrument (child focused)	**Intended outcome/s measured**
Child Behavior Check List (CBCL)	External and internal behaviour problems
The Vineland Adaptive Behavior-II	Socialisation
	Daily living skills
	Communication
	Motor skills
Coping with Children's Negative Emotions Scale (CCNES)	Perceived coping with child negative emotions
Parenting Stress Index (PSI)	Perceived parenting stress

experienced a decrease in depression and an increase in coping (Eloff et al., 2014).

The caregivers also completed a qualitative group evaluation form after attending the 24-weeks intervention. They indicated that their communication with their children improved significantly and they felt emotionally closer to their children. They enjoyed spending time with their children. The caregivers felt better equipped to discuss their HIV positive status with their children. They reported enhanced parenting skills (95%) and the use of more meaningful discipline practices. The majority (79%) of caregivers indicated that their children displayed better behaviour at home and school after the intervention (Finestone, 2013).

13.7 Self-Reported Experiences of Community Care Workers

In completion of the Kgolo Mmogo intervention study, the careworkers facilitated 12 groups of caregivers and their children for a period of 24 weeks each. They had thus each facilitated or co-facilitated on average 288 group sessions. The careworkers acquired an in-depth understanding of the groups and a remarkable repertoire of group facilitator skills. Their experiences are therefore of utmost importance to guide future training and planning for support groups to facilitate resilience and quality of life in families affected by HIV in a South African context.

They reflected on their personal experiences as careworkers, the effect of the sessions on group participants in their viewpoint, their views on the intervention and manual used and specific difficulties they experienced during the group sessions.

13.7.1 The Reflection of Careworkers' on Their Experiences as Group Facilitators in Intervention Groups

The careworkers indicated the importance of adequate knowledge and skills to empower them as group facilitators. The most important skills according to them were listening and communication skills "*With children one needs to listen to them and give them a chance to talk about their feelings and be able to help them, I think listening to them was the best option for the children*". The caregivers recognised their preconception of 'children are seen and not heard' and came to the conclusion that for a successful session with children mutual respect and understanding are important group intervention aspects. "*Working with this group made me realise that children also have feelings and emotions and we have to be careful how we talk to them and what we do to them*". They also recognised that child groups can only succeed if there is engagement in the child's world on his/her level of development. "*By giving them a chance and showing them you really appreciate what they are saying by so doing we came to their level*". The careworkers placed emphasis on the importance of meticulous observation of all behaviour during group sessions as they were able to identify from the children's behaviour the relationship of the caregiver and child. The careworkers felt their training in child development and identification of problematic behaviour empowered them.

13.7.2 Careworker Observations of the Effect of the Group Support Sessions on the Participants

The careworkers reported that during the sessions they experienced the participants to display a positive future perspective. This also motivated the careworkers for the sessions "*Most of the children do have high hopes in their lives*". They were definite multiple indications of improved caregiver-and child-relationships which were one of the main aims of the intervention "*… that after mothers allowed children to express themselves we noticed that communication between them was much better*". The careworkers stated that the support sessions helped the children to share their emotions with their caregivers "*… but after group the child could speak to her about his emotions*" The caregivers furthermore reported to the caregivers that their children's behaviour improved both at home and school "*the teachers want to know where the children go to therapy as their behaviour improved*".

13.7.3 The Careworkers' Evaluation of the Support Group Manual and Intervention Process

The opportunity was given to the careworkers to critique the content of the sessions and the intervention process. They were asked to indicate which activities in the manual according to their experience facilitating the groups needed to change. The general consensus was that the activities were appropriate and accepted in the community. The *masekitlana* indigenous game for the children's intervention and life-map for the caregiver intervention were highlighted as the most successful activities according to them. The joint sessions were furthermore described as the sessions with the most impact on the caregiver-child relationship.

The careworkers felt they made a difference to the community as they experienced the intervention having a positive impact on behaviour "*Children enjoyed coming to the group because at home there are problems like no food and domestic violence. When time gone by you saw positive changes in them. They talk more, smile more, are more caring and they talk about how they feel. The group accommodated each other*".

13.7.4 The Careworkers' Observations of Difficulties Experienced During the Support Group Sessions

The intervention groups for families affected by HIV were at times challenging for the careworkers to facilitate. They indicated that they felt anger and inadequately trained to cope with situations where group members reported that they were sexually molested "*…she didn't give me problems but I wanted to reach out but she did not allow me…*". Caregivers reported that external behaviour problems such as hyperactivity and aggression some of the child participants displayed were experienced as difficult to accommodate in the groups "*…he did not finish what he was doing and he wants to do something else and as a result he was disturbing the group*" and "*sometimes he bullied other children especially when we did not see him*". Many of the families who attended the intervention sessions lived in extreme poverty. The caregivers were able to identify with these families as they themselves experienced socio-economic difficulties "*we couldn't change lots of domestic problems*".

Adequate group facilitation training, basic counselling skills, comprehensive HIV knowledge, regular debriefing sessions, and adequate professional support are important for achieving optimal success in group interventions for children affected by maternal HIV.

13.8 Barriers to the Intervention Sessions

Specific barriers experienced in the intervention related to the unique South African context included school holidays, transport, social grant days, follow-up visits at clinics, illness, pregnancy, psychological disorders, employment, riots and in some cases the death of group members. Caregivers were weary to attend group sessions if they had not previously disclosed their status to their family and social network. The disclosure was, therefore, an issue that needed individual attention in the intervention sessions.

13.8.1 Absence Due to Holidays and Scheduled Appointments

Public and school holidays were a challenge to group attendance. Some of the children's biological fathers or extended family members stayed in different provinces and they only had the opportunity to travel during school holidays.

The December recess which is South Africa's longest school holiday in specific was a difficult time to arrange for group sessions as most of the group members were either not available or not interested. Sessions had to be arranged around these times to accommodate the group members. The researchers had to furthermore take into account days on which social grants were distributed to the caregivers and scheduled follow-up medical visits at the different clinics. The caregivers have to stand in long ques and wait for their turn. This caused them not to be able to attend the sessions.

13.8.2 Transport Difficulties

Transport was a concern and significant limitation for most of the caregivers and their children. South Africa does not have a reliable public transport system and caregivers had to depend on the informal taxi system. Children also attended school during the week and when they attended the group sessions directly after school, additional arrangements for transport had to be made for them.

Transport is expensive and although the caregivers did receive transport money they preferred to walk to the intervention sites to save the money. This preference meant that group attendance was poor during extreme weather conditions such as heavy rains or particular warm days.

13.8.3 HIV Related Health Problems and Pregnancy

The caregivers who attended the support sessions were selected for the intervention study because of their HIV positive status. This health problem did at times cause that the caregivers were unable to attend the sessions due to poor health. Some of the caregivers were pregnant which caused an added health stressor. In one instance a pregnant caregiver experienced health-related issues during a support session. She had to be stabilised and an ambulance was arranged by the careworkers. The careworkers also had to support a group of caregivers who underwent traditional 'cleansing' rituals. On their return to the group, they were usually very weak and needed to be referred to medical specialists. The careworkers had to be able to cope with an array of emergency situations and they had to be able to guide the group in their support of the caregiver experiencing health problems. Additional home visits were arranged for caregivers who experience health issues or need further support.

13.8.4 Employment of Caregivers

Most of the caregivers (78%) were not employed at the start of their support group cycle. Some of the caregiver participants succeeded to attain employment during the 6-month intervention. Although this had an effect on their support group attendance, it was encouraged by the research team. The consequence thereof was that some of the caregivers could not attend the joint sessions with their children and the careworkers had to stand in for them. This was not an ideal solution to enhance caregiver and child communication and interaction. It did, however, ensure that the children could complete their sessions. Some of the employed caregivers requested home visits and this action helped to ameliorate the intervention effect for both caregiver and child.

13.8.5 Riots and Unrest in the Communities

The group sessions were presented in the communities where the participants resided to ensure improved attendance as the venues were easily accessible. During some of the intervention sessions, riots and unrest prevented group members and careworkers from attending certain of the group sessions. The safety of both the group members and the research team was a high priority for the intervention planning and these sessions had to be repeated.

13.8.6 The Loss of Group Members Due to Illness and Death

The most difficult reality a support group focussed on HIV and other serious health problems face is the loss of a group member due to illness or death. The traumatic experience is further exacerbated in the Kgolo Mmogo support groups with the unique complicating factor of both caregiver and child groups. Both groups and the careworkers were immensely affected with the loss of a caregiver. Additional support and in some cases individual counselling sessions had to be arranged for group members after the death of a group member.

The children of the deceased caregivers received additional support and follow-up home visits. The group sessions were experienced as a source of support and some of the child participants attended the groups with their siblings after their caregiver passed away. Exceptional arrangements were made to accommodate the siblings in the groups and to ensure the child participant received optimal support.

13.8.7 The Impact of Psychological Distress or Disorders on the Intervention Group

Living with HIV has the potential to negatively impact a caregiver's sense of well-being and it could intensify existing mental health conditions. A support group is a small sample of reality and therefore it was expected that there could be evidence of mental health issues with some of the group members. The difficulties experienced by careworkers as group facilitators in cases of pre-existing mental health conditions or HIV-related mental health issues highlights the need for intensive caseworker training. An example of a psychological stressor on the group cohesion is a caregiver who displayed a mental disorder when she proclaimed herself to be a *sangoma.*[3] She was not trained as a traditional *sangoma*. She disrupted the group by making inappropriate references to hearing instructional voices indicating that all the group members' houses were burning down. This caused chaos and disruption in the group. The caregivers had to be able to defuse the situation and to make the necessary referrals.

A significant group of caregivers displayed depressive symptoms and inappropriate coping mechanisms at the beginning of the intervention. These participants were closely monitored by the careworkers and social workers. Some of the caregivers exhibited better coping skills as they intervention sessions progressed, but further referrals were made were necessary. During the sessions, a small group of child participants indicated that they were physically or sexually abused. Immediate action was called for where these children had to be counselled and the necessary steps were taken to report the abuse. The

[3] *Sangoma* refer to practitioners of traditional African medicine.

careworkers received training to deal with this type of trauma and to be able to calm the rest of the group after disclosure.

13.8.8 Disclosure of Parental HIV Status

An important issue when working with HIV support groups is disclosure. Almost 88% of the caregivers indicated that they have not disclosed their HIV positive status to their children or other family members. In the first intervention session, the caregivers were guided in setting up unambiguous group rules regarding disclosure of the HIV status of other group members to people outside of the group. Caregivers signed consent forms to indicate that they will not discuss the HIV status of the group participants outside of the support groups. There were incidences where caregivers shared the status of other group members outside the group and this breach of confidentiality needed specific intervention and mediation between parties.

The caregivers were supported throughout the intervention to disclose their status in a developmentally appropriate manner to their children, but it was not compulsory. The caregivers did receive regular feedback from the careworkers who facilitated the children groups. The careworkers indicated that many of the children experienced anxiety knowing their caregivers are ill and not knowing the reason for or prognosis of the illness. They see their caregiver going to the hospital, attending clinic check-ups and using medicine.

Some of the children mentioned that they saw their caregiver using the same medicine they saw television characters are using for HIV. The anxiety places the child in chronic trauma as the child in this age group comprehends the irreversibility of death. The children equated HIV with death and it was suggested to the caregivers that they disclose their HIV status and explain their prognosis to their children to alleviate their anxiety.

13.9 Added Advantages of the Group Support Intervention

The group sessions were planned with the aim to enhance the resilience and positive behaviour of children affected by parental HIV. A few unintended consequences were also reported and the need for supplementary referral services was indicted.

13.9.1 Unintended Consequences

More children attended the group sessions that were originally randomised to the groups. Reported reasons for this occurrence are that the caregivers could not leave their other children alone at home and some of the children told their school friends and brought them along to the sessions. A group of teachers in the nearby schools also contacted the researchers and enquired about the possibility of sending children in their classrooms to the support sessions as they experienced the positive behaviour changes the group attendees displayed.

Some children attended the sessions by themselves when their caregivers passed away, were hospitalised or employed. The children reported that the group sessions gave them support and helped them to cope with the daily difficulties they faced.

Many of the group participants experienced socio-economic difficulties, were single caregivers and not employed. In the initial planning phase of the intervention, it was recommended that sandwiches and cool drinks were given to the child participants before each session. Very early in the group sessions, it became apparent that most of the families attending the sessions lived in extreme poverty and they were in desperate need of support. Food parcels were given to families once a month and each of the sessions included cooked meals prepared by the careworkers for both the caregivers and children.

The careworkers themselves experienced the same type of hardships as the caregivers and could empathise with the difficulties they endured. The careworkers were empowered through their role as group facilitators. They reported enhanced parenting skills in their own families and all of the careworkers either started up with their own businesses or were permanently employed after completion of the Kgolo Mmogo project.

13.9.2 Supplementary Referral Services

An important consequence of the sessions was that caregivers and children were able to receive supplementary psychosocial support where it was indicated. The careworkers received basic counselling training and they were also guided to identify situations where external referral for participants was necessary. The South African psychological support systems are overloaded and interventions, such as the Kgolo Mmogo intervention provided the first point of support for participants. The useful advice from the group members themselves helped caregivers to access wider support more effectively. Socioeconomic constraints, a lack of social services and transport difficulties impact families where psychosocial support is desperately needed.

The careworkers and social workers of the Kgolo Mmogo intervention were able to refer participants in need of help to the necessary services and they were also able to do follow-up visits (Eloff, Forsyth, Finestone, Boeving, & Sikkema, 2011).

13.10 Discussion

Rigorous researched and documented theory-based support groups for young children affected by maternal HIV in South Africa are limited. The Kgolo Mmogo study aimed to provide support to HIV infected caregivers and their young children and to contribute to the scarce body of literature describing group interventions with HIV-affected children. The strengths and limitations of the intervention and the intervention implications for practice are highlighted.

13.10.1 Strengths and Limitations

The children's adaptive and non-adaptive behaviour were examined and risk and protective factors were identified. The risk factors identified in the intervention study were intra- and inter-family violence, abuse, maternal illness, poverty, broken families and negative caregiver-and-child relationships. The protective factors identified in the study after the 6-month intervention were a close caregiver-and-child relationship where they were able to play with one another, support from friends, enhanced communication skills, ability to share and identify emotions of self and others, the willingness to help others and to ask for help, showing respect, positive religious coping skills, adequate problem-solving skills, a positive future orientation, a supportive relationship with another adult other than the caregiver and life skills. The support groups provided an opportunity for the children to practice adaptive behaviour in a safe environment. They were thereby able to enhance their protective factors. This assisted them in coping with the risk factors they faced.

The caregivers reported that they experienced the Kgolo Mmogo support session as positive because they learned how to communicate positively with their children and these newfound skills helped them to get to know their children. They felt more comfortable in sharing their emotions with their children after getting to know them better through play activities.

Some caregivers could disclose their HIV status to their children because of their close bond. The group provided the necessary opportunities for the caregivers and children to develop effective relationships. Most to the caregivers indicated that their children's behaviour had improved significantly after attending the support sessions. The children displayed less aggressive behaviour (externalised behaviour problems) and they were better equipped to cope with problems.

A specific conclusion drawn from the support session study was that the children showed a definite need for order in their daily lives. The child participants in the intervention were exposed to a disordered milieu where one parent households, family unemployment, fluctuating relationships, persistent lack of resources and violence were part of their everyday lives. Their experience of an absence of control over their caregiver's illness added to this insecurity. The children in the groups displayed normative beliefs through their religious coping styles, their search for and demonstration of respect and their explicit assertion of what is right and wrong. The support group supported the child participants to create an inner protective domain of order through the ordered means in which the session, programme content and other sequential features were presented.

By creating the protective domain of order the children could order their life worlds which were thrown into disorder because of the presence of risk factors to which they were exposed.

Although the researchers went to great lengths to ensure that the child-focused questionnaires were culturally tailored and translated accurately, the questionnaires to measure the resilience outcomes for the children seems to be a limitation for the study. Possible explanations presented in the study of non-significant improvement indicated in most of the children's self-report questionnaires are that the participants in the study sample were not previously exposed to answering questions on a Likert-type scales or answering emotional-focused questions and that this was a learning experience for them. The questionnaires were furthermore mostly not standardised for the South African child population. The outcomes on the questionnaires stand in direct opposition to the significant behaviour and adaptive behaviour the caregivers indicated in the child-focused questionnaires and raises concerns regarding the applicability of self-report child-focused instruments that were not developed in South Africa for the South African population.

13.10.2 Implications for Quality of Life

Caregivers living with HIV have to deal with several challenging health and life issues. They have to cope with their own health concerns and also have the additional responsibility of being a parent. HIV infection was once feared a terminal disease but with the introduction of antiretroviral treatment (ART) options it is now dealt with as any other chronic illness, i.e. diabetes, where a normal life expectancy is anticipated (Torres et al., 2018). Interventions and support to caregivers who are HIV infected are needed in order for them to resume their normal daily life activities and to take up their parental responsibilities. The quality of life of families living with HIV is furthermore enhanced by their perceived satisfaction of family life and an important factor to take cognisance of when planning interventions for families. Quality of life is multifaceted and refer to the perception of an individual of how an illness (in this case HIV) or intervention affects their lives. This effect could be on a physical, emotional and/or social level (Mafirakurevaa, Dzingiraic, Postmab, van Hulstb, & Khozac, 2016).

On the whole, the Kgolo Mmogo intervention study provides convincing evidence of the support group programme's ability to enhance the quality of life of both caregivers and their children. The children's adaptive behaviour improved and the caregiver-child bond was strengthened.

The most important conclusions and recommendations to be drawn from the Kgolo Mmogo intervention are that the intervention programme was specifically tailored to address the identified needs of the community. The programme was delivered through a process of continuous monitoring, change of course and revised planning where necessary. The group sessions were delivered by members (caregivers) in the community who understood the cultural practices of the group participants, their language and barriers they faced. The caregivers received comprehensive training and mentoring that enabled them to facilitate the group sessions. The groups assisted in providing and enhancing peer support to both the caregivers and children. The parallel caregiver support groups maximised the positive impact of the group intervention. The group sessions were cost-effective to enable group facilitators in low-resource settings to repeat the intervention without major cost implications.

In addition, this evidence provides interventionists a foundation to plan for future interventions to enhance the quality of life of families. Important conclusions drawn from the intervention study are that communication between a child and caregiver is a key factor to ensure success and sustainable change in a family. The support sessions have to be perceived as culturally acceptable by the group members and specifically tailored to address the identified needs of the community where the intervention takes place. The planning and preparation for a support group in South Africa necessitate careful coordination and flexibility to ensure success. Transport, location, timing, caregiver illness, provision of lunch, limited childcare, disclosure, further individual psychosocial support referrals, and clinic visits are examples of factors to consider when planning for an HIV support group. The joint sessions need special planning to ensure optimal caregiver and child communication. Psychosocial support to families affected by HIV in South Africa is limited and group support sessions are the first level of intervention for families who experience difficulties. The support groups for young children affected by maternal HIV did not make any reference to HIV per se in the children groups. The structure, process, and content of the children groups and joint groups will, therefore, lend itself to other types of family interventions in South Africa.

Acknowledgments This principal research was supported by a grant from the National Institute of Mental Health (Grant Number: 5R01MH076442).

References

Arikawa, S., Rollins, N., Newell, M. L., & Becquet, R. (2016). Mortality risk and associated factors in HIV-exposed, uninfected children. *Tropical Medicine and International Health, 21*, 720–734.

Betancourt, T.S., Meyers-Okhi, S.E., Charrow, A., & Hansen, N. (2012). Research review: Mental health and resilience in HIV/AIDS-affected children: A review of the literature and recommendations for future research. The Journal of Child Psychology and Psychiatry, n. p. https://doi.org/10.1111/j.1469-7610.2012.02613.x

Boeving-Allen, A., Finestone, M., Eloff, I., Sipsma, H., Makin, J., Triplett, K., … Forsyth, B. W. C. (2014). The role of parenting in affecting the behavior and adaptive functioning of young children of HIV-infected mothers in South Africa. *Aids Behavior, 18*, 605–616. https://doi.org/10.1007/s10461-013-0544-7

Eloff, I., Finestone, M., Makin, J. D., Boeving-Allen, A., Visser, M., Ebersöhn, L., … Forsyth, B. W. C. (2014). A randomized clinical trial of an intervention to promote resilience in young children of HIV-positive mothers in South Africa. *AIDS, 28*(Suppl. 3), S347–S357.

Eloff, I., Forsyth, B., Finestone, M., Boeving, A., & Sikkema, K. (2011). Intervention groups for HIV-infected women: The need for additional services. *South Africa Journal of Psychology, 41*(1), 38–51.

Finestone, M. (2013). *An evaluation of a theory-based support group intervention for children affected by maternal HIV/AIDS.* Unpublished PhD-thesis. University of Pretoria.

Forsyth, B. (2005). *Promoting resilience in young children of HIV-infected mothers in South Africa.* Research proposal submitted to the National Institutes of Health. South Africa. Research proposal submitted to the National Institutes of Health, April 2005.

Goldberg, R. E., & Short, S. E. (2016). What do we know about children living with HIV-infected or AIDS-ill adults in Sub-Saharan Africa? A systematic review of literature. *AIDS Care, 28*, 130–141. https://doi.org/10.1080/09540121.2016.1176684

Mafirakurevaa, N., Dzingiraic, B., Postmab, M. J., van Hulstb, M., & Khozac, S. (2016). Health-related quality of life in HIV/AIDS patients on antiretroviral therapy at a tertiary care facility in Zimbabwe. *AIDS Care, 28*(7), 904–912. https://doi.org/10.1080/09540121.2016.1173639

Mundell, J. P., Visser, M. J., Makin, J. D., Forsyth, B. W., & Sikkema, K. J. (2012). Support group processes: Perspectives for HIV-infected women in South Africa. *Journal of Qualitative Research in Psychology, 9*, 173–187. https://doi.org/10.1080/14780887.2010.500350

Rochat, T., Netsi, E., Redinger, S., & Stein, A. (2017). Parenting and HIV. *Current Opinion in Psychology, 15*, 155–161.

Roux, S. M., Abrams, E. J., Nguyen, K., & Myer, L. (2016). Clinical outcomes of HIV-exposed, HIV-uninfected children in sub-Saharan Africa. *Tropical Medicine and International Health, 21*, 829–845.

Skerfving, A., Johansson, F., & Tobias, H. E. (2014). Evaluation of support group interventions for children in troubled families: Study protocol for a quasi-experimental control group study. *BioMed Central Public Health, 14*, 76. https://doi.org/10.1186/1471-2458-14-76

Torres, T. S., Harrison, L. J., La Rosa, A. M., Lavenberg, J. A., Zeng, L., Safren, S. A., … Huges, M. D. (2018). Quality of life among HIV-infected individuals failing first-line antiretroviral therapy in resource limited settings. *AIDS Care, 30*(8), 954–962. https://doi.org/10.1080/09540121.2018.1427207

UNAIDS. (2012). *Global report: UNAIDS report on the global AIDS epidemic 2012*. Geneva, Switzerland: UNAIDS. Available at http://www.unaids.org/sites/default/files/media_asset//20121120_UNAIDS_Global_Report_2012_with_annexes_en_1.pdf. Accessed 10 June 2018

UNAIDS. (2013). *Report on the global AIDS epidemic*. Available from: http://www.unaids.org/en/resources/campaigns/globalreport2013/globalreport. Accessed 10 Jun 2018.

UNAIDS. (2016). *AIDS by the numbers*. Switzerland.

Van Breda, A. D., & Theron, L. C. (2018). A critical review of South African child and youth resilience studies, 2009–2017. *Children and Youth Services Review, 91*, 237–247.

Decolonial Approaches to AIDS, Children's Wellbeing, and Education in Malawi

14

Zikani Kaunda, Nancy Kendall, and Upenyu Majee

Abstract

Children's and communities' quality of life in Malawi has been significantly and negatively impacted by the AIDS syndemic. Up to 10% of Malawian children now live with their grandparents in deeply resource-constrained households, where they face multiple threats to their wellbeing. International development organizations have responded to these threats with projects aimed at supporting vulnerable children's education. This chapter utilizes decolonial frameworks to describe the key normative assumptions that shape these school projects and limit their utility in improving vulnerable children's and AIDS-affected communities' quality of life; and provides two case studies of alternative program efforts that destabilize these assumptions and mobilize new modes of community participation to transform vulnerable children's individual, familial, and collective wellbeing.

Z. Kaunda
Institute for Participatory Engagement and Quality Improvement, Zomba, Malawi

N. Kendall (✉) · U. Majee
Department of Educational Policy Studies, University of Wisconsin-Madison, Madison, WI, USA
e-mail: nkendall@education.wisc.edu; majee@wisc.edu

14.1 Introduction

One of the greatest threats to human wellbeing in Southern Africa is HIV/AIDS and its multifarious consequences. The HIV virus has now raged for over 35 years in the region, and its effects are ubiquitous, diverse, and multigenerational. Every aspect of life—from the most intimate of moments and relationships to national production rates—has been impacted in heavily AIDS-affected countries like Malawi.

There have been significant community, national, and international efforts to address the consequences of what is commonly termed the "AIDS pandemic" on human wellbeing,[1] though these efforts have often been less effective than hoped (Dionne, 2017; Haacker, 2016; King, Burka, & Winchester, 2018). International devel-

[1]As Moller, Roberts, Tiliouine, and Lotschky (2017) note, the concepts of quality of life, happiness, and wellbeing are intertwined in Africa in ways that require an understanding of how basic measures of wellbeing interact with constructs such as "global happiness". Jirojanakul, Skevington, and Hudson (2003) note, Quality of Life (QOL) has been defined as "the individual's perception of their position in life, in the context of culture and value systems in which they live and in relation to their goals, expectations, standards and concerns" (WHOQOL Group, 1995, p. 1405). Efforts to conceptualize and measure children's QOL have been more limited than efforts to measure adult QOL, however. In this paper, we utilize the notion of wellbeing instead of quality of life, and more particularly the model of wellbeing developed in Friedson-Ridenour, Kendall, and DiPrete-Brown (2015).

I. Eloff (ed.), *Handbook of Quality of Life in African Societies*, International Handbooks of Quality-of-Life, https://doi.org/10.1007/978-3-030-15367-0_14

opment organizations' (IDOs') involvement in efforts to address HIV/AIDS is of particular interest and concern, because most of the countries[2] heavily impacted by AIDS are extremely dependent on IDOs for the financial resources deployed by governments in their responses to HIV/AIDS. For example, in 2016 86% of Malawi's HIV/AIDS response budget was provided by the international development community (Avert, 2018). As a result, IDOs often have an outsized say in determining how HIV/AIDS and its consequences are understood, the kinds of responses that are mounted against it, and the control and authority that local and national actors and institutions have in shaping these responses (Samoff, 1999).

Children—defined officially as all people under the age of 18—are perhaps the least-considered, heavily-impacted population in local, national, and international responses to AIDS. Children make up almost 50% of Malawi's entire population, and young women bear the highest proportional infection burden (UNAIDS, 2018). An estimated 15–20% of all Malawian children are orphaned, many due to HIV/AIDS. And, approximately 4,300 children are born infected with HIV each year (UNAIDS, 2018). Children are not just the country's future, as they are so often positioned in official discourse. They are the country's present, and yet their experiences, needs, wants, and wellbeing are generally decentered and even negatively impacted by current efforts to address HIV/AIDS.

For decades, the international community has positioned schooling as a panacea for improving children's rights and productive potential. Given international, national, and community understandings of schooling as a site in which the state invests in its citizens, and a site through which to provide essential knowledge to stop the spread of AIDS, it is not surprising that many IDO programs designed to support children affected by AIDS have focused on schooling as the central, or a central, mechanism for supporting vulnerable children and improving the outcomes for children affected by AIDS. The failure to secure educational opportunities and outcomes for children affected by HIV/AIDS is, therefore, viewed not only as a failure to meet children's basic rights and invest in each child's future, but also a failure that has ripple effects throughout development efforts—from undermining child survival goals, to decreasing political participation rates, to impacting environmental protection efforts (Vavrus, 2003). Not surprisingly, then, IDOs have focused a great deal of their (very limited) child-focused AIDS programming on children's access to and completion of formal schooling.

From the education sector's perspective, progress in reaching the access, equity, and quality goals of the Education For All movement, which is widely viewed as central to meeting children's rights and national human capital development goals (Mundy, 2016), is deeply threatened by AIDS and its system-wide effects (Kadzamira, Maluwa-Banda, Kamlongera, & Swainson, 2001; Kelly, 2001). Despite this recognition, however, there is remarkably little attention given to AIDS and its consequences on education policy, funding, or systems. Thus, AIDS programming in schools, and the consequences of AIDS on education policies and institutions, are too often uninterrogated by education scholars interested in learning about children's educational experiences and outcomes.

In this chapter, we provide a multi-level, critical analysis of IDO efforts to meet the rights and improve the wellbeing of children affected by AIDS by getting them into school and assuring they remain enrolled. We do so by carefully examining an IDO-funded project, namely the United States Agency for International Development (USAID)-funded Ambassador Girls' Scholarship Programme (AGSP). The AGSP serves as a case study that elucidates common features of many of the IDO-funded programs focusing on improving the wellbeing of children affected by AIDS. We argue that the conceptualizations of childhood, schooling, and

[2] Estimated adult (ages 15–49) infection rates of 7.1% (male)/11.2% (female), with youth (ages 15–19) rates climbing rapidly (UNAIDS, 2016). Data accessed at: http://www.unaids.org/en/regionscountries/countries/malawi

community participation embedded in IDO-funded programs aimed at children affected by AIDS are often imbued with understandings of social, generational, and economic relations that are rooted in neocolonial logics and that result in limited, and at times actively harmful, efforts to support these children. This was the case with AGSP, as it was first conceptualized and implemented. We then examine the second phase of the AGSP, during which a Malawian non-governmental organization (NGO) that had been subcontracted to implement the AGSP was allowed to change the programming and introduce what we argue were more decolonial approaches to educational programming. An examination of this second phase of AGSP points towards some of the principles that need to drive international development efforts to support the wellbeing of children affected by HIV/AIDS. We provide one other example of a community-driven education project that aimed to support children affected by AIDS to further illuminate some of the decolonial principles that might be enacted to improve the shape and consequences of efforts to improve the wellbeing of children affected by AIDS.

The chapter is organized as follows. We first describe prevailing notions of childhood; the role of schooling in international responses to the effects of AIDS on children; and the demographic and socio-economic consequences of AIDS in Malawi. We then turn to the AGSP case study: we describe the first phase of the AGSP project and explain why and how IDO-funded programs represent a neocolonial framework and the imposition of Western norms and rationales for conceptualizing and responding to children's and youth's wellbeing during an AIDS syndemic (Singer & Clair, 2003).[3] Then, we describe the second phase of the AGSP project, and the Participatory Approaches to School Improvement (PASI) project, to explore key components of community-driven approaches to supporting vulnerable children's schooling. Lastly, pulling back one more level, we lay out the primary components of a decolonial approach to improving Malawian children's wellbeing under syndemic conditions.

14.2 Notions of Childhood

Concern for children's wellbeing has been at the center of some, but certainly not most, global and national efforts to change the course of the AIDS pandemic. This is because HIV/AIDS has been conceptualized globally as an adult disease—and more than that, a disease associated with sex, which makes discussion of it in relation to children even more difficult and taboo for many actors and institutions. Most IDO resources for HIV/AIDS have focused on treatment and care of those already infected (an estimated 47% of resources), medical and public health interventions for adults who are at risk of HIV infection (23% of resources), and medical interventions to stop mother-to-child transmission of HIV (5% of resources) (Avert, 2018). Furthermore, there is an increasing focus on treatment to reach the UN 90-90-90 goals (Avert, 2018). While children may benefit from aspects of these foci, there is evidence that their adult-centeredness results in lower impacts for children than adults. For example, globally anti-retroviral (ARV) treatment coverage is estimated at 54% for infected adults, but only 43% for infected children (UNAIDS, 2016); researchers have recognized that this difference is due at least in part to the lack of attention given in policies and programs to the particular barriers that children face in accessing ARVs—including

[3] Singer describes the AIDS syndemic as follows: complex involving interconnected chains of disease causality nested in particular political economic and biosocial environments—what, in the case of southern Africa, might be called a perfect epidemiological storm (p. 9). This understanding of AIDS breaks down traditional medical approaches to understanding diseases in biological isolation from one another, and from the social, economic, political, and cultural environments in which they occur. Singer notes that from a public health perspective, in Southern Africa HIV/AIDS cannot be disentangled from malnutrition and poverty. Examining them instead as one syndemic emphasizes three key issues for understanding and acting to improve wellbeing: disease concentration, interaction, and social context (p. 10).

the requirement that they access medication and healthcare through adult caregivers (Avert, 2018).

When children are considered in IDOs' AIDS programming, they are usually conceptualized as children infected with HIV, children affected by AIDS (CABA), or children who are orphaned or made vulnerable by AIDS (OVCs). In all cases, and framed in large part by global conceptions of childhood and child rights, children are primarily positioned as victims of the disease who need and are entitled to adult protection and support to experience a childhood free of work and full of care and play. Thus, when children are centered in IDOs' understandings of and responses to HIV/AIDS, they are usually framed as twofold victims of the disease's impact on adults: first, children lose adult protection (a fundamental child right); second, they must take on adult roles (which often violate multiple child rights, such as the right to play). As Gillespie, Haddad, and Jackson (2001) describe:

> When parents fall sick, particularly in poor families, children come under intense stress that may continue in different forms for the rest of their lives. They may be taken out of school to farm land or to take part in income-generating activities. They may become caregivers themselves or even head of households. In many cases, such children become increasingly vulnerable to malnutrition, ill-health, abuse, and exploitation. There are psychosocial effects, under-researched but potentially very damaging, overriding these stresses, both in the short and long term. (p. 1)

USAID's understanding of the consequences of AIDS on children similarly emphasizes how the disease threatens and undermines international norms related to appropriate childhoods, and appropriate relations between adults and children:

> The consequences of the HIV/AIDS pandemic are catastrophic. One of the most tragic consequences is the toll on children. In 2001, more than 13 million children under age 15 had lost one or both parents to AIDS; that number will double by 2010. Along with the grief and dislocation that children of affected families experience comes the added burden of responsibilities that are far beyond the capabilities of young children: nursing a sick or dying parent, raising younger siblings, running the household or the family farm, substituting for a breadwinner, or scrounging for survival on city streets. In addition to these children who are affected by HIV/AIDS, there are more than 3 million children living with HIV/AIDS.
>
> But the pandemic's consequences go far beyond its effects on individual children's lives; it has devastated the families and communities where these affected youngsters live. Millions of mothers and fathers who would otherwise be raising the children and playing key roles in their families and communities have died, and the ability of the surviving adults, organizations, and institutions to nurture, socialize, educate, and support so many parentless youngsters is being overwhelmed. Beyond the emotional, educational, economic, and cultural harm to AIDS-affected children, the substantial gains made in child health and survival that countries attained in earlier years have begun to unravel. (2003, p. 1)

IDOs—and the international political community more broadly—conceptualize childhood as essentially different than adulthood, and child rights (to care, protection, play, and schooling) as essentially different than those of adults (Thangaraj, 2018). This approach to understanding appropriate childhood and its concomitant rights is reflected in language adopted by IDOs to explain the shape, scope, and intended impact of their efforts to address the effects of AIDS on children. For example, USAID (2003) declares: "The foundation of an effective USAID response must be to strengthen the capacity of families and communities to continue to provide care for vulnerable children and adolescents, and thereby reduce the number of children struggling to survive on their own" (p. 4).

This framing has some significant strengths, but the point that we wish to emphasize is that the primary focus of child-directed responses to HIV/AIDS largely still imagines children as needing adult protection and care, not as having rights, responsibilities, and experiences of their own that might differ significantly from adult assumptions and experiences. This is important not because children's rights claims on adults should be undermined, but because in practice many children can make few claims on adults in their families, communities, government, or the world (Ferguson, 2002). As a result, many children have adult responsibilities without concomitant rights, as opposed to having child responsibilities and rights.

14.3 HIV/AIDS in Malawi

In order to understand the care situations in which many children affected by AIDS find themselves, it is important to briefly review the effects of HIV/AIDS on socio-economic and familial relations in Malawi. Over the past 35 years, Malawi has been transformed by HIV/AIDS. At its peak, about 14% of Malawi's entire adult population was estimated to be living with HIV or AIDS. Following the widespread introduction of ARVs beginning in 2003, many key AIDS indicators began to turn around. By 2010, adult infection rates had fallen from a high of 14% to around 11%, and death rates plummeted to 24,000 a year in 2016. Yet by this time, 20% of Malawi's children were estimated to have been orphaned (NAC, 2010). Approximately half of all orphaned children in Malawi are estimated to be cared for by grandparents in grandparent-headed households. These data mirror the realities of children's household experiences in highly AIDS-affected countries throughout the region. Foster and Williamson (2000), for example, observed that the foster care of orphans is most often provided by elderly grandmothers with little or no assistance from other family members. According to Ainsworth and Filmer (2002), by the early 2000s more than one fifth of orphaned children were living with grandparents (almost entirely grandmothers).

The numbers of financially and socially marginalized elderly people who are now responsible for the care and upbringing of orphaned children is alarming (Help Age International, 2003). Grandmother-headed households largely depend on small-scale, rain-fed agriculture for their food security. The demographic changes wrought by AIDS, coupled with the heavy physical labor demands of agricultural survival, have by now rendered grandmother-headed households the poorest household category in Malawi. These households have also faced increasing social and financial marginalization as extended family and community care systems crumble under the weight of a lost parental generation, the continuing AIDS epidemic, and increasing food insecurity fueled in part by AIDS and in part by climate change (Joshua et al., 2016). Grandmother-headed households are often physically vulnerable and forced to face health and psychosocial struggles with little support (Rock et al., 2016). This again mirrors regional trends, where research indicates that "older people make up a significant proportion of the poorest of the poor, and even without the added threats created by HIV/AIDS, many older people struggle to survive and suffer poverty, social exclusion and age discrimination" (Barrientos, Gorman, & Heslop, 2003).

Orphans' peer networks and educational and health outcomes suffer when their households have such limited resources and become so deeply marginalized (Mashegoane & Mohale, 2016). Even as many orphans report that their grandmothers love and protect them, the depth of poverty and isolation many grandmothers and their charges experience undermines orphans' wellbeing (Munthali, 2002), fueling disproportionately high school dropout rates (Guo, Li, & Sherr, 2012) and food insecurity among orphans, and rising HIV infection rates among orphaned girls (Mkandawire, Tenkorang, & Luginaah, 2013).

14.4 Role of Schooling

For a variety of reasons related to colonial notions of childhood, colonial systems of labor (Thangaraj, 2018), and the international education movements that have sprung from these, schooling has been positioned—particularly since 1990—as the central international mechanism through which to address vulnerable children's immediate and future rights, needs, and realities. Indeed, many have now argued that schooling has been positioned as a development panacea (Vavrus, 2003), linked to improvements in almost all major development indicators. This notion of education's panacea effect predominates in the AIDS literature on children. IDOs—

and many other researchers and program and policy actors involved in international education and AIDS response efforts—often conceptualize schooling as the primary or only mechanism through which to:

- Prevent HIV (e.g., Vandemoortele and Delamonica's (2000) "education as a social vaccine" approach)
- Augment the fraying social safety nets on which children affected by AIDS depend (both by having the school play a service provision role, and by providing a site to organize community support for children, as the AGSP shows)
- Increase children's human capital and capabilities in preparation for adult roles
- Respond to international demands that children's rights be met (as the right to education is enshrined in multiple international declarations).

In response to the reality of fraying social safety nets and the vulnerability of many households caring for orphaned and vulnerable children, a few education sector actors have argued that issues of access, equity, and quality have to be rethought and expanded in the era of AIDS (Kelly, 2001). They view schools as environments that are particularly conducive—given the right resources—to supporting children affected by AIDS in multisectoral and integrated ways (Kendall & O'Gara, 2007). As the Association for Development Education in Africa explains this kind of positive, more expansive role schools might play in addressing AIDS:

> HIV and AIDS continue to pose a threat to the Education for All objectives, and researchers and analysts continue to be preoccupied with the extent of the assault of HIV and AIDS on education systems, particularly in high-prevalence countries of the sub-Sahara...Education systems in the region have had to face a 'first wave' of HIV infection, followed by a 'second wave' of AIDS mortality, and now face the challenge of the 'third wave': orphaning and family dislocation …
>
> Large numbers of vulnerable children in these AIDS-affected communities struggle to access resources and services they desperately need and are entitled to. Despite this, most children still attend school, making schools an obvious avenue through which to address the multiplicity of needs of vulnerable children.
>
> An example of a school-based response to the ever-increasing numbers of orphans and vulnerable children (OVC) is the **Schools as Centres of Care and Support** (SCCS), an innovative model built on the principles of a multi-sectoral partnership approach to tackling poverty, HIV and AIDS and other diseases. Schools are strengthened to provide quality education, and mobilised to function as hubs of integrated service delivery for children so that they have increased access to health and social welfare services and are able to access and benefit from this education…. (p. 3–5)

Most education systems in heavily-impacted countries have not, however, played this multi-sectoral and coordinating role. Instead, most developed some curricular materials in the late 1990s or early 2000s that addressed HIV/AIDS and distributed these to schools (teacher professional development to support these curricula was generally more limited). Some created new policies to address issues of teacher health (e.g., in Malawi, teachers were allowed to transfer to schools near health clinics if they needed to access regular health care services). Almost no education systems created policies or programs to directly address children's and families' experiences (Kendall, 2004).

The central role of schooling in international responses to children and AIDS can thus be viewed as a three-legged stool: schooling will provide multisectoral *support and protection* for children currently affected or infected with HIV, it will *prevent* HIV infection in the next generation by providing information and increasing children's human capital, and it will help *fulfil* national and international promises to uphold children's rights, and in so doing, improve children's wellbeing.

This international frame for understanding the role of education in improving children's wellbeing during the AIDS syndemic (and, indeed, improving all vulnerable children's wellbeing) fits easily within the educational plans and national AIDS responses of many countries in the region. In Malawi, for example, the government and many families talk about schooling as the primary mechanism through which all children—but particularly marginalized children—can overcome their current situations and fulfil their dreams of a bright future (Kendall & Silver, 2014). However, this apparently easy fit hides two issues: first, how the focus on schooling has resulted, de facto, in very limited government and IDO attention to vulnerable children's households and their material and social needs; and second, the complexities of AIDS-affected children's experiences in schools, and the deep limitations to the "add-orphans-and-stir" approach to schooling that has predominated in Malawi and many countries in the region. One quick example from fieldwork conducted in Zimbabwe can help explicate this issue: While interviewing a well-regarded grade 3 teacher about her experiences with children affected by AIDS, the teacher said to us (paraphrased): "You know, these children are really a problem. I do not know what to do! When you are trying to teach, they can just be crying—like this child here! (She pointed at a small boy in the back of the class who was bent over his desk in obvious distress). It is very difficult to know what to do with them." When we asked what activity the children were doing, the teacher responded that she had given them the activity of drawing their family. The little boy to whom she was pointing had very recently lost his mother. This teacher was not ill-intentioned, and she was visibly upset that she did not know how to handle the complex emotional responses that children were having as the grief and trauma of (often multiple) family deaths occurred. At the same time, her lesson plan was violently traumatic to some of her students—a reflection of the fact that she was never asked or required to reflect on how long-standing curricular practices and classroom activities might have to be changed in response to students' AIDS-related experiences.

Though arguments about if and how the effects of AIDS can be teased apart from the effects of poverty exist, there is growing consensus that in countries like Malawi, the likelihood of orphans and other children affected by AIDS dropping out of school is higher than non-orphan children (Bennell, 2005), and some orphans face additional challenges to gaining equal access to and maintaining equal retention and achievement in school (Ainsworth, Beegle, & Koda, 2002; Bennell, 2005). Some of the underlying factors affecting orphaned children's demand for and attendance of school include: economic difficulties, caregiving responsibilities, poor parental attitudes towards education, especially for girls, cultural practices and beliefs, illnesses, and disabilities (DeJaeghere, 2004). Other factors relate directly to the limitations that exist in current schooling models, and the stigmatizing and marginalizing experiences that children affected by AIDS have in many school settings.

This review of IDO assumptions about the role of schooling in supporting vulnerable children's improved wellbeing aims to raise questions about the common IDO and government assumption that schooling is an unquestionably positive force in the lives of children affected by AIDS, no matter what the daily policies and practices of schools are, and no matter the relationships among students, their guardians, and schools. It is evident that schools can play an incredibly important and positive role in supporting children's wellbeing; it is equally evident that many school settings fail to support or even harm children's wellbeing. This complexity is not surprising to anyone who has spent time in classrooms anywhere around the world: schools—like any complex social space—are productive and reproductive, generative and destructive, all at once, in different ways, for different people. But, importantly, beyond the evidently fallacious claim that any institution will impact everyone in the same (positive) way, formal schools in Malawi are colonial legacies, and the assumptions about appropriate behavior, about what can be taught to whom, about who belongs and why (Serpell, 2010; Stambach, 2013) that underlie these institutions also play an essential role in shaping the possibilities and challenges that formal schools represent to improving vulnerable children's wellbeing.

In order to explore these assumptions more fully, we turn to a case study of an IDO-funded, school-focused effort to improve vulnerable children's current and future wellbeing. The

Ambassador's Girls Scholarship Program's (AGSP's) main goal was to improve orphaned and vulnerable girls' retention in and completion of primary school, and thus to support their current and future wellbeing. AGSP was designed to accomplish these goals by providing scholarships to girls and boys who could have otherwise dropped out of primary school because of struggles directly related to their orphanhood. Girls who benefitted from the scholarship included orphans (90%), and girls born from physically disabled parents who lived in dire poverty (Samati, 2010). A small number of orphaned boys also received scholarships.

14.5 AGSP Phase 1

AGSP was funded by USAID, and the primary contractor was a U.S.-based organization that, as is often the case for USAID-funded projects, subcontracted to local NGOs for the project's implementation. One of the subconstrators was the Creative Center for Community Mobilization (CRECCOM), a Malawian NGO that had implemented IDO-funded, government-supported education programs aimed at improving girls' and orphaned children's education previously.

The process of centralizing initial planning, funding, and decisionmaking in the hands of IDOs is important, because this concentration determines the starting point of most projects like AGSP. In its initial design, AGSP embodied many of the more colonialist assumptions of which international development approaches have been accused: it focused purely on individual children, it made inappropriate assumptions about how families and communities understood orphanhood and vulnerability, and it imposed a particular understanding of gender inequalities, and therefore of gender equitable responsiveness, that did not examine the root causes of gender inequalities in education (Samati, 2010). It also assumed that the primary barrier to orphaned and vulnerable girls' schooling was the costs of schooling—an issue readily resolved through the provision of certain basic goods to reduce the cost.

Given this understanding of the problem (orphaned and vulnerable girls did not receive the material support they needed from their guardians, and without certain materials, girls were unable to attend school), the program's main activity initially comprised of procuring and distributing scholarship materials identified by girls and boys, parents, teachers, and other members of the community as important for AGSP scholars' success. The scholarship materials were distributed to individual children who were identified as orphaned or vulnerable and who were placed on a list of recipients. These individual children (and not their siblings, the children with whom they lived, or their guardians) then publicly received student school bags, exercise notebooks, writing materials, hurricane lamps and paraffin, mosquito nets, soap, blankets, school shoes, school uniform and other clothes, and sugar and maize flour.

Participating scholars indicated that the provision of school learning materials enabled them to be in a positive emotional state of mind as they had their material needs met through the scholarships. However, there were challenges when it came to utilization of the scholarship items. Most of the students lived in homes with foster parents, some of whom had children who were also in need. Follow-up supervisory visits by mentors, government extension agents and CRECCOM staff revealed that sometimes the materials given to the scholars led to their further marginalization and discrimination within the household. In other cases, the materials were distributed among all members of the household—a culturally appropriate use of the materials, but one viewed as wholly inappropriate—if not corrupt—by USAID. These findings have been echoed in other studies of projects that individuate support and make culturally inappropriate demands about sharing resources among family members (e.g., Bennell, 2005).

Thus, while the basic needs scholarship items handed out to program participants helped relieve the immediate pressures of poverty under which the AGSP recipients lived, the results of this relief were not what was expected. Just the opposite, in fact: one year after scholarships were first distributed, AGSP scholars' dropout rates increased to 17%, outstripping the 12.5% national dropout rate. More alarmingly, 90% of the AGSP dropouts were due to marriage and pregnancies (Samati, 2010). By comparison, nationally at the time, only 19% of dropouts were due to marriages and pregnancies (The Republic of Malawi EMIS, 2006).

Samati (2010) argues that the marriage- and pregnancy-linked dropout rates among participants rose because AGSP did not address the gender stereotypes that placed a low value on girls' education, including the common belief that girls should only go to schools to wait for marriage. The AGSP's focus on just providing scholarships for girls neglected the need for analysis and disruption of gender role inequities; as these were not disrupted, girl scholars continued to face an unequal division of labor, limited access and control of resources, and little control over decision-making within the households in which they were fostered. Guardians', girls, and broader social assumptions that gave low importance to schooling for vulnerable children's success were not disrupted.

CRECCOM staff argued that, within this environment, the provision of material goods actually backfired, in at least two different ways. First, many individual girls and boys who were identified as AGSP scholars paid a social price for the goods they received, often a price that was far greater than the benefit brought by the provision of materials. As has occurred with other programs utilizing individual child-targeted designs, faced with heightened inequities within their households, some guardians and siblings rejected individual scholarship recipients for having been targeted by an external organization and cut off familial support for them. CRECCOM staff reported that in some cases children were called "AGSP children", and were told that the project was now their guardian. Individual targeting also led to some children being told they were orphans for the first time ever, after they had been living with aunts or uncles who they thought were their parents. The AGSP's "beneficent" selection and public identification of the child as an AGSP scholar (that is, as an orphan) led to serious disruptions in their family units. These patterns have been noted in other programs targeting vulnerable children in the past (see Bennell 2005) and continue to be major issues facing IDO-led efforts because, despite their well-documented and known, harmful social consequences, IDOs continue to structure programs in this way.

Second, and relatedly, when AGSP girls received the materials distributed by the project, they were, for a short time, better-dressed, better-fed, and more visibly wealthy than many of their peers. This outcome would be short-lived, however, and many girls and guardians knew this. Some girls in the first year who became married or pregnant reported feeling increased pressure from guardians to get married while they were still "looking nice"; other girls felt they should leverage this one-time infusion of materials goods into a better marriage proposal than they might get later; still others reported receiving more male attention because of their improved outward appearance. And thus, the provision of materials could increase AGSP scholars' pregnancy and marriage rates (see Mojole 2018 for a related account in Kenya).

These outcomes should not have been a surprise to the IDOs involved in AGSP, as they were warned repeatedly about them by their local implementing partner, CRECCOM. Early on in the process of implementing AGSP, CRECCOM identified a core set of practices that were leading to unintended results. These included individual targeting of children, identification of orphans as opposed to AIDS-affected or vulnerable households, lack of community involvement in the project, a lack of support provided to AGSP scholars to help navigate the changes that the project brought to their situations, and a lack of engagement with the schools over how to integrate AGSP scholars more effectively and supportively.

CRECCOM staff had expressed concerns about a number of the AGSP programming components at the start of the project; these concerns were generally rejected in favor of the initial proposal and approved plan for the project. The poor scholar retention and achievement rates identified after the first year of the project created new openings to re-conceptualize the project and its core components. In this reconceptualization phase, the IDO that was the prime contractor for the project stepped back and allowed CRECCOM to develop and implement new project components to accompany the continued distribution of materials goods. The second stage of programming thus represented some significant shifts in the assumptions about society, childhood, and wellbeing that underlaid the project's main components. These shifts are described below.

14.6 AGSP Stage 2

Based on their extensive work with AGSP scholars and their communities, CRECCOM suggested introducing a mentoring program and community meetings to start addressing gender stereotyping directly; engaging families and communities in conversations about why individual children might need targeted material support and attempting to mobilize their support for such efforts; and bringing community leaders into the project in order to help assure that AGSP built scholars' social networks and support structures, instead of shrinking them.

One of the key components of the new programming was mentoring sessions, which were conducted by community members with each AGSP scholar. The mentoring sessions brought community leaders—often elder women—into regular and close contact with an AGSP scholar. These mentoring sessions included counseling and guidance from the mentor to the scholar, but they also provided the scholar with a broader adult social network, and more particularly, assured there was at least one adult outside of the scholars' home who had a sense of what was happening in the scholars' life and was made aware of any stresses the scholar was facing and any pressures they might feel growing on them to get married or become sexually active. The mentoring and these broader social connections helped improve the climate at home, and impacted scholars' wellbeing both socially and economically (as the mentors often helped out financially when the scholars' guardians could not or would not). AGSP scholars were also mentored by teachers. CRECCOM staff noted that, while teacher-student mentoring activities allowed AGSP scholars to express concerns they had with their schooling and to gain insights from teachers about how to navigate school, the school-based mentoring relationships did not appear to impact scholars' wellbeing as much as the community mentor relationships.

The second key component of the new strategy were the scholar retreats. At these retreats, AGSP scholars were accorded an opportunity to freely express the challenges they faced to their teachers, mentors, and fellow students. All of the retreat participants then jointly agreed on solutions and plans of action they would implement in order to address the issues. The retreats also included role modeling and counseling sessions. Girls that had achieved in education were called upon to give talks on what challenges they had met during their lives and how they had managed to succeed. The role models also gave the scholars advice about what course and exam subjects one had to pursue in order to undertake a particular career. The counseling sessions often included leaders from the community, and some life skills lessons, and provided spaces in which AGSP scholars had access to many of the adult leaders and their wise counsel—access that most AGSP scholars had not had previously because of their more marginalized positions in their families and communities.

AGSP scholars, their guardians, their community mentors, and their teachers reported that the retreats were powerful because they provided a space for guardians and their charges to hear each other—often for the first time ever, they reported. Guardians said that they realized that they were harming students without being aware of it. For instance, they said they woke the girls up very early to do household chores because they were afraid that otherwise the girls would become lazy and would not be seen as hard workers and good future wives. The girls, on the other hand, were able to express to their guardians that being woken up so early to do chores made them feel very resentful because waking up early to work prevented them from studying as their peers were doing.

Besides waking up early, the girls also raised concerns about their guardians shouting at them in ways that made the girls feel they did not belong in the households. This was part of the reason why the girls felt they should just go and get married quickly. In many cases, the guardians expressed their sorrow and concerns that the girls felt this way; and the retreat community together expressed the strong sentiment that girls should not feel this way, and that getting married before finishing school was ruining the girls' future. The community retreats thus provided a space in which girls and their guardians could listen carefully to one another and think together about how to resolve issues that the girls were facing. The retreats were also spaces in which new social norms counseling against early marriages for vulnerable girls were developed among guardians and local leaders.

The third key component was guardian training. This component was developed to address the problem (from the project's perspective) that, due to cultural norms, the scholarship items received were utilized by everybody in the household, and households were often quite large. Thus, the individual targeting imagined by the project did not, in practice, always happen. These challenges prompted the mentor teachers and community mentors in some districts to meet with community leaders to discuss how best this issue could be addressed. They decided to hold monthly educational retreats for AGSP scholars' guardians. The AGSP staff developed a 3-to-5-day, community-based training program and materials, which were utilized during the retreats. Guardians' training sessions looked at how the guardians could best care for the orphans, what challenges they met, and how they could solve them. Guardian training sessions thus helped turn the insights gained through the mentoring sessions into practicable actions that guardians could take to support their scholars. Remarkable results were achieved in the three zones where retreat-based education for the guardians was held as compared to where guardians were not included in the retreats as outlined below:

Zones with guardian education	**No of scholars dropped out over 3 years**	**No of scholars in std 8 selected to secondary school**	**Average performance of scholars each term**
Limbuli (Mulanje)	1	4 out of 5 scholars	95%
Kalonga (Lilongwe)	0	10 out of 11	95%
Mwazisi (Rumphi)	0	6 out of 7	95%
Zones with no guardian education			
Mathambi (Mulanje)	9	5 out of 15	75%
Mzumazi (Lilongwe)	8	3 out of 13	65%
St Peters (Likoma)	8	7 out of 12	65%

14.7 Decolonizing AGSP and Child Wellbeing

AGSP's three new activities reflect an Ubuntu approach to programming for children affected by AIDS. The activities decenter individual wants and needs, and re-situate scholars' individual experiences within the core social relations with guardians, peers, and community members, that give them moyo, or life, and that mark them as human. They shift power towards the community and away from the IDOs and their resources, and they shift focus from outcomes to process. The process of participation—of having people talk to one another about their experiences, needs, and fears—itself creates new ways of seeing each other and each other's experiences, and therefore new potential outcomes. AGSP scholars began to drop out of school for marriage or parenting less frequently. They felt more supported in their schools and by their peers, and felt more confident in their ability to navigate school. They also felt heard, respected, and listened to by their guardians and by the broader community. They felt they could point out times when they felt pressured to marry or be sexually active and receive broad community support to choose school over these options.

The improvement in scholars' wellbeing that resulted from the increased mentoring and social support included their academic outcomes. Their performance in various subjects and their persistence in school increased. Their daily attendance improved and their dropout rates declined. For instance, the number of girls who were in the program and dropped out of school was reduced from 2.8% (93 out of 3320) to 1.3% (43 out of 3320) by the fourth year (CRECCOM, 2006). The number of scholars that did well in exams improved tremendously over the course of the project, to the point that, by the last year, the number of AGSP scholars selected to secondary school increased to 33%, as compared to the national average of 23%. The students could also articulate what they wanted and had a voice in the type and quantity of the scholarship items they wanted to be provided to them by the program.

These improvements in academic outcomes reflect, we believe, significant, positive changes in multiple facets of AGSP scholars' wellbeing over the course of the project. By being reconnected to the community, by having opportunities to speak directly to adults (including leaders) about their experiences, their fears, and their goals; and by receiving the wisdom and support of their community to continue their education, AGSP scholars gained new allies and new connections among peers and adults. The success of AGSP II over AGSP I indicates the centrality of community relations and support to the wellbeing of children affected by AIDS. IDOs' belief that the provision of material resources was all that was needed to secure children's education was disproved: the material resources did indeed make a difference in scholars' lives, but the difference was often to increase pressure on them to shift from their social positions as children to become wives and mothers. As many of the scholars who made this shift said that they did not desire this shift, and as the international child rights frames also find these outcomes abhorrent, there is every reason to believe that AGSP I may have actually decreased the wellbeing of some participants. AGSP II had the opposite effect by simply recognizing scholars as social beings, whose social relations were, in fact, in danger of being negatively impacted if the project did not mobilize broader adult support for scholars, and community-wide social change around gender norms and relations, and around familial and community expectations of support for orphaned children by outside organizations.

While the second half of the project was widely deemed a success as measured by its own goals, and while many (including many scholars and community members) would argue that it increased the wellbeing of the majority of scholars by helping them gain agency and voice, gain social support, and increase their educational opportunities, the project was also limited in its impact by the continued focus throughout many of the project's components on individual children, their need for partiuclar material inputs (e.g., shoes, backpacks), and their educational success. For example, many scholars struggled to maintain their academic performance and enrollment in the face of extreme household-level uncertainties. Since most of the scholars supported were double orphans, they were often looked after by other guardians that were related to the deceased parents. There were a lot of changes in life that these orphans had to cope up with. Sometimes they were transferred from one relative to another due to various reasons such as divorce of guardians, transfers, jealousy because the supported scholar outshined the biological children in that family, and death of the guardian, just to mention a few. Most times the scholars ended up staying with grandmothers if they were alive. This greatly impacted the wellbeing and achievement of the scholars as they kept on changing schools and often ended up living in grandmother-headed households that were themselves financially and socially marginalized, and that often struggled with food insecurity.

The AGSP project's inability to address this broader level of family insecurity and the social disruptions caused by AIDS was not surprising: from the IDO perspective, AGSP was a school sector project whose goals were tightly organized around educational outcomes. While the project's initial failure created an opportunity to expand the IDOs' understanding of what was needed to achieve academic success, the resources put into this expansion were minimal—retreats and mentoring and guardian trainings were run on little to no budget, with the force of volunteer support. The notion that family units might need long-term support in order to stabilize scholars' home situations was never taken up seriously by the project for a number of reasons, including the individual focus it adopted from the start, concerns about "sustainability", concerns about "mission creep" outside of the education sector, funding constraints, and concerns about suppressing the volunteer "spirit" on which so many development projects rely.

14.8 PASI and Participatory Wellbeing

The AGSP II experience reflects a number of more recent experiments in how community-led participation might further decolonial approaches to education. One such experiment in Malawi, the Participatory Action for School Improvement (PASI) is described in detail in Kendall, Kaunda, and Friedson-Ridenour (2015). For the purposes of this comparison, what is important is that PASI's participatory planning and budgeting practices supported students and other marginalized groups in shifting roles, from being only spectators into being active participants in every stage of the project. PASI did so by creating supportive structures through which different groups of people in the community participated in every component of decision-making related to the project, which aimed broadly to improve the quality of the community's school, and in particular, to support vulnerable children's schooling.

PASI's model of community-led planning was designed to assure that the decision-making process was equitable along lines of gender, age, and social status. The group deliberation process—in which what might be termed affinity groups met to discuss the project and what they wanted it to accomplish—assured that no individual felt compelled or scared to participate. Each person could join a group in which they felt they belonged and where they felt they could express their opinions and have their experiences taken seriously. After each group met to plan, all of the groups met together to report out and discuss their ideas. Each group had an equal opportunity to speak, and the project required that the community adopt at least one idea from each group's goals and activities list. While this process was far from perfect, it did yield quite different results in each community than would have been the case without this process. For example, in many communities women were very quiet at the beginning of the process. They would not speak anything initially, but when it came to the planning and budgeting they were put in groups and this let them talk in a society where they are supposed to be quiet. It gave them a chance to voice out their thoughts and suggestions to each other. These thoughts and suggestions raised important points and ideas about project activities, processes, and outcomes that were not identified by the male leadership groups, but that significantly improved the project's plans in many communities and that stopped the project from causing harm to women's lives. For example, in one community, the male leadership planned for a large amount of sand to be brought to the school so that men could construct a classroom. The women's group pointed out that, while there were many resources allocated for the men's building activities, there were no resources allocated for women's transportation of sand to the school site—and the sand had to be carted from very far away. After the women's group voiced this concern, one of the male leaders agreed to have his bullock cart at the women's disposal so that they could load the sand but not carry it to the school.

The community-led planning process also helped improve the quality of life of teachers, because before the shared planning process, community members had seldom been aware of the issues that teachers faced at their school. The PASI planning and implementation process, as with the AGSP retreats, allowed groups from different social positions to hear each other reflect on a shared goal and recognize the different positions and experiences of other groups. The PASI process, unlike AGSP, was more flexible in that it placed few constraints on how communities needed to conceptualize educational quality and the social forces that impact it. By opening up the doors and asking diverse groups (including girls and boys) to identify what would improve the quality of school life for them, PASI placed fewer artificial sectoral limitations on the locus and scope of the issues communities decided to address in order to improve school quality. In this sense, PASI and AGSP, at their best, focused on community needs, goals, and practices; emphasized the centrality of marginalized community members' experiences; and actively sought to disrupt socio-cultural norms and economic relations that maintained inequities.[4] In so doing, they acknowledged and actively tried to support change in relations of power and social norms that negatively impacted the projects' "end users": vulnerable children.

14.9 Decolonial Responses to Improving Wellbeing in Malawi

In this section, we argue that support for decolonial approaches to addressing AIDS can have significantly different and better impacts on children's wellbeing than current internationally-funded models. However, as indicated in the review of the AGSP and PASI projects, such approaches require, by their very nature, both decentering IDOs' power and influence, and centering participatory models that recognize and actively respond to community relations of power and authority.

As both an epistemic and a political project, decolonial approaches seek the liberation and freedom of the people who experienced colonialism and who today continue to subsist and live under the reach of global coloniality (Ndlovu-Gatsheni, 2013) as masked under the rhetoric of progress, equality, fraternity, and liberty (Mignolo, 2011). Writing out of and about the continuous colonization and re-(or neo-)colonization of their everyday lives, decolonial scholars (who are often Indigenous or First Nations people) argue that "development" as a concept, process, discourse and practice remains caught up in the matrices of power that underpin coloniality and impede the formulation of possibilities for decolonized, democratic and inclusive development in Africa (Ndlovu-Gatsheni, 2012). Maldonado-Torres (2007) describes coloniality an invisible power structure that sustains colonial relations of exploitation and domination long after the end of direct colonialism. Thus, coloniality survives colonialism and is maintained alive in what gets accepted as common sense, in the self-image of peoples, and in aspirations of self.

Decolonial and critical development studies approaches to theorizing international development have revealed the continued neocolonial roots of IDOs' practices, policies, and resource distribution approaches (Crush, 1995; Escobar, 2011; Ferguson, 2015). These post-development theorists critique the very idea of development as a hegemonic discourse used to keep the targets of development as subjects of Euro-American power (Ndlovu-Gatsheni, 2013). These roots include, for example, the continued assumption that capitalist modes of production are the pinnacle of development and modernity, and thus the end-goal for all people in all places (Rojas, 2007); that rational individualism is key to the development process, and that individuals (and particularly their economic actions) are the primary unit of analysis and action in family, national, and global development (Portes, 1973; Quijano, 2007); that in capitalist societies wage labor should be the way people acquire purchasing power to the necessities of life (Ferguson, 2015); that development is best measured in relation to outcomes selected by IDOs, not by its processes or its consequences for "recipient" wellbeing; that human productivity is key to all progress and is imbued in the able bodies of adults; and that children's appropriate socio-economic roles are as learners in formal schooling and as (economi-

[4]This list of outcomes closely mirrors that developed by Cornish and Ghosh (2007) in their discussion of the complex power dynamics that must be balanced to achieve successful "community-led" health promotion outcomes.

cally) dependent members of family units (Thangaraj, 2018).

Reflecting this colonial ideology of modernity and development, IDOs' understanding of childhood, schooling, and community-based or participatory development approaches is often limited to individually-focused efforts to improve human capital development by enrolling and keeping children who are affected by AIDS in school. This approach views schools as inherently equity-promoting spaces that do not need to respond to diversity in children's needs and realities (the "add orphans and stir" approach), in which children automatically accrue both human capital and their own rights through their presence, and in which schooling is an inherent good that all community members and governments should support. This approach to participation, in other words, reflects many of the colonizing tenets of current international development approaches. As discussed in Kendall et al. (2015):

> Since the 1990s, the term participation has been increasingly mainstreamed into bilateral, multilateral, governmental, and non-governmental international development organization (IDO) discourses (Alejandro Leal, 2007). Though the term has liberatory and democratic philosophical roots, its use by IDOs has been described as co-opted and increasingly hegemonic (Cornwall & Brock, 2005). Common critiques include that IDOs may utilize participation simply as a means to their own predetermined ends (Hayward, Simpson, & Wood, 2004) and that their philosophical orientations may lead them to inappropriately account for (or fail to account for) power dynamics among and within funders and communities. Indeed, critical development researchers have shown how inequities (e.g., in wealth, geography, gender, education, language, age, social status, and disability) within and among groups shape participation patterns in development efforts to the detriment of socially just outcomes. (Kendall, 2008; Kothari, 2001; Rahnema, 2010)
> Similarly, in our work as critical development practitioners and researchers in Ghana, Malawi, Mozambique, and Zimbabwe, we observed that IDOs' participatory development education efforts commonly constituted a "participation-for-our-purposes" approach, which not only often failed to meet IDOs' stated goals of local "empowerment" and increased effectiveness, but in some cases, did active damage to people's sense of themselves, their knowledge, their rights, and their ways of being in the world. In this regard, we find useful the argument that international development efforts may constitute a form of abjection (Ferguson, 2002) and that abjection represents an always incomplete, but nonetheless powerful, reshaping of people's sense of self around the values of the colonizing other.

This critical approach to understanding community and participation provides an essential lens for reexamining IDO programs developed to support the wellbeing of children affected by AIDS. A critical analytic approach emphasizes that children's wellbeing can never effectively be conceptualized as an individual's wellbeing, and that wellbeing can never be solely or primarily understood in financial terms. Instead, children's wellbeing must be understood as situated within interwoven social, economic, political, and cultural relations that span levels of social organization from families and peer networks to transnational organizations; organize discourses, policies, and practices; and shape the consequences of efforts to improve wellbeing (Friedson-Ridenour et al., 2015). New approaches to supporting children's wellbeing that destabilize the aspects of international development practices that reify the individual and their economic wellbeing are essential, and have increasingly been addressed by IDOs through the discourse of "participation". IDO-led participatory efforts, however, have often been extremely constrained in their shape and scope, and have at times served to strengthen existing inequalities in relations of power and authority—among development institutions, community members, adults and children, communities and schools.

Decolonial participatory approaches require that ordinary people adjudicate over the issues that concern them, that they organize themselves and decide their fate, including by operating from their own meaning of concepts such as development, democracy, and human rights (Plaatjie, 2013). When implemented at the community level, such participatory models have great potential to engender collective transformative change through mobilizing and empowering whole communities, including marginalized groups, toward full local ownership and responsive development approaches (Samati, 2010).

AGSP's second phase and the PASI project offer examples of what these more decolonial approaches might look like and accomplish, even as both also clearly indicate the limitations to decolonial approaches that attempt to work within current IDO frameworks. For example, a key takeaway from both projects was that, despite their evident and publicly-lauded successes, IDOs were unwilling to cede control over the projects in such a way that the project's participatory processes could be maintained or expanded within communities. Since marginalized community members in marginalized communities have a difficult time maintaining projects that require significant resources, IDOs' unwillingness to provide resources to communities that have adopted strong participatory models results in the failure of these efforts to have a long-term impact (Kaunda, 2017).

14.10 Conclusion

In this paper we have argued that current international efforts to improve the wellbeing of children affected by HIV/AIDS are largely focused on improving these children's educational outcomes. Many of the projects created to achieve these goals reflect central tenets of coloniality, including individualization, a focus on material wellbeing, and the imposition of Western norms related to sharing and family structures. We have shown how such approaches fail—by their own measures and by more expansive notions of wellbeing. And we have also shown how relatively minor changes to programming that align projects more closely with what might be considered the values of Ubuntu (or Umunthu, in Malawi) and that pay careful attention to the power dynamics that shape relations among IDOs, NGOs, students, guardians, teachers, and community members can serve as decolonial moments in community relations and the development landscape alike. However, without more radical changes in who determines the distribution of resources, these efforts will always be limited and international efforts to support children's wellbeing will always be only partially positive in their effects.

References

Ainsworth, M., Beegle, K., & Koda, G. (2002). *The impact of adult mortality on primary school enrolment in northwestern Tanzania* (Africa region human development, working paper series). Washington, DC: World Bank.

Ainsworth, M., & Filmer, D. (2002). *Poverty, AIDS and children's schooling: A targeting dilemma* (Policy research working paper 2885). Washington, DC: World Bank.

Alejandro Leal, P. (2007). Participation: The ascendancy of a buzzword in the neo-liberal era. *Development in Practice, 17*(4–5), 539–548.

Avert. (2018). *Children, HIV, and AIDS*. Available via https://www.avert.org/professionals/hiv-social-issues/key-affected-populations/children#footnoteref60_r7i83jj

Barrientos, A., Gorman, M., & Heslop, A. (2003). Old age poverty in developing countries and dependence in later life. *World Development, 31*(3), 555–570.

Bennell, P. (2005). The impact of the AIDS epidemic on teachers in Sub-Saharan Africa. *Journal of Development Studies, 41*(3), 440–466.

Cornish, F., & Ghosh, R. (2007). The necessary contradictions of 'community-led' health promotion: A case study of HIV prevention in an Indian red light district. *Social Science & Medicine, 64*(2), 496–507.

Cornwall, A., & Brock, K. (2005). What do buzzwords do for development policy? A critical look at 'participation,' 'empowerment' and 'poverty reduction.'. *Third World Quarterly, 26*(7), 1043–1060.

CRECCOM. (2006). *AGSP report: Annual report*. Washington, DC: Winrock International.

Crush, J. (1995). *Power of development*. London and New York, NY: Routledge.

DeJaeghere, J. (2004). *Background paper for workshop 1: Quality education and gender equality*. Paper presented at the International Conference on Education: Forty-seventh Session, Geneva, Switzerland.

Dionne, K. Y. (2017). *Doomed interventions: The failure of global responses to AIDS in Africa*. Cambridge, UK: Cambridge University Press.

Escobar, A. (2011). *Encountering development: The making and unmaking of the third world*. Princeton, NJ: Princeton University Press.

Ferguson, J. (2002). Of mimicry and membership: Africans and the "new world society". *Cultural Anthropology, 17*(4), 551–569.

Ferguson, J. (2015). *Give a man a fish: Reflections on the new politics of distribution*. Durham, NC: Duke University Press.

Foster, G., & Williamson, J. (2000). A review of current literature of the impact of HIV/AIDS on children in Sub-Saharan Africa. *AIDS, 14*(Suppl 3), S275–S284.

Friedson-Rideneour, S., Kendall, N., & DiPrete Brown, L. (2015). *Gender, wellbeing, and the ecological commons: Towards a participatory framework of wellbeing for women and girls*. Madison, WI: 4W Initaitive.

Gillespie, S., Haddad, L., & Jackson, R. (2001). *HIV/AIDS, food and nutrition security: Impacts and actions*. Paper prepared for the 28th Session of the ACC/SCN Symposium on Nutrition and HIV/AIDS. International Food Policy Research Institute (IFPRI).

Guo, Y., Li, X., & Sherr, L. (2012). The impact of HIV/AIDS on children's educational outcome: A critical review of global literature. *AIDS Care, 24*(8), 993–1012.

Haacker, M. (2016). *The economics of the global response to HIV/AIDS*. Oxford, UK: Oxford University Press.

Hayward, C., Simpson, L., & Wood, L. (2004). Still Left out in the Cold: Problematising Participatory Research and Development. *Sociologia Ruralis, 44*(1), 95–108.

Help Age International. (2003). *Supporting older carers*. Available at http://www.helpage.org/resources/publications/?adv=0&ssearch=2003&filter=f.yeard&type=&region=&topic=&language=&page=4

Jirojanakul, P., Skevington, S., & Hudson, K. (2003). Predicting young children's quality of life. *Social Science & Medicine, 57*, 1277–1288.

Joshua, M., Ngongondo, C., Monjerezi, M., Chipungu, F., Liwenga, E., Majule, A., & Lamboll, R. (2016). Climate change in semi-arid Malawi: Perceptions, adaptation strategies and water governance. *Jàmbá: Journal of Disaster Risk Studies, 8*(3), 1–10.

Kadzamira, E., Maluwa-Banda, D., Kamlongera, A., & Swainson, N. (2001). *The impact of HIV/AIDS on primary and secondary schooling in Malawi: Developing a comprehensive strategic response*. Zomba, Malawi: Centre for Educational Research and Training (CERT).

Kaunda, Z. (2017). *Community participation in Community Day Secondary Schooling for orphaned and vulnerable students in Malawi in an era of shrinking community*. Dissertation, University of Minnesota.

Kelly, M. (2001). *Challenging the challenger: Understanding and expanding the response of universities in Africa to HIV/AIDS*. A synthesis report for the working group on higher education, Association for the Development of Education in Africa [ADEA].

Kendall, N. (2004). Global policy in practice: The 'successful failure' of free primary education in Malawi Dissertation, Stanford University.

Kendall, N. (2008). "Vulnerability" in AIDS-affected states: Rethinking child rights, educational institutions, and development paradigms. *International Journal of Educational Development, 28*(4), 365–383.

Kendall, N., Kaunda, Z., & Friedson-Rideneur, S. (2015). Community participation in international development education quality improvement efforts: Current paradoxes and opportunities. *Educational Assessment, Evaluation and Accountability, 27*(1), 65–83.

Kendall, N., & O'Gara, C. (2007). Vulnerable children, communities and schools: Lessons from three HIV/AIDS affected areas. *Compare: A Journal of Comparative Education, 37*(1), 5–21.

Kendall, N., & Silver, R. (2014). The consequences of global mass education: Schooling, work, and well-being in EFA-era Malawi. In *Globalization and education: Integration and contestation across cultures* (pp. 247–265). Lanham, MD: Rowman & Littlefield Education.

King, B., Burka, M., Winchester, M. (2018). HIV citizenship in uneven landscapes. *Annals of the American Association of Geographers, 108*(6), 1685–1699.

Kothari, U. (2001). Power, knowledge and social control in participatory development. In B. Cooke & U. Kothari (Eds.), *Participation: The new tyranny?* (pp. 139–152). London: Zed Books.

Maldonado-Torres, N. (2007). On the coloniality of being: Contributions to the development of a concept. *Cultural Studies, 21*(2–3), 240–270.

Mashegoane, S., & Mohale, N. (2016). Parenting AIDS-orphaned grandchildren: Experiences from Lephalale, South Africa. *Gender & Behaviour, 14*(1), 6931.

Mignolo, W. (2011). *The darker side of Western modernity: Global futures, decolonial options*. London, UK: Duke University Press.

Mkandawire, P., Tenkorang, E., & Luginaah, I. (2013). Orphan status and time to first sex among adolescents in Northern Malawi. *AIDS and Behavior, 17*(3), 939–950.

Moller, V., Roberts, B., Tiliouine, H., & Lotschky, J. (2017). Waiting for happiness in Africa. In *World happiness report*. New York, NY: Earth Institute.

Mundy, K. (2016). "Leaning in" on education for all. *Comparative Education Review, 60*(1), 1–26.

Munthali, A. (2002). *Adaptive strategies and coping mechanisms of families and communities affected by HIV/AIDS in Malawi*. Prepared for UNRISD Project: HIV and Development.

National AIDS Commission (NAC). (2010). *Malawi statistics*. Lilongwe, Malawi: NAC.

Ndlovu-Gatsheni. (2012). Coloniality of power in development studies and the impact of global imperial designs on Africa. *ARAS, 33*(2), 48–73.

Ndlovu-Gatsheni, S. (2013). Perhaps decoloniality is the answer? Critical reflections on development from a decolonial epistemic perspective. *Africanus, 43*(2), 1–12.

Plaatjie, S. (2013). Beyond Western-centric and Eurocentric development: A case for decolonizing development. *Africanus, 43*(2), 118–130.

Portes, A. (1973). Modernity and development: A critique. *Studies in Comparative International Development, 8*(3), 247–279.

Quijano, A. (2007). Coloniality and modernity/rationality. *Cultural Studies, 21*(2–3), 168–178.

Rahnema, M. (2010). Participation. In W. Sachs (Ed.), *The development dictionary* (pp. 116–131). London: Zed Books.

Rock, A., Barrington, C., Abdoulayi, S., Tsoka, M., Mvula, P., & Handa, S. (2016). Social networks, social participation, and health among youth living in extreme poverty in rural Malawi. *Social Science & Medicine, 170*, 55–62.

Rojas, C. (2007). International political economy/development otherwise. *Globalizations, 4*(4), 573–587.

Samati, M. (2010). *The Ambassador's girls scholarship program: Beyond access is attitude*. Master's Thesis, Brandeis University.

Samoff, J. (1999). *No teacher guide, no textbooks, no chairs: Contending with crisis in African education*. Paper presented at the 43rd Annual Meeting of the African Studies Association Philadelphia PA, November 11–14 1999.

Serpell, R. (2010). *The significance of schooling: Life-journeys in an African society*. Cambridge, UK: Cambridge University Press.

Singer, M., & Clair, S. (2003). Syndemics and public health: Reconceptualizing disease in bio-social context. *Medical Anthropology Quarterly, 17*(4), 423–441.

Stambach, A. (2013). *Lessons from Mount Kilimanjaro: Schooling, community, and gender in East Africa*. New York, NY: Routledge.

Thangaraj, M. (2018). *Silk, schools, special economic zones: The reconstruction of childhood, education, and labor in Kanchipuram, India*. Dissertation, University of Wisconsin-Madison.

The Republic of Malawi EMIS. (2006). *Education statistics 2006*. Lilongwe, Malawi: Education Management Information System (EMIS), Department of Education Planning, Ministry of Education and Vocational Training.

UNAIDS. (2016). *HIV fact sheet*. Available at http://www.unaids.org/sites/default/files/media_asset/UNAIDS_FactSheet_en.pdf

UNAIDS. (2018). *Malawi*. Available at http://www.udnaids.org/en/regionscountries/countries/malawi

USAID. (2003). *USAID project profiles: Children affected by HIV/AIDS*. Washington, DC: USAID.

Vandemoortele, J., & Delamonica, E. (2000). The 'education vaccine' against HIV. *Current Issues in Comparative Education, 3*(1), 6–13.

Vavrus, F. (2003). *Desire and decline: Schooling amid crisis in Tanzania*. New York, NY: Peter Lang Publishing.

WHOQOL Group. (1995). The World Health Organization quality of life assessment (WHOQOL): Development and general psychometric properties. *Social Science & Medicine, 46*(12), 1569–1585.

Part IV

Education

An EI Approach to Parent Communication Amongst In-Service Teachers

15

Giulietta Domenica Harrison

Abstract
This chapter looks at the concept of well-being and quality of life in relation to teacher education in ECCE and the Foundation Phase (FP), and how use of principles of emotional intelligence (EI) leads to improvement in well-being for teachers, parents and learners. Emanating from a call for help by in-service FP teachers who were studying for a B. Ed. (FP) qualification, came the realization that teachers were struggling to connect with learners and parents, resulting in a breakdown in quality of life. This research made use of a Vygotskian theoretical framework, coupled with application of the principles of EI and qualitative comments made by the aforementioned teachers. The result was improved communication between all parties and, in the process, the quality of life for the learner, parent and teacher improved through establishment of positive lines of communication and trust. Another study shows how QOL can potentially be enhanced through training teachers in ECCE to be professional, context adaptive and reflective individuals who place the child at the centre of learning.

G. D. Harrison (✉)
Africa A+ Schools, Grahamstown, South Africa

15.1 Introduction

Emotions and social relationships are central to human behaviour and have a profound impact on Quality Of Life (QOL) and well-being. The manner in which humans engage with one another has often been problematic in modern times, as seen in two world wars and many subsequent wars, up to the present day. Today the media, and especially online social media, provide a constant reminder of the crises that our societies and our planet are facing. In the South African context, QOL research conducted by Møller (2013) across three decades, measured QOL in terms of three categories, namely: Satisfaction, Happiness and Perceptions of life getting better. This study showed a marked upswing, post the new democracy, followed by a reality check in the 10 years following democracy and an additional improvement around the time of the 2010 Football World Cup, held in South Africa. This suggests that QOL is affected by political movement and international events, such as international sporting events, that undoubtedly foster national spirit, thereby accounting for an upswing in perception of QOL.

According to Moller, Roberts, Tiliouine, and Loschky (2017), African citizens expect much more from democracy than simple free and fair elections. They associate democracy with improved living conditions, basic services, such as water and electricity, and the freedom to

I. Eloff (ed.), *Handbook of Quality of Life in African Societies*, International Handbooks of Quality-of-Life, https://doi.org/10.1007/978-3-030-15367-0_15

criticize government. Furthermore, international research indicates that countries that enjoy good governance have accelerated development and consequently improved QOL (Moller et al. 2017).

The African continent has been scarred by the history of colonialism as well as many instances of weak democracies and poor governance subsequent to independence. Recent calls by students at higher education institutions (HEIs) have highlighted the need for change. Africanisation of the curriculum has been seen as one of the ways in which higher education can be made more relevant and consequently potentially improve the outcomes for students who would be able to identify better with the content (Gumbo & Msila, 2017). Since her new democracy in 1994, South Africa has been on a quest to improve academic results and the QOL of her citizens. This started with a drive to recognize the importance of Grade R and, most recently, the birth-to-4 phase of development, as key areas for improvement.

Research related to QOL and well-being with regard to Early Childhood Care and Education (ECCE) is sorely lacking. A review of current literature shows an emphasis on issues concerning health, with particular emphasis on mental health, HIV and AIDS, and autism (Mweete, West, Dave, Levitt & Lambert, 2014., Mwesiga et al., 2015; Schlebusch, Samuels, & Dada, 2016). A study on the mental health of patients suffering from HIV/AIDS showed that they had recurring bouts of depression which impacted on their quality of life (Mwesiga et al. 2015). The use of anti-retrovirals was shown to improve the quality of life of suffers with HIV/AIDS (Mweete et al., 2014). Having a regular family routine that incorporates cognitive therapy allows for a demonstrable improvement in QOL for families raising children on the autism spectrum (Schlebusch et al., 2016).

The contribution of education to QOL is usually couched in terms of the relevance of schooling to qualifications and vocational training as preparation for career, a working life and the ability to earn a living. While these are undoubtedly important considerations, they are by no means the only contributions that education makes to QOL. Acquisition of the basic skills of reading, writing and arithmetic alone do not equip the young person to be a full participant in society. This includes the capacity to be a life-long learner, with abilities to interpret and assimilate new information, including current news relevant to everyday life. It includes the ability to derive entertainment value and pleasure from reading in all of the arts, sciences and technologies. It also includes the tools to understand and use philosophical and practical ideas to apply in one's life and thereby enhance life's meaning, quality and even duration. All of these benefits from basic primary education can be amplified by effective secondary and tertiary education. If all aspects of education are considered, it is clear that it has an immeasurable impact on QOL, with potential for great good if the education is enlightened, and great ill if it is not.

When shifting focus to education and QOL, the state of teaching and teacher education is constantly called into question, particularly in South Africa where there is failure to reach desirable educational goals (PIRLS, 2017). Given how important teachers are in shaping the future of a child, it makes sense that, to achieve a positive outcome, teachers should have positive relationships with learners. A safe, happy learning environment is more likely to lead to learning (Fleisch, 2008). Furthermore, much of education emphasizes the holistic development of the child and teachers needs to work collaboratively with parents to achieve this (CAPS, 2011). Teachers must be able to communicate effectively with parents, as should parents with teachers. Both teacher and parent equally need to communicate effectively with the learner/child. The relationship between parent, child and teacher is seen as a triangle with the child as a central figure. A positive triangle of communication can only improve a child's sense of well-being and QOL.

All too often, research has shown that teachers are stressed, view parents as a threat, and spend much of their day doing little more than 'crowd control' (Harrison, 2014). Learners are subjected to inappropriate punishments, both at home and in the classroom, largely as a result of the stress that parents and teachers experience. It is understandable that much of the current research on

QOL and well-being has focused on health-related issues as it is often stated that humans are not capable of enjoying QOL if they do not have good health. This chapter will argue that the introduction of a communication system using EI, allowed for improved quality of life and well-being for teachers, parents and learners and that with this, children are able to learn in a positive environment consequently potentially allowing them to contribute to the well-being of society at large.

Before progressing further with this chapter, it is important to understand what is meant by quality and quality of life (QOL). Rapley (2003) suggests that QOL as a concept has been used to describe social and human science ranging from attempting to measure the state of population groups to that of specific individuals. A study of the literature has shown that it is both fragmented and contradictory in its descriptions making it too vast to arrive at one simple view point (Cummins, 1996). In order to achieve some semblance of understanding related to education I will focus on a national study which had at its heart the desire to improve quality of life through the way in which we train teachers in ECCE (Harrison, 2017). In so doing I am arguing that QOL in ECCE is determined by the way in which we educate our children as this will long term have an impact on the quality of life of the individual and on the society at large. In order to provide effective education of our children we need to ensure that our teacher training results in teachers who are capable, professional and empathetic.

A recent study for the development of a Diploma and Degree in the birth to four sector evidenced some useful information that can help to understand quality of life and what it means to implement a quality qualification in a South African context (Harrison, 2017). The aforementioned study was conducted nationally across ten Universities, three TVETS (Technical and Vocational Education and Training colleges) and five Non-Profit Organisations (NPOs). This research report served the purpose of informing the work of PIECCE which is specifically concerned with programme development at national level for an ECCE 0–4 year-olds Diploma/Degree. The work of the Project for Inclusive Early Childhood Care and Education (PIECCE) is unique in that it adopted a collaborative multi-stakeholder approach to understand how to achieve quality in ECCE. In addition, it recognised the importance of addressing diversity together with understanding what quality ECCE looks like, in order to bring about transformative pedagogy. In this respect it has a link to the Transformative Pedagogy Project (TPP). The TPP was designed to try and understand how to train ECE teachers and what might be transformative. The general consensus was that TPP needed to go beyond the boundaries of pedagogy to include context, historical background, equity and diversity. QOL research in Early Childhood would therefore need to include the contexts in which the teacher is operating, an appreciation of the historical background and understanding the needs of the individual learner/teacher/parent in order to realise a larger principle of equity in South African society.

The PIECCE report presents empirical data derived from three national surveys, together with collaborative literature reviews on four specific topics that were derived from an action research approach, adopted by the collaborative research team. The four agreed-upon areas were: academic support, work-integrated learning (WIL), recognition of prior learning (RPL), and norms and standards. The data were analysed quantitatively and qualitatively to benchmark current thinking and practices in ECCE.

All institution types acknowledged a need for academic support, with emphasis on mentorship at multiple levels. Mentorship is given in diverse ways, ranging from lecturers providing individual attention, to peer mentorship, to mentor teachers. What is suggested is that a community-of-practice (CoP) approach has potential to provide support at a variety of levels and should be encouraged. Extending mentorship beyond the confines of a training programme has direct implications for achieving quality, as without it there is minimal accountability and support for teachers/practitioners. Although the institutional surveys indicated an integrated approach to academic support, the student survey evidenced a non-integrated approach. It is apparent that a combination of both is most effective.

The concept of reflective practice was considered an essential aspect of learning for students/practitioners and for lecturers themselves. An analysis of a quality tool kit that focused on reflective practice showed that teachers found it to be beneficial, but seemed reluctant to apply it when there was no mentor present to guide the process. This raised questions around finding smart ways to ensure that reflective practice is achieved and thereby optimise quality implementation of ECCE programmes.

The importance of an adaptive approach to context emerged in the WIL component of this research. There was consensus that context is a key component of transformative pedagogy and that students/practitioners must be given the opportunity to work in a variety of contexts, but, most importantly, should be equipped with skills to be flexible and sensitive to context. There was some evidence of preparing student/practitioners to cope in a variety of contexts. These included providing specific training through dedicated modules, workshops, group discussions and efforts to expose students to varied teaching environments. There were, however, some marked constraints in the form of access, language difficulties, transport and, in some cases, inadequate exposure to 'best practice'.

A thorough examination of the policies that drive ECCE showed that a competency approach to programme development is a potential way forward. Ten competencies were isolated and considered in relation to quality and current institutional philosophies of training in ECCE. Three gaps were identified between policy and practice, namely, insufficient support for health, safety and nutrition; a need to provide more explicit training in leadership, management and administration; and a need for a stronger link between observation, assessment and development of the child.

RPL appears to have minimal uptake within HEIs because there is a sense that it may impact on institutions' reputations. There is evidence that RPL is gaining traction in the non-profit organisation (NPO) sector, but it is generally not sufficiently supported by training institutions because it is time consuming and costly when working with large cohorts. Given the present trend toward acknowledging that many in the ECCE workforce have considerable experience in the field, but limited financial resources and a need for a formal qualification, the suggestion is that deeper exploration of RPL is essential.

Finally, the issue of quality was examined through the lens of Bronfenbrenner's ecological model and Britto, Yoshikawa, and Boller's (2011) three-tiered pyramid, in order to unpack the levels of quality beyond the confines of classroom and pedagogy. It was determined that, while 'quality' is a term that is easily bandied about, it is not as easily defined or achieved. Empirical data in the PIECCE report suggested that providing academic support, mentorship at multiple levels, encouraging reflective practice, embracing diversity, and producing competent, adaptive educators who are able to lead, equals quality.

At the centre of quality ECCE is the teacher who is professional in her practice. It could be argued that teachers hold the key to unlocking the potential of children and therefore need to understand what it is to be professional and the impact they may have on the QOL of children they teach.

PIECCE sees professionalism embracing the following:

- The principles of inclusive education;
- The centrality and uniqueness of the learner;
- Development of a critically reflective workforce.

The next section of this chapter shares an example of how teachers can be inclusive, understand the uniqueness of the individual child and reflect on their practice in order to be a truly professional teacher who is contributing to QOL.

15.2 A Success Story

The study that follows arose from concerns of in-service teachers who were training on a B. Ed. (FP) programme and expressed their lack of connection to the learners that they taught, and their parents. There was a sense that these teachers were being reflective in so far as they had identified that they had a problem, but that they were not being sufficiently critical about what they might do to improve their situation and QOL for themselves and the children they taught. This was seen in their tendency to blame the parents for the situation, and the learners for being uncooperative. Learners were not seen as individuals, but rather lumped together as a collective problem that needed to be 'controlled'. This suggested that these teachers were not using principles of professionalism and EI, and that they needed support.

15.3 Literature Review and Context

EI is purported to be the gateway to QOL for both teacher and learner (Greenberg et al., 2003). While EI originated in a corporate environment, it was adopted by education to meet the demand for safe learning spaces and to assist teachers with classroom discipline (Goleman, 1996; 1998; 2001; 2007).

The teachers that were involved in this study worked in rural areas of Northern Cape and often in contexts of high learner-to-teacher ratios, coupled with poverty. The result of this context for teaching and learning was that parents did not have money to come to schools for meetings, drop off their children or engage with teachers on their children's progress. The teachers felt unsupported by the parents and complained that parents did not sign homework books, did not inform them of absenteeism or visit the schools. In addition, teachers noted that high class numbers meant that they spent their days doing little more than 'crowd control'. The result was that there was a lack of trust between parents, teachers and learners.

Bar-on (2003) is considered a pioneer in the field of EI, known for coining the term 'emotional quotient' (EQ) and arguing for the importance of studying human behaviour in terms of interpersonal relationships and coping skills. It was decided, as part of a Life Skills programme, to provide teachers with a research project that would establish EI principles and potentially build paths of communication between teacher and parent. It was hoped that in this way the QOL of all three parties (child, parent and teacher) would be enhanced. The teacher would be able to improve her classroom management and her relationship with parents. The parents could build a relationship of trust between themselves and the teacher, while learning how to support their children's relationships with the teacher and the school. The children could benefit from a more positive learning environment, validation from the teacher and their parents, and a resulting improved desire to learn.

By managing her relationships with learners and parents with an EI approach, the teacher builds self-respect and self-regulation, and potentially improves QOL (Harrison, 2011). EI was originally made popular by Daniel Goleman in 1996 who described it as the capacity to recognize one's own feelings together with those of others, motivating ourselves and regulating our emotions, particularly with regard to social relationships. These principles can be applied to build effective relationships between the teacher, child and parent (Elfenbeing & Maccann, 2017).

Karpov (2005) suggested, however, that educators must be conscious mediators who understand all aspects of the child's make-up, including cognitive, social, emotional and physical factors. Furthermore, the conscious mediator sets goals for the class as a whole and, perhaps more importantly, for each individual learner (Jahromi & Stifter, 2008). The goal, in this instance, was for the conscious mediator, namely the teacher, to inform the parents of their child's performance and behaviour, and to establish a line of communication through bonds of trust that would develop by using a message-book system that made use of specific EI-based principles and language. The second goal was to improve the teaching and learning environment through promotion of self-regulation in teachers and learners.

On examination of literature related to EI, Zeidner, Roberts, and Maccann (2003) indicated that EI consists of three main components, namely, the child's temperament, the child's rule-based learning, and competencies relevant to insightful understanding. As the child's temperament is inherited, the teacher can, at best, 'modulate' this aspect. However, she can assist the child to learn to self-regulate.

Salovey & Sluyter (1990) proposed a further conceptualizing of EI which adds more detail in relation to the teacher-child-parent triangular relationship. Salovey & Sluyter (1990) suggested four components of EI. The first has links to perception and refers to one's ability to identify how one is feeling within oneself and in relation to others. This is important in building relations of trust as teachers need to be authentic in their relationships with learners, something only achieved if teachers recognize their own emotions first (Salovey, 2004). This reduces potential for impulsive reactions so often seen in teachers who are stressed.

The second component of EI is grounded in emotional judgement whereby teachers prioritize information in order to problem solve (Salovey & Sluyter, 1990). This would clearly have a positive impact on the QOL or well-being of learners as they would learn to self-regulate through the conscious mediation and modelling displayed by teachers.

The third component of EI has implications in the South African multilingual classroom where language is frequently a barrier to learning. Salovey & Sluyter (1990) suggested that the labelling of emotions enhances understanding and interpretation, converting the complex to a level of simplicity that is potentially accessible to the parties involved.

The fourth element of EI has profound links to the work of the PIECCE report (Harrison, 2017), mentioned earlier in this chapter, which placed emphasis on reflective teachers who are able to critically evaluate their behaviour to temper their responses to learners.

15.4 Vygotsky and EI

The theoretical framework of a study can be described as the process of applying a particular lens of perception and understanding through which to discuss or analyse information. The choice of a Vygotskian approach to this study was fitting as Vygotsky's theories of learning interrelate with those of emotional intelligence (EI). Vygotsky (1978) suggested that we learn collaboratively, drawing from our existing knowledge to internalize new knowledge, and that this is most effectively achieved through use of cultural tools, the most important of which is language.

Lev Vygotsky, an eminent Soviet psychologist, made a profound contribution to the understanding of human behaviour (Moll, 2014). He saw humans as different from their animal relations in that they bring to their learning environment an ability to adapt and manipulate, resulting in production of cultural and historical tools (Van der Veer & Valsiner, 1991). The collective social history of the teacher and the learner is brought to the classroom and transferred from learner to learner, from teacher to learner and in this case, from teacher to parent (Vygotsky, 1997 & 1998). This process he referred to as mediation. Mediation should be goal directed and allow for a positive learning environment.

One of the most interesting aspects of Vygotsky's theories of learning is that he saw mediation happening with the assistance of signs and tools (Vygotsky, 1998). Language is considered the most important cultural tool for mediation. In terms of child development, language occurs at the same time as the child begins to use symbols and it is this language that opens the door to understanding the abstract (*sensu* Piaget, 2001). For example, an emoticon can be a tool to describe a child's behaviour and is instantly understandable to the child and the parent. This is particularly important in Foundation Phase where the child is beginning to acquire reading and writing skills. One of the first steps in learning to read is that of 'reading pictures' (CAPS, 2011). Consequently, the use of emoticons as a tool of communication between teacher, child and parent, allowed all parties to understand what was being conveyed.

In this instance, emoticons were directly linked to learners' performance and their ability to self-regulate. In order to address self-regulation, the teacher and parent, who are the child's key care givers, had to note the meaning of the emoticon and then respond. The outcome was a direct impact on the child's QOL, as the responses either validated or corrected the child's behaviour, encouraging continued self-regulation and promising the reward of receiving a positive reaction. When learners continue to self-regulate, they are more likely to be appropriately responsive to the teacher's requests and this results in a classroom environment that is happy and productive. The teacher is less likely to resort to draconian styles of classroom management as learners want to be validated for their self-regulation.

Given that the goal of this study was to improve communication and trust between teachers and parents, it is important to consider how Vygotsky's theory of mediation, together with EI, would interplay. The teacher, when mediating learner self-regulation through use of emoticons, self-regulated herself by ensuring that she placed a daily 'reflection' on how the child had behaved. The parents' responses to the daily reflections in the message book resulted in further self-regulation as they too were required to respond every day. The regularity of this process led to what Vygotsky termed 'practising a concept'. He suggested that it is only when one practises a concept that it becomes internalized. The act of the teacher placing an emoticon in the message book was a form of conscious mediation which allowed the child to temper her behaviour and her parents to respond. This built communication between the parties that comprised the 'sacred triangle', that is the parent, child and teacher.

15.5 Constructing Knowledge Socially and Collaboratively to Improve QOL

QOL research frequently suggests that it is collective endeavour that improves QOL (Zumbo, 2003). Vygotsky (1978) put forward the notion that we learn collaboratively, drawing from existing knowledge to construct new knowledge. Acceptance of language as the key socio-cultural tool for mediation when co-constructing knowledge, must take into account the context of teaching and learning.

EI suggests that learners be given the 'language of emotion' to understand and regulate their emotions. This is more important the younger the child is, particularly when working with second-language learners. The language of emotion is comprised of labelling emotions, discussing them and setting up care circles. The younger the child, the more basic the labels should be, for example, simple words such as 'happy, sad, tired or confused'. In South African classroom contexts, we are further challenged by multilingual classrooms where the Language of Learning and Teaching (LoLT) is often English and therefore not mother tongue. This situation frequently arises from pressure from parents who view English as the language of economic empowerment and, even though South African policy documents stipulate that children should learn in their mother tongue from Grade R to Grade 3, this is often not adhered to and this has a direct impact on QOL of teachers and learners.

As this study involved work with parents in rural settings who, according to the teachers, were considered uneducated and illiterate, it was essential to put in place a system of communication that would transcend the challenges of the multilingual classroom and the parents' limitations (Ruiz, 1984). A collaborative effort was established between the teacher who placed the icons in the book, the parent who responded to the message book icons, and the child who had to self-regulate, thereby determining which icon would be chosen to illustrate performance. The intention was to build a relationship of trust and communication between the three parties and, through collaborative effort, for learning to take place.

The use of icons/emoticons was the chosen method of mediation because, as a simple means of illustrating a child's behaviour, emoticons were quick to draw and easy to understand, irrespective of the literacy levels of parent or child. The parent responses ranged from a simple cross in place of a signature, to detailed sharing of deeply personal information that the parents now felt they could divulge because there was a relationship of trust and empathy. The language of communication was, therefore, a combination of an emoticon and short sentences expressing appreciation for the teacher's interest in each child. This collaborative effort facilitated learning at multiple levels and began the process of improving QOL for all concerned.

15.6 QOL and the Zone of Proximal Development

A key aspect of working collaboratively, according to Vygotsky (1978), is awareness of the Zone of Proximal Development (ZPD). Use of ZPD is defined by a goal, in this case regulating learner behaviour; the use of a mediational tool, namely language and an emoticon; and support of a more capable other. In this study, the more capable others were the teacher and the parent. The ZPD is essentially the development/learning space between present capabilities and potential achievement, mediated by a more capable other. At the heart of ZPD is the idea that the less capable learner should achieve independence in the set task or concept, through scaffolded steps of learning. This type of conscious mediation allows the less capable partner to internalise new learning and thereby set a new ZPD in a dynamic, evolving process of learning.

The researcher set an assignment for her in-service teachers that required them to make use of a message-book system to establish channels of communication between themselves and their learners' parents. In addition, the use of emoticons to describe learners' daily behaviour was intended to both communicate with the parents and to regulate learners' behaviour in the classroom. Through the work of the message book, as tool for mediation, multiple ZPDs were established. Firstly, the teachers were able to assist the parents in understanding their child's development as well as the work of the teacher, and thereby strengthen communication between teacher and parent. Thus, one of the ZPD relationships was between the teacher, the more capable other who scaffolded information through use of a message book, and the parents.

A second ZPD was established between parents and child when the parents checked the message book to determine their child's daily performance, and responded in a validating or supportive way. For example, if the child's message book showed that he/she had not had a good day (illustrated by a 'sad' emoticon), the parent could explore through discussion/language, why the child had struggled and then offer support. In this way, the QOL of the child was improved through the support of the parents. The teacher's QOL was improved as she feels supported by the parents, and the parents' QOL improved with the sense that the teacher cared enough about their child to communicate daily. The use of the message-book system was, therefore, a form of conscious mediation exercised by the teachers for the benefit of both child and parent. As the child's behaviour improved, a new ZPD, with new goals, was established.

15.7 Research Methods in QOL Study

A cohort of 29 B. Ed. (FP) in-service teachers were the subjects of this study which was designed to improve communication and QOL for teachers, parents and children in Grades 1–3 in rural schools in Northern Cape province. The lecturer wanted the teachers to experience the benefits of an EI approach to communication with parents and, in so doing, build positive relations between the teachers and their learners' parents.

Each in-service teacher was required to begin the project by running a workshop with parents to explain the new message-book system and what was required of participants. At the beginning of the assignment, each teacher was given a message-book template and sample emoticons that defined a set of basic emotions. The teachers were, however, encouraged to adapt the tools to their own individual teaching and learning contexts, including making use of emoticon stickers, adding columns to the template, or extra space for parents to respond. The system was then implemented over the course of one school term, followed by the teachers presenting a reflective piece on the use of the system and five sample pages taken from five different learners' message books.

As Vygotsky suggested, it is important to practise a concept to consolidate new learning (Smidt, 2009), it was decided to run the use of the message book over a full school term. This allowed teachers to scaffold the system with both parents and learners. It also allowed parents to scaffold their support of their children and, ultimately, for the child to begin to self-regulate. Additional support was given to the in-service teachers in the form of a set of lectures in how to use EI in the classroom, providing them with an open-source manual on the topic and a resource pack that facilitated immediate implementation of EI strategies once the teachers had returned to their classrooms. Strategies that were provided included the use of a 'care circle' to validate learners' performance; active discussion of emotions; the use of a 4-finger system to indicate how learners feel at the beginning of the day, and the use of a 'traffic-light system' to manage noise levels during focused learning times. The intention was to actively provide the teacher with tools to help them to create a positive learning space that would enhance QOL for both teacher and learner.

As described earlier, fostering reflective teachers is an important aspect of quality education because a reflective teacher is able to adapt pedagogy, based on reflection. With this in mind it was decided that each teacher would write a reflective piece describing how they had implemented the message-book system and how effective it had been. This would largely be measured against the goals of the project, namely to improve communication between teachers and parents, encouragement of learner self-regulation, and potential enhancement of QOL for all concerned.

The decision to use emoticons as the primary means of communication was a calculated one and derived from a desire to ensure that parents who were illiterate or non-English speakers, would be able to understand what was being conveyed. Emoticons are frequently used in the field of EI and are relatable for all levels of society, from young children through to adults. Emoticons are also quick to draw which was advantageous for teachers who had 35–40 learners in their classes and needed to put an emoticon in every learner's message book by the end of the day. It is fair to say that emoticons are not only a tool in EI, but have become part of the fabric of social communication as seen in Facebook, WhatsApp and other social media.

Below is an example of a basic grid completed by a teacher simply by using a pen to draw the emoticons (Fig. 15.1), followed by an example of a grid that was adapted through use of stickers (Fig. 15.2).

15.8 Data Analysis and Findings

Research has long made use of both qualitative and quantitative methods, but a combination of the two is a relatively new approach (Creswell, 2003). It was felt that this particular research project would be strengthened by what we now call a mixed-methods research design. In mixed methods, research is viewed as a set of interactive data rather than linear data (Creswell, 2003). The two types of data allowed for a strengthening of the analysis and triangulation of data (Burke, Johnson & Onwuegbuzie, 2004). Creswell (2003) clarified that quantitative data includes closed-ended information that may describe behaviours or attitudes. This is relevant to this study which sought to use the parent and teacher responses to the message book templates as a means of understanding how communication and QOL may be enhanced. The use of a reflective essay and analysis of parents' comments in the message book provided rich qualitative data, while quantifying positive responses, number of illiterate parents, adaptations of grids, etcetera, enabled a detailed picture to emerge.

The templates that were given to the in-service teachers are referred to here as 'grids'. A total of 145 grids were quantitatively and qualitatively analysed to answer a number of questions. These included:

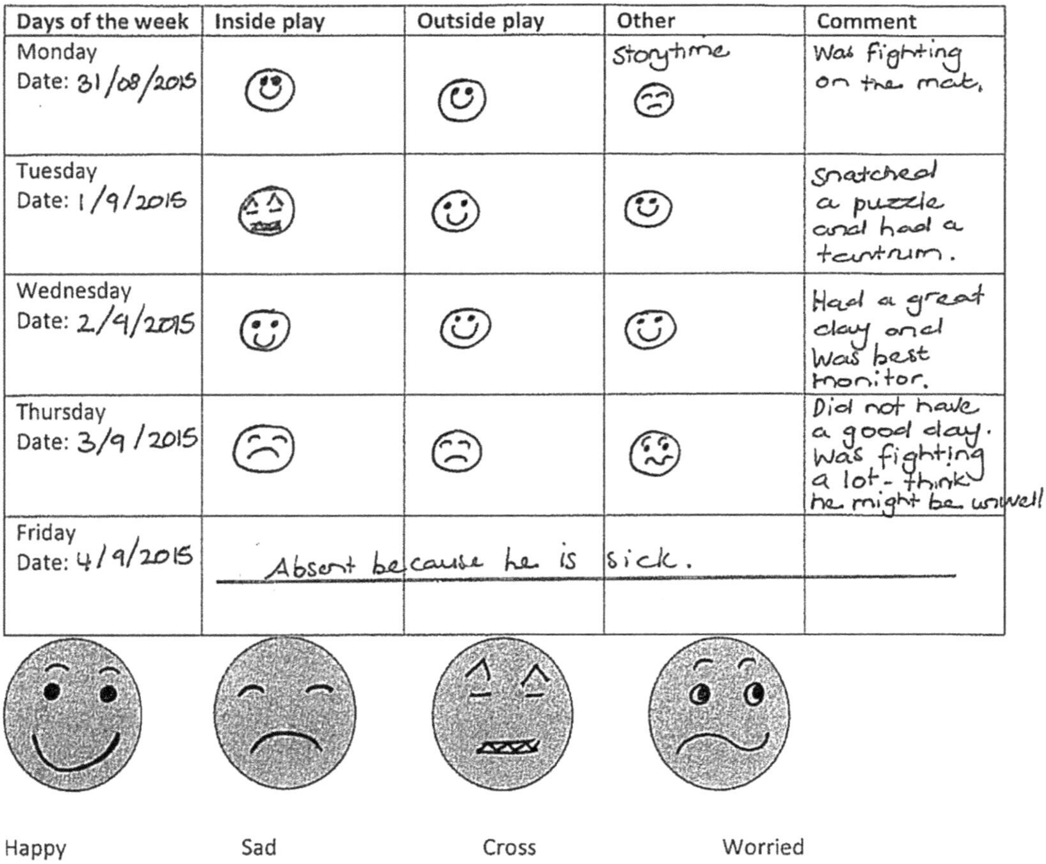

Days of the week	Inside play	Outside play	Other	Comment
Monday Date: 31/08/2015			Storytime	Was fighting on the mat.
Tuesday Date: 1/9/2015				Snatched a puzzle and had a tantrum.
Wednesday Date: 2/9/2015				Had a great day and was best monitor.
Thursday Date: 3/9/2015				Did not have a good day. Was fighting a lot- think he might be unwell
Friday Date: 4/9/2015	Absent be	cause he is	sick.	

Fig. 15.1 Example of a completed grid using the sample given

- How many teachers had adapted the grids to suit their individual contexts of teaching and learning?
- In what ways had teachers adapted the grids?
- What types of icons/emoticons were used?
- What types of comments were written by teachers and parents?
- What evidence was there that parents were illiterate?
- Had the parents responded to the system and its implementation?
- Can one surmise that there may be a shift in QOL for participants in the 'sacred triangle'?

The majority of teachers (78%) adapted the message book template to meet the needs of their own teaching and learning contexts. The types of adaptations included things like using emoticon stickers in place of drawing an icon; providing additional space for parents or teachers to comment; adding a place for a signature and cutting out emoticons to paste into the books rather than drawing them. These adaptations showed an understanding of the circumstances under which each teacher was operating. Some had access to photocopying facilities and therefore felt it beneficial to simply print emoticons to stick in books. Other teachers were able to get to urban areas and could therefore purchase stickers while those who could do neither were content to simply draw the emoticons.

It was interesting to note that many of the teachers did not write a comment or adapt the grid further to include a comment space for the teacher. The adaptation of extra comment space was mainly for the parent. When this was coupled

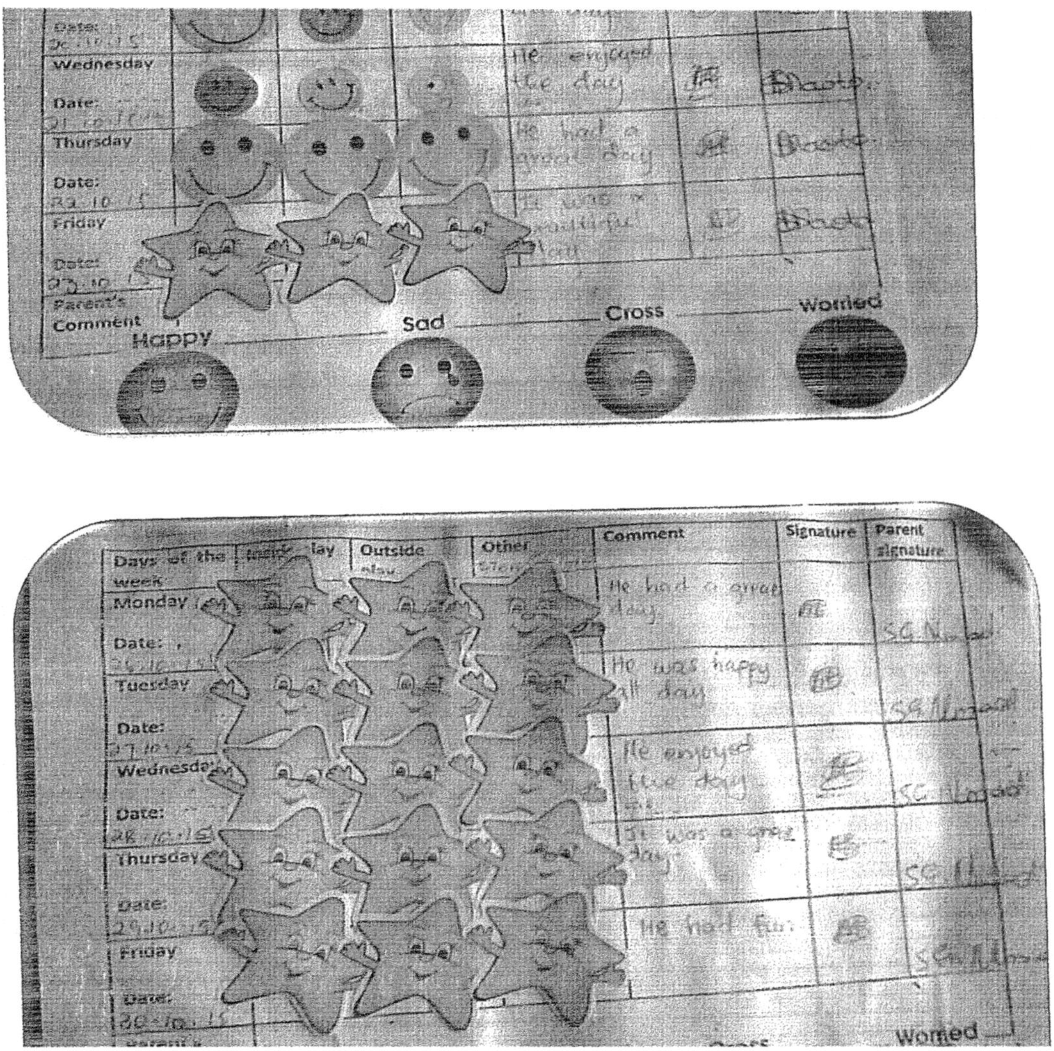

Fig. 15.2 Example showing modification of grid using stickers and adding a column for the signatures of parent and teacher

with evidence showing that most teachers did not comment, preferring to simply use the emoticons for the day, it can be surmised that many of the teachers simply did not have time to write comments. This is not surprising when the average class number is 35 learners per teacher. When a comment was made by the teacher in addition to the emoticon, it was interesting to note that the teachers tended to revert to the old style of commenting, namely only writing a comment when there was something negative to communicate. For example, "He was angry all day because he was feeling sick," and "He made a lot of noise in class, but he enjoyed the maths activity." Fortunately this was not true of all the in-service teachers and there were some positive comments too. For example: "He was excited to be at school," and "She had a good week and achieved in all learning areas". These affirming comments and emoticons were enough to convince the parents that the teacher cared about their child and the child's development thereby opening up the channels of communication between the respective parties.

It can be argued that QOL of parents is influenced by knowing how their child performed on any given day. Most of all, parents want to know that their child has had a positive school day and that the teacher cares enough to support their child in their role as surrogate parent and educator. It was, therefore, interesting to note that some of the comments that parents made showed a depth of understanding as to how they might support the teacher and the child and in so doing build an improved QOL for all concerned. "I will encourage him to learn and help him with all his school work"; "I was not aware of what you experienced at school but will observe her at home and will visit to share with you my experience"; "I am impressed to see that he enjoys being at school almost every day," and "I am happy to see that the teacher cares," or "I am so impressed to hear about the progress of my child at school".

The extent to which trust and communication had improved could be seen in the case of one parent who informed the teacher that she had initially thought that the teacher did not care about her child, but with the advent of the message-book system, she had realised she was wrong and now felt that she could share with the teacher that her child had been sexually abused. The weight of this deeply personal revelation could now be shared by both the parent and the teacher and could lead to improved support for all parties concerned. Another aspect of trust was shown by parents who were illiterate and who felt comfortable to simply put an 'x' as a signature, and then taking time to speak to the teacher about their child's progress.

QOL for the teacher is largely affected by her day-to-day interaction with the learners in her class, her colleagues and the occasional parent. When the teacher feels that she has gained control over her teaching environment, she is able to relax and enjoy the experience. Unfortunately many teachers express the opposite and would go so far as to describe their day being one of little more than 'crowd control'. This can be further exacerbated by a sense that parents do not engage with the school or their child, or that when they do, they bring with them a host of complaints. It was therefore relevant to determine if teachers' experience of the EI conceptualised strategy of a message-book system, had made a difference to their QOL. Teachers commented that, "What amazes me is that a week after I introduced the rubric, parents' attitude changed because every day the message book is signed and some parents even come to the school uninvited, which means they are showing an interest in their children." Another teacher noted, "The use of the message book helps us to show the parents that we value and respect the role they play in the child's life." The latter comment showed a marked shift in attitude from a teacher who had previously felt threatened by parents and did not have a positive relationship with them.

The use of icons had the additional knock-on effect of teachers realising that, "My children can also interpret what I am saying to their parents about them through using the faces," which meant that they were eager to be on their best behaviour in the classroom. Another teacher noted that, "Most of the learners are determined to do their best to keep their record clean and get smiley faces. This has helped me with my discipline." These comments show that the teacher felt more in control of her classroom environment and there was an air of optimism that had not existed before. It is, therefore, fair to say that the teachers' QOL had improved through positive communication with parents who showed appreciation towards the teacher and co-operated with her requirements for their child's studies. It was further improved by learners who became eager to please, were therefore self-regulating, leading to a situation in which the teacher was no longer expending negative energy, but was able to use her time and energy for positive teaching and learning (Durlak, Weissberg & Dymnicki, 2011).

It is interesting to note that the78% of the teachers who adapted their grids to their context had successfully applied the system (Table 15.1) in that the parents were responsive and the triad of parent, teacher and child was strengthened through positive communication. It is notable that only 28% of teachers made use of stickers with the rest preferring to draw the emoticons or cut them out and stick them onto the grid. This is

Table 15.1 Quantitative analysis of message book grids

Number of grids analysed	Number of grids with successful application	Number of parents (n = 145) who did not respond	Number of parents (n = 145) who were illiterate	Number of schools (n = 29) which continued to use the system
145 (100%)	113 (78%)	32 (22%)	5 (3%)	18 (62%)
Number of grids adapted to context	Number of teachers (n = 29) making use of stickers	Number of teachers (n = 29) who stated the system was useful	Number of teachers (n = 29) who said parents were actively involved and communication had improved	Number of teachers (n = 29) who thanked lecturer for exposing them to the system
113 (78%)	8 (28%)	26 (90%)	27 (97%)	10 (34%)

not surprising given that most of the teachers were in rural settings far from shops where they might purchase stickers. In addition, it was clear that the grids that were successful were also those that had been adapted to context. The data illustrated that, contrary to the teachers' assumptions, only 5% of sampled parents were illiterate, suggesting that this was, in fact, not a primary cause of poor channels of communication.

15.9 The Value of the Reflective Essay

Each teacher was asked to write a reflective essay as part of the strategy to develop reflective teachers and also to determine how effective the use of the consciously mediated tool of an EI message-book system had been in improving communication and development within the 'sacred triangle'. The 29 reflective essays were qualitatively analysed to determine how the teachers felt about:

- Implementation of the message-book system,
- Possible improvement in communication with parents,
- Continued use of the system,
- Possible improvements in classroom discipline,
- Any problems with the system as a whole,
- Evidence of improved QOL for child, parent and teacher.

Ninety-seven percent of teachers noted an improvement in parent involvement through the introduction of a system of communication (Table 15.1). This was seen in an improvement in parental attendance at class meetings, involvement in fundraising, and their coming to the schools to speak to the teachers about ways in which they could support the learning process. The in-service teachers had noted as particularly frustrating that parents did not let them know when a child was going to be absent from school. This meant that teachers were unable to plan for catch-up work or provision of emotional support. With the introduction and implementation of the message-book system, this aspect showed a marked improvement. Parents informed the teachers via the message books that their child had been sick or taken to the clinic for the day.

The reflective essay did yield open appreciation of the system, with 10% of the teachers thanking the lecturer for introducing them to the system. Statements such as, "If I had known this before, I could have achieved many things that hamper my daily teaching. With this system I have learned many things that I have never experienced before," illustrated the impact on the teachers' QOL. This showed that the teacher had not just improved communication between herself and her learners, but had experienced a shift in her pedagogic practice and consequently also her QOL.

Some of the in-service teachers involved in this research taught Grade R, which is often perceived in a negative light by teachers in higher grades. There tends to be a sense that Grade-R teachers are little more than glorified 'nannies' who are paid to mind children, not teach them. It was, therefore, interesting to note how the participating in-service teachers shared that they had gained credibility through their use of the message-book system and that teachers from higher grades had wanted to adopt the same system in their classrooms. In this way, the QOL of the Grade-R teachers had improved as the perception had shifted from one of low status to that of a reflective teacher capable of effectively managing her classroom environment. QOL for teachers in higher grades could also potentially improve with introduction of the system. The general consensus was that it was best to implement the message-book system at the beginning of the year and throughout a school, to maximize impact through consistency.

15.10 Limitations of the Study

It must be acknowledged that no research is completely successful or without limitations. An area of concern was the fact that 38% of the teachers indicated in their reflective essay that they would not continue with the system beyond the confines of the assignment. A further analysis of the data from these specific teachers showed that they had the largest class numbers and, often, were teachers who had particularly short school days. One can surmise that these teachers felt the constraints of having to fill in large numbers of message books within limited time and did not feel that it was worth their while. It was suggested to these teachers that they could limit message-book responses to once a week, rather than daily, thereby still providing regular feedback outside of a termly report and raising the potential for positive communication with parents and the learners.

Among the 38% of teachers who indicated that they would not pursue the message book system were those that cited learners' responses as problematic. This centred around the idea that learners were so excited by the prospect of sharing their performance with their parents that they tore pages out of their message books and damaged them. A few teachers additionally described how some learners lost their message books between home and school, resulting in the teacher having to provide a new book. As this was a very small percentage of teachers, the researcher felt that the teacher simply needed to socialise the learners into appropriate behaviour by using EI principles of validation of correct behaviour. In fact, more children returned their message books than damaged or forgot them. This was an improvement on what teachers had experienced before when sending homework and school notices home, thereby confirming that learners had the capacity to adopt appropriate behaviour. It could be argued that tearing out of the validating page is simply an indication of the enthusiasm of the learner and that rather than being frustrated or angry towards the learner, the teacher should acknowledge the enthusiasm and scaffold the appropriate behaviour. Generally, the teachers' responses were, "Most of the learners are determined to do their best, to keep their record clean and get smiley faces." This was an important statement as the teacher concerned had been vocal about her struggles with disciplining her class, and had experienced a significant improvement through introducing the message-book programme.

The reflective essays did evidence that some teachers were not prepared to change their pedagogic strategies and they reverted to their default position of phoning a parent whenever there was a perceived problem with a learner. The rationale given was that parents could not afford to visit the teacher to discuss the matter and therefore it made sense to simply have a telephonic parent-teacher meeting. It was unfortunate that these teachers did not see that part of the problem in the first place had been that parents were reluctant to communicate with the teacher because the only form of communication had been negative, leaving parents feeling that their child had been found wanting and that the teacher did not care.

Another area where there was evidence of the system not being entirely successful was that of parental response. The quantitative data showed that 32% of parents did not respond to the system. This resulted in their not signing the message books or attending parent-teacher meetings and school fundraisers. The reflective essays suggested that the parents who did not respond to the message-book system had not attended the initial workshop explaining the purpose of the system and how it would operate. This meant that these parents would not see the relevance of the exercise and therefore be reluctant to engage. It is also true that in every class there is a percentage of parents who do not support the teacher or the school, irrespective of their efforts. It could be argued that the teachers needed to make a special effort to inform parents who had not attended the workshop, but this may have been constrained by time and the cost of seeking out parents, together with their not having the means to attend school meetings. This is particularly true of the context of this study where many of the parents were unemployed and living inconvenient distances from the schools.

While it is evident that there were limitations in the study and that not all the teachers and parents could see the value in the system, it is important to realise that the system was implemented over only one term. This was not enough time to change entrenched habits. The in-service training programme that was the context of this study, had support in the form of a mentoring, on-site fieldworker who visited the teachers monthly. The fieldworker could work with individuals to assist those who were sceptical to iron out their issues and achieve a positive outcome over a longer period of time.

15.11 Conclusion

This chapter has endeavoured to examine how two very different projects have the potential to influence QOL in the field of ECCE. The PIECCE project demonstrated how institutions should respond to South Africa's crisis in education by professionalising the ECCE teacher training sector and developing quality educators who are reflective, have a sound knowledge of content, and are context adaptive (Harrison, 2017). The outcome of this should be that teacher-training institutions produce teachers who are able to step into ECCE contexts and provide children with appropriate learning that maximises their potential. In so doing, the QOL of the teacher is improved because she enjoys her job as she sees positive results. Equally, the manner in which the teacher engages with parents by showing empathy for the child, results in support for the parent. The support for parents and the use of the community to enhance ECCE teaching goals may improve QOL for all stakeholders in the field. Young children who have had the benefit of a positive learning environment prior to entering formal schooling are more likely to succeed on their academic path. It is obvious that a child who has succeeded in schooling will be able to continue training into tertiary education and consequently improve the QOL for themselves and their families.

A second research study was described to show how QOL can be improved at a more practical level through the apparently simple activity of introducing an EI-informed message-book system. This study stemmed from 'a cry for help' on the part of practising in-service teachers who were aware that they did not have a positive line of communication with parents. They were spending a lot of time performing 'crowd control' rather than teaching, and learners were not really learning. This was inevitably affecting the QOL of all parties that make up what I have termed the 'sacred triangle' that is responsible for holistic development of the child. The decision to use a message-book system as a conscious mediation tool for learning, enabled development of self-regulation in the child, the parents and the teacher. The children were motivated to manage their behaviour as they wished to bring home positive emoticons in their message books. The teacher regulated her behaviour by regularly communicating with the parents through use of emoticons in the message book. Parent regulated their behaviour through daily checking of the message book and appropriate responses to both child and teacher. This collaborative process shifted the channels of communication, building bonds of trust and understanding. These outcomes can be described as improved QOL.

It is important to acknowledge that QOL has not generally been discussed in ECCE terms or necessarily in the context of Foundation Phase classrooms; however, there is no doubt that the QOL of the average South African teacher and learner is not particularly positive. This results in poor matric results, teacher burnout and, perhaps most concerning, teacher apathy. It is essential that we provide teachers with practical ways in which they can engage with the 'village' that is involved in raising a child. Circumstances dictate that we cannot necessarily change challenging contexts, such as large class numbers, limited resources and impoverished parents, but we can provide teachers with the resilience and the practical tools that are founded in EI and that can improve QOL for all concerned.

There is definitely scope for future research into ways in which we can continue to enhance QOL of teachers by providing them with the type of training that allows for context adaptation, understanding of professionalism, having the courage to draw from the surrounding community, and adaption through reflective practice. PIECCE demonstrated that there is much work still to be done in improving how we equip teachers to face the challenges of their future classrooms (Harrison, 2017). Positive examples and experiences must be made available to incumbent and in-service teachers. Mentorship should be expanded beyond the confines of module or 1st-year course, and constructive support should be given to students who learn in a second language.

As teaching is fundamentally a practical profession, we must provide teachers with the tools of their trade that facilitate quality implementation. In this way, we can begin to redress the inequalities of the past and improve QOL for the most disadvantaged sectors of South African society.

References

Bar-on, R. (2003). How important is it to educate people to be emotionally and socially intelligent, and can it be done? *Perspectives in Education, 21*, 3–13.

Britto, P. R., Yoshikawa, H., & Boller, K. (2011). *Measuring quality and using it to improve practice and policy in early childhood development. Early childhood matters* (Vol. 126, pp. 83–90).

Burke Johnson, R., & Onwuegbuzie, A. J. (2004). Mixed methods research: A research paradigm whose time has come. *Educational Researcher, 33*, 14–26.

Creswell, J. W. (2003). *Research design: Qualitative, quantitative and mixed methods approaches* (2nd ed.). Thousand Oakes, CA: Sage.

Cummins, R. A. (1996). The domains of life satisfaction: An attempt to order chaos. *Social Indicators Research, 38*, 303–328.

Department of Basic Education. (2011). *Implementation plan of the National Curriculum and Assessment Policy Statements (CAPS) Grades R-12*. Pretoria.

Durlak, J. A., Weissberg, P., Dymnicki, A. B., et al. (2011). The impact of enhancing students' social and emotional learning: A meta-analysis of school-based universal interventions. *Child Development, 82*, 405–432.

Elfenbein, H. A., & Maccann, C. (2017). A closer look at ability emotional intelligence (EI): What are its component parts, and how do they relate to each other? *Social and Personality Psychology Compass, 11*, 2–26.

Fleisch, B. (2008). *Primary education in crisis: Why South African school children under-achieve in reading and mathematics*. Cape Town, South Africa: Juta.

Goleman, D. (1996). *Emotional intelligence*. New York, NY: Bantam Books.

Goleman, D. (1998). *Working with emotional intelligence* (lst ed.). New York, NY: Bantam Books.

Goleman, D. (2001). Emotional intelligence: Issues in paradigm building. In *The emotionally intelligent workplace* (pp. 13–27). San Francisco, CA: Jossey-Bass.

Goleman, D. (2007). *Social intelligence: The new science of human relationships* (1st ed.). London, UK: Arrow Books.

Greenberg, M. T., Weissberg, R. P., O'Brian, M. U., et al. (2003). Enhancing school-based prevention and youth development through coordinated social, emotional and academic learning. *American Psychologist, 58*, 466–474.

Gumbo, M., & Msila, V. (2017). *African voices on indigenisation of the curriculum: Insights from practice*. Wandsbeck, South Africa: Reach Publishers.

Harrison, G. D. (2011). *Mediating self-regulation in a kindergarten class in South Africa: An exploratory case study*. Cape Town: M.Ed. University of Cape Town.

Harrison, G. (2014). *Tools for learning: A socio-cultural analysis of pedagogy in early reading competency*. PhD dissertation.

Harrison, G. D. (Ed.). (2017). *Project for inclusive early childhood care and education (PIECCE): Output 2 baseline findings*. Grahamstown: Centre for Social Development.

Howie, S. J., Combrinck, C., Roux, K., Tshele, M., Mokoena, G. M., & McLeod Palane, N. (2017). *PIRLS literacy 2016 Progress in international Reading literacy study 2016: South African Children's Reading literacy achievement*. Pretoria: Centre for Evaluation and Assessment.

Jahromi, L. B., & Stifter, C. A. (2008). Individual differences in preschoolers' self-regulation and theory of mind. *Merrill-Palmer Quarterly, 54*, 125–175.

Karpov, Y. (2005). *The neo-Vygotskian approach to child development*. New York, NY: Cambridge University Press.

Moll, L. C. (2014). *Vygotsky and education*. New York, NY: Routledge.

Møller, V. (2013). South African quality of life trends over three decades, 1980–2010. Social Indicators Research, 113(3), 915 –940. Retrieved from http://www.jstor.org/stable/24719543

Moller, V., Roberts, B. J., Tiliouine, H., & Loschky, J. (2017). *World happiness report 2017*. Pretoria, South Africa: NRF.

Mweete, D. N., Sacha, J., West, J., et al. (2014). Quality of life in individuals living with HIV Aids attending a public sector antiretroviral service in Cape Town, South Africa. *BMC Public Health, 676*, 1–10.

Mwesiga, E. K., Nakasijja, N., Moore, S., et al. (2015). Depression with pain co-morbidity effect on quality of life among HIV positive patients in Uganda: A cross-sectional study. *Health and Quality of Life Outcomes, 13206*, 1–10.

Piaget, J. (2001). *Readings on the development of children: The stages of intellectual development of the child*. New York, NY: W.H. Freeman.

Rapley, M. (2003). *Quality of life research: A critical introduction*. London, UK: SAGE.

Ruiz, R. (1984). Orientations in language planning. *Journal of the National Association for Bilingual Education Vll, 2*, 15–34.

Salovey, P. (2004). Emotions and emotional intelligence for educators. In *Keys to educational psychology*. Cape Town, South Africa: UCT Press.

Salovey, P., & Sluyter, D. J. (1990). What is emotional intelligence? In *Emotional development and emotional intelligence: Educational implications*. New York, NY: Basic Books.

Schlebusch, L., Samuels, A. E., & Dada, S. (2016). South African families raising children with autism spectrum disorders: Relationship between family routines, cognitive appraisal and family quality of life. *Journal of Intellectual Disability Research, 6*, 412–423.

Smidt, S. (2009). *Introducing Vygotsky: A guide for practitioners and students in early years education*. London, UK: Routledge.

Van der Veer, R., & Valsiner, J. (1991). *Understanding Vygotsky: A quest for synthesis*. Oxford, UK: Blackwell.

Vygotsky, L. S. (1978). *Mind in society: The development of higher psychological processes*. Cambridge, MA: Harvard University Press.

Vygotsky, L. S. (1997). *The history of the development of higher mental functions*. London, UK: Plenum Press.

Vygotsky, L. S. (1998). *The collected works of LS Vygotsky. Volume 5 child psychology*. London, UK: Plenum Press.

Zeidner, M., Roberts, G., & Maccann, C. (2003). Development of emotional intelligence: Towards a multi-level investment model. *Human Development, 46*, 69–96.

Zumbo, B. D. (2003). *Advances in quality of life research 2001* (Social indicators research Series) (Vol. 17). Dordrecht, The Netherlands: Kluwer Academic Publishers.

Quality of Life Through Capacity Development in Junior Primary Teacher Education

16

C. B. Villet and J. Weiss

Abstract

"It's a dream come true." Over the last 4 years, this is a common sentiment echoed by two groups of teachers in Namibia: in-service teachers selected to participate in a university program designed to upgrade teaching skills, and teachers participating in a national research project who received a toolkit of educational resources as an intervention to address challenges in the classroom. A multi-disciplinary capacity building project in teacher education brought together Namibian educators from the University of Namibia (UNAM), United Nations Educational, Scientific and Cultural Organization (UNESCO) and the Namibian Ministry of Education, Arts and Culture (MoEAC), all sharing a vision to improve primary education in Namibia. The project began with a national needs assessment, involved pre- and lower primary school teachers, officials from the MoEAC and UNESCO, and UNAM teacher education lecturers in an action research study. The entire education community shared a common vision and sense of responsibility for improving the quality of teaching, especially for literacy and numeracy programs in Government pre- and lower primary classrooms. The 2-year action research project provided the foundation and model for a large scale national project aimed at elevating the qualifications for approximately 3000 un- and underqualified teachers teaching in the pre- and lower primary phase. This chapter describes the research, innovative practices and impact on the quality of life for the educators from varied educational sectors, who are participating in this national project.

16.1 Country Background

Despite the Namibian Government's large investment in the public education sector, it is well known that most Namibian children perform below average on national and regional reading, writing and mathematics' tests (Hungi et al., 2010). Namibia is also one of the African countries with the largest dropout and repetition rates in primary school. Less than 50% of all the children entering grade 1 will complete grade 12, the end of Secondary School in Namibia.

Namibia is officially ranked as a middle-income country, as evidenced by an average annual per capita in- come (2016) of $10,550

C. B. Villet (✉)
University of Namibia, Windhoek, Namibia
e-mail: cvillet@unam.na

J. Weiss
Pacific Lutheran University, Tacoma, WA, USA
e-mail: weissjm@plu.edu

I. Eloff (ed.), *Handbook of Quality of Life in African Societies*, International Handbooks of Quality-of-Life, https://doi.org/10.1007/978-3-030-15367-0_16

(Purchasing Power Parity/PPP) dollars. Nevertheless, Namibia remains one of the more inequitable societies in the world, with an income gini-coefficient of 0.572. The inequitable distribution of wealth and income mirrors inequities in education with the poorest children being the most disadvantaged (UNICEF, 2012).

In Namibia educational provision has been a priority for Government since independence in 1990. The sector (both Basic and Higher Education) continues to receive the largest budget, over 20% of the overall country budget since independence. This expenditure has increased and is expected to reach 25.3% in 2018/2019. Basic education (including pre-primary, primary and secondary, Arts and Culture) gets the largest share of the budget, between 74% and 79%. The remaining amount is allocated to Higher Education, training and innovation.

The World Bank Group on Early Childhood in Africa in their January 2011 Newsletter, states that the quality of education offered in a country is a strong predictor of its economic growth rates (Neuman, 2011). The Mo Ibrahim Foundation reports that Africa has one of the fastest growing youthful populations, about 46% of Africa's labor force are between the ages of 15 and 34 years (Mo Ibrahim Foundation, 2017). This situation requires innovative options for providing education and training to ensure that our youth are a social and economic asset and not a formidable challenge.

UNICEF asserts that giving children a solid foundation for future learning in the early years, is the best investment society can make in ensuring children succeed in life (Mzabalazo Advisory Services, 2016). However, for many young children in Namibia, getting a good start early in life is not always very possible. The early years of most children in Namibia is plagued by poverty, malnutrition, disease and lack of opportunities to play and learn the skills needed to do well in primary school. Regions in Namibia with the lowest coverage of Integrated Early Childhood Development (IECD) services, perform the poorest in standardized achievement tests, have the most over-aged learners in the school system, the highest dropout rates and the highest poverty rates (The Namibia Ministry of Health and Social Services & Namibia Statistics Agency, 2014; UNICEF Namibia, 2016).

The Government policy on Free Universal Pre-Primary Education in Namibia, increased the numbers of learners who enrolled for pre-primary from 22,000 in 2012 to 41,091 in 2016, an 86.7% increase according to the UNICEF 2016 report. However, only around 38% of school going children in Namibia attend pre-primary before entering grade 1. Access is often hampered by a shortage of classrooms, un- and underqualified teachers, and a general lack of understanding on the part of parents/caregivers and decision-makers about the importance of pre-primary education.

Several organizations focused on education are all in agreement on the impact formal education has on the quality of life of people:

> Investing in the early years is one of the smartest things a country can do to eliminate extreme poverty, boost shared prosperity, and create the human capital needed for economies to diversify and grow. Early childhood experiences have a profound impact on brain development—affecting learning, health, behavior and ultimately, income. An increasingly digital economy places even greater premiums on the ability to reason, continually learn, effectively communicate and collaborate. Those who lack these skills will be left further behind (The World Bank, 2017, http://www.worldbank.org/en/topic/earlychildhooddevelopment)

Participation in good quality preprimary programs has been shown to have beneficial effects on the cognitive development of children and the length of time they stay in the school system. The high dropout and repetition rates in primary schools in Namibia is therefore of concern. Reports on learner performance in primary schools in Namibia indicate that learners in the primary school phase often do not master the foundational skills, including literacy and numeracy, which would enable them to successfully continue in school. Mwabu and Ackerman (2013) state that a focus on early years' education is particularly important in Africa where many children face a multitude of disadvantages before they even enter schools. Preparing children to be all school ready will decrease repetition and dropout rates in the early grades, leading to higher primary completion rates. This is important in African countries where equity and learner performance in the higher grades lag far behind those in the developed countries. Literature on effective schools suggests that in low-income countries where children have all the socio-economic barriers stacked against them, one of the important variables that supports their learning performance, is the teacher and the quality of their teaching (Sammons & Bakkum, 2011). A recent study in Namibia on Positive Deviant Schools supports this notion that these schools most likely performed better than their neighboring schools because of the quality of the principal and the teachers and the provision of resources, as well as the relationship with the local community. In several developing countries, pilot projects in teacher training have achieved improvements in children's reading scores by adapting teaching approaches to address identifiable reading and numeracy deficiencies (Mzabalazo Advisory Services, 2016). Focusing on teachers and their teaching competence is a key step in solving the learning crisis in Namibia.

16.2 Project Background

A multi-disciplinary research project brought together Namibian educators from the University of Namibia (UNAM), UNESCO and the MoEAC to create a shared vision for improving primary education. The 2-year project, funded by the Chinese-Funds-in-Trust (CFIT), was part of a multi-country effort that focused on accelerating progress towards the attainment of quality education and the education-related Sustainable Development Goals (SDG 4(c)). The capacity building aspect of the project in Namibia, which focused on teacher education and teacher development, brought together the entire education community to create a shared responsibility for establishing an agenda to meet the goals for high levels of academic success. Educators from different sectors of society often work in isolation. This project minimized such isolation by drawing on the expertise of various stakeholders in the education sector to build a stronger, more unified foundation for educational achievement in Namibia.

16.2.1 Building Capacity for Delivering Quality Teaching and Learning

In 2012 the Chinese Government through the UNESCO Chinese-Funds-in-Trust project, availed funds to conduct a needs assessment study for capacity development of teacher education in Namibia. The purpose of the study was to identify capacity development needs in Namibian teacher education and training, so they could be addressed through a 3–4-year project (Ellis, 2013). The study recommended that UNESCO/CFIT should work with the Ministry of Education, the University of Namibia (UNAM), and other relevant stakeholder to develop a project, the strategic objective which would be to improve the quality of pre-school and lower primary education through enhanced teacher education and training. The 2014 project therefore focused on enhancing the capacities of teacher education institutions to prepare an adequate number of qualified teachers to achieve EFA goals at the time, now focusing on the SDG 4(c). The National Team of education experts who steered the design of the project, agreed to focus the interventions on improving the capacity of teacher educators to train students and teachers in teaching literacy and numeracy in pre- and lower-primary grades (Steukers & Weiss, 2015). What follows is a broad description from the last 5 years that continues to build a community of practice that assumes collective responsibility for improving the quality of early years' education in Namibia. The capacity development framework for the UNESCO-CFIT project brought together educational institutions in Namibia as well as teachers and administrators from all of the country's 14 regions. The project details were conceptualized by the National Coordinating Committee that consisted of three main partners in subdivisions of these organizations. At the University of

Namibia (UNAM) these included the Dean of the Faculty of Education (FoE), the Director of Continuing Professional Development, Teaching and Learning Improvement (CPDTLI) Center and lecturers from the relevant FoE departments. At the Ministry of Education, Arts and Culture (MoEAC) representatives from the various directorates relevant to the project included Higher Education, Programs and Quality Assurance (PQA), Planning and Development (PAD), and the National Institute for Educational Development (NIED). These varied sectors of the educational community set the stage for a countrywide collaborative endeavor that continues to this day in a variety of educational projects.

16.2.2 Understanding the Context for Quality Teaching and Learning

The project design incorporated a qualitative approach to collecting data that began with a yearlong action research process. The National Coordinating committee followed a cyclical action research model based on the works of Coghlan and Brannick (2015). Before identifying changes for classroom practices of primary teachers, the research team needed to know and understand existing practices to inform the intervention approaches that could benefit teachers and learners in Namibian classrooms. School selection was based on a set of criteria that included school setting, school size and language of instruction. Two classrooms in each school, generally pre-primary and Grade 1, comprised the study's sample group, resulting in an overall research sample of 56 classrooms.

Designed by a core research team of cross-organizational professionals, the February 2014 workshop aimed to build capacity and focused on protocols to help new and inexperienced researchers acquire and refine basic research skills. An initial 3-day training workshop on research protocol development brought together the stakeholders in the project and research: MoEAC key personnel; UNAM lecturers; and a selection of teachers, principals and regional junior primary subject advisors. Attendance records indicated strong participation which reflected high levels of engagement and commitment. Over 120 educators discussed the issues and challenges of teaching and learning at the junior primary level. Working groups, intentionally mixed to combine different educational expertise and perspectives, examined the status of literacy and numeracy instruction in Pre-Primary and Grade 1. Ultimately, a set of central questions emerged to propel the research agenda:

1. Which strategies are used by teachers to teach literacy and numeracy?
2. What kinds of factors support or hinder the learning of primary learners?
3. What kind of support is available and needed for teachers and learners to benefit at the primary level?

Based on the research questions, the core research team created a data collection resource binder to standardize and ensure uniform data collection procedures. The binder consisted of questionnaires for teachers, observation forms, journal templates for teachers, and above all, clear guidelines on conducting research. Researchers received tablets to advance the use of technology for research and teaching. The action research served as a capacity building exercise for the UNAM Department of Early Childhood and Lower Primary Education and MoEAC key personnel and also was the catalyst for the in-service diploma program that followed.

Participation in a large-scale national research project generated learning opportunities for practitioners while interacting with a variety of stakeholders in education. Over 70 inter-institutional and inter-disciplinary researchers afforded multiple learning opportunities for all team members. Researchers shared their own skills and knowledge during the research process and reinforced a dynamic collaborative learning environment.

Teams of four to six researchers that included two teachers, UNESCO key personnel, and at least one faculty member from UNAM's FoE

Lower Primary Department gathered data over a 2-month period. Classroom observations, interviews, and reflections provided data for case studies of each school. Research teams followed standardized guidelines to facilitate rich descriptions of the context and classrooms of the participating 28 schools. The final analysis and sharing of data brought together representative researchers from all regions that included participants from different education sectors and roles during a 2-day "National Consultative" meeting of rich conversations with varied perspectives. The group identified themes and patterns and generated a list of intervention strategies to address the findings. The first-year study provided a baseline for designing meaningful intervention activities and future in-service teacher training.

Analyses of the school reports identified various challenge areas in the Namibian pre- and lower primary classrooms. Overall, classrooms lacked materials to integrate instructional media and technology to enhance learning, and teachers displayed limited knowledge and application of effective learner-centered literacy and numeracy instruction and assessment. The findings led to the concept of a "toolkit of resources," a signature outcome of the project and currently a key resource for teachers enrolled in the DJPE-INSET program.

16.3 Interventions for Quality Teaching and Learning in Junior Primary Classes

16.3.1 Toolkit Development

The second year of the project focused on classroom interventions and technology integration training. In preparation for year two research, a group of educators gathered to develop a toolkit of teaching resources that responded to classroom challenges identified during the first year of the project. The group included researchers from the UNAM Faculty of Education, the National Institute for Educational Development (NIED), Senior Education Officers in the regions and teachers and principals from the participating research schools. Challenges included limited resources for activity-based teaching and learning, limited preparatory reading activities, few occasions where assessment informed instruction, limited ICT availability and utilization to enhance teaching and learning, and a limited range of questioning strategies (Steukers & Weiss, 2015).

The 46-member toolkit team met for a material development workshop to outline and assemble materials for the toolkit. Divided into five teams, toolkit developers received guidance from consultants in two Namibian organizations (Namibian College for Open Learning and the National University of Science and Technology). Teams identified potential toolkit materials and planned to use the 2-month school holiday to prepare relevant materials. After the holidays, the group met to share toolkit resources, receive feedback from colleagues, and make final revisions in preparation for production. The first toolkit was a collaborative effort by representative groups of Year 1 participants, who wrote teaching guides, developed teaching aids, and organized materials to improve instructional practices.

Communities of practice are viewed as groups of people who share a concern or a passion for something they do while they interacting regularly to improve their practice (Gotto, Turnbull, Ann Summers, & Blue-Banning, 2010). The collaborative opportunity for teachers, principals, lecturers, and Ministry of Education curriculum developers developed an understanding and respect for the different roles and expertise that support the quality of education for Namibian learners. It was a unique opportunity for professionals from different sectors to create a highly valued educational resource. Jimenez-Silva and Olson (2012) state that communities of practice have the potential to help educators acquire insights that will make them step out of national silos, single disciplines, and taken-for-granted understandings. It further reinforces a sense of belonging that has the potential to shape the individual's learning and development (Graven & Lerman, 2003).

16.3.2 Action Research Intervention

To prepare for the second phase of the project, researchers gathered for a comprehensive workshop that included sessions on conducting research using new materials, integrating technology, and using materials in the toolkits. Research teams received toolkits and laptops, the two main components of the intervention phase.

After this preparation, researchers revisited their respective case-study schools for a 4-day implementation of the intervention phase. Upon arriving at schools, researchers discussed the scope of the research project with the school principal and Head of Department. They shared findings and highlighted the five identified areas of particular challenge in pre- and lower primary classrooms. They also shared the toolkit contents. The research team met with teachers for a structured interview that guided teachers to make individual decisions about relevant toolkit resources for implementation during the intervention phase. Each teacher chose two of the five areas from the toolkit they wanted extra support to elevate learning.

During the 4 days, research team members supported teachers with the implementation of toolkit resources through a gradual release model, in which researchers modeled the use of toolkit materials and provided coaching and feedback. The inter-institutional character of the teams contributed to insightful discussions and reflections, and both teachers and researchers learned from one another. The reflective practice nurtured capacity building among ministry officials, lecturers and teachers who commented on the mutual respect and understanding of one another's knowledge and communication skills.

In addition to conducting research, the teams trained teachers and additional staff on ICT integration including using word processing software to create flashcards, puzzles and other teaching aids; creating digital stories to support storytelling in the language of instruction and learning basic internet skills.

The above-described intervention became a reflective practice for both teachers and UNAM staff members who modeled lessons for the participating teachers and coached them through teaching those lessons independently. One of the key rationales for reflective practice is that experience alone does not necessarily lead to learning; deliberate reflection on experience is essential (Priya, Prasanth, & Prince, 2017).

After the intervention phase, participants on the five UNAM campuses met as campus groups to share research experiences, discuss the report writing process, and identify the major highlights to include in the national report that would consolidate the action research intervention phase. Teams then completed their written school reports; relying on information from completed research forms, they detailed the implementation process and analyzed the influence of the toolkit and ICT training throughout the research week. A guiding question framed the writing of these school reports: "Does the toolkit, as an intervention strategy, influence teacher practices in Namibian classrooms?" Themes, conclusions and recommendations from all 28 school reports informed the contents of the national report.

An 8-week follow up activity that combined school visits and telephone communication supported teachers' implementation of practices aimed at improving the quality of education. Teachers and school administrators from the CFIT project reported noticeable changes in teacher practices. Learners became more engaged when teachers implemented learning centered-activities.

The UNESCO China Funds-in-Trust project provided a platform to bring together UNAM Faculty of Education, classroom teachers, government officials and other stakeholders to engage in a 2-year countrywide collaborative action research process. The research opportunity created an environment conducive to working collaboratively and learning from the experience and expertise of diverse professionals. Feeling empowered, researchers refined their skills, re-examined their perspectives of teaching and learning and adjusted their professional practice. Encouraged by the project's outcomes, UNAM continued strengthening instructional practices and expanded its efforts to elevate teaching practices and qualifications throughout Namibia.

16.4 Action Research and Quality of Life

Travel time, shared lodging and evening reflection sessions for research teams supported a sense of belonging and pride in being part of an important national work. Opportunities to collaborate on a large-scale research project added to several quality of life broad domains. These include achieving in life, emotional well-being and close relationships among educators from various backgrounds that would otherwise have been unlikely.

Researchers were influenced in a variety of ways through their participation in the intervention phase of the research process. Working alongside teachers, researchers increased their understanding of classroom practices and discovered ways to apply new knowledge in their endeavors to support students in the university classroom. Additionally, they gained greater confidence in their own practice, learned from team members and developed new perspectives related to teaching and research.

Researchers articulated a variety of ways in which their teaching practices were influenced by spending time in the classroom and actively participating in the research process. Gaining a sense of the realities in the classroom and interacting with teachers gave researchers insight into essential elements to emphasize in their teaching and strengthen in their students. Spending time in the classroom generated a repertoire of examples that lecturers have incorporated into their teaching to benefit students' professional development. The following quotations from two researchers describe their perspectives on achievement. "It helped me to be more aware of the reality on the ground. So when I teach, I now have a picture of what the circumstances are and what is going on [*sic* with learners]. It directed and redirected the way I teach. I changed the way I deliver my classes." Another researcher spoke collectively about her team: "We were not trained as lower primary teachers and we never had experience in those classrooms. It was good to go to the schools and know what is happening on a grassroots level. It helped me understand how teaching and learning takes place, and it enriched our practice."

Working collaboratively with colleagues and implementing a full action research cycle strengthened the feeling of belonging to a community of practice. The participation and sense of ownership and responsibility to the project facilitated feelings of confidence and empowerment. The researchers developed connections to their own practice, which translated into a feeling of efficacy for contributing to the educational profession and the process of teaching and learning. The following quotations from researchers, taken from the UNESCO/CFIT 2015 national report, highlight achievement, belonging and empowerment that developed during the 2-year research process:

> This process was once again an empowerment as theory and practice were brought closer. It was a 'live performance' that gave me an opportunity to experience teaching and children in a real life situation. The process of modelling, guiding and experiencing action research was felt!

> I was exposed to the practical part of research for my own growth. Many of the classroom areas became realistic to me because I was there. In the process, we were a team. I picked up a lot of skills on how to evaluate my students when they are out for practice. I picked them up from listening to my colleague from NIED when she was providing feedback.

> I learned about networking and learning from other people from different educational institutions. There was such team effort during the material development and the research. [Furthermore] the pre- and lower primary department really got to know each other's strengths and we benefitted from that. The lecturers have become closer and more of a team. (Steukers & Weiss, 2015)

16.5 Upskilling, In-Service Training and Quality of Life

The close collaboration between MoEAC officials and UNAM staff members during the CFIT project built professional relationships and trust that laid the foundation for the project that followed. After the national consultation workshop on the action research project results, colleagues from both the MoEAC and UNAM continued discussions on how the project findings could be cascaded to benefit more schools. One of the action research findings indicated that the majority of teachers in the pre-primary and grade 1 school phase were never formally trained as teachers. Many teachers indicated that their jobs were not secure due to their unqualified status.

The majority of teachers in this phase were working on annual contracts, which made it difficult for them to make long-term plans for their classes. Many were concerned about their job prospects and found it difficult to commit to programs aimed at improving the quality of teaching and learning in their schools. The teachers complained about not having enough money to continue their studies, not having much hope for their future, and constantly worrying about their job prospects for the next year. Their concerns were evident as researchers found that many of the teachers with whom they had worked the previous year were no longer employed at their schools. Officials from the Ministry also indicated that this transient situation made it difficult to engage unqualified teachers in continuing professional development aimed at improving their teaching practices. This situation, combined with the CFIT project research findings, sparked the idea of developing a specialized program for these teachers that would qualify them to become formally trained pre-primary and grade 1 teachers. This led to the development and implementation of a special Diploma in Junior Primary Education for In-Service teachers in Namibia called the DJPE (Inset). The rationale of the program in the Faculty of Education Prospectus 2016 states the following:

> The Ministry of Education, Arts and Culture believes that the upskilling of the competence of un- and under qualified teachers in Namibia, especially in the Junior Primary Phase (Pre-Primary to grade 3) could have long term positive effects on Namibian Learners' performance. Hence a request from the MoEAC to the UNAM/FoE to develop a program that can improve the competences of un- and underqualified teachers, particularly in the teaching of literacy, numeracy and other crucial subject content areas as reflected in the curriculum framework of this program (p.4) (Faculty of Education, 2015)

The 4-year in-service teacher education diploma program aims at upgrading the qualifications of over 3000 unqualified teachers at the Junior Primary Phase. The Diploma in Junior Primary Education (INSET) is a modular in-service program intended to equip the un- and underqualified serving/practicing teachers in Namibia with the necessary range of professional teaching knowledge, skills and attitudes to ensure quality teaching in schools. INSET students are taught by UNAM's Faculty of Education lecturers and supported in the field by mentor teachers, contracted and trained by UNAM. Additionally, the University hired 16 recent graduates, known as Staff Development Fellows (SDFs), to teach and support program implementation.

While the content of the teacher education in-service diploma is the same as the full-time program, the delivery mode differs from that of UNAM's full-time programs. Faculty content expert specialists developed the course syllabi and wrote and uploaded content modules to a learning management system (LMS). Collaboration with FoE staff members across campuses and access to content modules ensured program consistency. Staff members deliver course content during weeklong sessions at a vacation school that occurs during school holidays. Additional learning occurs during bi-monthly Saturday sessions with program mentors working through the interactive models on the LMS. Students gather during varied teaching sessions and the interpersonal interactions during these learning opportunities offer benefits such as depth and engagement with diverse perspectives as lecturers, mentors and students work together over time. Educational cohort models purposefully group students to enter a program of study together and develop a mutual commitment to an educational goal through shared experiences, interactions and collective efforts (Harris, 2006; Maher, 2005).

Since its inception in 2016, the INSET program has enrolled over 2700 teachers. All teachers enrolled in the program will not have their positions advertised if they make good progress in the program. The MoEAC also fully funds the program to the tune of 38 million Namibian dollars over 4 years. Participating teachers continue to teach fulltime in their schools. They receive a tablet and a toolkit of resources based on the toolkit developed during the CFIT project. As the teachers learn, they are encouraged to use the new knowledge in their classes and to reflect on it through practical and hands-on exercises. Saturday mentoring sessions are aimed at helping them reflect on their program module content, implement the required activities, engage with peers in deep discussions, and upload their assignments and short class teaching videos on the LMS for their lecturers. Although the teachers' participation in the program is aimed at obtaining a qualification, it is also promoting improvement in their teaching.

16.5.1 In-Service Teachers and Their Quality of Life

The majority of the un- and underqualified teachers who participated in the UNESCO/CFIT project (2014–2016) is enrolled in the DJPE (INSET) program. Students in the INSET program range in age and teaching experience. A representative sample from Khomas region includes teachers ranging in age from 23 to 50 years with between 4 and 8 years of teaching experience at the junior primary level.

For most of these students, this form of continuing professional development program contributes to their improved protection as un- and underqualified teachers and thereby impacts the quality of their lives. Kelchtermans (2004) defines continuing professional development (CPD) as "a *learning process* resulting from *meaningful interaction* with the context (both in time and space) and eventually leading to changes in teachers' *professional practice* (actions) and in their *thinking about that practice*" (p. 220). What follows is how these teachers describe the impact of their participation in both projects/programs on their personal and professional growth trajectory.

Gratitude and thankfulness for the opportunity to study and learn more about the teaching profession are echoed during the start of each cohort during vacation school sessions. The INSET program provides opportunities to gather as a group not only during vacation school but also during the bi-monthly Saturday mentoring sessions. The third-year students selected for the focus interview came from five different schools. During the focus group session this positive sentiment continued. One student stated, "I never believed I would be at UNAM. As a 36-year-old I am at UNAM. It's a dream come true." Other students used the phrase "a dream come true" in reflecting on finishing Grade 12, but never seeing the possibility of a University education. Participation in the program provided the opportunity for psychological and spiritual well-being; a sense of social cohesion, community and belonging; and opportunities for professional growth, all indicators reflected in the model of quality of life.

Prior to answering the question, "How has your participation in the INSET program impacted you from a personal and professional perspective? An older student stated:

> First of all, I want to thank the Namibian government and the Ministry of Education. This is a brilliant opportunity for us in the teaching profession without the qualification, and financially wise this really supports us because we don't take out money from our pockets to do the education that we are part of. To do something (teaching) without having the proper knowledge of it, it's *not easy*, but this program has put us at ease.

The students have less financial stress and worry since enrolling in the program. Many answered the government's call for those who had finished Grade 12 to apply for teaching posts to help manage the country's severe teacher shortage. As un- and underqualified teachers, they had to reapply for a teaching post each year. They worried about having a salary and enough money; receiving a 5-year contract for their enrollment in the program has relieved that stress. One student described increased family stability because she maintains an annual salary, in contrast to her previous domestic worker wages.

INSET students express a strong sense of hope for the future. They talk about the acquisition of knowledge about teaching and understanding students from a psychological perspective. They express pride and a belief they are more respected at their schools because colleagues know the challenges of being a teacher and a university student. Earning a qualification demonstrates commitment to the teaching profession and to their learners.

INSET students reported feeling valued by the Ministry of Education, Arts and Culture, which pays all university expenses and has committed to a 5 year teaching post that allows teachers to focus on studies and teaching and not worry about being moved annually to a new post. The INSET program allows them to articulate into UNAM's degree program which advances academic achievement, something many had dreamed about but didn't believe would happen.

Teaching, studying and raising a family are demanding tasks. Continuing to work while earning a degree benefits the participants. Students in the INSET program are able to support themselves and families while learning about teaching and earning a degree. They describe themselves as more humbled and open to learning, and they have also improved their time management skills. Multiple demands on their time help them be more disciplined, which adds to their positive sense of well-being.

Students describe their transition from being placed in a teaching position where they relied on personal experiences to guide their teaching to knowing something about children and classrooms because of their UNAM coursework in the vacation school and the Saturday mentoring sessions. However, they acknowledge that they "knew, but really didn't know," and expressed surprise at how much they have learned about the complexity of teaching. During the focus group interview, students demonstrated knowledge gained during 3 years in the program. They talked about the importance of responding to individual learner needs and unique family situations. They shared the benefit of using child centered learning aids to create an interactive learning environment that engages all in the learning process. These approaches are in contrast to how they taught before the program, which they say reflected a more teacher centered approach that emphasized standing in front of the class and telling learners what to do. In the third year of the program, INSET students speak with confidence about their teaching and hope for their future as teachers who will make a difference in the lives of Namibian children. The INSET students stated emphatically, "Kids depend on us," and they take that responsibility seriously.

They feel connected to the larger group of students and shared how they learn and work together. One student said, "being at your school and learning from people there is one thing. In this program, we are able to come together with other teachers, and the lecturers too, and learn from each other. We are a group of different teachers, and every time we come together we learn from each other. We share ideas [that we get] from each other and pass that onto our kids."

The large group has its own WhatsApp® community where they regularly share successes and challenges. They share a group identity as INSET students, and have also created sub groups with people at the same grade level. Collegiality among the focus group was apparent. One student explained his view of collegiality related to coursework and teaching. While pointing to different people, he said, "What I know, you might not, and what you know, I may not and that is how we learn from each other."

The group of students shared individual stories about their paths to becoming teachers. One teacher described her transition to becoming a teacher through this program. She said, "My son, who is studying at Poly [Namibia Institute of Technology] says this is a great opportunity for me. After matric, I was struggling to get a job. I was doing domestic work, but then from domestic work, I became a teacher. It was a great blessing."

Another student shared her interactions with her Grade 8 daughter. She explained that her daughter was experiencing challenges in mathematics but now "she sees her Mom at UNAM and I am achieving at 70 percent and showing her if I can do it, she can also do it. So now it's my job to get at least 70 percent and show her I can do it. It encourages and motivates her, too, and makes me work hard." Others also shared the encouragement they receive from others and how it benefits their performance as teachers.

16.5.2 In-Service Teachers' Mentors and Their Quality of Life

There are 80 mentors, appointed by regional administrators, associated with the INSET program. Approximately one third of the mentors are affiliated with regional Teacher Resource Centers in the capacity of Senior Education Officers, another third are Heads of Departments for Junior Primary Education and the other third are teachers, recognized for teaching excellence. Excellent teaching and the ability to support others professionally guided the selection of mentors. UNAM provided intensive mentor training and meets annually with mentors for program updates and additional specialized mentor training. The training goals for mentors were to:

- Gain strong knowledge about the DJPE INSET and recognize mentor roles
- Understand how to create effective professional growth environments for program participants
- Articulate effective practices in Junior Primary Education
- Create personal and collective vision for their work as mentors.

The concept of community, connection and belonging adds to life satisfaction for the mentors. Multiple layers exist within the community of mentors and students. Mentors develop relationships with other mentors and create their own affinity groups. Regions have unique WhatsApp® groups that include mentors and UNAM staff connected with the INSET program. The regional mentoring groups provide "another family." In one region, seven mentors gather bi-monthly as a large group of all students before breaking into smaller groups with their assigned mentees.

Mentors are part of a community of practice that extends beyond their Ministry appointed position. A sense of purpose underpins their work, and they embrace their bi-monthly mentoring sessions with INSET students. They believe they have a "huge responsibility" and a significant role in the transformation of teachers who teach at the junior primary level. They mentor with purpose and know they are changing teaching and learning in Namibia. They are part of a small community providing authentic learning opportunities for mentees, and at the same time part of a larger mission.

The Saturday sessions follow similar themes, and each group responds to the themes in ways that build knowledge and skills. One mentor describes her perspective of shared commitment to a common goal: "The sense, the power that you too are being changed, that you're part of the change to change motivates me and gives me courage to continue. Even though I am retiring at the end of the year, I will continue what I am doing as a mentor. What I do is important for the community, important for education."

Mentors report that participation in the INSET program as mentors has broadened their way of thinking and elevated their career paths. One mentor who has become a HOD during the project said, "My career path has changed. I've learned to listen to adults and to others' opinions. I was very stubborn, I was a one-way street and now I'm a two-way street. I've grown professionally."

What started as casual conversation during a mentor training became a reality for eight mentors from two regions. The regional mentor groups received a formal invitation to visit schools in Washington State and discuss the state's mentoring program with the Director of the statewide mentoring program. Eight of the 13 mentors took advantage of the invitation. Fundraising and personal money paid for the journey to the United States. Once in the U.S., money from an endowment at the sponsoring university funded the 10-day visit. The mentors summarized the highlights from the visit in a presentation to over 130 mentors. When addressing the group, a mentor said,

> This was once in a lifetime experience. We learned so much. We visited schools, met the university president, learned about the brain and learning, and many of us got to fly on a plane and experience snow for the first time. We saw how much learners can do. We visited high poverty schools and even the Grade 0 kids are reading and writing.

Observing learners in three schools triggered thinking related to personal ideas of what children are able to do. They observed pre-primary children writing without worrying about spelling and handwriting. They observed young children accessing word walls to help with writing and realized they want to change what they do with their own learners and also with students from the INSET program. They feel a deeper understanding about how the teacher and the classroom environment influence learning outcomes, and they are enthusiastic to make a difference in their schools and with their mentees. When sharing their experience and knowledge to INSET students during a Saturday session, they talked about being a group of mentors that came together from two regions to experience the trip. Before sharing their slides of learning content and supporting pictures, they acknowledged the funding and contextual differences between Namibia and the U.S. However, they urged the group to be part of the group, a community that positively influences the lives of Namibian children. They speak with passion and describe a sense of hope for the future. They find their lives already changed since returning from the U.S. One mentor, a primary grade teacher, was struck by the soft tones of American teachers. She adopted a quieter tone when speaking to learners and staff. One of her learners approached her husband and asked, "Is Miss sick since she came back from the U.S.? Her voice is so soft now." Modeling what she observed as consistent practice in all classrooms influenced her tone and language, and she already observes differences in the way learners respond to her and each other.

16.5.3 Staff Development Fellows and Their Quality of Life

Implementation of the DJPE (INSET) increased the need for recruiting academic staff on all the campuses where the program was being implemented. To teach at the University of Namibia, a relevant Masters' degree is a requirement. During the recruitment process it became clear that there was a very limited pool of qualified staff in pre- and lower primary education who could be recruited to teach at tertiary level. This was compounded by the fact that the newly recruited staff members on the different campuses should be able to teach mother-tongue in one of nine local Namibian languages. (All Junior Primary Education teachers are trained to teach one mother-tongue as a medium of instruction). The FoE management received permission to recruit 16 of their best bachelor degree graduates in the field of early childhood and lower primary education, to become staff development fellows (SDFs) who could assist with implementation of the in-service diploma, and at the same time obtain a Masters' degree in pre and lower primary education. The Faculty has been struggling for years to recruit students into the Masters' degree for early years' education. A study conducted by Moller and Villet (2014) discuss factors that influence the low intake into pre- and lower primary teacher education in Namibia. One of the major perceptions that negatively influenced choosing early childhood and lower primary teaching as career, was the low status and image of the profession.

Staff Development Fellows felt that their appointment at UNAM brought several benefits to their lives. Although many of them feel quite overwhelmed with the workload at the University, all of them feel grateful for the opportunity "to improve my academic qualifications as I am currently registered for the Master's in Education specializing in Early Childhood Development and Lower Primary Education. This will not only improve my qualification but will enhance my professional development and knowledge as the more I am involved in publication of journal articles, the more I will top up my knowledge," as stated by one of the SDFs on the Katima Mulilo Campus.

Other SDFs commented on the opportunities they now have for growing professionally, by attending meetings and workshops, being involved in material and course development at tertiary level, lecturing to students who are in many respects their peers, as well as to work alongside their former lecturers "of whom most of them have been my role models," stated a SDF based on the Khomasdal Campus.

Their comments also revolved around building collaborative relationships with teachers and school principals when they go out to observe their students' school-based activities; "Given an opportunity to interact with the community and more specifically with different schools through school based studies evaluation/visits." Further comments included the sense of independence they felt since teaching at the University, their new felt sense of confidence to stand in front of large University classes, their growth in the areas of using ICTs for teaching and ensuring they are up to date with University policies, student's assessment and posting of important information on students' e-learning portals: "Information here is communicated via email unlike at schools, one has to develop a culture of checking his/her email frequently. Policies and important documents are on the intranet and you have to read and understand them by yourself, unlike at school where things are explained to you during orientation week."

SDFs are enjoying the dynamic work environment of the University, feel a sense of "the joy of having to work at UNAM knowing that I am empowering students to became (sic) great teachers in the future." They also commented on the feeling of "appreciation that I have been able to get professional services like the medical aid which is actually really helping me and my family."

16.6 Conclusion

"Together we can do it, together we can do it." In a large hall, INSET students sing, sway and clap to the catchy tune at the closing of each vacation school. "Together" reflects the guiding principles embedded in Namibia's large-scale projects aimed at elevating quality education, a project that began with a collaborative multi-disciplinary/cross-sectoral process and is the framework for continued endeavors that include key players, who continue to build capacity and influence the quality of teaching and learning in Namibian classrooms.

The use of research to inform teaching and learning and the conception of an education community of practice contributes to Namibia's efforts in accelerating the progress towards the provision of high quality education. What started out as an action research project involving 28 schools and 56 school teachers, has grown in size and magnitude to involve over 2700 in-service teachers across Namibia, from all 14 education regions. The project provided a platform to bring together UNAM Faculty of Education, classroom teachers, government officials and other stakeholders to engage in a countrywide collaborative action research process. The action research findings are embedded in the in-service program, aimed at building capacity in teaching literacy and numeracy. In-service teachers receive toolkits that form the basis of their training, learn to use ICTs to access their training materials, record their progress, showcase their achievements, and build e-portfolios that will provide evidence of their personal and professional journey through the 4 years of their training in becoming qualified early childhood and lower primary school teachers.

While these are early days to report on the impact these major interventions have on learning in the classroom, the research on quality education points to the right "moves" being made in the Namibian education landscape to improve the quality of early childhood and lower primary education: interventions based on action research; teachers' involvement in their own learning and building of their capacity; resourcing classrooms with relevant teaching and learning resources; building communities of practice (Masino & Nino-Zarazua, 2016). This project created a conducive environment to learn about and participate in the research process, work collaboratively and learn from the experience and expertise of professionals. Feeling empowered, the researchers together with teachers and other colleagues, refined their skills, re-examined their perspectives of teaching and learning and adjusted their professional practice. The intentional design of combining the toolkit concept with a collaborative support framework and participants' ownership of the process bolstered the efficacy of the intervention phase and created a dynamic blueprint for professional development in the Namibian education community.

References

Coghlan, D., & Brannick, T. (2015). *Doing action research in your own organization*. Thousand Oaks, CA: SAGE.

Ellis, J. (2013). *Needs assessment for capacity development of teacher education in Namibia*. Windhoek, Namibia.

Faculty of Education. (2015). *Faculty of Education Prospectus 2015*. Windhoek, Namibia: University of Namibia.

Gotto, G. S., Turnbull, A., Ann Summers, J., & Blue-Banning, M. (2010). *Community of practice development manual: A step-by-step guide for designing and developing a community of practice*. Lawrence, KS: Kansas University. Retrieved from http://ktdrr.org/resources/rush/copmanual/CoP_Manual.pdf

Graven, M., & Lerman, S. (2003). Book review: Wenger, E. (1998). Communities of practice: Learning, meaning and identity. *Journal of Mathematics Teacher Education, 6*(2), 185–194.

Harris, B. A. (2006). The importance of creating a "sense of commitment". *Journal of College Student Retention, Research Theory and Practice, 8*(1), 83–105.

Hungi, N., Makuwa, D., Ross, K., Saito, M., Dolata, S., van Capelle, F., … Vellien, J. (2010). *SACMEQ III project results: Pupil achievement levels in reading and mathematics. Southern and Eastern African Consortium for Monitoring Educational Quality*. Paris, France. https://doi.org/10.1007/s11125-005-6819-7

Jimenez-Silva, M., & Olson, K. (2012). A community of practice in teacher education: Insights and perceptions. *International Journal of Teaching and Learning in Higher Education, 24*(3), 335–348. Retrieved from http://www.isetl.org/ijtlhe/

Kelchtermans, G. (2004). CPD for professional renewal: Moving beyond knowledge for practice. In C. Day & J. Sachs (Eds.), *International handbook on the continuing professional development of teachers* (pp. 217–237). Maidenhead, UK: Open University Press.

Maher, M. A. (2005). The evolving meaning and influence of cohort membership. *Innovative Higher Education, 30*(3), 195–211. https://doi.org/10.1007/s10755-005-6304-5

Masino, S., & Nino-Zarazua, M. (2016). What works to improve the quality of student learning in developing countries? *International Journal of Educational Development, 48*, 53–65. https://doi.org/10.1016/J.IJEDUDEV.2015.11.012

Mo Ibrahim Foundation. (2017). *Africa at a tipping point*. London, UK. Retrieved from http://allafrica.com/download/resource/main/main/idatcs/00101935:5129995725e8c4478bcf049bfcfa24ae.pdf

Moller, J., & Villet, C. B. (2014). Factors influencing the low intake into pre- and lower primary teacher education in Namibia. *NERA Journal, 12*(1), 20–38.

Mwabu, G., & Ackerman, X. (2013). *Focusing on Quality Education in sub-Saharan Africa*. Retrieved June 28, 2018, from https://www.brookings.edu/blog/education-plus-development/2013/05/28/focusing-on-quality-education-in-sub-saharan-africa/.

Mzabalazo Advisory Services. (2016). *We are the architects of our destiny: Study of positive deviant schools in Namibia*. Windhoek, Namibia. Retrieved from https://www.unicef.org/namibia/na.MoEAC_-_Positive_Deviant_Schools_Report_(2016)_-_web_quality(1).pdf

Neuman, M. (2011). Collaborative workshop promotes ECD in action. *Newsletter of the Africa early childhood care in development initiatiive*, pp. 1–2. Retrieved from http://siteresources.worldbank.org/EXTAFRREGTOPEDUCATION/Resources/ECCD-Newsletter-jan11-en.pdf

Priya, M., Prasanth, M., & Prince, J.P. (2017). Reflective practices: A means to teacher development. *Asia Pacific Journal of Contemporary Education and Communication Technology (APJCET), 3*(1). www.apiar.org.au

Sammons, P., & Bakkum, L. (2011). Effective schools, equity and teacher effectiveness: A review of the literature. *Profesorado: Revista de Currciculum y Formacion Del Profesorado, 15*(11), 9–26.

Steukers, G., & Weiss, J. (2015). *Quality teachers for EFA: capacity development for quality in pre- and lower primary teacher education in Namibia – 2015*. Windhoek, Namibia. Retrieved from http://unesdoc.unesco.org/images/0023/002348/234821E.pdf

The Namibia Ministry of Health and Social Services, & Namibia Statistics Agency. (2014). *Namibia demographic and health survey 2013*. Windhoek, Namibia. Retrieved from https://dhsprogram.com/pubs/pdf/FR298/FR298.pdf

The World Bank. (2017). *Early childhood development overview: Understanding poverty*. Retrieved June 28, 2018, from http://www.worldbank.org/en/topic/earlychildhooddevelopment

UNICEF. (2012). *UNICEF ANNUAL Report 2011*. Paris. Retrieved from https://www.unicef.org/nutrition/files/UNICEF_Annual_Report_2011_EN_060112.pdf

UNICEF Namibia. (2016). *UNICEF Namibia – Education*. Retrieved June 28, 2018, from https://www.unicef.org/namibia/education.html

Developing Capacity for Teacher Inservice Education in Rural Tanzania: Embracing Emergent Phenomena

17

Elaine Simmt, Andrew Binde, Florence Glanfield, and Joyce Mgombelo

Abstract

In this chapter the authors discuss a development project conducted in Tanzania which became known as "*hisabati ni maisha*"—mathematics is living/life. The goal of the project was to build capacity for mathematics teaching and learning in rural and remote communities. The work was based on lessons learned from research conducted in Tanzania prior to the project, Canadian indigenous perspectives and complexity thinking. Of critical importance was the building and nourishing of relationships between the team and participants and among participants, and ongoing openness to emergent ideas and strategies. This openness led to constant tinkering with the design and activities of the project which we believe led to a project that had better and unexpected outcomes. We pay particular attention to some of the ways in which we tinkered with the design of the project in light of interactions among the project team and participants in the project.

> When I was told that "we will be learning together," I asked myself, how is it possible to sit and learn together in the same class having a diversity of people? Because we were teachers, educational quality assurance officers, academic officers, adult educational officers, and teacher educators—from teacher colleges and universities. I thought the class would be complicated… This project … has helped us to know each other clearly. We are from different areas, but we love each other, and we learn together. (GAC project participant)

17.1 Introduction

Hisabati ni maisha (mathematics is living/mathematics is life) began as a development project, funded by Global Affairs Canada (GAC), that deliberately brought together people who have an impact on primary school teachers and teaching in an effort to create enhanced professional development for rural and remote teachers in Tanzania. *Hisabati ni maisha* has become a call to action among those educators and community members who participated in the project to support the mathematics teaching and learning of primary school children. *Hisabiti ni maisha* is the legacy of collaborative work among Tanzanian and Canadian educators to enhance mathematics teaching and learning in rural and remote primary schools in Tanzania.

17.2 Context

As the educational community knows well, the goal for all children to have a basic education must be met in two ways: access and quality

E. Simmt (✉) · A. Binde · F. Glanfield · J. Mgombelo
University of Alberta, Edmonton, AB, Canada
e-mail: esimmt@ualberta.ca; glanfiel@ualberta.ca; jmgombelo@brocku.ca

I. Eloff (ed.), *Handbook of Quality of Life in African Societies*, International Handbooks of Quality-of-Life, https://doi.org/10.1007/978-3-030-15367-0_17

(Bellamy, 2013; Kendall, 2007). It is widely reported that Tanzania, like many of the countries in sub-Saharan Africa has met the goals of access to basic education for all, however the quality of education has become a more difficult challenge (Hardman, Ackers, Abrishamian, & O'Sullivan, 2011).

Ongoing professional learning for teachers is an important means to enhance instructional practice (Darling-Hammond, Hyler, & Gardner, 2017) in primary school classrooms. In sub-Saharan Africa professional development opportunities for primary school teachers in rural and remote communities are difficult to access. In the project baseline survey of rural and remote teachers in six districts of two rural regions in Tanzania only 11% of the teachers responding indicate they had attended some form of professional development in their career.

Inservice education in Tanzania is commonly in the form of workshops offered either by the government and its agencies or international non-governmental organizations (INGOs). The Tanzania Institute of Education (TIE) and the Agency for Development of Education Management (ADEM) each offer professional development in Tanzania, the former as it relates to curriculum and the latter on educational management. Professional development opportunities also arise from programs offered by development partners and INGOs. In the time frame surrounding and including this project a range of opportunities were offered in Tanzania through support of development partners and INGOs including: Global Partnership for Education LANES, EQUIP, USAID TZ21, UNICEF and GAC Teacher Education Support Program.

In a discussion of the large scale project "Education for All" in Tanzania, Aikman (2010) points to the need for INGOs to work at the intersection of citizens and states, where citizen rights and government responsibilities are both addressed in programming and advocacy. She illustrates an advocacy model Oxfam proposed for a multi-layered one-program approach to education development work in Tanzania. The model proposes advocacy at multiple levels: global, regional, national, district and local. She discusses two programs that involved pedagogic innovation intended to feed into education policy advocacy. One of the programs was to enhance education quality through pedagogy. In that project MOUs were signed between the two implementing agencies and brought together a range of stakeholders: school inspectorate office, education officers, and officials from the local government authority. A review of the project revealed that, in spite of some success at the level of student-teacher relationships, problems in program efficiency, delays in implementation, and ability of decision makers to assert influence as needed impacted the overall success of the project. She explains that there was a lack of understanding of the INGO about the formal and informal political structure and decision-making lines which had implications for the project. Further, the project lacked shared purpose, neglected referencing the MOUs, and demonstrated poor understanding of the partner institutions values, beliefs and cultures. Addressing these challenges is critical to a project's success.

One thing we have noted is the rarity of local initiatives supporting teacher inservice development, whether it is a small learning community led by a master teacher or a professional development series facilitated by teacher educators, such as college tutors. We wondered how we might be able to leverage the human resources afforded by the proximity of local universities and teacher colleges to rural schools to contribute to inservice education to practicing teachers in rural and hard to reach communities. Further we knew that in the school system itself, master school teachers, school quality assurance officers and others within the communities also could be resources for ongoing teacher development. The presence of educators (with many different roles in the education sector) who could provide support in the communities close to their places of work and home suggested to us that they were resources which could be mobilized to support ongoing professional learning. We saw an opportunity with our project to create capacity for a culture of ongoing professional learning.

It is the case that in Tanzania there is some interaction between higher education institutions and schools. Schools are the sites for the placement of student teachers for teaching practice and they are sometimes the sites for research. Hence to some extent teacher educators and educational researchers are already involved in schools in some ways. Teachers and school communities benefit from this relationship however, there is a concern with this model that the relationship is one sided— it exists insofar as the universities need sites for their research or teacher colleges need placements for their student teachers; but there seems to be little reciprocity. For example, schools do not call on the universities or teacher colleges to do research needed by the school or to provide inservice education that might be needed for their teachers. On the other hand, we did identify a master of education program that demonstrates reciprocity. After completing advanced degrees, teachers had the possibility of becoming professional development teachers who facilitated inservice programming in their local communities (see Halai, 2001, Halai & Rarieya, 2004).

In this chapter we discuss the design and implementation of a 5 year development project (GAC project[1]) funded by Global Affairs Canada and led by a team of mathematics teacher educators from two Canadian universities and one Tanzanian university. The GAC project intended to build capacity for mathematics teaching and learning in rural and remote communities in Tanzania. Framing the study with scholarship about Indigenous ways of knowing and being, complexity theory, and research findings from a study done in collaboration with Tanzanian teachers and educational specialists provided us with a robust design that we were able to tinker with as challenges and possibilities emerged throughout the project.

17.3 Scholarship and Research to Inform GAC Project

The research on professional development suggests long term projects have more potential for enhancement of outcomes than short term ones. Professional learning that is ongoing, peer to peer, and embedded in context has better results than one-shot workshops and top-down sessions. Whereas bottom-up projects create a sense of ownership, top-down projects often allow for teachers to resort to their old ways of knowing (Wayne, Yoon, Zhu, Cronen, & Garet, 2008). Darling-Hammond, Hyler, and Gardner (2017) suggest seven characteristics of effective professional development (PD): it is content focused; it incorporates active learning; it is collaborative and embedded in context; it models effective practice; it provides coaching; it provides expert support; and it is sustained (p. 4). We are sensitive to these general research findings; they reflect our sensibilities and the professional development the Canadian team members do in our home communities. However most of the studies which led to those conclusions were conducted in contexts different from sub-Saharan Africa, and Tanzania in particular. We were also informed by research conducted in Tanzania with Tanzanian colleagues (Simmt et al., 2014; Glanfield, Mgombelo, & Simmt, 2016) in the 2 years prior to the implementation of the GAC project. That research asked, how can universities work with communities to provide professional development opportunities for rural teachers. Underpinning both that study and the GAC project are two complementary theoretical perspectives that shaped our conceptualizations, decisions and actions: Canadian Indigenous perspectives and complexity thinking. These two frames are important to us as we attempt to establish a collaborative and collective learning system.

[1] We use of the word development in two different ways— to refer to the development project and to refer to teacher professional development. To avoid confusion, we will use the phrase GAC project to refer to the capacity building project (or "development project" funded by Global Affairs Canada. We use teacher professional development (or PD) to refer both to the professional learning activities and the concept of development for professionals.

17.3.1 Canadian Indigenous Ways of Knowing and Being in Community

Canadian indigenous people's ways of knowing speak of the significance of reciprocity, respect, relationships, community knowledge, traditional practices, the wisdom of elders and communal concerns over individual ones. "Being with" others creates and nourishes relationships. Being with others involves respect for both the Indigenous knowledge of the local community and the academic knowledge of the university (Donald, Glanfield, & Sterenberg, 2011, 2012, 2013; Poirier, 2007). Being with others is listening with respect: from that listening communal interests, concerns and challenges are identified and possibilities emerge. Being with others fosters the possibility of shared work on communal concerns.

17.3.2 Complexity Thinking

From a complexity thinking perspective (Davis & Simmt, 2016) we know that a collective learning system demonstrates a number of conditions (Davis & Simmt, 2003). In particular, there is a diversity among agents (participants) which can satisfy the demands of a shared goal, at the same time there is redundancy—shared experiences, roles and skills—which ensures that people can work together, and that with the loss of any particular agents others can pick up the roles. Complex learning systems demonstrate decentralized and dynamic control; control is not centrally fixed but is dynamically assumed by participants and groups of participants in response to the emergent needs of the system. The diversity of participants within the collective learning system interact creating the processes and products. Those processes and products become part of the system creating new possibilities for interaction from which new products and processes emerge. In other words, the system grows and learns. A critical feature when thinking with complexity is that of emergence. From collective interactions emerge a way to proceed.

17.3.3 Universities Working with Communities

Universities and communities, academic and local knowledge, professional relationships and community relationships—there are many differences between what universities and communities can offer in a collaborative effort to address educational challenges in a region. We assert that it is those differences that constitute reasons to work together to shape and implement projects that can enhance mathematics education. However, those differences mean special attention needs to be paid to developing "working relationships" (Machimana, Sefotho, & Ebersohn, 2018; Donald et al., 2011). Such relationships must be founded on respect, shared concerns and goals, and an understanding of what each system offers. Aikman's 2010 analysis of development projects suggests a project without these will be impeded. We believe knowledge of context and existing relationships can serve to mitigate some of these issues. Simmt et al. (2014) investigated how universities could work with communities to enhance mathematics teaching. That study, conducted in Tanzania with Tanzanian collaborators prior to the GAC project, was formative to our conceptualization of the GAC project.

Simmt et al. (2014) conducted a series of interviews, observations and document reviews to understand governance, school, and curriculum structures and to identify stakeholders implicated in mathematics education. As well, they sought to learn about the successes and challenges teachers and local authorities experience in rural communities in Tanzania in relation to mathematics education. The professional introductions and conversations with a number of educational specialists in national, regional and district offices, and visits with ward coordinators and mathematics teachers were seen as critical to gathering the insights they needed to do work with Tanzanian educators. All conversations were valuable but the conversations with teachers (and some parents) in their classrooms and school yards raised awareness of context in a very nuanced way. For example, teachers in one school talked about how their school was supported at one time by an NGO but that was long ago and nothing remains but an abandoned well. In a school yard a couple of parents from a pastoral group approached the team with questions about what the foreigners were doing. The parents were quick to offer suggestions about what could be done to keep their children in school.

Intending to learn more than simply the results of school leaving examinations and avoiding a deficit perspective, Simmt et al. (2014) deliberately sought out success stories by asking district and regional authorities to recommend sites of promising practices. For example, a regional education officer recommended we visit a rural school that had some very high performing students in mathematics. Researching the village of which this school was a part, Ngalawa, Glanfield, and Simmt (2015) encountered people that valued the school and the education it provided their children. The villagers supported the local school through ensuring children were fed, teachers were assisted in their lives outside of school, and funds were provided for sample test papers (for example). In turn, the school teachers provided tutoring outside of school hours and sample test papers for children to practice. A master mathematics teacher served as a resource to other teachers. A second case recommended to the research team was to visit a district that was on a trajectory of increasing student performance on the school leaving examination. In that work Simmt et al. (2014) noted how the district education officer who had completed a master of education degree (from a university whose goals were educational development) had prioritized mathematics education within her district. She encouraged her team to think about themselves as all contributing to student success in mathematics. She also put funds into a traveling teacher who could provide rural teachers support for mathematics instruction. These and other promising practices led us to the point of imagining professional development in rural and remote communities in Tanzania.

The second contribution to the GAC project from the Simmt et al. (2014) study came from work in which study participants co-constructed criteria for professional development in rural and remote communities in Tanzania. These criteria emerged out of a set of sequential and staged prototyping activities that involved:

(a) Initial school visits;
(b) Study of promising practices;
(c) Document review of governance structures;
(d) A working session with educational stakeholders (ministry level to school level) to share the research team's learning from a – c above;
(e) Seek recommendations for developing an appropriate model for PD;
(f) Pilot a PD workshop developed and facilitated by a Tanzanian university lecturer alongside a college tutor and primary school teacher;
(g) A working session to evaluate and refine the prototype with the people who participated in it;
(h) And finally a symposium in Canada to share findings from the work.

The following suggestions that emerged from the PD prototyping and subsequent activities directly informed the development project (Table 17.1) (Glanfield, Mgombelo, & Simmt, 2015).

Table 17.1 Features of PD co-constructed by university researchers and community stakeholders

Content	Include primary school mathematics content
	Current Tanzanian curriculum
	Examples of student work
Teacher	Invite teachers to try ideas in their classrooms and use their experiences
	Attend to and encourage gender-sensitive teaching strategies
Assessment	Acknowledge and attend to national examinations
Learner	Pay attention to non-fluent Kiswahili speakers
Resources	Acknowledge there is a shortage of resources/teaching aids/books
Methodology	Participatory: develop understanding through communication and interactions
Sustainability	Involve decision makers in the workshops

Finally, dynamics of university and community partnerships uncovered in the Simmt et al. (2014) study provided us with a set of guiding principals for the work in our development project (Glanfield, Mgombelo, Simmt & Binde, 2016). We reflected on these throughout the GAC project.

- Establish and nourish personal **relationships** between university and community participants.
- Layer activity and interaction over time creating a dynamic of **recursivity**. With each activity and interaction past experiences are invoked and transformed.
- Pay attention to the nature of the partnership, who the people are and what role they play to sustain the collective work. The relationship must involve giving and receiving: it must be **reciprocal**.
- Recognize that perceptions of status and the ability to influence decision making speak to the **power** relationships that will emerge. Control needs to be distributed as demanded by the activities of the project.
- Ensure there is frequent and ongoing communication. This is achievable through commonplace technologies. **Communication** is critical to the success of the project.
- Expand the conception of **resources** to include among other things: human resources, monetary resources, academic knowledge, specialist knowledge and local community knowledge. Sharing of the resources among participants is an ongoing dynamic within a partnership.
- Work **ethically**—not in the sense of an *a priori* set of rules which come from a particular system to guide action but rather in the sense of ethics as enacted in situations based on what the person (or group) poses as relevant in the moment as they brings forth a world of significance together (Varela, 1999).

To illustrate, the GAC project was designed to build on a number of the relationships that were established in the research. The promising practices, criteria for PD and dynamics of partnerships were identified and conceptualized from some of the very regions that would come to be part of the project. The districts and people that we visited in the research study were prioritized as sites and participants of the GAC project. The research used to conceptualize the GAC project meant that it was built explicitly to include and engage use of local research, and ongoing and emergent local input, decision making and facilitation.

17.4 The GAC Development Project as Designed

Understanding of the importance of relationships for working with communities, the dynamics of universities working with local communities to enhance mathematics teaching and promoting the emergence of a collective learning community on the basis of complexity thinking we built a multi-faceted highly connected (or networked) project to build capacity for mathematics teaching in primary schools (Simmt, Binde, Mgombelo, & Glanfield, 2018). In this section we discuss the design of the GAC project and offer indicators of the challenges and success of the project. Permeating our project was an underlying premise, to build a project that uses the expertise of the university coalition, local educational specialists, and the local practices and knowledge of the community in ways that create the potential for sustainable support for primary school mathematics teaching in rural and remote communities.

We have found other projects that begin with commentary on instruction in mathematics classes where it is critiqued as traditional (Dembele & Lafoka, 2007) and/or teacher directed resulting in passive learners (Hardman et al., 2011) and then propose means for disrupting such practices through inservice education. This was not our starting place. We conducted this work with the premise that teachers are knowers (Davis & Simmt, 2006); teaching practice is impacted by the people who set educational policy and the people who administer and lead schools (Simmt et al., 2014); and that community context in which teaching takes place influences mathematics teaching and learning (Ngalawa et al., 2015).

With access to funding from GAC we saw an opportunity to create conditions for local experts in education (including ministry officials, district and regional education officers, school quality assurance officers, university and college tutors, adult educators and master teachers) to collaborate for the purpose of enhancing mathematics education in primary schools. In the proposal stage the Canadian team, with the advice of the Tanzanian Canadian Cooperation Office, identified a local country co-director. It turned out that we had previously interacted with him (Binde) in the context of the prior research study. With the proposal in the midst of development the local country co-director began to offer input into the design. He was particularly excited about the focus of the project that was to address primary school teachers in rural and remote communities.

A multi-faceted and highly networked design was proposed for the GAC project to build capacity for supporting mathematics teaching. It involved a range of stakeholders and activities to support mathematics teaching in multiple ways: teacher education, community awareness, and policy conversations and recommendations. These constitute what we refer to as three primary nodes of the project (Fig. 17.1). They each address a specific facet of support for mathematics teaching. We conjectured that if we had difficulties in delivering appropriate activities and interactions in one of the nodes that the overall project still could succeed with the other two nodes intact. Indeed, there was a moment in the project when we were concerned about potential

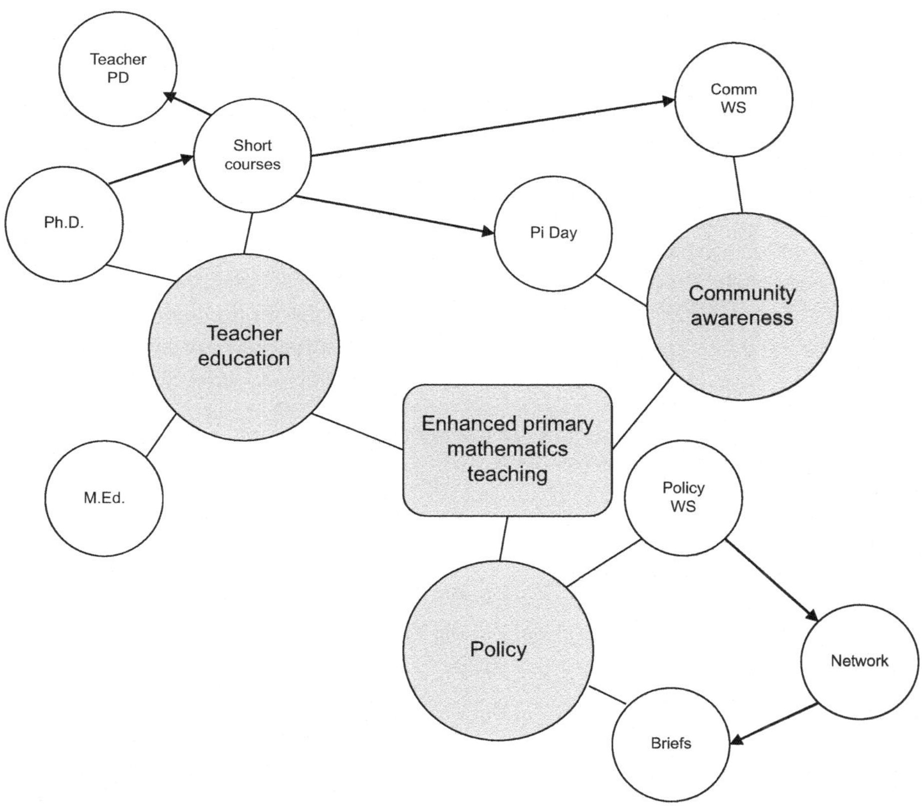

Fig. 17.1 Network design of the GAC project. Edges with errors indicates product from the work done in that node activity

failure of the policy node. However, because the work was informed by complexity theory and indigenous perspectives we were open to and invited perturbations that would enable us to tinker with the project design, keeping it organic and fluid to transform as needed. In the next part of the chapter we discuss the rationale and design of each node, and follow that discussion with examples of how the design was tinkered with given emergent concerns, ideas and resources.

17.4.1 Teacher Education Node

The teacher education node involved three forms of primary level activities and two forms of secondary level activities. First level activities were delivered by project team (except degree programs which were offered by one Canadian university and one Tanzanian university). Second level activities were delivered by local participants who participated in first level activities. First level activities included: doctoral studies for three education sector professionals; master level studies for 22 teachers and teacher educators; and short courses for 53 people whose work could be seen as either directly or indirectly contributing to teacher learning and development. The second level activities included professional development for 430 teachers and community mathematics awareness workshops for 245 community members. The teacher education node activities were the broadest and most time and human resource intensive of the GAC project. Table 17.2 describes participant involvement by type of activity and their role in the education sector.

Setting aside the advanced studies leading to M.Ed. and Ph.D. degrees (these were intended to build capacity for leadership in mathematics education and were offered through traditional programming of universities), what we refer to as short courses (9 weeks over 4 years) served as the site of building capacity for developing and facilitating teacher in-service and community awareness sessions. Selecting people on the basis of their role and potential influence in teacher development was a critical design feature of the GAC project. University lecturers educate future college tutors and secondary school teachers; college tutors educate primary school teachers; quality assurance officers monitor and advise in-service teachers; district academic officers coordinate the implementation of regional and national policies and practices; district adult educators work to provide community based adult education: and master teachers are viewed as knowledgeable colleagues whom are turned to by their colleagues for advice. We know that people in these positions have the potential either to work closely with teachers or to facilitate others who work closely with teachers to support them in their local school communities. Having identified communities in which to work, we invited people in these roles from each of the nine districts of the GAC project to the short courses. Identified from among the participants in the short courses professional development facilitators were invited to develop and deliver modules to rural and remote teachers of mathematics. We describe the short courses here as an illustration of the work in the teacher educator node.

Table 17.2 Participants by role and activity in teacher education node

	Form of participation				
Role in education sector	Ph.D	M.Ed.	Short course	Teacher PD	Community workshop
University Jr. Lecturer	x		x	x	
Government Curriculum Specialist	x			x	
College Tutor		x	x	x	x
District Academic Officer			x		
Quality Assurance Officer			x	x	
District Adult Education Officer			x		x
Master School Teacher			x	x	x

17.4.1.1 Short Courses

The intention of the short courses was to build capacity for locally developed and delivered in-service professional development in rural and remote communities in nine districts in four regions of central Tanzania. We agree that "Intensive, sustained, job embedded PD focused on content of the subject that teachers teach is more likely to improve teacher knowledge, classroom instruction and student achievement" (Wayne et al., 2008, p. 470). Hence the 9 weeks of short courses over 4 years focused on the mathematics that teachers use in their teaching (Davis & Simmt, 2006), resources for teaching and learning mathematics, and models for professional development. From Table 17.3 it can be observed that the short courses were multidimensional, at once attending to pedagogical, mathematical, gender equity and professional development concerns. Included but not noted in the table is how the short courses were used as a site to prepare participants for designing and delivering professional development opportunities to rural and remote teachers. The question of the value to the participants in the short courses (the vast majority of whom were not teachers of mathematics) of framing sessions around doing mathematics and addressing pedagogical knowledge might be asked. We have ample evidence of the high level of engagement the mathematical activities generated and the perceived value of that mathematical work. These are the words of GAC participants invited to reflect on the project:

> In reality when I started been part of this project, I had an idea that mathematics is a very hard subject to teach and learn, but from the knowledge drawn from part of this project, I came to realize how mathematics is not as hard as I thought to be. … I have realized this because in this project we have been involved in different learning and part of preparation different simple teaching tools and this has made me like this subject… the skills and knowledge drawn from this course has made me understand this subject very well and I am proud of this.
>
> I have been applied this in my business (because I am also a businessman). So, now I know how to effectively handle my business, like what to buy, price, how much profit will I make etc.
>
> In this project we have managed to learn other things like how we can come up with different school development plans, budgeting based on priorities, and also opportunities available even from within the surrounding environment.

Table 17.3 Short course descriptions

Theme	Mathematics focus	Professional development focus
Teacher as resource[a]	Number	Participatory
Assessment (formative)	Measurement	Workplace learning
Assessment (summative)	3-D geometry	Professional development models
Gender	General	Gender inclusivity
Algebraic thinking	Patterns and relations	Inclusive pedagogy
Community support for mathematics education	Statistics	Facilitating adult learning
Sustainability	Finance	Proposal writing
Mathematical proficiency and problem solving	Ethnomathematics	Planning lesson with "found" mathematics from the community

[a]2 weeks in duration

Each short course was a week in duration. The pedagogy was highly interactive and participatory drawing on the knowledge (both explicit and tacit) that the participants brought to the sessions and re-introducing them to mathematics, curriculum and teaching strategies from their experiences with school mathematics. This form of pedagogy provided ample opportunity for neighbouring interactions and relationship building. During the short course participants were also introduced to ways of working with teachers and facilitating teacher professional development. Having participants sit as district groups ensured there was a range of specialists at the table: college tutors, academic officers, master teachers, quality assurance officers and adult education officers. Complex systems require such diversity. It is through interactions among people that have different perspectives, skills and knowledge that the group can work towards a goal. At the same time, by having tablemates from the same geographical areas there was common ground among those present who were able to understand nuances that are place based in educational endeavours. In complexity terms, such redundancy in a group enables the group to function and work towards a goal. With specialists at the table and shared educational concerns among them control was distributed. There were moments over the course of a week where the school teacher was the expert and could direct the group, at other times policy became relevant and the district academic officer took the lead. Yet at other moments the college tutors or quality assurance officers took the lead. The reflection on the organization of the groups illustrates how complexity thinking and Canadian indigenous perspectives underpinned the GAC project at this finer level of detail.

Different from the cascade model, whose value has been critiqued by development specialists (Burns, 2014), the ways of working and the learning materials created in short courses were not intended for trainers to deliver to teachers. Rather they were developed for people who work with teachers. The materials and ways of working were to serve as exemplars for locally developed modules that would be created and delivered by members of the short courses. In the short courses participants did mathematics, examined curriculum, engaged in a variety of participatory instructional approaches, examined and discussed a variety of professional development models, and they raised and discussed issues about teacher learning and development pertinent to their own roles and districts. These short courses were the training ground for the cohort of teacher inservice educators who would develop and facilitate professional development in their own districts with the support of the project. Fundamentally we saw the work of the GAC project team to work with these education specialists so that post project they could find appropriate ways to support mathematics teaching and learning in their own communities.

Of the 50 some participants in the short courses approximately one half of them became professional development developers and facilitators for the project. In district teams of three people, all of whom had to have direct contact with teachers (either pre-service or in-service), three modules were developed and delivered over 2 years to more than 400 teachers in their local school communities. It was in those local activities for teachers that short course participants began to see themselves as teacher and educational resources in their own communities. They reflected on the impact of the project on themselves.

> Another thing, as a lead teacher, I have to set an example (be a role model) to invite mathematics teachers at my school come see what I do and teach them what I acquired from this project.
>
> This is very key to me and I am proud of being part of *Hisabati ni Maisha*. Also, before I had no experience in facilitation, and never worked as facilitator. But this project has given me facilitation skills, where I did teach my fellow teachers in different areas through PDs such as shapes, numbers, and algebra.
>
> Because I'm the Quality Assurance Inspector, I have been able to use knowledge and skills acquired through this project in my daily working plans. So, when I go to different schools I observe the way teachers teach mathematics and later we meet with all mathematics teachers for feedback. We discuss strengths and weakness and find ways to address these weaknesses.

The community awareness node also leveraged the work and participants from the short courses.

17.4.2 Community Awareness Node

Recognizing the important role that the village (community) plays in educational outcomes (Ngalawa et al., 2015) we understood the importance of including opportunities for parents, village councillors, religious leaders, elders and others to think about the value of mathematics education. The GAC project was designed to offer community members workshop opportunities to think about the relevance of mathematics education. We planned to deliver two community workshops within a 1 year time frame. To prepare for this aspect of the GAC project Adult Education Officers were ongoing participants in the short courses. With the support of three adult education specialists from the local country partner university, we specifically addressed issues of gender equity in mathematics education, mathematics awareness among non-educators within a community, the mathematics that may be useful to school committees, and principles of adult education. This work in the short course enabled us to have participants of the short course do the module development and facilitation of the workshops within this node of the GAC project.

Teachers, tutors and adult educators developed and delivered the community mathematics education awareness workshops. As well, it was short course participants who identified the categories of participants most suitable for the community workshops. Two workshops were offered: the first was to raise awareness of gender issues as they relate to mathematics education, and the second was to consider mathematics as it related to finance, in particular school budgets. These workshops were well received and helped some community members understand that supporting the mathematics education of their children or supporting the teacher did not mean having to do mathematics but instead it meant creating a positive attitude towards mathematics, recognizing that mathematics was appropriate for girls and boys alike, and seeing how with others they could teach their fellow villagers and children that mathematics has value in the community.

> One of the very important things I learned is that everyone can play a role in learning and teaching process. You don't have to hold a certain level of education, but just to build capacity to the community to play a role in helping children understanding mathematics.

A facilitator reflected on the community workshops.

> Another thing which I saw it really different, when we were education community including religious leaders, when I was preparing to go educate them, I had a wrong perception that they also don't see the importance of mathematics, but realized that they were all eager and see mathematics as part and parcel of their life.

17.4.3 Policy Node

The policy node was intended to establish a network of decision makers who have influence in the education sector. The plan for this node was to enhance decision makers' strategies for consulting with stakeholders when developing policies and to reflect on current policies and work on policy recommendations for inservice teacher education. The policy node involved high level officials representing: two government ministries (one responsible for education and the other for local government), two governmental agencies (responsible for programs and examinations), government gender specialists, teacher college principals, district and regional education officers, university lecturers, zonal quality assurance officers, national level organizations such as the teachers' union, the mathematical association, and an association of funders. The participants in the policy node met five times over the GAC project, with ward coordinators and head teachers joining the policy network for the final three sessions.

Believing that momentum and sustainable change require positive affect and social bonding we began the policy meetings with workshopping an approach known as appreciative inquiry (Cooperrider, Whitney, Stavros, 2008). The appreciative inquiry approach asks decision makers and leaders to value the best in people, to affirm strengths and possibilities and to make an effort to add value by encouraging the best around them. Using appreciative inquiry stimulates new ideas, stories and images that generate new possibilities for action. It assumes that systems move in the direction of the questions they most persistently and passionately discuss. In all phases of inquiry, effort is put into using works that point to, enliven and inspire the best in people.

In the GAC project appreciative inquiry created opportunities for the participants to think through the policies that impact teacher inservice education and mathematics teaching. Using the approach participants began by discussing educational policies regarding teacher education and related to their areas of responsibility. Then they "dreamed" of what good mathematics teaching in rural primary schools could look like. This was followed by an exercise that had them working with ward education coordinators and head teachers to practice the technique. The network participants were then asked about the policies that need to be in place for high quality mathematics teaching in rural primary schools. Their work through appreciative inquiry discussions of policy contributed to the development of five policy briefs.

A second contribution of the policy network to the GAC project was to support (in small but significant ways) the work of other nodes. Many of the participants in the policy node activities were responsible for the management and oversight of people in the teacher education node: the college principals have oversight over the college tutors; district education officers have oversight over district academic officers; and so on. The direct relationships between members of the network and members of the short course contributed to the success of the GAC project. For example, college principals released tutors to fully participate in the GAC project activities including 9 weeks over 4 years for the short courses and up to 4.5 additional weeks to deliver PD to teachers. District education officers provided the consent for personnel in their districts to participate in the GAC project. Ward coordinators organized the PD that was offered to teachers in the rural communities. Examples of unexpected forms of support include: a district education officer providing a small amount of funding to a small project a few of the short course participants did in their district; the president of the Mathematics Association of Tanzania became a strong advocate for the project and invited our participation in many of the association's activities. This advocacy resulted in national awareness of what became known as the *hisabati ni maisha* project (GAC project). We believe the relationships between the people (and roles) in the policy network node and the short course and community nodes helped mitigate against the disconnects between project organizers and local participants that Aikman (2010) found in other projects.

17.5 Emergent Awareness and Tinkering with the GAC Project Design

Complexity thinking has led us, as educational program and curriculum designers, to put in place particular conditions for groups of people to come together to work on shared goals. In this section, we illustrate how the planned GAC project design was tinkered with over the course of the activities as we as a collective system learned. To clarify, for us a collective learning system (in interaction with an environment) is self maintaining and transforming through its own activity. Triggered by our actions, a collective learning system emerged that took on a "life of its own". Throughout the planning, implementing and evaluating, the project was in a constant state of transformation that was not a result of preplanned actions or directives from the organizers but instead utilized the rich contributions that were available to it because of the environment with which it was coupled. Consistent with Canadian Indigenous perspectives we sought out to foster relationships and be open to counsel from the many people with whom we interacted: whether it was serendipitous interactions with people we met where we took lodging; or whether it was deliberate seeking of advice from our advisory group, and the other groups that contributed to the project.

17.5.1 Hisabati ni Maisha

The slogan *hisabati ni maisha* is an example of something that emerged out of planned advice seeking, not planned slogan seeking. In our work with the Canadian Cooperation Office we asked them to share development project success stories with us. As an aside they told us about an initiative that sought to have local communities become committed to keeping beaches clean. The project with very little funding had a great deal of success. Each person who volunteered was given a t-shirt identifying the project. We wondered what role that small token played in the people's commitment to the initiative. Later when we met with our advisory board for the first time we were discussing how we could raise awareness and commitment to the project. Talk of the beach project resurfaced and out of that discussion came the idea of a project slogan. *Hisabati ni maisha* (mathematics is living/life) was uttered and immediately there was consensus of the suitability of the slogan for the GAC project. It was much more poignant than the long title "Building capacity for mathematics teaching and learning in rural and remote communities in Tanzania." Indeed one day at the short course a facilitator seeking the attention of the people who were working in small groups called out in a big teacher voice, "*hisabati*" at which point some people in the room responded "*ni maisha*". From that moment on the chant "*hisabati*"—"*ni maisha*", "*ni maisha*"—"*hisabati*" permeated all project activities. Late in the project after community workshops had taken place, a participant from the GAC project encountered a villager with his hand-pulled utility cart which had been adorned with the slogan, *hisabati ni maisha*.

17.5.2 Tinkering with the Short Course

The members of the short course were the most active and stable of participants in the GAC project. Not only did they meet together with the GAC project team for a total of 45 days over the course of the project but (as already noted) some of them worked on the teacher PD and others of them on the community workshops. Some members became representatives of the project at various educational events in Tanzania such as the Mathematics of Tanzania Association annual conference. The stability of this group of participants might be in part due to the extensive commitments the GAC project team made to them and in turn the commitments they made to the project. Fostering this reciprocity and distributed control required we continuously tinkered with the project. We invited their ongoing participation by giving participants things to do between sessions, involving them in decision making, and giving them responsibility for aspects of the project. Nominating teacher PD providers, selecting topics to work on with teachers, doing small projects between meetings, becoming the teacher PD and community workshop providers are but some of the ways in which reciprocity was fostered and control was distributed.

17.5.2.1 Nominating Professional Development Teams: Distributed Control

We planned for participants (members of the district groups) to use their short course experiences to identify professional development needs of teachers in their districts, and then develop and facilitate professional development training modules for teachers. However, we had not planned for the composition the PD facilitator group would take, nor what form the final PD activities with teachers would take. It was clear to us as that all nine participants from each district could not do the PD sessions (both for pedagogical and financial reasons).

A local practice helped us formulate a strategy to select teacher PD developers and providers. The nomination and election of a head student is common in Tanzanian classrooms. Two of the project leaders from the Canadian universities experienced this in the advanced studies, when working with master of education students. We felt this strategy of nominating members of the group to lead the teacher PD could be useful, however we had some concerns ensuring our project goals for gender equity and developing local capacity for sustainable inservice education would be met by the composition of the teams. Most of the women in the short courses were master teachers. In the district groups, they might be viewed as holding the lowest ranking roles and were at risk of not being nominated. Further, we felt it was particularly important that people whose roles included working directly with and educating teachers, as well as having close geographic proximity to schools was important to the sustainability of the work. The Tanzanian project coordinator recommended we use a nomination process with some constraints. District groups were told that the PD teams would include only three members of the district: two members would deliver the PD and the third member would be an alternate. Then the district groups were asked to nominate four people for this work, one of whom must be a woman and all whom must interact with teachers as part of their regular duties. This meant adult educators and district academic officers could not be nominated (Again, these were roles many of the women in the group held). From the four nominations made by the district groups the project leadership team was able to select the teacher PD teams. We did have some concern that we may have trouble keeping the non-PD participants interested in the short course, and over the duration of the project there was some grumbling from a couple of people that they did not get selected for the PD. Neither of these turned into problems for the project. Indeed participation in the short course was very high and stable. Teacher PD facilitation triads consisted of some combination of university instructors or college tutors, master teachers and school quality assurance officers. Those people developed and delivered teacher PD modules in the local school communities of the GAC project.

17.5.2.2 Module Development: Fostering Reciprocity

The planned design of the GAC project involved teacher educator training (short courses) which was to create capacity for developing and facilitating teacher PD. The GAC project required PD facilitator teams to develop and facilitate modules specific to the perceived needs of their local school teachers. In this aspect of the project the planned approach required only a little tinkering but it required support. The project team knew the modules would have to be conceptualized and developed in Swahili, however, two of the Canadians did not speak Swahili. Over the life of the short course we took advantage of both English and Swahili to help all of us work through mathematics concepts, pedagogical practices, cultural differences (even between indigenous groups within Tanzania), and ways of interacting with each other. Knowing the full load of supporting the development of modules could not be placed on the shoulders of the two project team members that spoke Swahili, we made a decision to have the three doctoral students from Tanzania (who were studying in Canada as part of the project) become the mentors/facilitators to the teacher PD development teams. Each doctoral student was assigned three districts to mentor through the development of the modules. This emergent idea and the subsequent decision benefited both the teams and the doctoral students. Further it placed responsibility for this work in the hands and hearts of the Tanzanians whose teachers it would impact. The network design of the project became more highly linked internally connecting the Ph.D. students to the short course participants. Offering opportunities for short course participants to engage their learning in their communities extended our project directly out into the community. This could be conceptualized as adding new nodes of activity to the planned GAC project.

17.5.2.3 Work Place Assignments and Micro-projects: Recursivity

Reaching out into the districts and school communities with the GAC project participants was further extended as we sought ways to keep all participants engaged in the project outside of short course periods. After the very first short course we realized two things: (1) people needed to try out ideas they were being introduced to in the short courses in their schools, colleges and workplaces; (2) there was so much time that would pass between short courses that interest in the GAC project may not be sustained. Our first decision was to take the 2-week short courses that were to be offered once per year, split them into two 1-week sessions and scheduled them every 6 months thus reducing the length between short course sessions. The second decision was to ask teachers and college tutors to do an activity in their classrooms and bring the results of that back to their district groups to share at the subsequent short course meeting. This turned out to be very valuable. Not only did it keep people interested in the project, but the use of materials created by the children or student teachers in schools and colleges from their own communities was very educative. The third benefit was how the position of the primary school master teachers began to be reframed—the teachers were indeed "masters" in this domain.

After the second short course a new idea emerged: the GAC project would provide funding (just a token, as the local country director was found of saying) to cover expenses for district teams to work together on something between the sessions. To get that funding the district teams wrote small proposals describing what they would work on, why and how much money they needed to do the work. Although, it is common for people to get an allowance for doing things outside of their normal duties the project was not prepared to pay allowances. It would only covered receipted expenses for things like supplies, bus tickets and refreshments. There was a bit of pushback by participants but this did not stop them from writing the proposals and carrying out small activities related to mathematics teaching in their local schools.

In the last phase of the project, district teams were given an opportunity to propose something much more ambitious, a small research project, a teacher PD, or a community workshop. For this micro-project the participants had to write a much more formal proposal including rational, literature review, activity description and evaluation. They were provided support from the GAC project team to write those proposals. All of the projects reported back during the short course and at least one of the projects used this micro-grant as leverage for another funded project.

Each of these emergent activities recursively invoked and built upon the work done in the short courses in some way, and each of them contributed contextualized experiences from which we could all move the project forward.

17.5.3 Tinkering with the GAC Network

Unlike the short course, participation in the policy node meetings was not stable over the GAC project. In the second meeting we planned for the network we found participants coming and going. We observed multiple times when participants would be distracted from the meeting by telephone calls. In one particular case, a number of government representatives all left at the same time; the minister was to make an announcement and they all had to immediately return to their posts. We reflected on this phenomenon and made changes to our invitation list.

17.5.3.1 Modifying the Invitation Lists: Fostering Relationships

In the second meeting we noticed that a number of the people who attended the first meeting did not return. Among the new group of participants we noticed some participants were "representing" the person we had invited, and other new participants included people who were newly transferred into their positions. Working with these new people meant we had to start over with introductions, explanations of the GAC project, the role of the policy node in the project, re-explain appreciative inquiry and re-establish a participatory way of working in the meeting. It took almost a full day simply to prepare for new activities. This second meeting happened to involve ward coordinators and head teachers who attended the policy meeting as focus group participants. It was after the meeting was over that we realized the ward coordinators and head teachers may be very suitable participants for the policy node activities since: (1) they are responsible for implementing policy in the schools; (2) they seemed to be more stable in their positions (less likely to be transferred to a new community); and (3) they do not have the same emergent and urgent demands on their time that the high level decision makers and officials have. In addition to the original invitees, we invited the ward coordinators and head teachers to all subsequent meetings of the policy node. An unexpected benefit of their participation was the direct link they were to the schools from which teachers were being selected for the teacher PD. The relationships between them and the people providing and taking the PD sessions enhanced the GAC project logistics and sustainability. Such building of relationships among participants in the GAC project built robustness into it that served the project well.

17.5.3.2 Policy Recommendations: Facilitating Communication

With the change of members who participated in the policy node, the expected products of that node also morphed. The GAC project intended to have participants in the policy node write policy recommendations. However, by the fourth (of five) policy node meetings we were concerned that policy recommendations were not shaping up as we expected they would. However, we had been challenging the policy node participants to think about how they could make a difference for mathematics education. Many ideas came forth and were strongly supported but there was a recognition that the ideas had to move beyond the walls of the room. They had to be brought forth into various conversations across the sector about education and teacher education. A representative of the ministry stood up and suggested that the project prepare policy briefs reflecting the work of the policy node meetings. So rather than prepare simple policy recommendations, five policy briefs were prepared addressing: teacher resource centres, empowering primary schools, teacher led professional learning, encouraging girls to study mathematics, and engaging parents. These policy briefs reflect the GAC project team's deliberate attempt to communicate the work the participants of this project did to consider how mathematics teaching and learning in rural and remote communities can be supported.

17.5.4 Tinkering with the Community Node: Reimaging and Leveraging Resources

When we first began work in Tanzania a common refrain we heard was "we need more resources". The refrain continues today but we hope that to some extent the project has helped participants think more deeply about the resources they do have and how those resources can be leveraged. The University of Dodoma, the project's local country partner, was a resource to the GAC project. It provided office and meeting space and staff from the College of Education was released to attend project programs and events. The local country project manager and accountant were both seconded from the University of Dodoma and the local country co-director was a faculty member in the college. When we approached the point in our project to do the work for the community node we realized how much work was being placed on the small local country team. Discussions among the GAC team led us to invite adult education lecturers to join us in the project work. Specifically, they would take on preparing and leading the short course participants to work with community members to enhance their awareness of the value of mathematics education for children. Seriously considering the University of Dodoma as a resource for the project beyond the initial contributions had a positive impact on the project and built more capacity at the University of Dodoma for working alongside communities to enhance the education of children.

An other example of tinkering with the community node is demonstrated by how some funds that became available when we re-designed the community workshops were redeployed. Initially, funds had been set aside for child care. However, the redesigned from full day workshops to 2 h sessions meant the amount of funding set aside was not needed. Because this money was to go to math activities when children were being cared for while their parents where in sessions we wanted to ensure the funds were directed to math activities for children. In the end these funds were used to participate in and support a national initiative by the Mathematical Association of Tanzania "pi day. "Pi day" celebrated world wide raises awareness about the importance of mathematics among children. Posters about mathematics illustrated by children (whose teachers were in the short courses) and mathematical songs and game sheets were distributed to almost 100 schools across the project, along with 35,000 buttons for the children to wear declaring *hisabati ni maisha*.

By leveraging resources in Tanzania, the University of Dodoma and the Mathematics Association of Tanzania were part of the tinkering with the project to raise awareness in the community about the importance of mathematics for girls and boys.

17.6 In Conclusion

The GAC project, which became known locally as *hisabati ni maisha,* was designed to build capacity for supporting mathematics teaching in rural and remote communities in Tanzania. The activities were conducted in 27 wards in 9 districts. It was designed as a set of networked activities involving three primary nodes: teacher education; policy discussions and community awareness training. Over the course of the project these primary nodes became more highly connected within the network through the interaction of secondary nodes. Remarkably, emergent tertiary nodes of activity extended the network outward. The local country director, who is very familiar with educational development, confirms the project took on a life of its own. "*Hisabati ni maisha* as not just a project. It is a movement," he claimed. We know by anecdotal reports that a number of the GAC project participants (especially those from the teacher education node) are working on subsequent projects because of their work on this project. We believe this is evidence of the capacity the GAC project built.

We attribute the success of the project to the Tanzanian educators who committed themselves to it. We also believe that the design itself, which was highly networked and open to ongoing tinkering, accounts for some of the success. This model and orientation to development projects could be taken up by educators doing development work not only in Sub-Saharan Africa but in their local contexts as well. Sustained, content focused active learning that is collaborative and embedded in context, that models effective practice and provides coaching and expert support does have the potential to transform the lives of mathematics teachers, learners and those that support mathematics teachers and learners. We close with the reflections of one of our master teachers. Our dream is that professional learning grows in these communities that have had some capacity building through the GAC project.

> I have learned a lot of things from this project which are very important when someone is teaching mathematics: earlier numeracy... how to encourage female students to like mathematics... how to use simple techniques to help students acquire knowledge of the subject matter and be able to like/love the subject... to involve community so they can also be part of the learning process... the use of research... [T]his started from the school itself to see which techniques did not work well and apply other better techniques.... [and] within our wards to make sure that everyone gets involved. [I also learned to] to set plans in different levels from school, village, ward, and district just to make sure that the teaching of mathematics become part of their plans.

References

Aikman, S. (2010). Marching to different rhythms: International NGO collaboration with the state in Tanzania. *Development in Practice, 20*(1), 498–510.

Bellamy, C. (2013). *Education access or quality? We don't have to choose*. Retrieved from the Global Partnership for Education blog: https://www.globalpartnership.org/blog/education-access-or-quality-we-don%E2%80%99t-have-choose

Burns, M. (2014). *A tale of two teachers: how the cascade approach fails teachers like Ismail*. Retrieved July 27, 2018 from https://www.globalpartnership.org/blog/tale-two-teachers

Cooperrider, D., Whitney, D., & Stavros, J. (2008). *Appreciative inquiry handbook: For leaders of change* (2nd ed.). Brunswick, OH: Crown Custom Publishing.

Darling-Hammond, L., Hyler, M., & Gardner, M. (2017). *Effective teacher professional development*. Palo Alto, CA: Learning Policy Institute.

Davis, B., & Simmt, E. (2003). Understanding learning systems: Mathematics education and complexity science. *Journal for Research in Mathematics Education, 34*(2), 137–167.

Davis, B., & Simmt, E. (2006). Mathematics-for-teaching: An ongoing investigation of the mathematics that teachers (need to) know. *Educational Studies in Mathematics, 61*(3), 293–319.

Davis, B., & Simmt, E. (2016). 17 Perspectives on complex systems in mathematics learning. In L. English & D. Kirshner (Eds.), *Handbook of international research in mathematics education*. New York, NY: Routledge.

Dembélé, M., & Lefoka, P. (2007). Pedagogical renewal for quality primary education: Overview of trends in Sub-Saharan Africa. *International Review of Education, 53*(5–6), 531–553. https://doi.org/10.1007/s11159-007-9066-8

Donald, D., Glanfield, F., & Sterenberg, G. (2011). Culturally relational education in and with an indigenous community. *Education: Exploring our Connective Educational Landscape, 17*(3). http://www.ineducation.ca/article/culturally-relational-education-and-indigenous-community

Donald, D., Glanfield, F., & Sterenberg, G. (2012). Living ethically within conflicts of colonial authority and relationality. *Journal of the Canadian Association of Curriculum Studies, 10*(1), 53–76.

Donald, D., Glanfield, F., & Sterenberg, G. (2013). *Enacting miyo-wichitowin through culturally relational research practices*. Paper presented at the annual meeting of American Educational Research Association, April 2013.

Glanfield, F., Mgombelo, J., & Simmt, E. (2015). *Conceptualizing and actualizing international partnerships for training and support for mathematics teaching*. Washington, DC: Comparative and International Education Society.

Glanfield, F., Mgombelo, J., & Simmt, E. (2016). *Primary mathematics teacher development in rural communities: Lessons learned from a multi-organizational, interdisciplinary, international research partnership*. Vancouver, Canada: Comparative and International Education Society.

Glanfield, F., Mgombelo, J., Simmt, E., Binde, A. (2016). *Primary mathematics teacher development in rural communities: Lessons learned from an international research partnership*. 13th International Congress of Mathematical Education, Hamburg Germany.

Halai, A. (2001). On becoming a "Professional Development Teacher": A case from Pakistan. *Mathematics Education Review, 13*, 31–43.

Halai, A., & Rarieya, J. (2004). *Impact: Making a difference*. Karachi, Pakistan: Aga Khan University, Institute for Educational Development. Retrieved from https://ecommons.aku.edu/books/5

Hardman, F., Ackers, J., Abrishamian, N., & O'Sullivan, M. (2011). Developing a systemic approach to teacher education in sub-Saharan Africa: Emerging lessons from Kenya, Tanzania and Uganda. *Compare: A Journal of Comparative and International Education, 41*(5), 669–683.

Kendall, N. (2007). *International Review of Education, 53*, 701. https://doi.org/10.1007/s11159-007-9058-8

Machimana, E., Sefotho, M., & Ebersohn, L. (2018). What makes or breaks higher education community engagement in the South African rural school context: A multi-partner perspective. *Education, Citizenship and Social Justice, 13*(2), 177–196.

Ngalawa, A., Glanfield, F., & Simmt, E. (2015). Exploring the emergence of community support for school and encouragement of innovation for improving rural school performance: Lessons learned at Kitamburo in Tanzania. *Global Education Review, 2*(4), 101–125.

Poirier, L. (2007). Teaching mathematics and the Inuit community. *Canadian Journal of Science, Mathematics and Technology Education, 7*(1), 53–67.

Simmt, E., Binde, A., Mgombelo, J., & Glanfield, F. (2018). *Building complexity into development projects: A case study*. Paper presented at the Fields Research Symposium, Toronto, Canada, January 2018.

Simmt, E., Glanfield, F., Ngalawa, A., Mgombelo, J., Makombe, I., Msabila, D., …, Kajoro, P. (2014). *Partnership development to research possibilities for primary mathematics teacher development in rural and remote communities*. Paper presented at the International Research Symposium, Edmonton, Canada, July 2014.

Varela, F. (1999). *Ethical know-how: Action, wisdom, and cognition*. Stanford, CA: Stanford University Press.

Wayne, A., Yoon, K., Zhu, P., Cronen, S., & Garet, M. (2008). Experimenting with teacher professional development: Motives and methods. *Educational Researcher, 37*(8), 469–479.

18 Improving *Quality of Life* Through Teaching and Learning Innovations in Multilingual Contexts: Lessons from Sub-Saharan Africa

Margaret Funke Omidire

Abstract
Education contributes to the quality of life in many countries including those in sub-Saharan Africa. Individuals are not considered educated unless they are able to communicate their thoughts and ideas meaningfully to others. Language is the means by which this is done and once language becomes a barrier to learning, there's a snowball effect that negatively impacts the quality of life. Problems and challenges are further exacerbated when there is unequal access to education either directly or indirectly and where inequitable practices prevail. This chapter discusses language-in-education in multilingual contexts and innovations that have been implemented in different sub-Saharan countries to enhance teaching and learning in these contexts and ultimately to improve the quality of life. The chapter utilises and elucidates multiple purposefully selected studies and projects, conducted in Uganda, South Africa, Nigeria and Ethiopia to illustrate the benefits of multilingualism and mother tongue/home language instruction in terms of educational outcomes and quality-of-life at the individual and systemic levels.

M. F. Omidire (✉)
University of Pretoria, Pretoria, South Africa
e-mail: funke.omidire@up.ac.za

18.1 Introduction

In this chapter we discuss how to improve quality of life through innovative teaching and learning strategies in multilingual contexts. An initial discussion of education pathways to quality of life and the connection of language-in-education to the process is followed by an analysis of the various stages in achieving the desired quality of life in sub-Saharan Africa. The nature of the multilingual contexts and the advantages and challenges of such contexts will be discussed before an analysis of a cross-section of the innovative strategies used in various communities.

18.2 Education as a Pathway to Improved Quality of Life

Quality of life can be viewed from two main dimensions: objective quality of life (societal and cultural expectations in terms of wealth, status and well-being) and subjective quality of life (personal satisfaction). Both of these dimensions are currently intricately connected to education and the ability to excel in school, obtain a qualification and be gainfully employed, and thus be classified as 'an educated individual'. The first dimension dealing with societal and cultural expectations in terms of wealth and status is usually deemed attainable with a good education and qualifications. It is also assumed that once the

I. Eloff (ed.), *Handbook of Quality of Life in African Societies*, International Handbooks of Quality-of-Life, https://doi.org/10.1007/978-3-030-15367-0_18

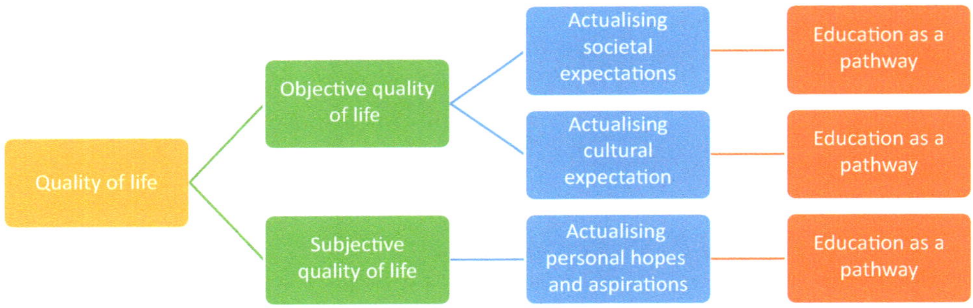

Fig. 18.1 Linking quality of life to education

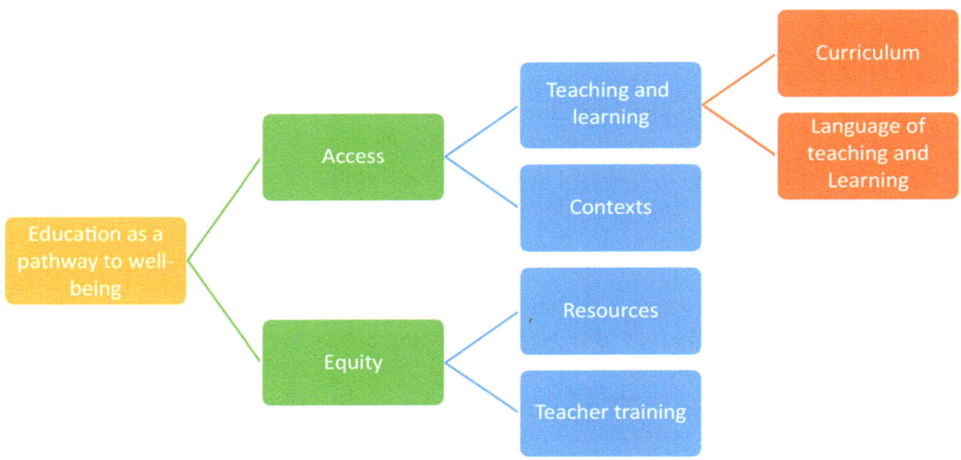

Fig. 18.2 Education pathways to quality of life

objective quality of life has been achieved, the subjective quality of life follows, controlling for unexpected life stressors.

Deriving an education and the percentages of educated people within a given society is often associated with the rate of development of such societies and one could assume that this has a direct relationship to individuals being functional members of their societies who can either seek gainful employment or become entrepreneurs themselves and provide employment opportunities for others. However, success in education and schooling largely depends on the ability to learn effectively. Learning effectively cannot, however, be expected in contexts where language constitutes a barrier to learning. The reality for many societies in sub-Saharan Africa is that this is the case. The societies are largely multilingual, have students that are usually taught (and have to learn/demonstrate knowledge) in a second language (L2) or an additional language (AL). Research has shown that students often lack academic proficiency (sometimes even basic proficiency at a social level) in the language of instruction (Omidire, Bouwer, & Jordaan, 2011). Research has also shown that the students' languages and culture are often devalued and an attitude of immersion in a dominant culture promoting subtractive multilingualism is the prevalent strategy adopted (Heugh, 2015). Under such circumstances, the quality of life at the personal level is negatively affected.

Figures 18.1 and 18.2 above attempt visually represent the close relationship between education and quality of life.

Figures 18.1 and 18.2 above show the link between quality of life and education. Within Fig. 18.2 access to education and equity constitutes key constructs in the attainment of quality of life through education. Access to quality education is critical and directly related to having conducive environments and contexts where teaching and learning can be effectively conducted. Of critical importance is also equity in provision of the necessary tools for ensuring education as a pathway to wellbeing; guaranteeing resources are allocated according to need, to provide a level playing field for the teachers and learners. Each of the factors related to equity and access such as teaching and learning contexts, availability of resources and the adequacy of teacher training could be linked to language in education.

Where English, French or Portuguese are used as the medium of instruction, teacher proficiency in the language of learning is important, otherwise the teacher becomes a poor model of the language and may transfer incorrect usage of language to the students. This is frequently compounded by a lack of adequate training to teach in multilingual settings. Availability of resources to facilitate teaching and learning or lack thereof constitute challenges. Education pathways to improving the quality of life has to consider the language in education dilemma created by the contexts.

18.3 Promoting the Use of Multiple Languages

The United Nations is one world organisation that recognises the importance of language in society and language in education. Language is intricately linked to culture and identity. The loss of a language has far reaching consequences in terms of the loss of the culture, norms and value of the group. Students are quite often asked not to use their home languages in school and this leads to confusion especially at a younger age. Often leading to the belief that, for some reason, the home languages are not good enough for the school environment. The practice of devaluing the languages of students has been shown to have devastating effects on children whose culture and identities are portrayed, sometimes inadvertently, as inferior; thus, affecting the learners' self-esteem and well-being. Most sub-Saharan countries have plurilingual communities so whether or not recognised by government policies, multiple languages are a reality of daily existence.

Students having their languages denied on entry into schools have to grapple with the reasons for this type of subtractive multilingualism that requires them to assume a new identity and culture, leaving prior knowledge and current experiences from the repertoire that could be drawn on to make meaning of their learning. Even while research has shown the benefits of mother tongue instruction, parents and teachers are sometimes opposed to the idea. Mother tongue instruction refers to the use of a learner's first/home language for teaching and learning across the curriculum. United Nations Educational, Scientific and Cultural Organisation (UNESCO) advocates mother tongue/home language instruction and also value multilingual education from the early years for the following reasons

> It lays a solid foundation for learning – It improves access to education, especially for girls – When used at home and/or at school, it promotes literacy in the mother tongue (L1) and later in the second language (L2).
>
> It facilitates learning both of academic subjects as well as the second language (L2). At school, children can concentrate on the subject matter instead of struggling to understand the language of instruction as well.
>
> It improves learning outcomes as it promotes dialogue and interaction between learners and teachers by means of better communication and understanding.
>
> It raises the quality of education by emphasising understanding and creativity rather than repetitive memorization. (UNESCO, 2014:2)

Communities across the African continent have found strategies for communicating with each other regardless of the multilingual nature of such communities. They also respect the various cultures represented and are able to co-exist despite differences in language, culture and identity. This acceptance of language realities and mutual respect is, however, not transferred into the education system where one language is often times imposed on learners as the language of instruction notwithstanding the low levels of proficiency in the language by both the teachers and the learners. The situation is often complicated by political, economic and historical considerations.

The world is multilingual and many communities are multilingual. We need to come to terms with providing education that reflects the linguistic diversity of the society. Very few countries are linguistically homogeneous and with the rate of current migration and urbanisation it continues to change. We can therefore safely assume that multilingualism is the norm and not the exception. Providing education that caters to the linguistic diversity of the learners should be top priority.

Learning in the mother tongue/home language and multilingual education are by no means devoid of challenges. Quite to the contrary, there are a number of challenges associated with mother tongue instruction and those who oppose this form of instruction tend to focus solely on these challenges, despite empirical evidence that show the benefits of investing in mother-tongue instruction. There are merits in the arguments that point at the challenges of mother-tongue instruction, but focusing exclusively on problems is not the solution.

Some the challenges include:

- There may be variations of the same language.
- Home use of a language may be different from the standardised version.
- The orthography might not be well developed or there might be no written form of the language yet.
- There might not be appropriate terminology for educational purposes.
- There could be as many as four or five mother tongues represented in a single classroom or school.
- Teachers might not be competent users of some or even all of the languages.
- Teachers might not be trained to teach in the languages they are able to speak.
- Teaching and learning materials might not be available in the target languages, making them difficult or impossible to adopt for teaching and learning.
- Historical, political and economic reasons may cause resistance to the use of local languages for teaching and learning in schools.
- Learners not being literate in their home languages.

18.4 Considering the Benefits of Multilingualism and Multilingual Education

Quality of life is often affected by an individual's perception of self-esteem and as discussed earlier, self-esteem can be eroded by the devaluation of people's culture, language and identity. Research has shown that learning in a language which is not one's own provides a double set of challenges. The first challenge being learning a new language and the second is learning new knowledge *contained* within that language. If we factor in the possibility of learners having specific learning disabilities then challenges are more pronounced. Cultural and linguistic diversity is a reality and there's a need to integrate support systems for linguistically diverse learners within the education sector. Opportunities should be created for learners to learn in their own languages, integrating their cultures and experiences. There's a need for a shift in terms of the attitude of parents, teachers and even some learners' views of indigenous languages. Those who oppose multilingualism and multilingual education focus solely on some of the challenges highlighted above. In this chapter, however, an argument is presented that the benefits (as discussed below) of mother tongue instruction and investment in multilingualism outweigh the challenges.

According to UNESCO (2014), "*Language is not only a tool for communication and knowledge but also a fundamental attribute of cultural identity and empowerment, both for the individual and the group. Respect for the languages of persons belonging to different linguistic communities therefore is essential to peaceful cohabitation.*" Oftentimes parents are not even aware of the consequences of their language decisions and only focus on the projected economic and social value of subtractive multilingualism.

18.4.1 Benefits of Multilingualism

Okal (2014: 227) highlights several benefits of practicing multilingualism in the education sector. These have been summarised here as follows:

- Knowledge of more than two languages allows us to communicate with many people in both personal and professional contexts.
- Traditions and culture are passed down orally in some communities and indigenous language are believed to provide an access to a vast reservoir of wisdom, expertise, knowledge and skills contained in the bodies of speakers of the languages concerned. The more languages are transmitted the more cultural resources are available.
- When one knows the official language and perfectly speaks the indigenous languages then the person will be able to synthesis knowledge and express it accordingly. It is therefore necessary to include indigenous languages in education so as to realise the benefits of synthesizing and clearly expressing knowledge in its full diversity.
- Thus, multilingualism opens doors for quicker and easy communication. To remove the notion of 'fixity of reference', entrenching multilingualism in education will enable one to avoid restrictions in communication thus enabling movement to another stage of communication.
- Multilingualism practices enhance intellectual flexibility and creativity. Recent studies have indicated that children who grow up in a supportive environment speaking more than one language from an early age are more perceptive and intellectually flexible than those who speak one language (Mwololo, 2008).
- Children with parents constantly speaking different languages grow up being equally fluent and comfortable with the two home languages and can even learn a third and fourth language.
- Students who are exposed to many languages will tend to be intellectually flexible.
- Enhancement of intellectual flexibility is corroborated by various viable findings. Thus, many children who are fluent in more than one language are superior lateral thinkers, have strong social adaptability, their thinking and reasoning skills as well as their cognitive abilities are better (Okal, 2014).
- Multilingualism provides an insight into the understanding of different cultures and experiences.
- Multilingualism enhances an automatic understanding and appreciation of cultural values of the societies that are contained in the concerned languages. The experiences gained from learning different languages automatically tend to change the attitudes, skills, beliefs of the people, society and create an expansion of world views. All these attributes are formally taught in the classroom and informally in the daily communication outside the classroom.
- Multilingualism provides a competitive edge in today's job market. Besides the academic and professional credentials, employers also look for fluency in the desired languages as an added advantage. Therefore, being a multilingual is a plus to any job seeker in this millennium.
- Multilingualism is also a form of human capital.
- Multilingualism helps in national unity especially if people learn national languages besides their indigenous languages and lingua franca. In the process, the people concerned will automatically embrace the value of togetherness.
- The consequences of multilingualism are numerous – ranging from the linguistic to the socio-political domains. Linguistic consequences of multilingualism include, among others, the creation and growth of *lin-*

gua franca that normally develops because of the need for cross group communication.

- Multilingualism practice creates the development of mixed languages mainly due to intense language contact. As a result, speakers therefore tend to involve a mixture of languages during verbal communication. This contact may also result into the creation of slangs.
- Multilingualism practice generally develops cross linguistic communication strategies like code switching and code mixing. When people switch from one language used at homes to the other outside the home environment then code switching occurs.
- Multilingualism creates an aspect of diglossia whereby when there are two official languages, there is always one language that tends to dominate the other. This is generally referred to as the subordinate language. This happens when viewed from a functional point.
- Multilingualism practice tends to create the development and general acquisition of cross-cultural communication skills. In this regard people tend to learn different skills of the languages in place, especially speaking, reading and even writing. These cross-cultural communication skills enable one to gain both the communicative and discourse competencies (Okal, 2014:227).

18.5 Teaching and Learning Innovations in Multilingual Contexts

Multilingual education refers to the use of two or more languages as mediums of instruction. *However, UNESCO adopted the term 'multilingual education' in 1999 in the General Conference Resolution 12 to refer to the use of at least three languages, the mother tongue, a regional or national language and an international language in education. The resolution supported the view that the requirements of global and national participation, and the specific needs of particular, culturally and linguistically distinct communities can only be addressed by multilingual education. In regions where the language of the learner is not the official or national language of the country, bilingual and multilingual education can make mother tongue instruction possible while providing at the same time the acquisition of languages used in larger areas of the country and the world. This additive approach to bilingualism is different from the so-called subtractive bilingualism which aims to move children on to a second language as a language of instruction* (UNESCO, 2003).

In the field of language and education, the reports and recommendations of the International Conference on Education (ICE) have emphasized the importance of:

- mother tongue instruction at the beginning of formal education for pedagogical, social and cultural considerations;
- multilingual education with a view to the preservation of cultural identities and the promotion of mobility and dialogue;
- foreign language learning as part of an intercultural education aiming at the promotion of understanding between communities and between nations (UNESCO, 2003: 34).

UNESCO further states that questions of identity, nationhood and power are closely linked to the use of specific languages in the classroom. Language itself, moreover, possesses its own dynamics and is constantly undergoing processes of both continuity and change, impacting upon the communication modes of different societies as it evolves. Educational policy makers have difficult decisions to make with regard to languages, schooling and the curriculum in which the technical and the political often overlap (UNESCO, 2003: 34).

There are however lessons to be learned from those areas where progress has been made. The innovations discussed below are a few examples of strategies that could be used in multilingual environments.

Figure 18.3 below, details five main innovative practices aimed at facilitating teaching and learning, improving student achievement, involving whole communities and ultimately improving

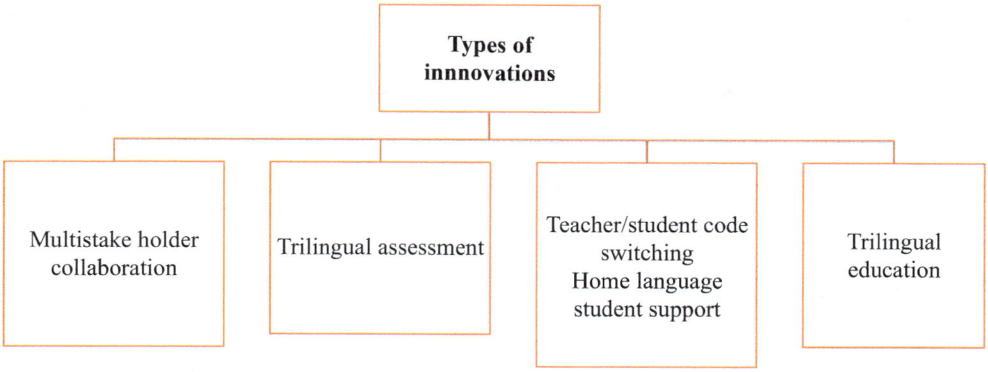

Fig. 18.3 Teaching and learning innovations in multilingual contexts

the quality of life. The first is multi stakeholder collaboration, teachers' communities of practice, trilingual assessment, teacher/student code switching/translanguaging, home language use as a student support strategy and a current project – primary learners' multilingual intervention.

Different communities across sub-Saharan Africa have found ways to embrace the multilingual nature of their communities. There has been a shift from viewing local indigenous languages as undesirable within the learning environments. In recent years, across sub-Saharan Africa we have seen a rejuvenation of African culture, arts, music, and entertainment in African languages. Individuals and communities expressing their identity in these artistic forms, thereby promoting music and drama in indigenous languages. Similar strategies could potentially be embraced in the education system to promote psychological well-being.

The above-mentioned teaching and learning innovations will be discussed individually.

18.5.1 Multi-stakeholder Collaborations

Stakeholders:

- Learners
- Teachers
- Parents
- Community members
- Specialists (educational psychologist, remedial teachers, speech therapists)

In communities where there is cooperation and partnerships between teachers/parents, community members and individuals in specialist fields, it is more likely that progress can be made in terms of achieving education objectives. There will be trust in situations where parents feel that their opinions and inputs are valued. Teachers communicate with parents, specialists are involved where necessary, parental suggestions are valued and incorporated, and there is strong parental presence.

Community and government or non-governmental organisations (NGOs) conduct joint initiatives for adult education and the provision of out-of-school educational opportunities. An example of this type of initiative is the Literacy programme in Uganda.

Community involvement in Education – Literacy programme Uganda (Heugh, 2013; Heugh & Mulumba, 2014).

The multi-stakeholder collaboration, NGO-led rural project in Uganda involved parents, community leaders, teachers, teacher educators and Language Boards. The programme was aimed at building the stakeholder capacity. It involved using local language as medium of instruction. It also involved setting up a centre that afforded adult learners and school children spaces to work after hours. The MTE project has involved parents and in some instances grandparents and communities in school learning, through joint parent-child classes each week and through adult literacy classes. Other initiatives include, parents sharing learning with children; villages establishing Home Learning Centres (HLC), homework support, early child care, pre-school/kindergarten, adult education -adult literacy and numeracy, village saving schemes and micro-economic enterprises. These also led to the finalisation of an implementation handbook, and a national use teacher development handbook.

Some of the achievements of the project include

- Improvement in enrolment,
- Improved learner achievement in literacy and numeracy
- Increased community and parental awareness of the value of local languages in education
- Community collaboration
- Interdependence and support
- Increased capacity of language boards which has played a significant role in capacity development, orthographic development of languages
- Production and use of sample reading materials
- Production of children's magazines which contain learners' stories written in local languages, drawings and other artefacts, and these have been well-received by school children.
- Teacher education
- Dissemination of experiences to policy makers and maintaining a participatory and collaborative approach with district and national levels of government and in the Multilingual Education Network.

Studies like this illustrate that teaching children in the language that they know best, is undoubtedly the best policy and approach for effective learning, but it also indicates that it has to be well-resourced. In particular, parental involvement in the joint sessions and Home Learning Centres in the villages seem to have had a positive impact on student achievement in this project.

Of course, projects such as these experience challenges such as the provision of essential resources. Inadequate supplies of reading and learning materials in the schools, and high incidence of children without pencils and paper to use for reading, writing and numeracy tasks, are risk factors to the implementation of any intervention (Heugh, 2013).

In terms of multi-stakeholder collaborations, it seems that the vision and leadership should come from schools and NGOs where there is capacity to mobilise other community members.

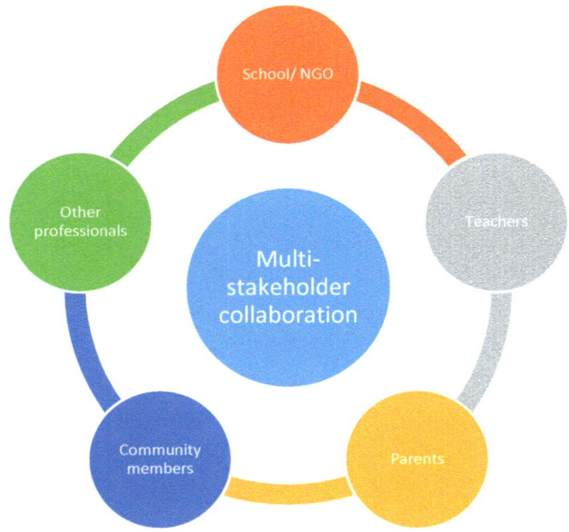

The positive effect on quality of life is visible. Everyone is working together to promote their local languages, adult literacy, providing sustainable employment, promoting partnerships, building relationships, improving teacher awareness and giving access to further professional development. Another outcome of this type of innovation, is individual enablement and collective empowerment, mother tongue instruction and learning is used, community literacy levels are improved, parents and community leaders have a say, and the stakeholders are able to contribute to the development of stories and books. Their opinions and suggestions are valued and incorporated, thereby leading to enhanced self-esteem and a sense of collective self-worth.

18.5.2 Trilingual Assessment Project: Cape Town

The experimental trilingual assessment project in Western Cape South Africa aimed at using multiple languages for assessment and was initiated out of the quest for linguistic equity in circumstances where the dominance of English was often regarded as inequitable practice. The languages used were Afrikaans, English and Xhosa. The fact that multiple languages are presented constitute the future possibility of equity regarding language in education. Learners whose home languages feature alongside English in an examination are likely to feel a sense of belonging regardless of the outcome of the assessment. It symbolises an acknowledgement of existence and importance.

While this project was experimental in nature it also demonstrates that though political will and commitment to removing language as a barrier to learning, embracing the reality of linguistic diversity and creating equitable education that utilises assets to achieve goals and objectives, can be achieved in contexts with significant challenges.

Heugh (2015) highlights the implications of a trilingual assessment study for future system-wide teaching and assessment:

- It is possible to accommodate linguistic diversity in system-wide assessment
- Test development needs careful consideration in terms of types of items appropriate for this type of assessment. Multiple choice items, for instance, were found to have limited value in contexts of weak literacy for assessment across the curriculum
- Literacy/language assessment needs to be conducted in both language learning area *and* across the curriculum to offer more penetrating diagnostic information
- Teacher development potential/value in the marking/coding process
- Diagnostic feedback is possible at student, parent, class teacher, school, district and provincial office levels.

18.5.3 Nigeria Teacher Support Using Code Switching, After School Support in HL, Peer Tutoring in HL

Research conducted in Nigeria, (Omidire, 2009), involving non-participatory classroom observations of grade 8 students in two schools demonstrated how learners embraced the use of their home languages as a learning support strategy to make progress in their school work. Students revealed that they had tutorial and support sessions at home during which their home languages were used to explain the content of the school subjects. Indeed, code switching was used systematically by some of the top achieving students in their private lessons at home.

In the same way, teachers opted to use code switching and code mixing to break down and explain difficult concepts. This was more visible during Integrated Science lessons. Code switching refers to a switch of language that occurs between sentences to carry the full statement and is otherwise known as inter-sentential switching. It is the use of more than one language in a single phrase, sentence or speech act. Code mixing is a switch in language that occurs within one sentence to utilise appropriate words or phrases and it is also known as intra-sentential switching (Brock-Utne & Holmarsdottir, 2004; Nieman, 2006; Omidire, 2009). The use of code switching and code mixing oftentimes supports learning because the learners get a clearer picture of the subject matter and are also able to express their own understanding and questions more readily. Code switching and code mixing can be used for cognitive purposes, to reformulate questions and instructions, it can be used to facilitate group work by learners and it can also be used to give general information to learners. Code switching and code mixing are also used for affective purposes in the classroom, as their use can create a warm atmosphere devoid of tensions. In addition to this, there are instances where code switching has been used for classroom management, to ensure discipline and also as an inclusive strategy to reduce alienation of learners.

Code switching functions on two levels, the receptive and the expressive levels. At the receptive level it aids comprehension and means that the teacher can act as mediator of understanding and at the expressive level it helps one to convey one's knowledge and understanding (Brock-Utne & Holmarsdottir, 2004; Nieman, 2006). In the study, the implication of code switching where practised, was that the learners were able to achieve some measure of comprehension of the lesson content. However, achieving some understanding did not ensure any communicative competence at the expressive level. English was still the medium of expression of whatever had been learned. Code switching to convey understanding was not permitted – instead, learners frequently were stringently penalised for the slightest of errors. During the mediation, the students were accommodated through code switching that they could actually convey their knowledge and understanding.

The teacher's use of code switching during the observed Science lessons was an indication that she understood that the learners in her class lacked proficiency in the language even at BICS level – and wanted to maximise the learning experience by ensuring that comprehension of the lessons was achieved. The use of Yoruba and particularly code switching on the part the Science teacher appeared to initiate and promote interaction. The teacher used code switching/ mixing as an inclusive strategy to get the learners engaged in set activities. Each time she followed up her statements with a Yoruba translation the learners responded well and contributed to the discussion. This strategy was effective in the sense that the learners, at least, responded in the classroom. It seemed to encourage learner participation and interaction but that per se did not seem to translate into greater achievement for the learners. They all still perceived Integrated Science to be a difficult subject.

18.5.4 Trilingual Education in Ethiopia

In Ethiopia multilingual education systems embraces the use of three languages – the mother tongue/home language, the national language and the international language. This was a change of policy from promoting *English mainly* education to continued development and retention of primary/home language alongside English (Jha, 2013). While not everyone agrees that the implementation of multilingual education and the prominence given to indigenous languages is the best approach in the twenty-first century, the initiative has resulted in the development of orthographies of local languages and the development of writing materials, which results in more job creation at different levels of society.

Arguments against this approach, cite low achievement in English as a deterrent. However, low achievement in English can be addressed in other ways such as teacher training and specialized language teaching tools.

18.6 Reflections on Language, Literacy, Multilingualism and Quality-of-Life

Language is a key factor in learning on three levels: knowledge construction, reconstruction and reproduction (and/or application). At each of these levels, language plays a pivotal role. In the classroom, for appropriate learning to take place, the learner has to be able to construct knowledge, and apply meaning to those concepts and units of learning he comes across. Post classroom encounter, the learner must then reconstruct what he has come across, identifying main points, memorising and internalising them using various strategies to ensure adequate learning in preparation for assessment (Omidire, 2009). Research has shown that there is a relationship between academic proficiency in the language of teaching and learning (English), and achievement; and also, that lack of proficiency impacts assessment and progression (Howie et al., 2012).

The Department of Education 2007 Annual School Survey indicated that 65% of South African learners used English as the language of teaching and learning (DoE, 2007) and that figure has been on the increase. Of the South African learners in grade 4 tested in PIRLS 2006 only 13% could achieve the lowest benchmarks for reading as opposed to 94% of the grade 4 international peers (Howie et al., 2008).

Howie et al. (2012) in the prePIRLS 2011 found that 29% of grade 4 students in South Africa were completely illiterate in the language of teaching and learning, there is little or no opportunity for language development and enrichment. Classroom environments encourage chorusing and collective answering and shallow responses (Hoadley, 2010). Based on the statistics above, the language of teaching and learning can be viewed as a barrier or a risk factor to successful academic achievement of most learners who participated in PIRLS 2006 assessment. However, statistics indicate success of some learners in spite of existing language barriers. It is for this reason that understanding of factors that contribute to the success and failure of learners are understood to motivate for resilience processes within the teaching and learning domains as antecedence for enhanced quality of life.

Spaull (2015) confirms other earlier research of a strong relationship between fluency and comprehension. But he also found that 60% of grade 5 learners in rural schools were reading at grade 1 level and assumptions of very low literacy and comprehension levels can safely be made. This outcome links to multilingualism in the classroom where there are as many as three or four languages represented in a given classroom apart from the language of instruction that is different from the learners' home languages/mother tongue. This situation creates a challenge for teachers who have to ensure that irrespective of language of instruction, high level learning with comprehension and student engagement takes place as opposed to mere rote learning.

As stated earlier, multilingual classrooms are no longer features of education in Africa alone, but have become commonplace in developed countries as well. The multiplicity of languages is often compounded by the fact that the language of teaching, learning and assessment differs from the learners' home languages. The negative implications of learning in a language in which one lacks adequate academic proficiency has been well documented (Barry, 2002; Cummins, 2000; Omidire et al., 2011). Teaching and learning pedagogies can no longer ignore the complexities and dynamics of multilingual classrooms because that would continue the reinforcement of past worldviews and prolong the attainment of the future we aspire to; access to education for all as a pathway to improved quality of life.

From the examples in this chapter, it seems that a fundamental way of facilitating learning is to support teachers who are in multilingual classroom situations to rise above the complexity of the circumstances and to adopt strategies that enable learners to maximise the opportunities to learn. Research has shown that barriers to learning are exacerbated by low levels of literacy, as well as challenges to teaching in a second language (L2) (Spaull, 2015). Learners often struggle to cope with the linguistic demands of academic study when the language of learning and teaching (LoLT) is an additional language (AL) (Guglielmi, 2008; Hugo, 2006; Levin & Shohamy, 2008).

It is critical to acknowledge that all learning areas are intrinsically related to language proficiency and a high level of language proficiency is therefore seen as an essential aspect of the learning process in schools (Brock-Utne & Holmarsdottir, 2004; Cummins & Swain, 1986; Heugh, 2009; Levin & Shohamy, 2008). As a result, access, retention and performance, especially in rural and remote schools, are hindered by L2-barriers where neither teachers, nor learners are first language speakers of English. Oftentimes, the multiplicity of languages represented in the classroom is deemed a hindrance to teaching and learning. Where the above hindrances of language in education exist, what kind of quality of life can be expected? Inadequate education is one of the factors constitutes a barrier to social advancement. Intrinsic, extrinsic and systemic barriers to learning create challenges in the education sector that affect the quality of life of those concerned. The two dimensions of quality of life: objective quality of life which includes societal and cultural expectations in terms of wealth, status and well-being; and subjective quality of life, personal satisfaction, are impacted by these barriers. There is no meaningful way to effectively tackle improving quality of life through education pathways without confronting and addressing the issues surrounding multilingualism and language in education. A bottom-up approach is required to peel through the layers to ensure that individuals have access to equitable education and a hope of being gainfully employed and functional members of their communities. Cramm, Møller, and Nieboer (2012) in a study conducted in the Eastern Cape province of South Africa found that unemployment had a significant correlation with subjective well-being. Even in situations where, the subjective quality of life is at an adequate level, it is still relative because in such instances, individuals concerned might have various coping strategies and networks that create a state of complacency and a sense of satisfaction in the face of adversity. Regardless of this state, the objective quality of life still falls below expectation.

18.7 Implications of the Various Innovations for Quality of Life

Moller (2013), found that inadequate provision of education was associated with subjective well-being where respondents (black South African youth) rated their lives worse than average on all indicators of subjective wellbeing used. Access to education was identified as one of the criteria which could make individuals happier. This fact was seen as a consequence of the old Bantu education system which "prepared black pupils only for menial occupational stations in life" (Moller, 2013: 921). Proper education creates opportunities for individual enablement, skills to find gainful employment and achievement of better quality of life. Addressing the challenges of language in education in multilingual contexts is one of the first steps in the right direction. The phenomenon of multiplicity of languages in a classroom is now a permanent feature so there is a need for a closer examination of avenues by which the languages can be used to facilitate learning. There's a need to rather move towards viewing indigenous languages as assets and *resources* within classrooms.

Most people agree with the position of UNESCO (2003) that learning another language opens up access to other value systems and ways of interpreting the world, encouraging intercultural understanding and helping to reduce xenophobia. The fact that various initiatives are springing up and that there are pockets of excellence emerging means that there is hope for multilingual education on the continent of Africa. Education that incorporates the home languages of the learners incorporates their culture, identity and values the prior experiences they bring to the classroom. We can include the majority of learners who come to school being only aware of their mother tongues and who are excluded from the learning based on the language of instruction. There are also learners who are labelled or misclassified because of language being a barrier and yet others who are not diagnosed with learning disabilities and simply categorised as lacking proficiency in the language of learning. The studies and projects shared in this chapter indicate that reflexive linguistic approaches can provide supportive learning environments for a diversity of children in African classrooms and ultimately contribute to their quality-of-life over a lifespan.

18.8 Conclusion and Way Forward

Multilingualism and multilingual education are the way forward in a diverse global context. It captures entire knowledge systems and creates pathways to increasing quality-of-life. To facilitate the process there's a need for focused directed strategies to be embraced. According to Okal (2014) multilingualism in education calls for the involvement of language education communication skills which is an essential tool for the development of the learner's speaking and writing abilities. Application of communicative language teaching focusing on linguistic, sociolinguistic, discourse, socio-cultural, social and strategic competences and drama can help in the achievement of multilingualism in education. Encouraging the use of indigenous languages in education besides the national and official languages enhances multilingualism. Developing multilingual dictionaries and publishing grammar and story books in local languages provide resources and reference materials to support learning. This also contributes to the development of the vocabulary in multiple languages. Furthermore, writing and staging drama and poetry in indigenous languages can ensure that there is no stigma associated with the use of the indigenous languages and it can facilitate its acceptance in the education settings.

Official documents in indigenous languages provides important platforms for language development. South Africa which is an official multilingual country with its constitution translated into 11 recognized indigenous languages, serves as an example in this regard.

Finally, specialised language teachers are important and training should be provided for language teachers. These teachers would be the model for languages and would be experts in teaching the languages and promoting the use of multiple languages across the curriculum. Additive multilingualism and outright multilingual education has to be given priority not just at the policy making level, but it has to be seen as a way of life in schools and communities.

Education can be a successful pathway to improving the quality of life in sub-Saharan Africa but only if there is a paradigm shift in attitudes to the multilingual nature of the communities. Communities are multilingual, that is the reality. This reality should be embraced and extended to the education system. Individuals cannot thrive if their language, culture and identity is devalued in any form. Effective learning cannot take place where language is a barrier to teaching and learning. Multilingualism is an asset and a step in the right direction to improving the quality of life of all.

References

Barry, D. (2002). Language equity and assessment in south African education. *Journal for Language Teaching, 36*(1), 105–111.

Brock-Utne, B., & Holmarsdottir, H. B. (2004). Language policies and practices in Tanzania and South Africa: Problems and challenges. *International Journal of Educational Development, 24*, 67–83.

Cramm, J. M., Møller, V., & Nieboer, A. P. (2012). Individual- and neighbourhood-level indicators of subjective well-being in a small and poor eastern cape township: The effect of health, social capital, marital status, and income. *Social Indicators Research, 105*(3), 581–593.

Cummins, J. (2000). *Language, power and pedagogy: Bilingual children in the crossfire*. London: Multilingual Matters Ltd.

Cummins, J., & Swain, M. (1986). *Bilingualism in education: Aspects of theory, research and policy*. London: Longman.

Department of Education-SA. (DoE). (2007). *Annual school survey 2007*. Pretoria: Government Printers.

Guglielmi, R. S. (2008). Native language proficiency, english literacy, academic achievement, and occupational attainment in limited-english-proficient students: A latent growth modeling perspective. *Journal of Educational Psychology, 100*(2), 322–342.

Heugh, K. (2009). Contesting the monolingual practices of a bilingual to multilingual policy. *English Teaching, 8*(2), 96.

Heugh, K. (2013). An evaluation of the Literacy and Basic Education (LABE) Mother-Tongue Education (MTE) Project, UGANDA Final report.

Heugh, K. (2015). Multilingual education, knowledge systems & community participation: What we know from southern experience & research. *Transatlantic Forum on Inclusive Early Years* 8–10 July 2015 Washington, DC.

Heugh, K., & Mulumba, B. M. (2014). *Implementing local languages medium education in the early primary curriculum of Ugandan schools: A literacy and adult basic education (LABE) intervention in six districts in North and North West Uganda*. Kampala, Uganda: LABE. http://labeuganda.org/reports/LABE%20MTE%20Evaluation%202013%20Final%20SEPS%20jan.pdf

Hoadley, U. (2010). *What do we know about teaching and learning in primary schools in South Africa? A review of the classroom-based research literature. Report for the grade 3 improvement project of the University of Stellenbosch*. Cape Town: Western Cape Education Department.

Howie, S., Venter, E., & Van Staden, S. (2008). The effect of multilingual policies on performance and progression in Reading literacy in south African primary schools. *Educational Research and Evaluation, 14*(6), 551–560.

Howie, S., Van Staden, S., Tshele, M., Dowse, C., & Zimmerman, L. (2012). *South African children's reading literacy achievement: PIRLS 2011 summary report*. Pretoria, South Africa.

Hugo, A. C. (2006). Overcoming barriers to learning through mediation. In M. M. Nieman & R. B. Monyai (Eds.), *The educator as mediator of learning*. Pretoria, South Africa: Van Schaik Publishers.

Jha, S. K. (2013). Multilingual education: An emerging threat to quality english education in Eastern Ethiopia. *Theory and Practice in Language Studies, 3*(10), 1737.

Levin, T., & Shohamy, E. (2008). Achievement of immigrant students in mathematics and academic Hebrew in Israeli schools: A large-scale evaluation study. *Studies in Educational Evaluation, 34*(1), 1–14.

Mwololo. M. (2008). Are you fluent in your mother language? In *Daily nation, living, February 20th, nation media group, Nairobi, 3.*

Moller, V. (2013). South African quality of life trends over three decades, 1980–2010. *Social Indicators Research, 113*(3), 915–940.

Nieman, M. M. (2006). Using the language of learning and teaching (LoLT) appropriately during mediation of learning. In M. M. Nieman & R. B. Monyai (Eds.), *The educator as mediator of learning*. Pretoria, South Africa: Van Schaik Publishers.

Okal, B. O. (2014). Benefits of multilingualism in education. *Universal Journal of Educational Research, 2*, 223–229. https://doi.org/10.13189/ujer.2014.020304

Omidire, M. F. (2009). *Investigation of dynamic assessment (DA) as a means of addressing the assessment dilemma of additional language learners*. Unpublished Ph.D. thesis. Pretoria, South Africa: University of Pretoria.

Omidire, M. F., Bouwer, A. C., & Jordaan, J. C. (2011). Addressing the assessment dilemma of additional language learners through dynamic assessment. *Perspectives in Education, 29*(2), 48–60.

Spaull, N. (2015). Examining oral reading fluency among rural grade 5 English Second Language (ESL) learners in South Africa: An analysis of NEEDU 2013. *South African Journal of Childhood Education, 5*(2), 44–77.

UNESCO. (2003). *Education in a multilingual world*. Paris, France: UNESCO.

UNESCO. (2014). *Multilingual education: Why is important? How do we implement it?* Paris: UNESCO.

Van Avermaet, P. (2015). *Functional multilingual learning*. Presentation at TIFEY, 8 July, Washington, DC.

The *Quality of Life* of Teachers in Sudan

19

Amani Ibrahim Abdelgafar

Abstract
This chapter reports on the quality-of-life of teachers in Sudan. The study investigates the factors that contribute to quality in the life of teachers, as indicated by factors such as travel distance to and from their place-of-work, teacher accommodation, community engagement, and parental involvement in the teaching and learning environment. Inadvertently, the study also indirectly alludes to the quality of life of the pupils and the parents involved in Sudanese schools, as reflected by access to safe water, infrastructure and the availability of basic learning materials. The chapter uses direct quotes by teachers to create a conversational narrative that illustrates the realities of life for teachers in Sudan.

19.1 Introduction

Good teachers stay in our memories for a long time. We define good teachers in a multitude of ways. Good teachers can be humorous, serious, and charismatic, but whichever it is, we usually recognize them easily.

In this chapter we focus on the teachers in Sudan in the Gabalmura mountains in west Sudan. The scenes when the large band of teachers set out, carrying their blackboard on their backs, sometimes using it as shelter, is unforgettable.

Teachers working in rural areas tend to have closer professional and personal relationships with the community than those who are working in urban areas. Likewise, rural communities tend to be more involved in school life. In some cases, the proximity between schools, teachers and communities can provide opportunities that enhance the learning experience of pupils, reduces the pressure of the teacher's workload and contributes to community development in a wide variety of ways. This proximity, combined with the relative isolation and poverty that can cause tensions between schools and communities, can potentially also stifle learning and motivation.

This chapter explores the teacher's relationship with the pupils' parent and with the wider communities in which they live. It looks at the teacher's understandings of their pupil's families, and how they adapt and extend their activities outside the classroom and school in line with these understandings. It highlights the value and the value of positive relationships between the school and the community, the factors that contribute to such relationships and to what extent the impact of these relationships can develop teachers' motivation, local perceptions of education and the teaching profession, and pupil learning.

A. I. Abdelgafar (✉)
Open University of Sudan, Khartoum, Sudan

I. Eloff (ed.), *Handbook of Quality of Life in African Societies*, International Handbooks of Quality-of-Life, https://doi.org/10.1007/978-3-030-15367-0_19

19.2 Participants in the Study

Twenty-five teachers participated in the study (n = 25). There were 15 female and 10 male teacher participants. All participants had completed a degree and certificate in education. It is compulsory for all teachers in Sudan to hold a degree and a teaching qualification.

The data for the study was collected by means of a focus group and interviews. The focus group and interviews were conducted by the author and two experienced teachers. Data was captured by field notes and audio recordings. The data was collected from seven states in Sudan, e.g. North Sudan, South Sudan, North West Kordofan, South Kordofan, East Sudan, Kartoum, Elgazera. The interviews were conducted in Arabic and translated into English for the purpose of reporting in this chapter.

19.3 Physical Isolation

In Sudan, you don't have a choice in where you work as teacher. A teacher has to agree to work where he or she has been sent in the republic. You have no choice where you go. The rationale behind this policy is to equip teachers with the skills and experience to work in different environments.

One of the main problems of rural schools is their physical isolation and the frequent shortage of accommodation. Where there is no housing provision for teachers, or where teachers would prefer to live in more built-up areas with their families, the journey to school can be long, expensive and arduous.

Moreover, working in different areas equips the teachers, especially the younger's ones, towards more experience and to also exercise some influence at the place of their posting. Mhadi (Sudan, White Nile State, Elgazeera Aba) began his career teaching in a farm school, but requested a move to a township school after staying 5 years there.

A Sudanese teacher, who is used to move from an extremely isolated school to the village school posting demonstrates this problem. She worked in the White Nile State, in Sudan. She said "I work in a place which was not so enjoyable, actually. It was a hardship area. I have been posted where there no houses, no accommodation, no transport, there were many difficulties. You go to school in the morning, and it is the same on the way home……. We walked for almost 7 km each way. This may reduce the ability of the teachers to achieve the learning objectives successfully".

It is rare for teachers in the rural areas of Sudan to have their own means of transport. Some of them are able to walk to and from school, but the others are reliant on public transport. Schools that are close to the road, and in an area that is served by public transport are incredibly attractive to these teachers.

The teachers working at farm schools face particularly long journeys. Mukawi walks for 20 min from his house to the main road. From there he travels in a local, shared taxi for half an hour. A car- share scheme then takes him from the side of the road for 20 min into farmland. He then walks for half an hour up an unpaved farm track to reach the school. "It was expensive to move to and from the farm and it was really exhausting me financially as I am a single parent with one kid, so it was stressful for me" (Mukawi, South Sudan).

Where housing is provided, teachers themselves can become isolated. Amal lives in a room adjoining a house. If she wants to visit the bank, the doctor or friends, she has a 90-min walk to the main road from where she has to hitch a ride into town. Of all the challenges she faces in such a rural school, Amal finds the distance from the road the "hardest thing".

The isolation of rural schools in Sudan is a major concern for the teachers in this study. While the provision of teacher housing makes life easier in some respects, teachers still have difficult decisions to make in terms of balancing their family and work commitments.

> Yes ……. Travelling is difficult, but we can't do otherwise because we don't have houses here to stay. But even if there were houses here at the

> school, we have our own kids to look after at home, so if we stayed here our own kids would be disadvantaged! So we must stay in town with families. It's hard, especially when it's raining or cold and you must be here. (Amal, South Sudan state)

The teachers are also concerned about their pupils' long and difficult journeys to school, and the effect this has on their learning. "At the farm school, children walk up to 3 km and when they get to school they are already tired, so it was a challenge for us to motivate them. When it comes to, let's say, rainy season, you see that, in the morning when it's raining, the majority of children won't come to school, just a few, then whatever you teach them, the rest of the children won't benefit and so you have to go back over it all, then it's very difficult".

In addition to tiredness and absenteeism, Amal and Mukawi highlighted a more serious issue concerning their pupils' journey to and from school.

> … there is a terrible problem with learners on the farms starting to leave school for doing other things. (Muhideen Amed, South Sudan)

Muhideen and other teachers try to protect these learners by occasionally accompanying them part of the way home, but they have to balance this with their own arduous journey in the opposite direction, and a desire to be at home to spend time with their own children before nightfall.

According to what has been mentioned above, one could say that moving from one area to another (especially for the new teacher) and to the rural areas specifically is an essential factor in helping to contribute in solving several problems that may face students in terms of learning issues. Yet, it is also clear that there are significant additional problems involved in such a movement.

19.4 A Closer Look at Rural Schools

To deal with the problems that may exists in rural schools in Sudan, a clear and serious approach is needed for these schools. The schools in this study range from a one-room structure with no water, electricity or no seats for the students to sit on to a multi-building site with flushing toilets and a computer lab. All of the teachers in the study felt that their school was lacking in amenities. A good head teacher has to have a deep understanding of what is needed at the school.

Thatalntageen in South Sudan has changed beyond recognition since Mrs. Amal became head teacher 12 years ago. She described the condition of the school when she arrived:

> Of course the school was in a bad state – there was no fence around the school. All the windowpanes were broken. The toilets were unusable, which is very unhealthy. Also, the classrooms were health hazards, broken cement floors with potholes,

Mrs. Amal and her staff have worked tirelessly to raise funds to improve the condition of the school. It now has an administration block, two new teaching blocks, modern toilets and a computer lab. There is a fence around the school grounds to keep the buildings safe from vandals and trespassers.

> … there is no windows and that other classroom is not good, so fencing for security, and looking after school because there's no glass it is too cold to teach in, very cold winter and too hot in the summer. (Sara, South Darfour State, Sudan)

Several teachers think that overcrowding is a problem in a lot of Sudanese schools and this meant that the head teachers had to implement a split-shift teaching system which causes a lot of disturbances for the teachers.

The problems with classrooms result in pupils dividing into groups because there are not enough rooms for them to study in. "Some schools would put them in the sun under a tree and teach them there, but they would get so tired. So we decided that one class takes over from morning till 11.00 a.m., the others come in at 11.00 a.m. and take the some room" (Tarig, Kadogli, Sudan).

Headteachers has to apply for the government to build new classrooms, which was recently approved for crowded schools. It is clear that funding should be made available for additional classrooms in rural schools.

Another challenge relates to the teachers' shortages in Sudan. According to some recent statistics of educational organizations in Sudan, numerous classes have over 70 pupils. So there are a lot of challenges related to rural schools in Sudan.

In Gafa village, in the White Nile State, there is no water supply. Teachers have concerns about the effect this has on the children's hygiene.

Amal thinks that such problems make her job particularly difficult and she is not alone. The lack of water in this village was the key reason the teachers did not want to be there in the village.

The remoteness of some schools means that the children's health suffers in other ways too. The teachers in the rural schools in Sudan are angry that their pupils miss out on government health campaigns for schools because they are so far away from the main road.

> We don't have good hospitals like other schools, or even nurses. Other schools have a nurse to visit once a month but they stop at the tar road. Our Schools here do not receive this service. (Mobarak dongula outskirt, Sudan)

What frustrates teachers more than infrastructural problems, however, is the lack of teaching and learning resources. Several teachers admitted to using their own money to supplement government rations of textbooks and exercise book.

> No we don't get enough textbooks, or especially stationery, so we must buy them books for next year. (Yagoop, Elgazeera Aba, Sudan)

> The children are overpopulated at my school, so each teacher has no room for rest. There are no facilities, no teaching material – at times, the teacher has to get these themselves. So it is difficult for the teacher. (Ahmed Omer, Sudan)

Supplementing students' learning resources is an additional burden faced by teachers in rural areas, but a burden that all of the teachers in this study accept, and in many cases they embrace the challenge inventively as individuals or collectively. Esther, for example, collects old, food packets from her neighbors and has set up a "shop" in her classroom to help with Math and English teaching. In the township, the teachers take advantage of the high density of schools and have developed a resource borrowing system: "If you don't have a book here, you send a child to borrow it from the neighboring school. It is not like that in the farm school, because schools are so far apart – it is difficult to send children to other school".

According to the data from this study, head teachers and government has to carefully assess the basic needs of the rural schools so as to solve the problems that result from the lack of these basic resources.

19.5 Deep –Rooted Relationships and Long-Standing Ties

The researcher tries to mention some of the examples that provides evidence of the positive learning outcomes that can be achieved when there is a good relationship between teachers and the community that predates their teaching role. Marim Ahmed, who lived in the North Kordfan state, Obied, moved to her husband's home village,; Bara's outskirt when they got married. She lived there for 20 years raising her five children before she started working at the local school.

> All students and parents in the village know where we live! My house is a reference to the people of the village in many Ways. (Marim, Sudan)

The village of Teriat Elbigia consists predominantly of members of the Khwala tribe. Most of the villagers are related to each other. When Marim walks in the village, she points out who lives where, revealing a rich and complex network of cousins, sisters, uncles, brothers-in-law, mothers-in-law and husbands. This knowledge of the kinship networks in the town where she teaches, creates a web of support for the children and the school at the same time.

Another sample in the study of a teacher who could be considered as an established member of the community simply through the longevity of their teaching role is Raja. When Raja was posted to teach at the government school outside Khartoum State in one of the outskirts of the White Nile State, she was considered to be an outsider teacher.

> I was considered to be as the newcomer of the Gafa village, ten kilometres North east of Rbak, the capital of the White Nile State. Very much so.

> People don't tend to move very much in this area and to be together for a lot of social issues' was a real link between them after ten years of work as teacher. (Raja, Sudan)

However, after 10 years of work as the teacher among the small members of the village, she now stands in front of the grandchildren of her first pupils and she feels that she is accepted as 'local member'.

Moreover, at Mona's school in Shakan, the south Kortofan state, only one of the teachers is from the village. The rest of relatively young staff, including Mona, either stay in a teacher's house and travel home at weekends in Kdogli, which is the Kapital of the state, or even more arduously, travel to the school from their home towns each day.

The teachers who have a historical or familial tie to the communities in which they teach appear to have a markedly different relationship with both their and the pupil's families as opposed to the teachers who are seen as outsiders. These connections also appear to affect how teachers feel they are perceived by the community. An example of this can be seen in how the teachers spoke about their salaries, and how they felt their income affected their reputation in the community.

Teachers are relatively poor in Sudan especially during the late decade of twentieth century. They sometimes also *look* poor, even in the eye of the children they are teaching and the families in the community. Pupils, in turn, then don't want to become teachers, because they think it makes you poor. But this was seen as a less important impact factor by the teachers who had close ties with their communities.

> A lot of people especially in the rural areas in Sudan see teachers {teachers} as responsible people!" (Abdelrahman, Sudan – Khartoum), so they respect them! Because they teach their children, they are the custodians of the children when they are in school, so they respect them. (Alam, Sudan Kosti)

> Even though we live in this house [the teachers' boarding house] and it is old and small, it is not too bad because we are close to the school and we live here because we are teachers – everyone knows we are teachers. (Focus group, Sudan)

The community in Teriat Elbigia make regular contributions to the school to cover the electricity costs at the boarding house. In addition, informal contributions of food and clothes are regularly donated to the teachers who are there.

For Marim and her colleagues in Sudan, things are very different. They first present to the villages as teachers. They try to go to the markets for shopping themselves but later on they begin to avoid shopping at the village market because the market women overcharge them. Marim explained that the majority of the villagers make their living from crops. They reap from their own farms. The teachers have a weak salary and they are considered to be poor. Marim and her colleagues now do their grocery shopping in their home towns at weekends. The situation is such that when the head teacher of the school requested contributions from the community to assist those living at teachers' house with their bills, a community member reported him to district education office for fraud. While he was able to prove his innocence and his honest intention, the damage to his reputation, during the inquiry had him out of the school and into early retirement.

19.6 Communication Between the School and the Community

The relationship between the teachers and the community has a noticeable effect on the way information travels between the school and the community. Where the relationship is strong and positive, there is a constant flow of information through informal channels.

> The relationship is very cordial, so they can come to you at home, they can come to you at school, they are free! They are not restricted! (Sumiya, Sudan)

> Yes! [The parents] come and meet me sometimes in my home! Sometimes we will talk there and sometimes I will ask them to come back and meet at the school. (Head teacher, rufaa)

The physical proximity of the teachers to the community appears to play a key role in developing the learning outcomes:

> The community? Ah... Since I'm not staying here, ah, I used to visit them, but I'm not all that close to them. Like, I'm coming with a vehicle, when I see them I only greet them... So far as I am not staying here I do not go to them. (Head teacher)

The situation at a lot of schools in different villages and towns in Sudan suggests that the distance between the school and the community does not need to be vast. If so, it will affect the relationship between them. The head teacher at Elmostagbal school in Sudan has experimented with different ways of overcoming the communication gap between the school and the community. The school now addresses school notes and messages to their pupils' elder siblings. The pupils' parents are mostly farmers and builders who spend long hours away from the family home and a lot of them are illiterate. Sending messages to siblings and visiting them at their farms and building sites have proved to be a more successful communication channel and ensures that information is received and understood.

The teachers in this study also highlighted the importance of more formal channels of information exchange between the school and the community through bodies such as the Parent Teacher Association (PTA). This is discussed in the next section.

19.7 Parents' Involvement in Their Children's Learning

Parents' involvement in their children's learning plays a very crucial role in enhancing their learning outcomes. Teachers working in local farming communities appear to have less involvement with pupils' parents than those in towns which raise the responsibility of the teachers who are working in villages. It seems from this study that many of these parents working in a farm school community, compared to a township school, lack an interest in their children's education.

> This made me feel less supported because when we used to call parents, whenever you want to solve a problem, the parents were not able to come because they are busy working in the fields. They would be harvesting. Here, if you call parents, some don't work, they are stay-at home mothers, so if you need the assistance of a parent they will be quick to get here. (Amal, South Sudan)

For other teachers in the study, these challenges are ongoing:

> Yes, we have to involve the parents in the learning process of their children, because we would not be able to run the school without them, although at times we call them for meetings and they are very busy, and they find it hard to come. They are working on the farms and no one can give them permission to leave their work, so we have to do without them. We have to go where they work and ask for their help. Or we try to hold them in the evenings so they will have been freed from their work. But if we want something done, it is up to us to communicate with them. (Abaker Sudan, port Sudan outskirt)

Some teachers feel that it is not just a lack of interest, but a lack of understanding or confidence. Illiteracy is widespread in many of these teachers' communities and some teachers believe that parents are not comfortable discussing their children's education with teachers because they feel insecure about their own educational backgrounds. Other teachers interpreted this as a lack of interest in or appreciation of education more generally:

> Most of the community members in rural areas are farmers. It is difficult for them to respond to your call in the school to discuss a certain matter that related to educational matters. If they come, they will come, and they do respect the teachers, but the weakest part is that they don't force their learners to come to school daily. If the child is saying, 'No, I don't want to go to school,' the parents they are rarely forcing them or showing them the need of education. They don't say, 'It is a part and parcel of you.' They don't say, 'GO to school.' That is their weakest part... Most of them are illiterate. That is the main problem... So they don't know what their children are missing. They usually say, 'Go to school.' But they don't show them the need of education, nothing more than telling them, they don't elaborate on why. (Mohammed, South Sudan – Dmazeen)

The teachers in this study, in collaboration with local education authorities, are working hard to combat these attitudes. One key method appears to be raising awareness of education issues through Parents Teachers Association PTA meetings, which are held at all the schools in this study:

> The basic job of headmaster is for the community to know the importance of education. He or she has to spread to them. That is why you call PTA meetings. So that if they are not aware of the future of their children, you tell them. And you can compare other areas to them… say… look at this person, they are from a poor house, now look at the position. Wouldn't you like your child to be of that nature? (Head teacher, Gazeera State, Sudan)

> I would say [the greatest challenge is educating the semiliterate parents with the importance of talking their children to secondary school… it is a challenge for us to convince the parents to get their chances at making something of their lives, it will be enhanced by furthering their learning. (Asha, Kordufan)

Many of the parents referred to by this study's participants did not attend school, but they do know that their children should be put in school. It seems that rural parents are increasingly interested in their children's education and are keen to see what their children are doing in school.

> Also, some are nervous about PTA meetings so we encourage them to come to us any time, there is no specific time… we want them to know that any parent can walk up to a teacher and say, 'Look, I want to know what my child is doing.' They are free to do that.

The establishment of the PTA is therefore very important in villages as well as towns in Sudan, because it helps teachers to have a good and fruitful relationship with the school communities that help in enhancing the learning outcomes of their children. As attested in many developing African countries, the importance of education can be communicated to parents through such associations.

19.8 Parents' Involvement with School Life

Parents' involvement with school life supports the learning outcomes of students. Regardless of their overall perceptions of community interest and involvement, every teacher in this study had a story to tell about how the school had received generous gifts and contributions from parents in times of particular need. For example:

> In some villages in Sudan, the time the toilets sunk, the school was about to be closed. We called the committee and decided to ask the parents for help. These were donated and helped fix the problem and this is how parents can contribute to the problem solving in rural schools. (Adam Isag, Gazeera State, Sudan)

> Some others schools have other schemes … one of them is that the children; have porridge in the morning and soup at lunch. Children are encouraged to have funds, the teachers touch people; for example, one lady, once a week or month she busy the school 25 litres of peanut butter and 25 kilograms of soup that we give to the children with bread. Instead of the jam and marge snack, which is not nutritious, we give them soup. We also take money from the school fund, with the approval of the government body of course. But we do have people who support the school, most are businessmen. (Mss. Ameira – Kassla, West of Sudan)

> Really parents have great contribution to local schools. They are trying to help us in achieving our job. They are raising money for our things like, chalk, we don't have… enough chalk, we don't have brooms for sweeping, sometimes they come and furnish our classes, help us with the chairs… and so on and so on. We use the money for… all that. (S, Heauaad head teacher, Sudan)

While the teachers expressed gratitude for these generous donations, they are aware of the tensions that come with asking communities for money, and make difficult decisions about how additional funds are used:

> The parents will always see that the help that they do could be considered as responsibility of the government. So the government should do that. So what we are interested in, from the parents, is getting them their books and writing materials. If we ask for more, they will think we are asking too much. We have to prioritise. (Ahmed Basheer, head teacher, Shandi, Sudan)

> This time is very difficult because everything being done by the parents. Chalk was provided by the parents, watch-man, books, they had to buy the books for their children, pens, what have you… So it was a bit difficult getting the money from the parents. Taking into account the school environment and that of the parents themselves, they were just squatting in a farm here, just doing casual jobs, so it was even difficult to put food on the table for their children. (Mrwa, Sudan)

According to the international standard, the school has to pay for the all learning needs such as, printing of exam papers. We have two terms in the year, the government says it is not going to pay for them. They should be paid by the students' families. So this time around we call the parents and then we talk to them and tell them this is what the government is going to do. So... if the parents allow the teachers to write everything on the board during the end of the term, it's not... it will not be enough. Because, let's say, if there is one board... writing all the questions. Some [pupils] are slow writers and by the time they are finished writing the questions, there is no time to write the answers... so they tell the parents they should pay some amount of money for the printing... so teachers will use it to buy official papers for the children. (Rasha, Sudan)

Recent government initiatives, such as the abolition of school fees and increased spending on school resources, have dramatically eased the burden on these teachers, ensuring that they do not have to act as debt-collectors in their communities. This has had a positive effect on the relationship between them and the communities in which they teach.

"Then, until 1990, everything was available in the schools and the money was provided [by the government]. Since then, everything has been running smoothly, because we never have to come into contact with the parents for finance unless it is an emergency" (sbuliman, Elgazeera Aba, Sudan), so this created a respectful relation between the teachers, students. The children are no longer paying school fees. The government said they should not pay school fees because their education is free.

When students do not pay for the school to learn, this makes it easier for the teachers because they don't have to make decisions about who can come to school and who cannot... even if they have not paid, everyone can come to school! We also found out last week that we have a cheque account that they will pay into monthly, so we can help the school and rely less on parents and our own pockets! Some students had to be outside the class room because they don't pay. (Radi, South Sudan)

Not all schools are as fortunate. Parents of pupils at in South Sudan must pay for their children's education, a contribution that, for some families, is crippling. Mrs. Maha has explored a variety of ways to reduce this burden:

... the kitchen volunteers are from the community. They are parents. They could not afford to pay school fees and they came to me and offered to clean classes once a week, but I said, 'No, I can't allow that; the children should learn to clean the classes themselves.' But you help us to prepare meals and clean out the admin block. (Mrs Sami, Sudan Kassala)

The most remote schools in this study were the farm schools. The teachers from these schools described high levels of involvement and support from their local communities:

Yes, of course, the parents, they do support. The children are small to clean, so their parents, they come every week to clean the windows and sweep the floors because the children are too young. They volunteer to do that.

Yeah, the community is playing a big role, they are helping us in everything. Like if we are going to have a concert they come along and ask, 'What can we do to help you?' Even if there is a workshop and all the teachers are going, a parent will come along and say, 'Don't close the school, I am going to be here and be with and supervise the kids.' Also, if we are going to do activities outside town, like excursions, ... they volunteer to help, and if the kids have to walk to the road to catch a taxi, the parents will volunteer to escort them to the place, and when they are coming back, they will be there to fetch them to their homes. Even if we are away, they will phone us and ask, "How are you doing, are you OK? So they are very much involved. (Soma, South Sudan)

According to what has been mentioned by participants in this study parents has to be involved in the life of the schools, because the role of the government has been reduced and schools are in a great need of the help of the community and also the students' contribution. The study suggests that, in remote and rural environments, where teachers are poorly supported, some of the most valuable contributions from communities may involve the gift of time, and not necessarily money.

19.9 Teachers' Extended Role

A teachers' role in the teaching process should be more focused on the job that they do *in the school*. None of the teachers in this study, however, believe that a teacher's work ends when the school bell rings at the end of day. Most believe that being a teacher in a rural area goes hand in hand with a responsibility for and involvement in the community.

Sumiya, who is referenced in a national teaching policy, documented that community involvement is part of the teacher's role. It is clear, that she considered helping local families to buy school uniforms and books to be both a professional and a moral duty:

> … I see my role as caring for these children, and that means I care for them like my own children. There is no difference. And this means helping their families too… Being a teacher extends to the families of the students too; it is not just an academic job. And because they are my relation too, I do not hesitate.

Many of these teachers work in communities where parents spend long hours working on, and travelling to and from, their farms. The teachers felt an important part of their role was the pastoral care and discipline of pupils when their parents were not around. Many teachers referred to themselves as the second parents of their pupils:

> If they are outside the school and I see them doing something wrong, or going to a place I know could harm them, I will prevent that. I think, by doing so, I am teaching and guiding them outside school. (Sumiya, west Sudan)

> We found ourselves playing a big role like a parents, even more than that sometimes. That child has been sent to the school in the morning. They are sent to us very early and this is every day. We notice more problems than the parents. If a child is lacking books, or a pencil, we sometimes give them ourselves, so it is easier than contacting the parents to solve such problems. (Eman, Kosto, -Sudan)

Sometimes the teachers feel this additional responsibility can be a worrying burden to shoulder alone. They need to know the importance of this additional job to achieve their work properly:

> One time I had permission to be out of school. In town, I saw the children in the river; they were swimming. I keep on hearing about children drowning and I was worried, so I called the parents and most of the parents did not come, so I feel it is my challenge, that parents [leave] the burden to you alone, and if you can't solve it, it is just hanging. I was not able to solve it alone, but we should – parents and teachers – be solving these problems together. (Amna, S, South Sudan)

In terms of the quality-of-life of a teacher in Sudan, the above-mentioned indicate the importance of the work of the teacher outside the classroom. This work has been emphasized by numerous experts in the field of education, but for a teacher in Sudan, it seems particularly acute.

The teachers also take responsibility for the children's welfare on a more official basis. The following quotation explains the crucial role of the teachers outside the classroom:

> We have a big role to play because, as I said, they are raised by grannies and the grannies might not be aware. They only know the child's behavior is different to what it used to be. The granny does not know where to go. So we have to refer them sometimes, for evaluation, and some cases are sent to the social workers. And, if you notice, we are cooking here, because there is a lot of poverty, so there are a lot of challenges besides teaching in the classroom. (Amna, South Sudan)

Mrs. Yagoop strongly believes that nurturing the link between school and home has a positive role in enhancing the students learning outcomes. It also has great benefits for children's learning in rural areas. As he said "… my responsibility should not be confined within the school yard, I should go beyond the school yard into the community where those children come from. I cannot expect to have effective learning from a child who comes from an unhappy home situation."

"The gulf between the school and the parents was large then! In 1 day we crossed it! I didn't have to persuade them! Vision crafting did everything for me! I don't know how it happened… but when they saw we were trying to reach out to them, relations between us and them became quite good.

She further explains that [I used to be a] "… no-nonsense principle. But after, I became more accommodating, still strict, but more willing to listen to my staff members and also… of course I have always respected parents but… before that, none of the principals knew they had a role to play in the community, but after our involvement with nongovernmental organization I began to see things differently, I became fully involved in the life of the parents, as far as helping them with some of their problems, especially with government officers, you know?"

19.10 The Impact of Rural Environments on Teaching and Learning

The teachers in this study were not simply concerned about their own challenges of living in a rural area, they were also deeply concerned about the effect a rural environment has on the children they teach. The teachers described how, for a variety of reasons, the children rarely left their home area. Many had never travelled to the nearest town, let alone beyond it. They feel that this isolation from the outside world has severe implications for the children's behaviour, learning, their ambition and future prospects. Many believed that working against these constraints to inspire and motivate their pupils was central to their role as a rural teacher.

Mukawi, for example, is particularly concerned that the children in the township have limited social skills, especially when faced with unfamiliar environments:

> Yes, it was my choice to be involved in these things. I like interacting and I like to bring a different culture to them because we find out that they don't know how to handle themselves… and that worries me a lot. How can I put this, we are not isolated anymore, we play sport with schools from the other side of town. They will say things they are not supposed to say; if the learner knows an English word they are not allowed to say, if it's a very rude word, they will say it and how are the other visitors going to feel when they say that? So I am saying they must change, but they must understand these other cultures. (Mukawi, South Sudan)

Sumay (Sudan) thinks that the combination of a small school in a relatively isolated area fails to inspire a sense of competition among her pupils and gives them a chance to enhance their learning: "…there's no competition here. We don't see the essence of competition. It's like … nobody is more intelligent than them so they don't care…." (Noha, Obiet outskirt, Sudan).

Noha tried to raise the motivation of her class with a point system, but this has not been a great success. Being top of the class has few tangible benefits for children who expect to leave school at the end of the year to work on their parents' fields.

> …if, let's say, you are doing well, and then all of a sudden they down, they don't care about that.

She feels this is due in part to the low expectations of the children's parents, but also due to a lack of role models in a village where almost everyone works on a farm. She continued:

> Yes, because when you compare their lives to those in the town, they really need help. The children themselves, they don't see… they don't worry about the future…some will be sitting there laughing – they don't know. Some will want to be a taxi driver, but they will not know how to go about it. Just a few will mention a nurse, maybe two will be a teacher! One guy says he wants to be president! One wants to be an engineer! But most will sit there looking at you. Some just want to sell salt. I think that is just what they see around. That is all they see as opportunities for jobs… Even when they tell you they want to do this, you don't see it in their performance, because it is not a real option for them and they know that.

The head teacher at Noha's school is well aware of this issue, and believes it is rooted in several generations of isolation and subsistence:

> [Even when people from the village finish their education] "…they don't come here to work, they go to, Khartoum, and so children here don't have role models, they don't see. And parents also, they don't realise the importance of enabling their sons and daughters to go to school. (Sahih Adam), Head Teacher, Kadogli

Mr. Mensah feels strongly about this. He sees PTA meetings as an opportunity to inspire parents to have ambitions for their children beyond the village. He invites wealthy education officials and religious leaders to the meetings and uses them as examples. He also sees himself as a living, breathing example of what education can do for rural people.

In addition to the effect of low expectations, some of the teachers feel that their pupils' prospects of further education and a career are also limited by their language skills:

> Also, teaching in English is a challenge because they never go into town and never come into contact with people, so the only English they speak is in school. (Sabah, South Sudan)

The teachers in this study were not simply concerned about their own challenges of living in a rural area, they were also deeply concerned about the effect a rural environment has on the children they teach. Their quality-of-life were therefore affected at the personal level, but it was also affected by their concern for those in their care.

19.11 Extra –Curricular Activities

Education outcomes and objectives cannot be achieving depending only on the school curriculum. It needs additional activities of skilful teachers. The teachers in this study participate in or lead a wide range of extra-curricular activities. They are passionate about the benefits of these activities for the pupils involved, but also for their families, and for their families' futures.

The teachers in the farm schools saw these activities as a distraction from deprivation of their pupils' home lives and a way to combat the isolation and insularity of the farm environment. They also saw the after-school clubs as a way of protecting the girls from the advances of male farm workers.

> We do activities to make the students feel free and happy. We've got traditional dances, they can do ballroom dances, they can sing, they can do all such things … they can do poetry … they are so … these farm school kids are so popular because we go to a place with them to do these activities like traditional dances… and sport. They are also involved in sport. I like sport very much. We are playing volleyball, football, both boys and girls, netball, chess, and also doing indigenous things. (Sahih Adam, Head Teacher, Kadogli)

Participating in cultural events and sports competitions gives the children otherwise unlikely opportunities to travel outside the farm and meet other children. Gada spoke nostalgically about her early years as a teacher, and the importance of these events for both teachers and children:

> I do agree with what has been said by Gada from South Sudan that emphasizes the role of additional activities rather than depending on the curriculum of the school. Teachers have to be creative to bring their own activities that help them to solve a lot of problems that may face them. (Sabh, South Sudan)

> I loved it then, there were so many schools then, there is a farm there, and there, and there, and also there, there were so many farms and schools. After school we enjoyed ourselves! We did concerts. We had many children then – I had 55 when I came here, and it was fun. [But now] the numbers have gone down because… many people are moving from the farms to the towns. (Gada, Sudan)

Now, nearing retirement and being the only teacher for miles, Gada struggles to find the energy, resources and support for any extra-curricular activities:

> I like to bring a different culture to them because we find out that they don't know how to handle themselves. How can I put this, we are not isolated anymore, we play sport with schools from the other side of town. So you find out that they don't know how themselves, and that worries me a lot. They will say things they are not supposed to say; if the learner knows an English word they are not allowed to say, if it's a very rude word, they will say it and how are the other visitors going to feel when they say that? So I'm not saying they must change, but they must understand these other cultures." (Sabh, South Sudan).

Solutions to this concern are manifold. She draws on the support of a wide range of organisations to help her with these projects:

> I use for example, on Monday and Wednesday, I have a reading club. Kids here have a problem with classrooms, we don't do that in our homes- reading is not encouraged. So in the classroom we have 55 minutes, and if you are going to do a comprehension, those that are slow at reading, you cannot reach them, so I created this opportunity for those, so we have a whole hour, or an hour and a half, where the children have one-on-one tuition; we have volunteers that come in. We have games and activities so they can learn.

> …I'm also responsible for other activities. There is a dance programme at school and the kids from

> townships started socializing and I intervened to see if the girls from here can be taken, and even the boys, so they can socialize. So that was arranged and they were taken by bus, it was one of their social outreach projects. So they speak English. It improved their language and understanding. (Sabh, South Sudan)

To ensure the sustainability of these clubs, teachers have sought donations to pay for a small snack for each child that attends:

> Yes, they do go when you introduce it. You say, 'Do you think you need it?' and they say, 'Yes,' and they join. But when it's after hours, they want to go home and you have to chase after them. So I asked the ladies [volunteers from the community] to prepare a slice of bread that they can have before they start reading. I understand that they have been away from home since the morning – some of them didn't even have breakfast – so it's not easy for them to stay at school with empty tummies. And the volunteer students bring biscuits and juice so the children don't go hungry. (Sabh, South Sudan)

Sabh is extremely grateful that she works with a head teacher who feels similarly about the dramatic benefits these extra-curricular activities can have for the children's learning and behavior. Gada, who also teaches at school, described how she is involved with the school volleyball team and the (award-winning) school choir. Mila credits the success of the school teams with the head teacher. The head teacher of Munyaka School in Kenya takes a similar approach to arranging activities and persuading volunteers from the community to help out. A particularly popular activity is the Farm Club, in which children are taught about the skills and science of agriculture. Esther teaches Class Three and so is not involved in this scheme, which is open to pupils in Class Four and above. However, she feels that the basic principles of farming should be understood even by the younger pupils and so has set up a small farm in her classroom.

In some remote areas in Sudan children leave the school and do not come back and instead continue to work on the farms. They might have some skills from their parents, but then again some of them are orphans. So teachers' role here is crucial to bring them back to school:

> I have an experience of setting up a plan to help these children to work in the farm and to study as the same time. If they drop out, then at least they will have the skills to be employed and feed themselves and it will save them from being away from schools. (Suzan Gazeera state, Sudan)

19.12 Turning Challenges into Opportunities

These stories paint a pretty bleak picture of what life and work is like for these teachers. However, despite the adverse conditions, rather than to sit back and complain, most of the teachers are involved in the improvement of their schools through fundraising or outreach schemes. They do not appear to accept passively what they believe to be inadequate working conditions for themselves and unfair and under-resourced learning environments for their pupils. Instead, they are active in challenging the constraints of these environments to enhance their pupils' learning experiences.

The isolation of the schools, for example, means that there is a lot of open space. The teachers make the most of these space and offer extra-curricular sport lessons. For instance, Adam from North Sudan, explains that:

> "a lot of teachers and students in rural areas do not enjoy being in the classroom because of the challenges they have, so they might come to school thinking, well, I'll bear with the teachers for a few hours and then it will be fun. I know they do like sport to be involved in learning effectively". Much of this land I farmland. Teachers believe this is like being surrounded by a giant science laboratory and they supplement their lessons with real-life example from the farms. Many teachers in the study also highlighted the relative safety of rural areas and the benefits children gain from being able to roam freely in their spare time without fear for their safety.

Some teachers commented that there were some aspects of living in a rural area that made up for the resource shortages, for example the fact that parents and grandparents are less likely to be at work during the day and therefore more available to be drawn on as a teaching resource:

> If, for example, you are going to teach drama and you ask a parent to come in and tell a story, they will listen attentively. Stories are being told by elderly women. I invite a particular parent. (Amal, South Sudan)

It would be easy for their teachers to accept the potentially limited futures of the farm school children, but some teachers refuse to do this. Instead, they work especially hard to build up the confidence of their pupils and persuade them that they can be anything they want to be, if they put their minds to it.

One teacher feels that it is an important part of her role as a rural teacher to ensure the children are as confident as possible when they leave her school. She feels that although there are some challenges to multi-grade teaching, this actually helps to build the children's confidence and improve their ability to learn:

> And what I also enjoy is that when I'm teaching grade two. The one who is in grade one, when she is coming to grade two, she already knows a lot. (Sabh, South Sudan)

19.13 Conclusion

It appears, from this study, that the more remote a school is in Sudan, or the more deprived the children are, the more likely teachers will involve themselves in community work, take on additional responsibilities concerning their pupils' welfare, be involved in future prospects, and support extra-curricular activities. The teachers' voice suggest that there is a clear moral purpose to their work, and one that draws on their individual experiences, family ties, religious beliefs and community life expectations. The teachers also feel that their contributions in community life help to build and maintain positive relationships between the school and the community, which enhances communication and problem solving. It also appears that, in remote environments, teachers benefit from the opportunities for social interaction that these activities provide.

This study also suggests that *relationship* is reciprocal. The school in this study, depends heavily on contributions of money and time from the community. The study also found that for the most rural schools with the fewest staff, the physical presence and assistance of the community in the school is as valuable, if not more so, than fiscal support.

For many people living in an environment like the ones these teachers are working in, the realities of rural life may be insurmountable. The teachers are critically aware that the future prospects of many of their pupils are bleak. For these children, the additional support offered to their families by teachers, and the provision of additional learning opportunities and extra- curricular activities are invaluable.

> The extra activities, being involved in them, it really does enrich my job. That's when I feel my presence as a teacher. (Sara, Sudan)

It is not an exaggeration to say that a great teacher can change a student's life. There are an endless amount of great teacher stories that attest to the benefits of a strong relationship between an educator and a pupil.

As some of the most influential role models for developing students, teachers are responsible for more than just academic enrichment. If you want to be a great educator, you must connect with your pupils and reach them on multiple levels, because the best teachers are committed to their students' well-being both inside and outside the classroom. By forging strong relationships, educators are able to affect virtually every aspect of their students' lives, teaching them the important life lessons that will help them succeed beyond term papers and standardized tests. In doing so, they are enhancing their own quality-of-life.

References

Berliner, D. C. (2001). Learning about teaching from expert teachers. *International Journal of Educational Research, 35*, 463–482.

Cruickshank, D. R. (1990). *Research that informs teachers and teacher educators*. Bloomington, IN: Phi Delta Kappa Educational Foundation.

Duncan, J. S. R. (1952). *The Sudan, accord of achievement*. Edinburgh, UK: William Blackwood & Sons Ltd.

HyattsVille, M. D. (1986, May). *A nation prepared: Teachers for the 21st century*. Carnegie Forum on Education and the Economy (USA). Task Force on Teaching as a Profession.

Moon, B. (2013). *Teacher education and the challenge of development – Global analysis*. London, UK: Routledge.

Ross, J. A., & Regan, E. M. (1993). Sharing professional experience: Its impact on professional development. *Teaching and Teacher Education, 9*(1), 91–106.

Sudan country profile. Library of Congress Federal Research Division, December, 2004. Library of Congress Country Studies Ministry of Education – Sudan. Access at: http://www.moe.gov.sd/

Sylvester, A. (1977). *Sudan under Nimeri*. London, UK: The Bodley Head.

Thakrar, J., Wolfenden, F., & Zinn, D. (2010). *Open educational resources to the challenges of teacher education in Sub-Saharan Africa*. Carnegie Forum on Education and the Economy's Task Force on Teaching as a Profession.

Part V

Family

Traditional Views of Black South Africans on Quality and Successful Family Life

20

Motlalepule Ruth Mampane,
Selogadi Ngwanagwato Mampane,
and Sylvia Ocansey

Abstract

This chapter aims to illuminate the various connotations about quality-of-life within successful family life in black South African families. The exploration includes the African social divide, the historical antecedents that impacted on families and its implications for the black South African family in particular. Successful family life is a desired life asset for most individuals and widely viewed as an accomplishment. Human beings desire success broadly to attract prestige, status and recognition in society. The *meaning* of a successful life has, however, remained contentious, given that it continues to be defined in diverse ways. Ideas of a successful life and quality life appear to be interrelated and are frequently measured in terms of successful family life. *Medical* literature abounds with research on patients' quality-of-life, most of which relates in some way to family life. The varied opinions on what black South Africans regard as successful family life will be explored in this chapter. Given that human life commences in some way within a family system, the exploration of features of the black African family, as a key focus of successful and quality life, will be central to this discussion. Conceptual parameters will include quality-of-life, successful life, African or South African family life and broader family life and family structures.

20.1 Introduction

A family represents the basic unit of universal human communities (McAdoo, 2007). The social unit of the family is identified by unique norms, beliefs and practices (Ocholla-Ayayo, 1997) which underscore the singular responsibility of the African family. According to Franklin (2007), the family is one of the most robust and key traditions in the African community. In concurrence with this fact, Clark (2015) defines the family as the basic human institution that shapes the personal identity, social roles and overall future focus of the individual. Haar and Roche (2010) also agree that the family is key to the individual's development. As elsewhere in the world, the African family transmits values and acceptable norms as well as beliefs and cultural practices of the society to its young ones (Ocholla-Ayayo, 1997). By implication, every African person portrays the culture and 'training' received from the family of origin. The family therefore serves as the primary system of development and economic sustenance for its children, particularly during their tender years. There are multiple

M. R. Mampane (✉) · S. N. Mampane · S. Ocansey
University of Pretoria, Pretoria, South Africa
e-mail: ruth.mampane@up.ac.za

I. Eloff (ed.), *Handbook of Quality of Life in African Societies*, International Handbooks of Quality-of-Life, https://doi.org/10.1007/978-3-030-15367-0_20

family structures and systems in the world, for example: the nuclear family with biological children, single parent family, stepchildren family, grandparent-headed family, extended family and child-headed family. Mampane (2018) (in her inaugural lecture) reported that, black South African families from a township in Mamelodi, East of Pretoria defined a family as: *a group of people living together, it can either be the father, mother and children, or father and mother, or a mother and her children, or it can be orphaned children living alone or a man/woman living alone.* In their definition of family, it is defined by residence (occupying a particular home/house), cohabitation (living together) and blood bonds.

Additionally, research indicates that African cultures are collectivist when compared to individualist Western cultures (Eaton & Louw, 2000). In the African context, the basis of the family relies on the principle of collectivism and interdependence, hence the emphasis on a much wider membership network (Siqwana-Ndulo, 1998). The extended family system is relied on for security and social support. Similarly, Mberengwa and Johnson (2003), confirm that collectivism is key to the survival of the African family system while individualism is destroying the African family system. There is a dearth of literature on the traditional views of black South African families, including what constitute to them, a quality and successful family life. Quality of life is most important in health care practices and focused literature on the construct dates as far back as 1948 (Testa & Simonson, 1996). According to Testa and Simonson (1996:835), the World Health Organization (WHO) in their definition of the construct quality of life they focus on the medical conditions as the "absence of disease and infirmity," and on the psychosocial aspect of the individual as "the presence of physical, mental and social well-being". Therefore, literature frequently view the construct of quality of life more from a philosophical, rather than a scientific perspective; and ultimately the construct contains many subjective elements (Slevin, Plant, Lynch, Drinkwater, & Gregory, 1988). Diener and Suh (1997) confirm three major approaches that determines quality of life, namely: subjective well-being derived from individual experiences, satisfaction of one's performance (economic resources and desires) and finally, good life as guided by normative ideals of, for example, religion, philosophy and other systems. Thus, quality of life is subjective and guided by normative and cultural experiences.

One of the many cultural practices of ancient traditional black families is polygamy (mostly polygyny). A review of literature on African family structures brings to the fore polygamous marriages. Traditionally, polygyny ensured that every female is married off (as arranged marriages) by their family because being a spinster and bachelor was undesirable and discouraged. Thus, marriage was a necessary developmental outcome. It could be understood that, polygamy represented of quality of family life, an achievement and expected developmental outcome. Thus, marriage was considered as a quality of life and a developmental outcome envisaged for all individuals of marriable age (as determined by the practices and norms). A study by Hayase and Liaw (1997) confirms that polygamy in Sub-Saharan Africa is still prevalent. The authors concur that the purpose of polygamy has always been to "maintain the endless line of births and rebirths and to strengthen the power of the family as well as the status of the old patriarch through the growth in family size and the expansion of conjugal linkages to other clans" (Hayase & Liaw, 1997:296). It can be assumed that polygamous (especially polygyny) marriages, by the standard of the times, represented the quality of life because these marriages ensured that every female was married off (by the family). However, the rights of those females were insignificant, instead the collective culture was more significant and enforced as the family determined the conditions and the nature of the marriage.

In essence, this chapter aims to encapsulate the views of literature on traditional black South African families regarding quality and successful family life. Suldo and Huebner (2004) report that the psychological influence of life satisfaction is potent enough to minimize stress and anxiety later in life. Layard, Clark, Cornaglia, Powdthavee and Vernoit (2014) pronounce that significant childhood experiences ultimately fortify future emotional health. The mentioned effects of satisfying life equally generate immense psychological rewards to the individual via an improved self-concept, a robust resilience towards life's issues and an overall well-focused personality. Ultimately, a family that values quality of life and successful family life is ideal for every country, race and nation.

20.2 Background on the Traditional African Family

Family is central to human development and learning. In every nation, a family represents an interface between its individual members and the society (Sewpaul, 2014), it is the backbone and basic unit of society (Yankuzo, 2014). Traditionally, some African family structures have maintained a distinctive element of family when contrasted with that of the Western society, especially extended and polygamous families. The traditional African family is thus comprised of a man and his wives, many children, nieces and nephews, grandparents, granduncles among many others (Ocholla-Ayayo, 1997; Siqwana-Ndulo, 1998). The strength of traditional families is enhanced by their numbers. Sometimes, non-kins also formed part of the African family (Siqwana-Ndulo, 1998). Considering shared values and beliefs, culture is important in traditional black families. Such traditional African families are characterized by understanding, unity and oneness (Yankuzo, 2014). Additionally, Mberengwa and Johnson (2003) confirm that relationships, communication and household responsibilities are key characteristics to the strengths of African traditional families. According to Mampane (2018), communication and relationship was seen as the panacea for resilience. About the significance and type of communication that allows the family to experience quality family life this is what the participants in her study (Mampane, 2018: 13) said:

> The other important issue to note is when we go out, and are having discussions communication must be good. Communication plays a very important role. If we can teach each other how to communicate. Communicate at all times and be patient with each other, listen to what the other one is saying. Good communication, understanding, thanking each other, forgiving each other, are one of the things that create a decent home. I should not keep secrets from my husband, where there is honesty there is love and everyone loves such a home. Where there is truth there is harmony, the communication is also respectful the home will be liked by all.

About the significance of relationships in promoting quality family life, the participants said the following:

> Love keeps the family together. Respect also keeps a family together and strong. Being loving and respectful to your husband can work wonders for women. The way a person behaves, if you behave well and are submissive at all times, if we are all submissive and respectful to each other our children can also learn from this. Families are dynamic in the sense that we cannot all be alike, one of us will have some weak points and we must take that into consideration. We cannot say this person has no say because of his/her weak points. We must show respect to all individuals. The way we behave towards each other and being together also strengthens the bonds of a family and ensures that there's a lot of love in the family.

Matrimonial linkages enhance the strengths of families. Marriage or multiple marriage system, childbearing, gender roles and intergenerational relationships are core to sustainable traditional African families (Oheneba-Sakyi & Takyi, 2006). Family is often seen in the context of relationships, economic prospects and culture. Traditionally, polygamy has been a preferred African family system and structure. According to Budlender, Chobokoane and Simelane (2004) polyandry is rare (if any) in South Africa and polygamy is thus often associated with polygyny. Indeed, the polygynous family, where a man was legally entitled to more than one wife was the ideal in traditional Africa (Mair, 2013). Polygyny as a patriarchal marital system, denigrated the women's status as much lower to that of men (Welch & Glick, 1981). Polygyny exacerbates the vulnerability of women who are spouseless and childless to that of shame and loneliness

(Hayase & Liaw, 1997). Thus, polygamy in its traditional form as explained above, does not allude to life satisfaction or quality of life especially by oppressed females within the marital system. Saxena, Orley and the WHOQOL Group, (1997:263) suggest that though the concept of quality of life is broad and complex, it encompass the person's "physical health, psychological state, level of independence, social relationships and their relationship to salient features of their environment."

Even though the polygamous tradition is no longer the norm, it is highly practiced in South Africa and Swaziland (especially by powerful traditional males), for example former President Jacob Zuma (Andrews, 2008; Ras, 2010), King Mswati III (Tobias, 2001) and King Zwelithini (Ras, 2010). It is true that age connected to wealth and power promotes and sustains polygamous marital systems (Andrews, 2008; Delius & Glaser, 2004). On the issue of the protection of women, the South African government is a signatory to the Convention on the Elimination of All forms of Discrimination Against Women (CEDAW), which requires the state to eliminate various forms of discrimination against women. The constitution of South Africa is also strong on the protection of the rights of all its citizens (Higgins, Fenrich, & Tanzer, 2006). As indicated previously, polygamy is associated with the age of male partners (mostly older men marrying younger females), thus making these men more powerful and in most cases of high economic status. The power and economic imbalance in polygamy make many females highly vulnerable to this form of family structures and partnerships. Since CEDAW, states that women should enjoy the "same rights and responsibilities as men during marriage and its dissolution" (Higgins et al., 2006:1659). Therefore, polygamy according to the General Recommendation 21: Equality in Marriage and Family Relations "contravene a woman's right to equality with men and can have serious emotional and financial consequences for her and her dependents that such marriage ought to be discouraged and prohibited". However, in the event that all these legal documents are usually unable to empower and protect women against abusive partners and males in marriages and relationships (Higgins et al., 2006), women's quality of life and successful experiences of marriage and family life are often threatened. Thus, quality of life becomes a relative construct which is dependent for example, on the individual's status on: health, economic, power, education and vulnerability.

History shows that besides economic factors, security was the main reason for maintaining polygamous marriages. The most cited reasons that sustained polygyny, as a system of marriage was that: it created more children that signified greater wealth, a bigger family and therefore a stronger defense against the enemy (Mair, 2013). Polygyny above all also yielded the much-desired increased hands to meet the labor demands on the family's farmlands. The strength of a family was measured by not only economic and security factors but, the number of family members who contributed to the economic and security prospects of the family through physical labor. The patrilineal or matrilineal system also established the key kinship feature in the traditional African family (Hill, 2003; Mair, 2013). In the patrilineal system, the entire larger group of relatives living and sharing the same economic means of livelihood can be traced to the father but in the matrilineal, the mother remains the key source. Kinship represented a unique feature of low-income black families, given that rather than relying on paid labor; the entire family participated in the farming process (Hill, 2003). According to Hill (2003), kinship involves accepting children of distant relations into the family for various reasons. Accordingly, the traditional African family was maintained through marriages and kinship. Oheneba-Sakyi and Takyi (2006) claim that since the move from the traditional African family to the modern twenty-first century family, they have observed that the differences between the traditional and the modern family lies in the following four key factors: the *distribution of power*, *decision making*, *communication* and the *division of labor*. The demise of the traditional African family structure and polygyny, bring to question how these key factors are enacted within the family system.

Literature confirm that economic migration, especially in South Africa, significantly contributed to urbanization (Reed, 2013; Smit, 2001) and as a result destabilized and weakened traditional families and its matrimonial practices. Specifically, in the South African context, Siqwana-Ndulo (1998) reports the disorganization and gradual crumbling of the traditional family system. In reference to early reports by Krige (1936) and Phillips (1953), emergent family features like late marriage among women, the disintegration of larger households and the dissolution of marriages, is attributed to modernization and exposure to western culture (Siqwana-Ndulo, 1998). Smit (2001) and Reed (2013) refer to urbanization which resulted with the massive move of migrant workers from rural to urban residential areas. This move increased mobility of mostly employable men within with the country. Economic migration during the Apartheid era led to the rise of urbanization and the destabilization of the traditional family system, including the extended family, as a result of separation of husbands from their wives while in search of employment. Since husbands and men moved without their families it encouraged cohabitation resulting in increased incidents of births outside wedlock due to parental relocation to urban settings in search of better employment opportunities. In the isolated village of Ngcingwane in the Eastern Cape Province for example, reports of new household formations and the high incidence of female-headed families evidenced the extensive migration of family heads and father figures to urban centers for enhanced employment. In part, the inevitable result of this trend is the current loss of parental control over children and its associated weakened protection for female children in the family (Hill, 2003), thus derailing successful family life and an overall life satisfaction among such family members. However, research indicates that a circular migration was maintained by migrant workers between rural to urban areas (Reed, 2013; Smit, 2001) which helped to maintain strong ties with families and kins.

Other apparent transformations within the traditional South African family system include the decline of the extended family pattern (Hill, 2003) and the degeneration of the fertility and economic trend and polygyny (Siqwana-Ndulo, 1998). Literature confirms the importance of fertility and economic life facets among traditional South African natives, hence their uncompromising adherence to polygyny (Boserup, 1970; Lesthaege, Kaufmann, & Meekers, 1989). Recent literature alludes to a different family and marital system in South Africa traced to the institutionalization of the migrant labor system during Apartheid. Because the marital system was disrupted by the Apartheid systems through the institutionalization and enforcement of migrant or economic labor systems, as migrant laborers were not allowed to move with their families, married couples were forced to live apart (Hosegood, McGrath, & Moultrie, 2009). Husbands left wives and their homes, mostly in rural areas, to form new residences around their areas of employment, mostly hostels (Wilson, 1972), leading to sometimes cohabitation and informal marriages. However, this meant that because of strong family ties, a circular migration was observed between rural and urban areas. Other literature maintain that this was positive as families enjoyed financial benefits from migrant workers (Reed, 2013; Smit, 2001) which in turn contributed towards their family's sustenance. However, the weakening of marital and family bonds and relationships, the removal of emotional support and security that the wife, children and extended family needed is not accounted for in such discussions. Neither is the lack of reciprocal emotional support offered to the breadwinner by the family members due to geographic distances. The quality of life was severely disrupted since family bonds were weakened and since farming was no longer within the family, central poverty set in. Smit (2001) confirm that because economic and migrant labor affected young men and sometimes women at the prime and critical years of their youth, it affected their decisions and prospect of marriage.

A study by Hosegood et al. (2009) on marriage and partnership patterns in KwaZulu-Natal in South Africa, confirm high rate of non-marriage among Africans in South Africa especially in urban areas. This claim is supported by Smit (2001) who confirmed that the circular migration from rural to urban areas occurs in prime and critical years of youths. Traditionally, this could be equated to the 'marriageable age'. The result is the postponement of marriage while prioritizing economic, educational and social needs. Mhongo (2013) also confirms that research has shown the decline of marriages among African males and females in South Africa between 1921 and 2001. Hosegood et al. (2009:293) report that there is little national data available on marriage in South Africa, but their findings confirm other forms of cohabitation and non-marital partnering, where between 2000 and 2006, the majority of unmarried women (63%) and men (63%) aged 18 years and above were reported to have a regular or casual partner. Therefore, the study shows that even though marriage has declined, other forms of relationships are still maintained. The initial undermining of the marital and family system by the Apartheid government has also resulted in dire consequences for the African family and marital system, as children had to be raised by females while males were working far from home. The situation endorsed and instituted the female-headed family structure in South Africa. Despite the reported decline in the traditional South African marriage, institution (Hosegood et al., 2009) research evidenced an increase in cohabitation, regular non-marital partnership and sometimes multiple sexual partnerships (Delius & Glaser, 2004). The trend indisputably hinders fruitful and stable family life.

The firm association of the family to the social institution of marriage is equally key to this review. Marriage undeniably can establish the family and can fortify its scope. The type of marriage often prevails over the existing interactions of family members, to overcome the overall home atmosphere. Happy marriages thus radiate warmth, acceptance, joyful and caring homes and the contrary exists when marriage is sour. Indeed Carr, Freedman, Cornman and Schwarz (2014) corroborate the observation that marital satisfaction positively correlates with an overall life satisfaction and momentary happiness. South and Spitze (1986) similarly confirm the report by underlining some key divorce factors that affect the home environment. The benefits of a rewarding family life are intertwined with the quality of foundational social life experiences and the prevailing marriage characteristics that occupy the home.

Equally important are the reports on the immense adulteration of the authenticity of the traditional South African marriage custom. The desertion of certain marriage processes has reportedly compromised the tradition, resulting in a disregard for marital obligations and responsibilities both between the couple and the entire South African society (Siqwana-Ndulo, 1998). Many African city-dwellers, for instance, increasingly evade the payment of the famous 'lobola' (bride price) which constitute customary marriage to adopt the western-style civil marriage (Siqwana-Ndulo, 1998). Customary, lobola is recognized and without it there is no marriage custom only (Mberengwa & Johnson, 2003). To indicate the significance of the lobola marriage custom, most native South Africans, would settle for customary marriage through lobola payment and a civil union (what is referred to as the Western marriage or union), thus both marriages will be done.

The above-mentioned alterations to the original traditional South African norms have therefore come with immense repercussions, not only to the very fabric of the African society, but also to the quality of life of native South Africans. It cannot be ignored that marriage and extended family (including kinship) was the cornerstone of the traditional African family system.

20.3 Family and the Quality of Life

The definition of family in this chapter encompasses the primary system of human development and learning, interfacing between its individual members and society at large; the marital system; an emerging and multidimensional relational system with complex kin and non-kinship relationships, as well as an evolving and ever-changing microsystem. Thus, family is a relational and comprehensive human system. Walsh (2016) confirms that the family needs resilience to flourish and rebound from the various forms of adversity it experiences. Every family accordingly encounters adversity, and for it to advance and remain united, family resilience is key. Black and Lobo (2008) define family resilience as successful coping of family members under adversity, which enables them to flourish with warmth, support, and cohesion. Similarly, Walsh (2016) defines family resilience as healthy family functioning in situations of adversity. South African resilience researchers like, Theron, Theron and Malindi (2012) and Mampane and Bouwer (2011) equally concur that resilience is contextual and is not uniform across all contexts. Theron et al. (2012) infer that African conceptualizations of resilience refer to collectivist philosophies, thus ensuring the interdependence between the individual and the family. The survival and wellbeing of families is crucial for its sustenance and is dependent on its resilience, which also determines the quality of life and success experienced by all its members.

Similar to resilience, definitions of quality of life remain fluid, subjective and contextual (Lawford & Eiser, 2001). According to Alriksson-Schmidt Wallander and Biasini (2006) definitions of quality of life can focus on health – medical or disease (addressing symptoms) as well as a generic broader view of life (for example, family, friends, job, school or goals in life). Reviewed research on resilience and quality of life focuses on disease and health, psychological adversity and family protective factors to enhance resilience (Alriksson-Schmidt et al., 2006; Lawford & Eiser, 2001). Alriksson-Schmidt et al. (2006) found that increased life stressors (adversities) were associated with poor quality of life and that enhancing the resilience of adolescents in their study might enhance their perceived quality of life. Studies of resilience have shown that not all individuals who are exposed to adversities (stressors) in life experience negative developmental trajectories (Mampane & Bouwer, 2011; Masten, 2001; Theron et al., 2012). Thus Alriksson-Schmidt et al. (2006) confirm that positive outcomes in the face of adversity also indicate quality of life. This implies a close relationship between quality of life and resilience, as they both conform to positive outcomes in the context of stressors.

According to Phaladze et al. (2005), the concept of quality of life is multidimensional and difficult to define, as a result, researchers have agreed to a health-related focus on quality of life. The World Health Organization Quality of Life Group (1998:1570) defines quality of life as "individuals' perception of their position in life in the context of the culture and value systems in which they live and in relation to their goals, expectations, standards and concerns". The concept of quality of life first emerged in the 1950s when the first director of the National office of health statistics, Dr. Halbert, attempted its explanation. The director simply equated quality of life to 'high level wellness' (Land, Michalos, & Sirgy, 2011). His elaborate definition of the concept described quality of life as 'an integrated method of functioning which is oriented towards maximizing the potential of which the individual is capable, within the environment where he or she is functioning.' (Land et al., 2011; p. 2). Sen (1998) on the other hand describes the resource as depending largely on a combination of physical and social conditions. He further highlights key social factors like reliable health care services, education, insights into healthy living conditions among the less educated, and better living conditions as aspects of quality life.

Andrews and Withey (2012) on the other hand categorize social quality life conditions into the objective and subjective facets of life. The objective elements focus mainly on specific observable social indicators comprising health, education, home or living conditions, crime rates, wealth or affluence, among many others (Andrews & Withey, 2012; Sen, 1998). Essentially, the major physical, social life influences emerge as the objective quality of life indicators, though they simply present as social mortality factors (Sen, 1998).

Contrary to the objective elements are the subjective factors that are mostly idiosyncratically defined. Individuals normally vary in their personal desires and satisfaction factors. The quality of life indicators thus diverge to accommodate the several unique individual human needs that may or may not be satisfied by personal experiences (Diener & Suh, 1997). The focus lies on the psychological influences the individual derives from the met need or experience. Diener and Suh (1997) opine that the subjective approach to quality life centers on 'people's choices' and may be more related to 'modern economic thinking' (p. 190). Examples of the subjective quality of life factors include feelings of contentment, satisfaction, confidence and reassurance that usually endorse the psychological well-being of the individual (Clark, 2015).

Interestingly, many of the subjective factors directly emerge from the home environment where the individual was nurtured. The warm home atmosphere that radiates comfort, love, peace, reassurance and a promising future, often shapes the child's understanding and guides him into responsible adulthood (McAdoo, 2007). According to Beuhler, Rhodes, Orme, John and Cuddeback (2006), a successful home reflects a secure and nurturing environment, discipline and progressive education, that promote a robust social and emotional development in the youth. The interactive communication, optimism, meaningful instruction, constructive criticism, feedback and reinforcement opportunities from the home environment efficiently draw the growing child onto the family's recognized social path (Clark, 2015).

The focus of quality of life in the current study indeed relates both to the physical social elements and subjective personal evaluations of Black South Africans in general. The subjective references of quality of life refer mostly to the individual's perceptions on satisfaction with life. The patterns and settings of shared personal human relationships, established in the home, depict the quality of life. Experiences of love, sense of belonging, hatred, respect, responsibility, and dependency among many others, define individual estimations of quality of life. Diener (1984) in this regard sums up the meaning of subjective well-being as contentment, life satisfaction, and positive affect. Yet the objective factors seem to hinge more on broader societal issues. Health, housing, nutrition, education and religion depict the primary physiological human needs that many societies and the family in particular, require to promote life.

Family quality of life refers to how family members collectively live their lives as a unit (Poston et al., 2003). Barnes and Olson (1982) in Summers et al. (2005:779), define family quality of life as the "family's sense of the fit between themselves and their environment". Summers et al. (2005:779) declare that when the quality of family life is assessed, the family's health, financial wellbeing, relationships, support from other people, support from services, careers and preparing for careers, spiritual and cultural life, leisure and community and civic involvement are measured. A study measuring the quality of life in families of children with disabilities found that, family relationships, spiritual and cultural life and careers and preparing for careers as strong contributors for their families' quality of life (Summers et al., 2005). Another study conducted by Poston et al. (2003) found that quality of family life was reported as: financial wellbeing (source of income, financial security, health care and paying for basic necessities); parenting (teaching discipline and parental guidance); family interactions (positive interaction an environment, communication, supporting each other and flexibility) and daily family life (satisfaction in everyday family activities and care). Figure 20.1 below gives an encapsulation of what the literature above defines as +quality of life.

Therefore, family quality of life self-report enables families to assess their satisfaction with family life and functioning, the available opportunities they have to participate in their environment, the attainment of their goals and the initiatives created for them to attain life satisfaction (Summers et al., 2005). Family quality of life is focused on the quality of family functioning. Everyday family activities, including family

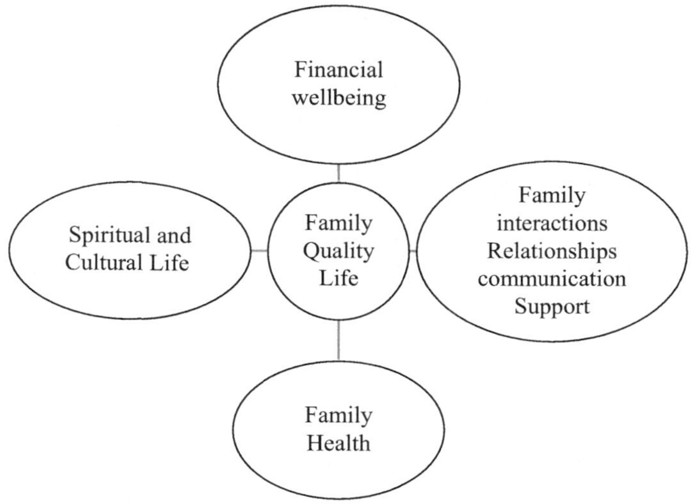

Fig. 20.1 Family quality of life

interaction, communication, cohesion, family support and access to resources contribute to their quality of life.

20.4 Successful Family Functioning

Peterson and Green (2009), posit that family communication is key to successful family functioning. The authors define family communication as "the way verbal and non-verbal information is exchanged between family members" (p. 1). Olson and Barnes (2004:1) define family communication as "the act of making information, ideas, thoughts and feelings known among members of a family unit". Communication according to Peterson and Green (2009) also refers to the ability to "pay attention to what others are thinking and feeling" (p. 1). Family communication is a meaning making process which is dynamic, interactive, interactional and a collaborative part of everyday activities within a family unit. Communication is intended to transmit a message and evoke emotions in the process. The important part of communication is to listen to the communicated (verbal and non-verbal) message which can be presented as directly or indirectly, a clear or a masked message (Epstein, Bishop, & Levin, 1978). Accordingly, Epstein et al. (1978), identified four types of communication namely:

1. Clear and direct communication is seen as a healthy and desired form of communication because it presents a plain and direct message
2. Clear and indirect communication presents a clear message but does not direct the message or address the relevant or intended person
3. Masked and direct communication present an unclear message which is truly directed to the relevant persons, however, the content of the message remains unclear
4. Masked and indirect communication presents an unclear message which is also not directed to the relevant or intended person.

Walsh's (2003, 2016) family resilience framework, refers to the three key resilience processes that families need to function well, be resilient and flourish. The three key resilience processes as identified by the Family Resilience Framework of Walsh (2003:7) are:

1. Family belief system which is made up of three substructures – making meaning of adversity, positive outlook and transcendence, and spirituality;

2. Family organization patterns, which is defined by three substructures – flexibility, connectedness and social and economic resources; and
3. Communication and problem solving with three substructures – clarity, open emotional expression and collaborative problem solving.

Epstein et al. (1978) refers to McMaster's model of family functioning which is an objective assessment questionnaire measuring structural, organizational and transactional characteristics of family functioning using the following variables: communication, affective responsiveness, problem solving, behavior control, affective involvement and roles. According to Epstein et al. (1978), depending on the severity of the variables, family functioning can be measured as functional (experiencing success) or dysfunctional.

The impetus on family operations motivated Beavers and Hampson's (2000) development of the Beavers Systems Model of Family Functioning. The tool measures family competence (measured by family structure, available information and adaptive flexibility of the system). Beavers Model of family functioning uses health-competence dimensions ranging from (Beavers & Hampson, 2000:130–133):

- Severely dysfunctional family (severely deficit communication);
- Borderline family (chaotic overt power struggle alternating with ineffective efforts to establish power and dominance);
- Midrange families (these are clustered as three groups of dysfunctional families containing functional but vulnerable children, with parents who are susceptible to psychological problems);
- Adequate family (uses control and intimidation to achieve optimal functioning); optimal functioning families (effective functioning)

Beavers' Model of family functioning dictates what successful family functioning should look like (effective – optimal functioning) and what unsuccessful family functioning entails (dysfunctional families). When families are successful, their functioning is effective. Based on Peterson and Green (2009), Beavers and Hampson (2000), Epstein et al. (1978), and Walsh (2003, 2016), communication is a key intersecting factor to effective family functioning. The above-mentioned family functioning models dictate that family function varies based on the identified variables, which are all interactional and relational. Thus, how family members relate to each other, communicate and function, can lead it to experience success or not. Successful family functioning is varied, contextual and relational. Families have the capacity to experience successful functioning based on how they deal with the adversity they are experiencing. However, it seems communication is key in all the mentioned family functioning models. Effective communication can help families to work together in resolving the stressors they are encountering and thus experience a successful life – or thus experience successful lives.

Communication is also key in other contexts of development, especially the work environment. According to Tangiuri and Davis (1992), clear identification and communication of company goals to employees efficiently guides their behavior and development over time. Effective communication skills are beneficial to adults who function in both the family and work environment. Accordingly, Tangiuri and Davis (1992) conclude that the family's efficient transmission of societal goals and purposes to the individual, ultimately promotes a rewarding family life. Indeed, socialization processes define the child's understanding and construction of fruitful relations with significant others in the society and thus validates the worthwhileness of the home, by meeting both the child's physiological and psychological needs. The combination of met needs and the satisfaction the individual derives from the reflection of personal definitions highlights features of successful life to the individual. Though focused on needs achievement and satisfaction overall, the meaning of a successful life remains subjective as individuals and families may perceive them differently.

20.5 The Quality of Life Among Black South Africans

The trauma of apartheid South Africa in the past years deeply affected the lives of black South Africans in particular (Möller, 1998). The violence that characterized the period at the time engendered severe discontentment, high levels of poverty, insecurity, anxiety and fear among the general populace. South Africa was described as a nation of 'stark contrast and social turbulence' owing to evidence of 'abject poverty amidst plenty for the dominant white group' (Möller, 1998:28). Living conditions among the black population was deeply disheartening thus emphasizing the need for poverty alleviation to remedy the situation.

In April 1994 when the first democratic elections were held, democracy was celebrated and people shared a remarkable experience that possibly turned around the lives of many South Africans. Improved living conditions became apparent even among black South Africans and the better life for all agenda of the new government, restored a more favorable quality of life in the country. The 'livability' theory targeted enhanced living conditions towards a more satisfying life (Veenhoven, 1995). In her research, Möller (1998) found that, health, education and employment rates improved significantly, but the elements easily faded away within a space of 2 years. The ensuing decline in living conditions especially among black South Africans was deeply alarming (Moller, 1998). Eventually the need to ascertain the extent of political change in the life quality of black South Africans in particular, necessitated further research on the subjective well-being of the public.

The Quality of Life Trends Research Project conducted during the late 1990s documented the change factors in the living conditions of black South Africans. The research revealed stark truths about the deprived conditions under which the majority of black South Africans resided (Möller, 1998). Continuous reports of decline in contentment levels among the native poor, coupled with an even deeper socio-economic demarcation between poor black South Africans and the white elite group, were recorded. Statistics South Africa (2017) has shown that due to unemployment (23% in 2015), poverty levels among South Africans rose to 30.4 million in 2015. As a result, the government social grant, which is the only source of income among the poor majority in black South African communities and families, is a much-needed social relief. The Social protection expenditure (of which social grant is a part) has increased exponentially to R164.9 billion for the period of 2015–2016 (Statistics South Africa, 2017).

Møller and Devey (2003) additionally confirmed that a greater proportion of older South Africans are still living in poor, multi-generation households during this much-heralded democratic rule. Many households reportedly comprised at least an over 60-year-old member though with limited access to potable water, hydroelectric power and home entitlement (Mampane, 2017). Pension contributions typically served as a main economic source for such families (Mampane, 2017), but the elderly tended to be more pleased with their reasonable living conditions. Ferreira, (2006) underscored the critical economic role pension incomes play, especially among the aged and poor households in Black South Africa. Pension incomes often served as the pivot of social and economic advancement in many households by reducing their vulnerability statuses, meeting key human needs, sustaining lives and providing essential resources (Ferreira, 2006). The situation demanded immediate attention to outline novel strategies to improving living conditions for the general populace (Møller & Devey, 2003).

The Minister of Health, Dr. Aaron Motsoaledi, revealed the National Health Insurance (NHI) Bill which is reported to introduce changes to medial aid rules in South Africa. The intention of the Bill is to improve the well-being of South Africans, by making health services accessible to all (Government Gazette, 21 June 2018). However, although the bill is designed to ensure that all South Africans can access quality health care and thus improve their lives, it is not yet clear how the NHI Fund will be financed.

Within the realm of healthcare, the historical announcement made on 1 December 2009 by President Jacob Zuma (The Presidency, 8 April 2010) about fast-tracking the plan to roll out HIV/AIDS antiretroviral drugs, was seen as a victory for the populace and a move towards improving the quality of life for South Africans, especially women and children suffering from HIV/AIDS. Subsequent to the President's announcement on expediting HIV/AIDS antiretroviral rollouts, sentiments expressed by the current Minister of Health, Dr. Aaron Motsoaledi, regarding the alarming rates of HIV/AIDS and his emphasis on the urgency for change to salvage life, was an acknowledgement of the poor quality of life among South Africans in general. In his address, Dr. Motsoaledi alluded to the four additional quality of life priority areas targeted by the former President, Jacob Zuma, namely: employment, education, public safety, and economic development (Coovadia, Jewkes, Barron, Sanders, & McIntyre, 2009). Thus, quality of life is achieved when the impact of stressors on families and individuals is minimized and more protection and resources are made available. When family stressors are buffered to increase protection and support, the quality of life in the family increases with the family's experience of successful developmental outcomes. Indeed to date, the poverty levels encountered by many black South Africans cannot be equated to successful family or quality life.

Lack of education, single parenting and unemployment are equally considered among the most prevalent social indicators of poverty in South Africa (Statistics South Africa, 2017). Acquiring and creating access to education is perceived as an assurance to future quality and successful life. For this reason, Rychen & Salganik, (2003) describe education as an indispensable asset for individual and social advancement. Governments' growing concern regarding the adequacy and quality of public education and the Organization for Economic Co-operation and Development's (OECD) interest in the discipline, firmly validates the versatility of education (Rychen & Salganik, 2003).

Emphasis on academic attainment and skills development in the area of science, computer studies, reading, writing and mathematics in particular, are also considered essential competencies that equip the individual to confront future social life challenges, thereby facilitating progress towards a successful life (Rychen & Salganik, 2003). In their research, Proctor et al., (2010) discovered self-gratified adolescents scoring highly at school and in relation to inter and intra-personal variables. Suldo et al., (2008) also associate students' satisfaction to specific school-related factors like school grades, classroom behavior and overall school social experiences. Indeed, the dire effects of academic stress on the mental health of high-achieving adolescents globally attests to the importance of education in predicting overall life satisfaction (Suldo et al., 2008). In effect, education, and high academic attainment in particular, resonated social prestige and self-confidence among the youth, thereby promoting the possibility of a successful and quality life.

Trank et al., (2002) further pronounce that students' job preferences and organizational attributes are often influenced by their special abilities and academic achievement. Students with higher cognition and attainments usually displayed preference for job flexibility, high pay and promotion systems that often inclined them towards interesting and more challenging employment opportunities. The above-mentioned elements basically endorse the influence of education on students' future life satisfaction (Trank et al., 2002). Considering the collectivist African culture, it is expected that students will probably share their success and financial resources with their families. This justifies the African proverb that 'no one can succeed without help from others' (Above Whispers, nd), likewise the South African proverb that suggests that 'children are the future of the nation' (Above Whispers, n.d.). In effect, the African society sanctions her youth to accept their immediate familial and societal responsibilities once they reach adulthood and in reciprocation, every traditional society yearns for a successful and quality life for its youth.

Until recently, higher education in particular also served as a primary passport to accessing high-paying employment. Graduates were then mostly assured of reliable employment once they completed their accredited degree programs. According to Harvey (2000), university graduates at the time often earned more than their non-graduate counterparts and the graduates' careful selection or preference for specific employment opportunities, reflected the immense influence of their academic training on their quality of life. High pay means more affordability and better living conditions, that also culminates in a satisfying life (Harvey, 2000). Clarke and Lunt (2014) subsequently observe that the high earning premiums of higher degree holders led to a substantial increase in the demand for post-graduate education. The simple justification was that a higher education degree was symbolic of critical and analytic thinking, high level knowledge and intellectual ability (Harvey, 2000). Lately, the changing trends of higher education have raised worldwide concerns regarding the difficulties of education at a higher level (Clarke & Lunt, 2014).

In most African black families, traditional beliefs, culture and spirituality are a source of strength. As mentioned, Walsh (2003) concurs that family beliefs, of which spirituality is a part, are key to family resilience and an enhanced quality life. Most literature, when referring to spirituality in African culture, also include ancestral beliefs (Masango, 2006; Mazama, 2002). The stark contrast between spirituality and religiosity is not differentiated in such literature on appeasing the ancestors and worshiping them. Nevertheless the concepts used in appeasing the ancestors vary significantly from the adopted ones in worshipping God as conceptualized within Christian traditions. However, the concepts are often confused in the literature thereby promoting the belief that black South Africans worship ancestors as part of their religion. This, however, remains a misconception even though ancestors are important to the African culture and part of the lineage of every family. A clear distinction therefore exists among black South Africans between ancestral worship and the reverence for God. For example, Ross (2007) stresses the black South Africans' socio-cultural meanings of illness and disability to be centered on religion. This assumption by Ross (2007), should be interpreted in context as it cannot be assumed that acceptance and knowledge of disability as a medical condition is absent. Similarly, Cocks and Møller (2002) claim that treatment approaches like prayer and rituals are often adopted, *as well as* the use of natural substances for healing. These belief systems and practices of black South Africans are not deficits but rather an acknowledgment of the traditional and cultural practices of elders who grow and use medicinal herbs for healing and acknowledging that Western medicines are not the only valid and reliable resources for healing. African herbs and medicines can be reliable and are trusted by the families and communities who use them. Thus, knowledge of herbs and their healing properties is key to African culture, which is one traditional practice that most black South Africans do not want to lose. Cocks and Møller (2002) likewise confirm the above report with the revelation that over 27 million South Africans adopt indigenous medicines and herbs for treatment. The basis of these treatment approaches stems from the belief that 'good health is holistic and extends to the person's social environment' (Cocks & Møller, 2002:387). Many South Africans thus rely on herbal and traditional medicines not only for cultural purposes, but also to improve their overall personal well-being and to further treat some physical health conditions (Cooks & Moller, 2002). Richter (2003) concur that traditional medicines are important and key to treating some ailments. Spirituality and religion should therefore be seen as distinct concepts where the native black South African is concerned.

20.6 Conclusion

Family is key to human developmental and is a primary system for the education of the child. It can be assumed that family is not static, but developmental in nature and continuously consists of a cycle of birth, growth and death. Marriage in most instances is intertwined with family life. However, literature has shown that family is complex and is not always about marital couples and that relationships and communication are key to the quality and success of family life. There are no explicit 'traditional views' or practices that are documented in literature on black South Africans' quality and successful family life. However, family resilience literature indicates that a resilient family experiences success and a better quality of life. Thus, a relationship between successful and quality family life and resilience can be assumed based on positive developmental outcomes the family may experience. Every family experiences adversity or stressors. When a family is able to overcome adversities and experiences successful developmental outcomes, it is viewed as resilient and resilience is key to experiencing successful and quality family life. Black South African families need resilience to flourish and experience quality of life.

This chapter has shown that the African family as it was known traditionally (in terms of polygamy, extended family systems) has evolved and changed drastically over time. In addition, globalization has influenced the development of family structures and systems and has, in some instances, contributed to the replacement of traditional African cultural values with global values (Yankuzo, 2014). Culture, economics and politics are more central in globalization debates (Yankuzo, 2014) and has subsequently manifested in the quality of life of black South African families.

References

Above Whispers. (n.d.). *African proverbs sayings*. http://abovewhispers.com/2016/02/21/south-african-proverbs-and-sayings/. Accessed 27 June 2018.

Alriksson-Schmidt, A. I., Wallander, J., & Biasini, F. (2006). Quality of life and resilience in adolescents with a mobility disability. *Journal of Pediatric Psychology, 32*(3), 370–379.

Andrews, P. E. (2008). Who's afraid of polygamy-exploring the boundaries of family, equality and custom in South Africa. *Journal of Law & Family Studies, 11*, 303.

Andrews, F. M., & Withey, S. B. (2012). *Social indicators of Well-being: Americans' perceptions of life quality*. New York, NY: Springer Science & Business Media.

Barnes, H., & Olson, D. H. (1982). *Parent-adolescent communication, family inventories. Family social science*. Minneapolis: University of Minnesota.

Beavers, R., & Hampson, R. B. (2000). The Beavers systems model of family functioning. *Journal of Family Therapy, 22*(2), 128–143.

Black, K., & Lobo, M. (2008). A conceptual review of family resilience factors. *Journal of Family Nursing, 14*(1), 33–55.

Boserup, E. (1970). *Women's role in economic development*. London, UK: St. Martin's Press.

Budlender, D., Chobokoane, N., & Simelane, S. (2004). Marriage patterns in South Africa: Methodological and substantive issues. *Southern African Journal of Demography, 9*, 1–25.

Buehler, C., Rhodes, K. W., Orme, J. G., & Cuddeback, G. (2006). The potential for successful family foster care: Conceptualizing competency domains for foster parents. *Child Welfare, 85*(3), 523.

Carr, D., Freedman, V. A., Cornman, J. C., & Schwarz, N. (2014). Happy marriage, happy life? Marital quality and subjective well-being in later life. *Journal of Marriage and Family, 76*(5), 930–948.

Clark, R. M. (2015). *Family life and school achievement: Why poor black children succeed or fail*. Chicago: University of Chicago Press.

Clarke, G., & Lunt, I. (2014). *International comparisons in postgraduate education: Quality, access and employment outcomes*. Bristol, UK: Higher Education Funding Council for England (HEFCE).

Cocks, M., & Møller, V. (2002). Use of indigenous and indigenised medicines to enhance personal well-being: A South African case study. *Social Science & Medicine, 54*(3), 387–397.

Coovadia, H., Jewkes, R., Barron, P., Sanders, D., & McIntyre, D. (2009). The health and health system of South Africa: Historical roots of current public health challenges. *The Lancet, 374*(9692), 817–834. https://doi.org/10.1016/S0140-6736(09)60951-X

Delius, P., & Glaser, C. (2004). The myths of polygamy: A history of extra-marital and multi-partnership sex in South Africa. *South African Historical Journal, 50*(1), 84–114.

Diener, E. (1984). Subjective well-being. *Psychological Bulletin, 95*(3), 542–575.

Diener, E., & Suh, E. (1997). Measuring quality of life: Economic, social, and subjective indicators. *Social Indicators Research, 40*(1–2), 189–216. https://doi.org/10.1023/A:1006859511756

Eaton, L., & Louw, J. (2000). Culture and self in South Africa: Individualism-collectivism predictions. *The Journal of Social Psychology, 140*(2), 210–217.

Epstein, N. B., Bishop, D. S., & Levin, S. (1978). The McMaster model of family functioning. *Journal of Marital and Family Therapy, 4*(4), 19–31.

Ferreira, M. (2006). The differential impact of social-pension income on household poverty alleviation in three south African ethnic groups. *Ageing & Society, 26*(3), 337–354.

Franklin, J. H. (2007). African American families. In H. P. McAdoo (Ed.), *Black families*. Thousand Oaks, CA: Sage.

Haar, J. M., & Roche, M. A. (2010). Family supportive organization perceptions and employee outcomes: The mediating effects of life satisfaction. *The International Journal of Human Resource Management, 21*(7), 999–1014.

Harvey, L. (2000). New realities: The relationship between higher education and employment. *Tertiary Education & Management, 6*(1), 3–17.

Hayase, Y., & Liaw, K. L. (1997). Factors on polygamy in Sub-Saharan Africa: Findings based on the demographic and health surveys. *The Developing Economies, 35*(3), 293–327.

Higgins, T. E., Fenrich, J., & Tanzer, Z. (2006). Gender equality and customary marriage: Bargaining in the shadow of post-apartheid legal pluralism. *Fordham International Law Journal, 30*(6), 1653–1708.

Hill, R. B. (2003). *The strengths of black families*. Lanham, MD: University Press of America.

Hosegood, V., McGrath, N., & Moultrie, T. (2009). Dispensing with marriage: Marital and partnership trends in rural KwaZulu-Natal, South Africa 2000–2006. *Demographic Research, 20*, 279.

Krige, E. J. (1936). Changing conditions in marital relations and parental duties among urbanized natives. *Africa: Journal of the International Institute of African Languages and Cultures, 9*(1), 1–23. London: Oxford University Press.

Land, K. C., Michalos, A. C., & Sirgy, M. J. (Eds.). (2011). *Handbook of social indicators and quality of life research*. Berlin: Springer Science & Business Media.

Lawford, J., & Eiser, C. (2001). Exploring links between the concept of quality of life and resilience. *Pediatric Rehabilitation, 4*(4), 209–216.

Layard, R., Clark, A. E., Cornaglia, F., Powdthavee, N., & Vernoit, J. (2014). What predicts a successful life? A life-course model of well-being. *The Economic Journal, 124*(580), F720–F738.

Lesthaege, R., Kaufmann, G., & Meekers, D. (1989). The nuptiality regimes in sub-Saharan Africa. In R. Lesthaege (Ed.), *Reproduction and social organization in Sub-Saharan Africa*. Berkeley, CA: University of California Press.

Mair, L. P. (2013). *African marriage and social change*. London, UK: Routledge.

Mampane, M. R. (2017). Resilience of the socio-educational afterschool and community intervention drop-in centre. *Perspectives in Education, 32*(2), 126–141.

Mampane, M. R. (2018). *Resilience processes of families in economically depressed environments*. Inaugural Lecture, 21 June 2018, University of Pretoria, Faculty of Education, Groenkloof Campus.

Mampane, R., & Bouwer, C. (2011). The influence of township school on the resilience of their learners. *South African Journal of Education, 31*(1), 114–126.

Masango, M. J. (2006). African spirituality that shapes the concept of Ubuntu. *Verbum et Ecclesia, 27*(3), 930–943.

Masten, A. S. (2001). Ordinary magic: Resilience processes in development. *American Psychologist, 56*(3), 227.

Mazama, M. A. (2002). Afrocentricity and African spirituality. *Journal of Black Studies, 33*(2), 218–234.

Mberengwa, L. R., & Johnson, J. M. (2003). Strengths of Southern African families and their cultural context. *Journal of Family and Consumer Sciences, 95*(1), 20.

McAdoo, H. P. (Ed.). (2007). *Black families*. New York, NY: Sage.

Medical Schemes Amendment Bill. (2018). Government Gazette, Republic of South Africa: Government Notices, Department of Health, No. 636 No. 41726. www.gpwonline.co.za. Accessed 21 June 2018.

Mhongo, C. (2013). Declining rates of marriage in South Africa: What do the numbers and analysts say? *Acta Juridica, 2013*(1), 181–196.

Møller, V. (1998). Quality of life in South Africa: Post-apartheid trends. *Social Indicators Research, 43*(1–2), 27–68. https://doi.org/10.1023/A:1006828608870

Møller, V., & Devey, R. (2003). Trends in living conditions and satisfaction among poorer older south Africans: Objective and subjective indicators of quality of life in the October household survey. *Development Southern Africa, 20*(4), 457–476.

Ocholla-Ayayo, A. B. C. (1997). The African family between tradition and modernity. In A. Adepoju (Ed.), *Family, population and development in Africa* (pp. 60–67). London, UK: Zed Books Limited.

Oheneba-Sakyi, Y., & Takyi, B. (2006). Introduction to the study of African families: A framework for analysis. African families at the turn of the 21st century (pp 1–24). In Y. Oheneba-Sakyi & B. K. Takyi (Eds.), *African families at the turn of the 21st century*. Greenwood Publishing Group.

Olson, D. H., & Barnes, H. (2004). *Family communication* (pp. 1–9). Minneapolis, MN: Life Innovation. Available on: www.laviecounselling.org/vfh/vfhasm/FACESIV.FamilyCommunicationscale.pdf

Peterson, R., & Green, S. (2009). *Families first-keys to successful family functioning*. Communication. Virginia Cooperative Extension.

Phaladze, N. A., Human, S., Dlamini, S. B., Hulela, E. B., Mahlubi Hadebe, I., Sukati, N. A., … Holzemer, W. L. (2005). Quality of life and the concept of living well with HIV/AIDS in Sub-Saharan Africa. *Journal of Nursing Scholarship, 37*(2), 120–126.

Phillips, A. (Ed.). (1953). *Survey of African marriage and family life*. London, UK: Oxford University Press.

Poston, D., Turnbull, A., Park, J., Mannan, H., Marquis, J., & Wang, M. (2003). Family quality of life: A qualitative inquiry. *Mental Retardation, 41*(5), 313–328.

Proctor, C., Linley, P. A., & Maltby, J. (2010). Very happy youths: Benefits of very high life satisfaction among adolescents. *Social Indicators Research, 98*(3), 519–532.

Ras, J. J. (2010). Polygamy (polyandry & polygyny): Yes or no? *Inkanyiso: Journal of Humanities and Social Sciences, 2*(2), 108–114.

Reed, H. E. (2013). Moving across boundaries: Migration in south Africa, 1950–2000. *Demography, 50*(1), 71–95. https://doi.org/10.1007/s13524-012-0140-x

Richter, M. (2003). Traditional medicines and traditional healers in South Africa. *Treatment action campaign and AIDS law project*, 17, 4–29.

Ross, E. (2007). Traditional healing in South Africa: Ethical implications for social work. *Social Work in Health Care, 46*(2), 15–33. https://doi.org/10.1300/J010v46n02_02

Rychen, D. S., & Salganik, L. H. (Eds.). (2003).*Key competencies for a successful life and well-functioning society*. Boston: Hogrefe Publishing.

Saxena, S., Orley, J., & WHOQOL Group. (1997). Quality of life assessment: The world health organization perspective. *European Psychiatry, 12*, 263s–266s.

Sen, A. (1998). Mortality as an indicator of economic success and failure. *The Economic Journal, 108*(446), 1–25. https://doi.org/10.1111/1468-0297.00270

Sewpaul, V. (2014). A structural social justice approach to family policy: A critique of the draft south African family policy. *Social Work/Maatskaplike Werk, 41*(4), 310–323.

Siqwana-Ndulo, N. (1998). Rural African family structure in the Eastern Cape Province, South Africa. *Journal of Comparative Family Studies, 29*, 407–417.

Slevin, M. L., Plant, H., Lynch, D. A., Drinkwater, J., & Gregory, W. M. (1988). Who should measure quality of life, the doctor or the patient? *British Journal of Cancer, 57*(1), 109.

Smit, R. (2001). The impact of labor migration on African families in South Africa: Yesterday and today. *Journal of Comparative Family Studies, 32*, 533–548.

South, S. J., & Spitze, G. (1986). Determinants of divorce over the marital life course. *American Sociological Review, 51*(4), 583–590. https://doi.org/10.2307/2095590

Statistics South Africa. (2017). *Poverty trends in South Africa an examination of absolute poverty between 2006 and 2015* (Report No. 03-10-06). Pretoria, South Africa: Statistics South Africa. http://www.statssa.gov.za/publications/Report-03-10-06/Report-03-10-062015.pdf. Accessed 23 Aug 2017

Suldo, S. M., & Huebner, E. S. (2004). Does life satisfaction moderate the effects of stressful life events on psychopathological behavior during adolescence? *School Psychology Quarterly, 19*(2), 93.

Suldo, S. M., Shaffer, E. J., & Riley, K. N. (2008). A social-cognitive-behavioral model of academic predictors of adolescents' life satisfaction. *School Psychology Quarterly, 23*(1), 56.

Summers, J. A., Poston, D. J., Turnbull, A. P., Marquis, J., Hoffman, L., Mannan, H., & Wang, M. (2005). Conceptualizing and measuring family quality of life. *Journal of Intellectual Disability Research, 49*(10), 777–783.

Tangiuri, R., & Davis, J. A. (1992). On the goals of successful family companies. *Family Business Review, 5*(1), 43–62.

Testa, M. A., & Simonson, D. C. (1996). Assessment of quality-of-life outcomes. *New England Journal of Medicine, 334*(13), 835–840.

Theron, L. C., Theron, A. M. C., & Malindi, M. J. (2012). Towards and African definition of resilience: A rural South African community view of resilient Basotho Youth. *Journal of Black Psychology, 39*(1), 63–87.

Tobias, B. Q. (2001). A descriptive study of the cultural mores and beliefs toward HIV/AIDS in Swaziland, Southern Africa. *International Journal for the Advancement of Counselling, 23*(2), 99–113.

Trank, C. Q., Rynes, S. L., & Bretz, R. D. (2002). Attracting applicants in the war for talent: Differences in work preferences among high achievers. *Journal of Business and Psychology, 16*(3), 331–345.

Veenhoven, R. (1995). The cross-national patterns of happiness. Test of predictions implied in three theories of happiness. *Social Indicators Research, 34*, 33–68.

Walsh, F. (2003). Family resilience: A framework for clinical practice. *Family Process, 42*(1), 1–18.

Walsh, F. (2016). *Strengthening family resilience* (3rd ed.). New York, NY: Guilford Press.

Welch, C. E., III, & Glick, P. C. (1981). The incidence of polygamy in contemporary Africa: A research note. *Journal of Marriage and the Family, 43*(1), 191–193.

Wilson, F. (1972). *Migrant labour in South Africa*. Johannesburg, South Africa: Ravan Press.

World Health Organisation Quality of Life Group (WHOQOL). (1998). Development of the World Health Organization WHOQOL-BREF quality of life assessment. *Psychological Medicine, 28*(3), 551–558.

Yankuzo, K. I. (2014). Impact of globalization on the traditional African cultures. *International Letters of Social and Humanistic Sciences, 4*(1), 1–8.

21 "Whatever Small Thing I Have, I Should Be Grateful for": Gratitude as Understood and Experienced by African Adolescents

Tharina Guse and Tshiamo Matabane

Abstract
Gratitude is a psychological strength associated with several positive outcomes for adolescents, including increased well-being and having satisfying interpersonal relationships. Research suggests that culture could play a role in the experience and expression of gratitude. This qualitative exploratory study aimed to examine how Black adolescents understood and experienced gratitude. Six Setswana-speaking adolescents (three females and three males) participated in a focus group. Semi-structured questions explored how they defined gratitude, what they were grateful for, and how they expressed gratitude. The data was transcribed and analyzed using thematic analysis. Results indicated that the participants' understanding of gratitude was broad and generalized, with the connective nature thereof salient. The adolescents were thankful towards family and God, in line with existing research. Novel themes included gratitude for having had negative experiences and for own abilities and opportunities to excel. They also expressed gratitude through showing good behavior towards parents and others in the community. This group of African adolescents' understanding and expression of gratitude therefore seems similar to existing research, yet also be influenced by contextual variables such as culture and socio-economic context.

21.1 Introduction

Being thankful for that what we have received is a virtue universally valued across most cultures. From a psychological perspective, experiencing and expressing gratitude is important to strengthening social relationships (Wang, Wang, & Tudge, 2015) and has consistently been linked to positive psychological outcomes in adults (Wood, Froh, & Geraghty, 2010), adolescents, and children (Froh, Emmons, Card, Bono, & Wilson, 2011; Renshaw & Olinger-Steeves, 2016). However, there is increasing evidence that ethnicity and culture are important to understanding positive psychological characteristics and experiences (Oishi & Gilbert, 2016) including gratitude (Layous, Lee, Choi & Lyubomirsky, 2013; Naito, Wangan, & Taini, 2005; Tudge, Freitas, Mokrova, & Wang, 2015). To date, most research on gratitude emanated from the global north, particularly the American-European context, and cross-cultural studies focused mainly on differences

T. Guse (✉)
Department of Psychology, University of Pretoria, Pretoria, South Africa
e-mail: tharina.guse@up.ac.za

T. Matabane
Department of Psychology, University of Johannesburg, Johannesburg, South Africa

I. Eloff (ed.), *Handbook of Quality of Life in African Societies*, International Handbooks of Quality-of-Life, https://doi.org/10.1007/978-3-030-15367-0_21

between Western and Eastern participants in experiencing gratitude (e.g. Layous et al. 2013). Taking a new direction, Tudge and his colleagues (2018) investigated the development of gratitude among children from countries in the majority world, including Brazil and Guatemala, finding evidence for the importance of cultural context in the expression of gratitude. However, there is still a paucity of research on gratitude in the African context in general, and among youth in particular. In this study, we explored gratitude as understood, experienced and expressed by a group of Black South African adolescents.

21.2 What Is Gratitude?

Broadly speaking, gratitude involves an acknowledgment of having benefited from someone else's actions. Gratitude can differentially be defined as an enduring trait, a fluctuating state, or as a persisting mood (McCullough, Emmons, & Tsang, 2002; Watkins, 2014). Emmons & McCullough, (2003) viewed gratitude as a positive trait, universally found across cultures and integral to most religions. Klein (1957) asserted that the capacity for gratitude was present from birth and developed further during childhood. Later Rosenberg (1998) developed a framework for understanding gratitude as either a fluctuating state or an enduring trait. Gratitude can also extend to a transcendent source, something larger than the self, like God or a Higher Power (Wood et al., 2010). However, Lambert, Graham, and Fincham (2009) argued that defining gratitude only in terms of benefits received might be too narrow and provided evidence that lay people conceive gratitude in broader, more generalized terms.

The bulk of recent research on gratitude has followed the conceptualization offered by McCullough, Kilpatrick, Emmons, and Larson (2001), viewing it as a moral affect. This implies that an individual would be inspired to act prosocially in the future after having benefited from an act by a benefactor. According to this view, gratitude has three moral functions: as a moral barometer, moral motive, and moral reinforcer. As *moral barometer*, gratitude gives an indication of the moral climate one finds oneself in (Watkins, 2014). When we feel grateful, the moral climate is positive, and we feel good. As a *moral motive*, emotions of gratitude prompt individuals to behave pro-socially towards others. In other words, one is motivated to do good to others. Third, through expressing grateful emotions to a benefactor, whether through words or actions, gratitude becomes a *moral reinforcer* (Emmons & Shelton, 2002; McCullough et al., 2001) and may also motivate the benefactor to engage in pro-social acts again in future. Viewed as a moral affect, gratitude has a strong social element and is important to promoting connection with others (Froh et al., 2011; Yoshimura & Berzins, 2017).

As a dispositional trait, gratitude involves an individual tendency to experience thankfulness in everyday life. When this trait is present, one would experience gratitude frequently, intensely and across a wide range of eliciting situations (Emmons & McCullough, 2003). Following on the earlier work of McCullough et al. (2001, 2002), Wood et al. (2010) proposed a broader view on gratitude, describing it as a life orientation whereby the positive aspects of life, people, and the world are noticed an appreciated. Renshaw and Olinger-Steeves (2016) put forward a broad behavioral definition of gratitude as a positive response to receiving a benefit. Alternately, Tudge et al. (2015) considered gratitude to be a virtue, rather than an emotion, criticizing contemporary scholars' focus on gratitude as an emotion and life orientation.

Gratitude also implies some reciprocation (Tudge, Freitas, O'Brian, & Mokrova, 2018). Yet, research on how gratitude is expressed seems limited (Yoshimura & Berzins, 2017), despite the fact that gratitude's association with well-being not only lies in the fact that it is experienced per se but also because it is expressed (Algoe, 2012). Following on the classic work by Baumgarten-Tramer (1938) on children's expressions of gratitude, Tudge et al. (2018) embarked on several studies regarding the expression of gratitude among children and early adolescents in various cultural contexts, but knowledge on gratitude expression among older adolescents, and specifically African adolescents, seems scarce.

In a review of varied conceptualizations of gratitude, Gulliford, Morgan, and Krustjánsson (2013) concluded that there were several incompatible sub-conceptualizations of gratitude. Naito et al. (2005) further argued that the definition of gratitude is dependent on cultural context. Thus, more research is needed on what gratitude means to lay people, and how it is understood in different populations (Gulliford et al., 2013; Lambert, Graham, & Fincham, 2009).

21.3 Gratitude in Adolescence

There is increasing evidence that gratitude is positively related to subjective well-being in adolescence and negatively related to emotional distress and somatic symptoms (see Renshaw & Olinger-Steeves, 2016, for a review). Accordingly, gratitude seems to be a protective factor in positive youth development and serve as a buffer against high-risk behaviors such as drug and alcohol abuse (Ma, Kibler, & Sly, 2013). Further, being grateful has been associated with social integration and higher levels of satisfaction with self, school, friends, family community and life in general (Froh et al., 2011; Guse, Vescovelli, & Croxford, 2017; Renshaw & Olinger-Steeves, 2016). Gratitude may motivate adolescents to engage in future benevolent behaviors towards others, serving as a critical social skill in the successful navigation of developmental challenges (Froh, Bono, & Emmons, 2010). Additionally, feelings of gratitude could support identity development in adolescence (Poelker, Gibbons, Hughes, & Powlista, 2016).

Experiencing positive mental health in adolescence is key to successful developmental transition to young adulthood (O'Connor, Sanson, Toumbourou, Norrish, & Olsson, 2017) and contribute to optimal functioning in adulthood (Richards & Huppert, 2011). Since gratitude is strongly correlated with positive psychological functioning, it is important to understand its nature and mechanisms during adolescence, and in particular, in the context of culture.

21.4 Gratitude and Culture

Research on human well-being needs to consider cultural variations related to positive psychological experiences and characteristics (Oishi & Gilbert, 2016). Until recently most research on gratitude, an important correlate of well-being, has been conducted in the global north and predominantly the United States (Merçon-Vargas, Poelker, & Tudge, 2018). There is increasing evidence that the expression and experience of gratitude may be influenced by cultural variables (Diener, Oishi, & Ryan, 2013; Guse et al., 2017; Mendonça, Merçon-Vargas, Payir, & Tudge, 2018).

Some authors (e.g. Mendonça et al., 2018; Wang et al., 2015) argue that gratitude is learned through socialization processes of the culture in which individuals grow up. This is particularly important in the exploration of gratitude among youth, as adolescents constantly interact with others whose behaviors and rules inform cultural beliefs and practices (Jensen, 2012). Further, Nsamenang (2011) proposed that, in African cultures, development of the self is not only understood in terms of individual psychological and physical processes, but also in terms of social, ancestral and spiritual aspects. Therefore, Black African adolescents, growing up in the global south, may understand and express gratitude differently to adolescents in western countries.

Further evidence for the role of culture in expressing and experiencing gratitude can be found in studies examining the positive effects of engaging in gratitude activities. Layous et al. (2013) reported that American participants benefitted more from writing a gratitude letter than South Korean participants. The researchers concluded that South Koreans may be more likely to experience mixed emotions (indebtedness and gratitude) when engaging in these activities, as they experience contradictory emotions simultaneously based on Eastern philosophical tradition. More recently Mendonça et al. (2018) reported differences in the expression of gratitude among children from seven different societies. They found that children in two Asian societies (China and North Korea) were more likely to express connective gratitude (which involves reciprocity and taking the benefactor's needs into account). Conversely, children from Brazil, Guatemala, and the United States were less likely to do so.

21.5 The Current Study

It is evident that there is a need for further clarification on how gratitude is understood among ordinary people, and specifically in cultural and developmental context. Despite findings which indicate that the experience and expression of gratitude may differ across cultures, (Layous et al., 2013; Mendonça et al., 2018) most of published gratitude research seems to be based on the implicit assumption that findings obtained in the North-American context, implemented among European Americans, are equally applicable to other populations (Merçon-Vargas et al., 2018). Indeed, with the exception of recent work among youth in Brazil (Palhares, Freitas, Merçon-Vargas, & Tudge, 2018) and Guatemala (Poelker & Gibbons, 2018; Poelker, Gibbons, Maxwell, & Elizondo-Quintanilla, 2017), most studies among adolescents have been implemented in the global north. Only one study focused on gratitude among African adolescents (Guse et al., 2017), but this quantitative study also implemented questionnaires developed in the United States. Through qualitative inquiry, we aimed to address this gap in knowledge and explored how gratitude is understood, experienced and expressed by a group of Black South African adolescents.

21.6 Method

21.6.1 Participants and Procedure

Six adolescents (three female, three male), were obtained through purposive sampling and participated in a focus group. One participant (Nthabiseng) was 15 years old, while the others were 16. All the participants lived and went to school in Soweto. Information regarding each participant, using pseudonyms, is presented in Table 21.1.

Table 21.1 Demographic information of participants

Name	Gender and birth order	Background
Bakang	Male, eldest	Lived with grandmother and uncle. Mother was alive but father deceased. Had two sisters
Lesego	Male, eldest	Lived with mother, father was alive. Had one brother and one sister
Tshepiso	Male, eldest	Lived with father and stepmother. Mother was deceased. Had two sisters
Nthabiseng	Female, eldest	Lived with mother and grandmother, father was alive. Had one brother
Tshegofatso	Female, eldest	Lived with grandmother. Both parents were alive. Had one stepsibling
Naledi	Female, youngest	Lived with mother, father was alive. Had one brother and two sisters

The second author conducted a focus group using semi-structured questions, in the participants' native language (Setswana) and used audio-recordings to store the data. Questions explored how they defined gratitude, what they were grateful for, and how they expressed gratitude.

21.6.2 Data Analysis

Data was first transcribed and then analyzed using an inductive approach, following Braun and Clarke's (2006, 2013) six steps of thematic analysis. We analyzed the data mainly on a semantic level, focusing on surface level meanings (Braun & Clarke, 2006), from a realist/essentialist stance. After analyzing the data, the second author used member checking (Creswell, 2014) to provide the participants with the opportunity to authenticate their views and experiences and to enhance confirmability.

21.6.3 Ethical Considerations

The University of Johannesburg's Faculty of Humanities Research Ethics Committee approved the research. Prior to conducting interviews, parents provided written informed consent and the participants gave assent. Participation was voluntary and pseudonyms were used to ensure anonymity.

21.7 Findings

21.7.1 What Is Gratitude?

We extracted two main themes related to participants' understanding of gratitude: Gratitude is about being thankful and has to be shown or expressed.

21.7.1.1 Being Thankful

The participants all indicated that gratitude is about being thankful and appreciative. This thankfulness revolved around three sub-themes: being thankful in general, being grateful towards others, and being grateful to a Higher Power.

All the participants stated that gratitude is about *appreciating and being thankful,* for everything, including good or bad, big or small, tangible or non-tangible things around them: Bakang mentioned "…being thankful for everything you have", while Tshegofatso stated: "Gratitude is being thankful for the things that you have." Thus, for these participants, gratitude was about the 'things' they have.

Tshegofatso further stated that the quantity of what one has was irrelevant when it came to experiencing gratitude and being grateful. She said: "The little that I have, whatever small thing I have I should be grateful for it." Naledi mentioned: "For me it's being able to accept and cherish what you have, not focusing on what you don't have but focusing more on what you can do with what you have". Similarly, Tshepiso voiced that one should be grateful for what one has, irrespective of monetary value and possible status ascribed to the item:

> Like people who are wealthy they can go to a store and buy expensive items then you knowing that you are less wealthy you come with the very same thing. That wealthy person is going to tease you about having a 'fong kong' [fake goods] item and stuff. You must just be thankful that you also have such an item, even if they tease you.

The participants' expressions of being thankful for 'things' and 'everything' an individual has, reflects an attitude of being grateful, similar to the conceptualization of gratitude by Wood et al. (2010) who referred to it as "a wider life orientation towards noticing and appreciating the positives in the world" (p. 2). Their descriptions also point to a broader, generalized view of gratitude (Lambert, Graham, & Fincham, 2009) as they did not refer to a specific benefit received from a benefactor.

The second subtheme revolved around being *thankful towards others.* While the question put to the group was to define gratitude, most of the participants explained it in relation to others, and often, close relationships. Lesego encompassed both family and peers, by stating: "I'm grateful for my little brothers" and "…grateful for my friends." For Naledi and Bakang, it was their mothers. Naledi stated: "I am grateful for my mother" while Bakang reported: "I'm grateful for having a single parent (mother)." Nthabiseng, on the other hand, said she was "…grateful for my parents." These experiences indicate that, for these participants, gratitude was other-directed (Emmons, 2004; McCullough et al., 2001), and again, more generalized (Lambert, Graham, & Fincham, 2009) than associated with specific benefits received.

Nthabiseng was the only one who stated: "… we appreciate our parents for being there for us", upon which all the participants nodded and smiled. Since they defined gratitude in the context of others, the participants' understanding reflects the connective nature of gratitude (Wang et al., 2015) as they valued others' presence, existence, and availability. Further, the adolescents' understanding of gratitude in the context of others supports the notion that gratitude is a moral affect, with a strong social element, which can promote connection with others (Froh et al., 2011; Yoshimura & Berzins, 2017).

In the third sub-theme, the participants defined gratitude as an acknowledgment of a *Higher Power*. Nthabiseng stated: "we appreciate God", while Bakang stated that he was grateful towards God because of "everything that God gives you." In various other studies (Chun & Lee, 2013; Emmons & McCullough, 2003; Froh, Kashdan, Ozkowski, & Miller, 2009; Hlava & Elfers, 2014; Krause, Evans, Powers, & Hayward, 2012) participants expressed gratitude towards God. This understanding of gratitude seems to be religious in nature and refers to a sense of connection with something larger than the self (Hlava & Elfers, 2014; Wood et al., 2010). The participants' responses thus reflect the centrality of understanding gratitude through the lens of religion, similar to existing research (see Allen, 2018 for a brief review).

Taken together, the participants' understanding of gratitude seems to be broader than only a reaction to a benefit, similar to Lambert, Graham, & Fincham's (2009) view of generalized gratitude. For these adolescents, gratitude is also positioned in the context of other, mostly close relationships and contains a transpersonal element of connection to a Higher Power (Hlava & Elfers, 2014; Wood et al., 2010). While the participants' view of gratitude is similar to some existing literature, it is also possible that the centrality given to others and God may implicate culture-specific aspects such as the importance of the community, spiritual traditions and a collectivist cultural orientation (e.g. Adams, Van de Vijver, & De Bruin, 2012; Eaton & Louw, 2000; Nsamenang, 2011).

21.7.1.2 Gratitude Is the Expression of Thankfulness Towards Others

Three participants mentioned that gratitude is not only about being thankful but also about showing this gratefulness. Bakang said: "...gratitude, in another way, is how we appear to people....showing them how you appreciate by expressing yourself but like with words, words are so important for me". Nthabiseng stated: "We appreciate our parents for being there for us but what are we doing to make them see that we are appreciative?". Lesego referred to how he used his talent to show gratitude: "How you use what you are given mam. Like I was, I've been given music so it depends on how I use music mam".

Bakang's description of gratitude as a verbal expression is indicative of verbal gratitude (Baumgarten-Tramer, 1938; Freitas, Pieta, & Tudge, 2011), the simplest form of gratitude (Wang et al., 2015) which may not necessarily involve reciprocation (Mendonça et al., 2018). On the other hand, Nthabiseng's understanding reflects connective gratitude, a sense of relatedness and reciprocation (Mendonça et al., 2018) which is more common among older children and adolescents. It also points to gratitude as a moral affect, through engaging in prosocial behavior (McCullough et al., 2001). Lesego's definition points to finalistic gratitude (Baumgartner-Tramer, 1938) which refers to actions that promote personal development as a way of repaying a benefactor (Freitas et al., 2011). Since only three participants referred to the expression of gratitude as part of its definition, it seems plausible that, for this group at least, the generalized experience of being thankful was more salient than its expression.

To conclude, the adolescents in our study viewed gratitude in broad terms, as appreciation that towards others that is both experienced and expressed.

21.7.2 What Are Black South African Adolescents Grateful For?

Our second question to the group was: What are you grateful for? Four main themes emerged: (a) grateful to be part of a family, (b) grateful for friends, (c) grateful for own abilities and opportunities to excel and (d) grateful for negative experiences.

21.7.2.1 Grateful for Having Family

All the participants explained that they were grateful for their family as a whole and/or for specific family members. This included both nuclear and extended family members as well as siblings.

The first subtheme relates to *family in the broad sense*. Tshepiso said: "I'm grateful for having my family", explaining that he referred to both his nuclear and extended family. Similarly, Bakang stated that he appreciates "the whole family… my mother's family." Tshegofatso and Naledi identified specific family members for whom they were grateful for. While Naledi was grateful towards her mother, Tshegofatso spoke about gratitude towards her great-grandmother:

> She is like my mother … everything that I want and need I get it from her … even when I don't get what I want, I know that she will do something for me. So that's what I'm most grateful for … my great-grandmother.

Tshegofatso lived with her great-grandmother at the time of the research and her statement reflects the maternal role her grandmother played in her life. Bakang also lived with extended family members and expressed his gratitude towards them: "…my grandmother because I live with her and not my mother who lives in [referring to his mother living at her place of employment]". This type of living arrangement and support is common among Black African communities in South Africa (Amoateng, Heaton, & Kalule-Sabiti, 2007; Bray, Gooskens, Kahn, Moses, & Seekings, 2010). Through these practices, extended family members play multiple roles and therefore become involved in the character development, including instilling moral virtues such as gratitude, of Black adolescents. Family and family members can assist in the cultivating of gratitude, good character and overall development (Padilla-Walker, Harper, & Jensen, 2010), which seems to have been the case for these participants.

The involvement of family may also point to the experience of social support, which may be a precursor of gratitude (Reckart, Huebner, Hills, & Valois, 2017). One participant, Bakang, who is an aspiring musician, reflected on how he receives support from his family when he goes to perform: "…every time there is [a] performance at … they [are] always there, and they show me that what I'm doing is highly appreciated." This experience also supports social identity development, through feeling cared for and supported (Poelker et al., 2016).

Previous studies on gratitude among children have also found relationships to be a prominent theme (Gordon, Musher-Eizenman, Holub, & Darymple, 2004) and in particular gratitude towards family (Oros, Schulz-Begle, & Vargas-Rubilar, 2015; Poelker et al., 2017). For our participants, having parents and extended family clearly contributed to their experiences of gratitude.

The second sub-theme was being grateful for having *siblings*. Lesego mentioned that he was grateful for his "…little brothers … [as] they taught me responsibility." However, it was not easy for him in the beginning. As the first-born child, he was accustomed to receiving everything and this changed when he had siblings since they also became a priority. Tshepiso, Nthabiseng, and Bakang did not explicitly indicate that they were grateful for having siblings, but their statements alluded to it. Bakang said: "my little sisters... they taught me how to be responsible… I have to show and be a good example as I am my mother's firstborn child, so I have to guide them through the obstacles of life." Furthermore, they saw themselves as positive role models, showing good behavior such as advising and sharing with their siblings.

Within the African culture and across ethnic groups caring for siblings is a common practice (Bray et al., 2010; Nsamenang, 1992). It is possible that this source of gratitude is specific to these cultural contexts as siblings were not mentioned in earlier studies (e.g. Gordon et al., 2004; Oros et al., 2015) on what children were grateful for. The participants' comments also point to the function of gratitude as a moral reinforcer (McCullough et al., 2001), as they are showing prosocial behavior towards their siblings in exchange for the benefits they have received when they were younger.

21.7.2.2 Grateful for Friends

The second main theme relates to gratefulness towards peers for bringing, playfulness, positive emotions and support to their lives. While only

Naledi and Lesego mentioned gratitude towards friends, the other participants recounted their positive experiences with friends in response to Naledi and Lesego's statements during the interview.

Naledi was grateful for having friends as they cheered her up, making it easier for her to attend school. She said: "Another thing that I appreciate is my friends. I have 'crazy' friends… They give me a reason to come to school". Furthermore, she stated that when she experienced confrontations and was upset by life's demands, she found comfort in her friends' humor: "I sometimes leave to go and chill with my friends. They will pull a joke one has never thought about." Naledi seemed to be grateful for friends since they provided emotional support through sharing positive emotions such as humor, which may, in turn, facilitate her experience of positive emotions, including gratitude, thus contributing to an upward spiral of well-being (see broaden-and-build theory, Fredrickson, 2001, 2013).

Lesego explained how he was grateful for making friends as he used the be socially inept: "I'm also grateful for my friends mam because I'm socially awkward… I cannot make friends easily but this year mam I've changed, I can make friends." In this case, being with friends was a more challenging experience. He stated: "But mam my friends like making jokes… they can turn you into a stronger person, making fun of you. You accept it mam and then you use those jokes to make a better person of yourself." Lesego's gratitude indicates that peer influences can still be positive, even if experiences are challenging (Allen & Antonishak, 2008), and become a source of appreciation.

Earlier research (Gordon et al., 2004) also reported gratitude towards friends among children. In our study, gratitude towards friends developed not only due to positive experiences, as Naledi reported, but also through challenges in friendship experiences, as evident in Lesego's account. Thus, being grateful towards friends not only stems from experiencing their actions as benevolent (cf. McCullough et al., 2002) but also from finding the positive in the world (cf. Wood et al., 2010), including challenging situations, through using positive interpretations (Wood, Joseph & Linley, 2007).

21.7.2.3 "I Am Grateful for My Brain": Gratitude for Opportunities Due to Own Abilities

Two participants were grateful for opportunities they had to excel. Naledi said "…when I was in grade 4 or 5 I got a scholarship… [and] last year I got … a bursary … that is an opportunity I am grateful for. I'm receiving a lot of opportunities."

Lesego stated more colloquially:

> I am grateful for my brain. "Cause I was never a cool kid mam but mam, I made friends using schoolwork mam. My primary school science teacher liked placing me in science competitions, mam…so I made friends that way mam… they used to come to me and say 'can you help me with such and such?'"

He linked his intellectual abilities to the opportunity to compete and to strengthen peer relationships. Through these engagements he has also been able to help fellow learners and peers with schoolwork, illustrating prosocial behavior, which is widely associated with gratitude. (Froh et al., 2010, 2011; Tsang, 2006).

According to Wood et al. (2016), appreciating one's own abilities, as well as the environment which may have facilitated the individual's success could foster the development of gratitude. Naledi and Lesego focused on academic interests, good academic performance, and participation in extra-curricular activities which have been associated with moral gratitude (Ma et al., 2013) and finalistic gratitude (Baumgarten-Tramer, 1938). Although Poelker et al. (2015) viewed such expressions of gratitude as indicative of individualism and the need to stand out from others, the participants' experience of gratitude could also be understood against the backdrop of concerns about basic education and resource-constrained contexts in South Africa. Many children, especially those living in less affluent areas, do not have access to good education (Spaull, 2015). Thus, access to academic opportunities may be particularly valued and be a source of gratitude for South African adolescents from disadvantaged backgrounds.

21.7.2.4 "We Should Also Be Grateful for Bad Things": Gratitude Towards Negative Experiences

Several participants referred to being grateful for negative events in their lives. These negative experiences included occurrences at home, at school as well as experiences in the community.

Bakang and Naledi indicated that they were *grateful for being disciplined, by parents*, often through physical punishment. Bakang said: "The one thing I'm most grateful for that stands out, was being disciplined through being beaten". He continued to explain how he made sense of this physical punishment through the years:

> If my mother didn't discipline me the way she did, I would not be here. I wouldn't be speaking English so fluently. I would just be a person who was uneducated. So I had to understand that she has reasons why she disciplined me through beating. So that's key for me, it's important…our parents are also young and they are learning to be parents. Now she is proud of me cause of the things I do music, schooling. And every time I come with a report, she always carries a smile so for me, it's so nice me, to see that."

Naledi did not experience physical discipline but said:

> My mother is always tough on me. When we used to live with my father and we would all go to the stores I used to cry for things and my father would buy them. My mother didn't want that. If she said that you not getting it she meant that you were not getting it… [through that experience] I have learned to be patient and… to accept what I have.

Naledi also referred *to negative experiences at school*. First, she referred to friends teasing her: "We shouldn't be grateful for only the good things, we should also be grateful for bad things. You know, you can tease me but … you are strengthening me… I'm thankful for you having strengthened me". She alluded to becoming emotionally stronger through the experience.

Naledi and Bakang further spoke about being exposed to and receiving corporal punishment at school: "Grade 9, that was the best class, we used to get beaten, the whole class" (Naledi). Looking back she and four of the other participants referred to this as a positive experience, in the sense that it strengthened their friendship. Similarly, Bakang stated: "They beat us as a form of discipline, it's fine… afterwards, we can all laugh together." The researcher questioned these responses during the focus group and asked: "So you are grateful for being beaten?" to which all the participants nodded. Lesego reported more specifically on the benefits of receiving corporal punishment. He said: "It helped because you did not fail maths."

To summarise, three of the participants reported being grateful for having experienced disciplinary measures, including corporal punishment at school or at home, which could be seen as possible abuse (Dawes, de Sas Kropiwnicki, Kafaar, & Richter, 2005; Kemme, Hanslmaier, & Pfeiffer, 2014). These responses were unexpected and not reported in existing literature on what individuals are grateful for. The participants' references to being grateful for these negative experiences could be interpreted in two ways. First, it brings to mind Wood et al.'s (2016) caution about harmful gratitude. This can occur in situations that are abusive, where an individual feels powerless or compelled to feel grateful because others have either sacrificed for them or provided for them. Wood et al. (2016) argued that, if one views gratitude as a moral virtue, being grateful for experiencing physical abuse is not a virtuous reaction at all and even inappropriate. Jackson (2016) referred to propositional gratitude, which occurs when individuals find the good in malevolent or oppressive contexts and but which could be detrimental. However, earlier Fitzgerald (1998) argued that experiencing gratitude in the context of harm could prevent further harm, and promote interpersonal relationships (for our participants, strengthening friendships). Still, these instances of abuse cannot be condoned and the possibility that harmful gratitude developed cannot be ruled out.

Another possibility is that the participants made sense of these negative experiences through positive re-appraisal, gaining a more positive perspective and thus coping better (Lambert, Graham, Fincham, & Stilman, 2009). Accordingly, gratitude could have resulted from benefit-finding, a sense of personal growth which occurred following challenging events (Lechner, Zakowski, Antoni, Block, & Block, 2003). This may have been particularly relevant for Naledi, who experienced strict parenting yet reaped the benefits later, as well as Lesego and Bakang, who ascribed scholastic success to being physically punished by parents. The participants in our study, therefore, reported gratitude for experiencing physical punishment, possible bullying and strict parenting due to reframing these events as benefitting them in some way. Taken together, gratitude for the "bad things" reflects a sense of personal growth and possibly positive identity achievement (Watanabe, 2017) for these participants in our study. However, more research is needed to explore possible harmful gratitude in African contexts.

21.7.3 How Do Black South African Adolescents Express Their Gratitude?

Two main themes emerged regarding the expression of gratitude: The participants indicated that the show their gratefulness through excelling and utilizing opportunities coming their way. Second, they behave well, thus showing appreciation towards parents and family members.

21.7.3.1 Utilizing Opportunities and Excelling

Two of the participants elaborated on the various ways they use opportunities and performed well at school and extramural activities to express gratitude. Nthabiseng said:

> …I show it by going to school but not only like just going to school. There are those who come to school just to accompany others. They come to school because at home they told them to come to school…my parents can see that, OK my child is performing… which means she appreciates what we do for her.

Bakang added that he shows gratitude through "studying music … and every time there is a performance at … XX auditorium they [family] are always there, I show them how I appreciate them." These comments reflect the reciprocity associated with gratitude (Froh et al., 2010; McCullough et al., 2001). Their responses are also indicative of connective gratitude, through creating a sense of relatedness (Mendonça et al., 2018) as well as finalistic gratitude since the participants' expressions of gratitude reflect their personal growth and achievement to their families (Freitas et al., 2011). In a study among Guatemalan youth living in a low socio-economic context, Poelker et al. (2017) similarly found that the participants showed gratitude by doing well and trying their best. Therefore, expressing gratitude through performing well may be more prominent in contexts were opportunities and resources are scarce, which may also have been the case for the adolescents in our study.

21.7.3.2 "I Show Them by the Way I Behave": Expressing Gratitude Through "Good" Behavior

Four of the participants reported that they showed their gratitude by doing what was requested of them in the family context. Tshegofatso stated: "I show my appreciation by doing anything that is asked of me to do at home," while Lesego reported "…I show my gratitude to my family mam, in any way possible mam. I can babysit my little brothers mam… My parents are divorced mam so my father gives me an allowance mam so if my mother works late I can buy bread you know".

Naledi referred to applying values and principles she has been taught at home as her way of showing her gratitude towards the family. She said: "I show them by the way I behave. What they have taught me at home." Enacting these values also went wide than her immediate family, as she also helped her neighbors: "So I would be coming back from school tired of carrying my heavy bag and my neighbor, a woman, would send me somewhere…I don't complain I just take the money and go buy what she has asked me."

Tsepiso said:

> I show my appreciation by being respectful. Like at home sometimes they ask you to do your chores like cleaning and you cheat and hide things under the bed and stuff so sometimes you must show that you are thankful, so I would start 'spring cleaning' by shifting the beds so that they can be happy.

Nthabiseng expressed gratitude by looking after her cousin, who lived with them and who was a bit of a troublemaker: "For me, it's by taking responsibility. Like when my mother wants to go somewhere I would say to her, go ma, go I will keep an eye on him."

These expressions of gratitude reflect its function as a moral motive and moral reinforcer, where feelings of being grateful can motivate individuals to engage in pro-social behavior (Emmons & Shelton, 2002; McCullough et al., 2001) through doing good deeds and reciprocating through morally valued "good" behavior.

21.8 Conclusion

The main aim of our study was to explore gratitude as understood, experienced and expressed by a group of Black South African adolescents. Our findings suggested that their understanding of gratitude support a broader, generalized (cf. Lambert, Graham, & Fincham, 2009) view of being thankful in general for what they have, and for the presence of significant others in their lives. They further described gratitude in the context of a connection to a Higher Power, as previously suggested by Wood et al. (2010). The participants also described gratitude in terms of its expression. In other words, gratitude is not only an emotion but has to be enacted (Tudge et al., 2018) which could ultimately enhance well-being (Algoe, 2012). Taken together, the responses of the adolescents who participated in the study support the view that gratitude is found and valued across cultures (Emmons & McCullough, 2003). However, the fact that the adolescents in our study made specific reference to the presence of family members, without receiving a tangible benefit, also alludes to the importance of cultural context in the understanding of gratitude. In the African context, adolescent identity development is characterized by an evolving awareness of the self as being interconnected to others (Nsamenang, 2008; Ramakgopa, 2001). Further, the collectivistic nature of African culture, which places emphasis on interdependence and interpersonal relationships (Adams et al., 2012), may facilitate an understanding of gratitude as being connective, a way of recognizing others and a communal experience for these African adolescents.

Our second objective was to establish what the participants were grateful for in their lives. They referred to being grateful towards others (family and friends), opportunities, and also, negative occurrences in their lives. While previous research has also pointed to the prominence of family (Gordon et al., 2004; Oros et al., 2015) and friends (Gordon et al., 2004) in the experience of gratitude, it was evident that our participants also experienced gratitude in the context of community. In other words, the importance ascribed to the wider community, as characteristic of collectivistic societies (Adams et al., 2012), implicates that being thankful is not only experienced towards close family but also towards others in the community (friends, community members). Being grateful for opportunities is possibly also unique to this study and could be seen against the backdrop of the resource-constrained contexts in which many young Black South Africans grow up. The fourth aspect for which the participants in our study were grateful for, was somewhat unexpected. Being thankful for negative events, some of which could be seen as abuse was not reported in existing literature. Although this may reflect harmful gratitude (Wood et al., 2016), it is also likely that the adolescents used positive re-appraisal to make sense of negative events. Therefore, they were able to experience personal growth, which is expressed through being thankful for the event. Nonetheless, more research on possible harmful gratitude among adolescents is needed. Our findings thus suggest that, while some sources of gratitude (e.g. family) may be universal, cultural context, as well as socio-economic realities, could contribute gratitude for specific aspects of adolescents' lives.

The third aim was to investigate how the adolescents expressed gratitude. Their responses broadly indicated that they engage in prosocial behaviors (McCullough et al., 2001) such as helping others or showing 'good' behaviors. These acts reflect connective gratitude, which is more common among older children and adolescents (Freitas et al., 2011). However, these expressions of gratitude are also indicative of the importance African societies place on altruism and cooperation (Ramokgopa, 2001). In addition, some of the participants indicated that they express their gratitude, mainly towards parents, by excelling at school or in extramural activities. While this may reflect finalistic gratitude (Baumgarten-Tramer, 1938), in the African context this may also be a way of recognizing others (Nsamenang, 2008: Ramakgopa, 2001) and being mindful of the opportunities that many others in the greater community may not have. Thus, the expression of gratitude by the adolescents in our study includes both universal and culture-specific aspects.

While our study does bring some new insight into gratitude in the African context, it does have limitations. Using a focus group may have limited the responses of some of the participants. In-depth interviews may yield richer information and are recommended to further explore the unique aspects of gratitude among African adolescents we found in our study. In particular, it may be beneficial to explore gratitude in the context of negative occurrences and harmful contexts. Another limitation is that concerns that fact that the finding only reflects the view of one language group, living in a particular socio-economic context. Further research could include adolescents from other ethnic groups, as well as those living in rural areas.

To conclude, our findings suggest that, overall, gratitude may indeed be a universal virtue, but its experience and expression may be influenced by contextual variables, such as culture and socio-economic context. It is therefore important to consider these variables in planning and implementing interventions to enhance gratitude.

References

Adams, B. G., Van de Vijver, F. J., & De Bruin, G. P. (2012). Identity in South Africa: Examining self-descriptions across ethnic groups. *International Journal of Intercultural Relations, 36*(3), 377–388.

Algoe, S. B. (2012). Find, remind, and bind: The functions of gratitude in everyday relationships. *Social and Personality Psychology Compass, 6*, 455–469.

Allen, J. P., & Antonishak, J. (2008). Adolescent peer influences: Beyond the dark side. In M. J. Prinstein & K. A. Dodge (Eds.), *Understanding peer influence in children and adolescence* (pp. 141–160). New York, NY: Guilford.

Allen, S. (2018). *The science of gratitude* [White paper]. Retrieved August 23, 2018, from https://www.templeton.org/wp-content/uploads/2018/05/GGSC-JTF-White-Paper-Gratitude-FINAL.pdf

Amoateng, A. Y., Heaton, T. B., & Kalule-Sabiti, I. (2007). Living arrangements in South Africa. In A. Y. Amoateng & T. B. Heaton (Eds.), *Families and households in post-apartheid South Africa: Socio-demographic perspectives* (pp. 43–59). Cape Town, South Africa: Human Sciences Research Council Press.

Baumgarten-Tramer, F. (1938). "Gratefulness" in children and young people. *Journal of Genetic Psychology, 53*, 53–66.

Braun, V., & Clarke, V. (2006). Using thematic analysis in psychology. *Qualitative Research in Psychology, 3*, 77–101. https://doi.org/10.1191/1478088706qp063oa

Braun, V., & Clarke, V. (2013). *Successful qualitative research: A practical guide for beginners*. Los Angeles, CA: Sage.

Bray, R., Gooskens, I., Kahn, L., Moses, S., & Seekings, J. (2010). *Growing up in the new South Africa: Childhood and adolescence in post-apartheid Cape Town*. Cape Town, South Africa: Human Sciences Research Council Press.

Chun, S., & Lee, Y. (2013). "I am just thankful": The experience of gratitude following traumatic spinal cord injury. *Disability and Rehabilitation, 35*(1), 11–19. https://doi.org/10.3109/09638288.2012.687026

Creswell, J. W. (2014). *Research design: Qualitative, quantitative and mixed methods approaches* (4th ed.). Los Angeles, CA: Sage Publications.

Dawes, A., de Sas Kropiwnicki, Z. O., Kafaar, Z., & Richter, L. (2005). *Corporal punishment of children: A south African national survey*. Cape Town, South Africa: Human Sciences Research Council Press.

Diener, E., Oishi, S., & Ryan, K. L. (2013). Universals and cultural differences in the causes and structure of happiness: A multilevel review. In C. L. M. Keyes

(Ed.), *Mental well-being* (pp. 153–176). Dordrecht, The Netherlands: Springer.

Eaton, L., & Louw, L. (2000). Culture and self in South Africa: Individualism/collectivism predictions. *Journal of Social Psychology, 140*, 210–218. https://doi.org/10.1080/00224540009600461

Emmons, R. A. (2004). The psychology of gratitude: An introduction. In R. A. Emmons & M. E. McCullough (Eds.), *The psychology of gratitude* (pp. 3–16). New York, NY: Oxford University Press.

Emmons, R. A., & McCullough, M. E. (2003). Counting blessings versus burdens: An experimental investigation of gratitude and subjective well-being in daily life. *Journal of Personality and Social Psychology, 84*, 377–389. https://doi.org/10.1037/0022-3514.84.2.377

Emmons, R. A., & Shelton, C. M. (2002). Gratitude and the science of positive psychology. In C. R. Snyder & S. J. Lopez (Eds.), *Handbook of positive psychology* (pp. 459–471). New York, NY: Oxford University Press.

Fitzgerald, P. (1998). Gratitude and justice. *Ethics, 109*, 119–153.

Fredrickson, B. L. (2001). The role of positive emotions in positive psychology. The broaden-and-build theory of positive emotions. *American Psychologist, 56*, 218–226. https://doi.org/10.1037/0003-066X.56.3.218

Fredrickson, B. L. (2013). Positive emotions broaden and build. In P. Devine & A. Plant (Eds.), *Advances in experimental social psychology* (Vol. 47, pp. 1–53). Burlington, VA: Academic.

Freitas, L. B. L., Pieta, M. A. M., & Tudge, J. R. H. (2011). Beyond politeness: The expression of gratitude in children and adolescents. *Psicologia: Reflexão e Crítica, 24*(4), 757–764. https://doi.org/10.1590/S0102-79722011000400016

Froh, J. J., Bono, G., & Emmons, R. (2010). Being grateful is beyond good manners: Gratitude and motivation to contribute to society among early adolescents. *Motivation and Emotion, 34*, 144–157.

Froh, J. J., Emmons, R. A., Card, N. A., Bono, G., & Wilson, J. (2011). Gratitude and the reduced costs of materialism in adolescents. *Journal of Happiness Studies, 12*(2), 289–302. https://doi.org/10.1007/s10902-010-9195-9

Froh, J. J., Kashdan, T. B., Ozimkowski, K. M., & Miller, N. (2009). Who benefits the most from a gratitude intervention in children and adolescents? Examining positive affect as a moderator. *Journal of Positive Psychology, 4*, 408–422. https://doi.org/10.1080/17439760902992464

Gordon, A. K., Musher-Eizenman, D. R., Holub, S. C., & Dalrymple, J. (2004). What are children thankful for? An archival analysis of gratitude before and after the attacks of September 11. *Applied Developmental Psychology, 25*, 541–553.

Gulliford, L., Morgan, B., & Kristjánsson, K. (2013). Recent work on the concept of gratitude in philosophy and psychology. *The Journal of Value Inquiry, 47*, 285–317.

Guse, T., Vescovelli, F., & Croxford, S.-A. (2017). Subjective well-being and gratitude among South African adolescents. *Youth & Society*. https://doi.org/10.1177/0044118X17697237

Hlava, P., & Elfers, J. (2014). The lived experience of gratitude. *Journal of Humanistic Psychology, 54*(4), 434–455. https://doi.org/10.1177/0022167813508605.

Jackson, L. (2016). Why should I be grateful? The morality of gratitude in contexts marked by injustice. *Journal of Moral Education, 45*(3), 276–290.

Jensen, L. A. (2012). Bridging universal and cultural perspectives: A vision for developmental psychology in a global world. *Child Development Perspectives, 6*, 98–104. https://doi.org/10.1111/j.1750-8606.2011.00213.x

Kemme, S., Hanslmaier, M., & Pfeiffer, C. (2014). Experience of parental corporal punishment in childhood and adolescence and its effect on punitiveness. *Journal of Family Violence, 29*, 129–142. https://doi.org/10.1007/s10896-013-9564-3

Klein, M. (1957). *Envy and gratitude: A study of unconscious sources*. New York, NY: Basic Books.

Krause, N., Evans, L. A., Powers, G., & Hayward, R. D. (2012). Feeling grateful to God: A qualitative inquiry. *The Journal of Positive Psychology, 7*, 119–130. https://doi.org/10.1080/17439760.2012.656691

Lambert, N. M., Graham, S. M., & Fincham, F. D. (2009). A prototype analysis of gratitude: Varieties of gratitude experiences. *Personality and Social Psychology Bulletin, 35*, 1193–1207.

Lambert, N. M., Graham, S. M., Fincham, F. D., & Stillman, T. F. (2009). A changed perspective: How gratitude can affect sense of coherence through positive reframing. *The Journal of Positive Psychology, 4*, 461–470.

Layous, K., Lee, H., Choi, I., & Lyubomirsky, S. (2013). Culture matters when designing a successful happiness-increasing activity: A comparison of the United States and South Korea. *Journal of Cross-Cultural Psychology, 44*, 1294–1303. https://doi.org/10.1177/0022022113487591

Lechner, S. C., Zakowski, S. G., Antoni, M. H., Greenhawt, M., Block, K., & Block, P. (2003). Do sociodemographic and disease-related variables influence benefit-finding in cancer patients? *Psycho-Oncology, 12*, 491–499.

Ma, M., Kibler, J. L., & Sly, K. (2013). Gratitude is associated with greater levels of protective factors and lower levels of risks in African American adolescents. *Journal of Adolescence, 36*, 983–991.

McCullough, M. E., Emmons, R. A., & Tsang, J. (2002). The grateful disposition: A conceptual and empirical topography. *Journal of Personality and Social Psychology, 82*, 112–127.

McCullough, M. E., Kilpatrick, S. D., Emmons, R. A., & Larson, D. B. (2001). Is gratitude a moral affect? *Psychological Bulletin, 127*, 249–266. https://doi.org/10.1037//0033-2909.127.2.249

Mendonça, S. E., Merçon-Vargas, E. A., Payir, A., & Tudge, J. R. (2018). The development of gratitude

in seven societies: Cross-cultural highlights. *Cross-Cultural Research, 52*, 135–150.
Mercon-Vargas, E. A., Poelker, K. E., & Tudge, J. R. (2018). The development of the virtue of gratitude: Theoretical foundations and cross-cultural issues. *Cross-Cultural Research, 52*, 3–18.
Naito, T., Wangwan, J., & Tani, M. (2005). Gratitude in university students in Japan and Thailand. *Journal of Cross-Cultural Psychology, 36*, 247–263. https://doi.org/10.1177/0022022104272904
Nsamenang, A. B. (1992). *Human development in cultural context: A third world perspective*. Newbury Park, CA: Sage.
Nsamenang, A. B. (2008). Culture and human development. *International Journal of Psychology, 43*, 73–77. https://doi.org/10.1080/00207590701859093
Nsamenang, A. B. (2011). The culturalization of developmental trajectories: A perspective on African childhoods and adolescences. In L. A. Jensen (Ed.), *Bridging cultural and developmental approaches to psychology: New syntheses in theory, research, and policy* (pp. 235–254). New York, NY: Oxford University Press.
O'Connor, M., Sanson, A. V., Toumbourou, J. W., Norrish, J., & Olsson, C. A. (2017). Does positive mental health in adolescence longitudinally predict healthy transitions in young adulthood? *Journal of Happiness Studies, 18*, 177–198.
Oishi, S., & Gilbert, E. A. (2016). Current and future directions in culture and happiness research. *Current Opinion in Psychology, 8*, 54–58. https://doi.org/10.1016/j.copsyc.2015.10.005
Oros, L. B., Schulz-Begle, A., & Vargas-Rubilar, J. (2015). Children's gratitude: Implication of contextual and demographic variables in Argentina. *Revista Latinoamericana de Ciencias Sociales, Niñez Y Juventud, 13*, 245–262. https://doi.org/10.11600/1692715x.13213160315
Padilla-Walker, L. M., Harper, J. M., & Jensen, A. C. (2010). Self-regulation as a mediator between sibling relationship quality and early adolescents' positive and negative outcomes. *Journal of Family Psychology, 24*, 419–428. https://doi.org/10.1037/a0020387
Palhares, F., Freitas, L. B., Merçon-Vargas, E. A., & Tudge, J. R. (2018). The development of gratitude in Brazilian children and adolescents. *Cross-Cultural Research, 52*, 31–43.
Poelker, K. E., & Gibbons, J. L. (2018). The development of gratitude in Guatemalan children and adolescents. *Cross-Cultural Research, 52*, 44–57. https://doi.org/10.1177/1069397117736518
Poelker, K. E., Gibbons, J. L., Hughes, H. M., & Powlishta, K. K. (2016). Feeling grateful and envious: Adolescents' narratives of social emotions in identity and social development. *International Journal of Adolescence and Youth, 21*(3), 289–303.
Poelker, K. E., Gibbons, J. L., Maxwell, C. A., & Elizondo-Quintanilla, I. L. (2017). Envy, gratitude, and well-being among Guatemalan adolescents with scarce economic resources. *International Perspectives in Psychology: Research, Practice, Consultation, 6*, 209. https://doi.org/10.1080/02673843.2015.1067895
Ramokgopa, I. M. (2001). *Developmental stages of an African child and their psychological implications: A comparative study.* (Unpublished Doctoral dissertation.) Rand Afrikaans University, Johannesburg, South Africa.
Reckart, H., Huebner, E. S., Hills, K. J., & Valois, R. F. (2017). A preliminary study of the origins of early adolescents' gratitude differences. *Personality and Individual Differences, 116*, 44–50.
Renshaw, T. L., & Olinger Steeves, R. M. (2016). What good is gratitude in youth and schools? A systematic review and meta-analysis of correlates and intervention outcomes. *Psychology in the Schools, 53*, 286–305.
Richards, M., & Huppert, F. a. (2011). Do positive children become positive adults? Evidence from a longitudinal birth cohort study. *The Journal of Positive Psychology, 6*, 75–87. https://doi.org/10.1080/17439760.2011.536655
Rosenberg, E. L. (1998). Levels of analysis and the organization of affect. *Review of General Psychology, 2*, 247–270.
Spaull, N. (2015). Schooling in South Africa: How low-quality education becomes a poverty trap. In A. de Lannoy, S. Swartz, L. Lake, & C. Smith (Eds.), *South African child gauge* (pp. 34–41). Cape Town, South Africa: Children's Institute, University of Cape Town.
Tsang, J. (2006). Gratitude and prosocial behaviour: An experimental test of gratitude. *Cognition and Emotion, 20*, 138–148. https://doi.org/10.1080/02699930500172341
Tudge, J. R. H., Freitas, L. B. D. L., Mokrova, I. L., Wang, Y. C., & O'Brien, M. (2015). The wishes and expression of gratitude of youth. *Paidéia (Ribeirão Preto), 25*, 281–288.
Tudge, J. R. H., Freitas, L. B. L., O'Brien, L., & Mokrova, I. L. (2018). Methods for studying the virtue of gratitude cross-culturally. *Cross-Cultural Research, 52*, 19–30. https://doi.org/10.1177/1069397117737017
Wang, D., Wang, Y. C., & Tudge, J. R. H. (2015). Expressions of gratitude in children and adolescents: Insights from China and the United States. *Journal of Cross-Cultural Psychology, 46*, 1039–1058. https://doi.org/10.1177/0022022115594140
Watanabe, H. (2017). The mediating effects of benefit finding on the relationship between the identity centrality of negative stressful events and identity achievement. *Identity, 17*, 13–24. https://doi.org/10.1080/15283488.2016.1268536
Watkins, P. C. (2014). *Gratitude and the good life: Toward a psychology of appreciation*. Dordrecht, The Netherlands: Springer.
Wood, A. M., Emmons, R. A., Algoe, S. B., Froh, J. J., Lambert, N. M., & Watkins, P. (2016). A dark side of gratitude? Distinguishing between beneficial gratitude and its harmful impostors for the positive clinical psychology of gratitude and well-being. In A. M. Wood &

J. Johnson (Eds.), *The Wiley handbook of positive clinical psychology* (pp. 137–151). Chichester, UK: Wiley.

Wood, A. M., Froh, J. J., & Geraghty, A. W. A. (2010). Gratitude and well-being: A review and theoretical integration. *Clinical Psychology Review, 30*, 890–905.

Wood, A. M., Joseph, S., & Linley, P. A. (2007). Coping style as a psychological resource of grateful people. *Journal of Social and Clinical Psychology, 26*, 1076–1093. https://doi.org/10.1521/jscp.2007.26.9.1076

Yoshimura, S. M., & Berzins, K. (2017). Grateful experiences and expressions: The role of gratitude expressions in the link between gratitude experiences and well-being. *Review of Communication, 17*, 106–118. Wiley.

22 Researching Children's Subjective Well-Being in South Africa: Considerations for Method, Theory, and Social Policy

Shazly Savahl, Sabirah Adams, Elizabeth Benninger, Maria Florence, Kyle Jackson, Donnay Manuel, Mulalo Mpilo, Umesh Bawa, and Deborah Isobell

Abstract
In the current South African socio-political framework children have been afforded the highest priority within government. Not only have the rights and needs of children been entrenched in the development strategies of the government, but children themselves have been guaranteed socio-economic rights and protection from abuse, exploitation, and neglect. Subsequently, knowledge and information on the well-being of children have become important pursuits. It has also become increasingly important to obtain an understanding of what children regard as important to their well-being. The current chapter explores the importance of researching children's subjective perceptions of well-being. It considers the current methods of engaging with children about their subjective perceptions of various aspects of their lives, outlines the status of theoretical advancement, and importantly, considers the implications for social policy. The authors motivate for a focus on participatory methodologies and argue for the increased investment in research using these methodologies. Finally, they recommend that an effective child indicator system should include a consideration of subjective well-being and should follow a 'rights based' approach.

22.1 Introduction

The history of children and childhood in South Africa is that of adversity, characterised by social oppression, inequality, poverty, and exposure to various forms of violence, abuse, and neglect. Owing to apartheid, the prohibition of equal access to the law, property, and freedom of movement centrally impacted on families and their capacity for providing a healthy, oppression-free life for their children. The disparate and stratified allocation of resources across the racial classifi-

S. Savahl (✉) · E. Benninger · M. Florence
K. Jackson · D. Manuel · M. Mpilo · U. Bawa
D. Isobell
Department of Psychology, University of the Western Cape, Cape Town, South Africa
e-mail: ssavahl@uwc.ac.za

S. Adams
Language Development Group, Centre for Higher Education Development, University of Cape Town, Cape Town, South Africa

I. Eloff (ed.), *Handbook of Quality of Life in African Societies*, International Handbooks of Quality-of-Life, https://doi.org/10.1007/978-3-030-15367-0_22

cation system enforced during apartheid, had a deleterious effect on the development of children. The discriminatory unequal spend on the education and health of the 'Black child' resulted in a loss of investment in the well-being and development of a generation. This ongoing underdevelopment has persisted post-apartheid, with the transgenerational transmission of trauma, internalised inadequacy, poverty, and inequity. Several theorists (see e.g. Biko, 1978; Bulhan, 1985) suggest that the legacy of social oppression manifests in chronically high levels of violence, trauma, and social inequality among the youth who display negative behaviours emergent from the vestiges of internalised apartheid oppression. They bear the mark of an 'apartheid of the heart'; where healing from the trauma of prolonged oppression has not taken place. Following the advent of democracy in 1994, the newly-elected South African government instituted a range of legislations to redress the atrocities that children experienced in the past, and to improve the overall quality of life (QoL) and developmental trajectories of children. The first of these legal commitments is evident in Section 28 of the Bill of Rights (South African Constitution, p. 1255) which details children's basic human rights and advances the notion that "A child's best interest are of paramount importance in every matter concerning the child". This was complemented by the ratification of the United Nations Convention on the Rights of the Child (UNCRC) on the 16th of June 1995, which is guided by four principles: the first, 'non-discrimination/equity', ensures that all children, groups of children, and children in general are entitled to the same rights as adults without discrimination. The second principle safeguards that all actions concerning children take into account 'the child's best interests'. The third guiding principle outlines children's right to 'survival and development' and the State's responsibility to ensure that all children are able to reach their potential to its maximum extent. The fourth principle refers to 'participation/inclusion' and children's right to express their own views in all matters pertaining to children, and that these opinions are given due consideration as it relates to their maturity and evolving capacities. There is thus an obligation to listen to children and to facilitate their participation in all matters that concern them within the family, school, public services, institutions, communities, government policies and judicial procedures.

Further legislative advancement is evident in child-specific legislation, including the Children's Act (No. 38 of 2005), the associated Children's Amendment Act (No. 41 of 2007), and the Child Justice Act (2008). Furthermore, through the Social Security Agency Act of 2004 the government has ensured that children are the beneficiaries of social grants to mitigate against vulnerability and poverty. Acceding to these legal contracts has entrenched the rights and needs of children in the development strategies of the government, as well as guaranteeing children's socio-economic rights and protection from abuse, exploitation, and neglect. Co-ordinated by the Office on the Rights of the Child (ORC), the National Programme of Action (NPAC) was put in place to provide "an holistic framework for the integration of all policies and plans developed by government departments and civil society to promote the well-being of children" (2012, p. 9). With children elevated to the legal status of rights holders, and the government ultimately accountable as the principal duty-bearer, children's well-being and QoL are ostensibly afforded the highest priority within government.

Over the past two decades, the South African government has also made significant progress in developing strategies to measure the state and well-being of children. These initiatives highlighted the development and collection of objective indicators, which refer to observable measures that assess a range of pre-determined objective standards of living. However, after 25 years of democracy and despite the legislative advancements, the QoL for South Africa's children remains compromised (Savahl & Adams et al., 2015). This to a large extent is reflective of the high levels of social inequality in South Africa, which is regarded as an important indicator of children's well-being. Notwithstanding the fundamental premise of equality in the South African Constitution, inequality remains pervasive in the country. With a Gini Index of 0.63 (World Bank, 2018), considered to be one of the highest in the world (in terms of wealth and income), it demonstrates a great dispersion of both wealth and income between the privileged and the disadvantaged. Although this inequality is experienced by the majority of the population, the burdens of these multiple overlapping layers of inequality are often endured by children who necessitate care and supervision from adults for both safety and basic tenets of their well-being (Hall, Woolard, Lake, & Smith, 2012).

22.2 *Quality of Life* of South African Children: Key Objective Indicators

When considering objective standards of children's QoL in South Africa (SA), it is incumbent to acknowledge the historical 'situatedness' of childhood that has resulted in a plurality of childhood experiences. This 'plurality' is best understood if the objective QoL indicators are examined from the position of social inequality, whereby unequal social backgrounds in general have reinforced unequal conditions (Bray Gooskens, Kahn, Moses, & Seekings, 2010). Regardless of the fundamental premise of the South African Constitution, high levels of social inequality remain prevalent, where a great dispersion of wealth and income between the privileged and the disadvantaged exist (Savahl, Casas, & Adams, 2015). This has resulted in the disparity between the privileged and underprivileged communities (Savahl & Malcolm, et al., 2015). While high socio-economic status (SES) communities are characterised by high income, high educational attainment, high levels of employment, and low incidence of violence; underprivileged communities are characterised by low educational attainment and income, high rates of substance use, unemployment, crime, and violence (Savahl & Malcolm, et al., 2015). Further, access to basic resources such as water and sanitation, electricity, formal housing, food, and nutrition and health care are limited. These burdens are often endured by children, who depend on adults for care, supervision, safety and basic tenets of well-being (Hall, Woolard, Lake, & Smith, 2012).

Children living in low SES communities in South Africa experience deficiencies in nutrition, environmental health, and care. Research has shown that children who experience deficiencies in these three domains have a 30% higher likelihood of stunting (United Nations Committee on the Rights of the Child, 2016). In South Africa, 27% of children under 5 years old and 25% of those aged 6 months to 2 years old are stunted (Jamieson, Berry, & Lake, 2017). Additionally, the under-five mortality rate is reported at 42 per 1000, and the infant and neonatal mortality rates are 32.5 per 1000 and 12.4 per 1000 respectively. Furthermore, 62% of South Africa children live below the upper bound of the poverty line, whereas 13% live in extreme poverty with, 29% living below the food poverty line. Additionally, 13% of households report child hunger, with as many as 77% of children aged 6–23 months fed inadequate diets (Jamieson et al., 2017). To mitigate the unfavourable living conditions and the adverse effects of malnutrition, the South African government introduced the Child Support Grant which catered for approximately 11.7 million children in 2015. The grant aims to provide a safety net for poor households and improve the child's welfare and nutrition.

In relation to education, school enrolment is reasonably high at 97% for 7–17 year olds (Jamieson et al., 2017). In 2015, 12,814,473 learners were registered in primary and secondary schools, attending 25,691 schools with 416,093 teachers (Department of Education, 2017). South Africa has a school fee exemption policy, in compliance with Article 11 of the UNCRC, whereby school fees are waived for families who are unable to afford it. In terms of school completion, there is great variation with 90% of children completing primary school and 40% completing secondary schooling (UNICEF, 2017). Further, children from low SES communities are three times less likely to complete school. Given the high levels of inequality, many township and rural schools are poorly resourced, which impacts on children receiving quality education. Grade repetition and incomplete schooling are a common phenomena in low SES schools, with pregnancy and disability accounting for 11% of incomplete schooling (Jamieson et al., 2017).

Violence against children is a pervasive problem in South Africa. The majority of the perpetrators of child sexual and physical abuse are people closest to them. Unsafe school environments pose a significant risk for children who may be exposed to corporal punishment, cruel and humiliating forms of psychological punishment, sexual and gender-based violence, and bullying (Jamieson et al., 2017). Violence at school is considered a barrier to both quality education and ultimately QoL. Between January and March 2017, most reported child victims of crime in South Africa were female (84.7%) (and 15.3% males) (South African Police Statistics, 2017). Specifically, 4028 children were victims of rape; 704 children were victims of sexually assault; 2742 experienced common assault; 40 cases of attempted murder were reported; 2248 children fell victim to assault (grievous bodily harm); and 196 children were murdered (Statistics South Africa, 2017). More than double the global average, the child homicide rate is 5.5 per 100, 000 (Jamieson et al., 2017). Children younger than 5 years are at risk of fatal child abuse by someone close to them, and teenage boys are most likely to be killed in the context of male-on-male interpersonal violence (Jamieson et al., 2017).

Children are at a greater risk of experiencing or perpetrating violence when: parents are absent; they are subjected to domestic violence in the home; they live in underprivileged households; and when they are exposed to alcohol or drugs and crime within their community (Jamieson et al., 2017). This poses a greater threat to children living within impoverished communities as low levels of income, high rates of substance use, unemployment, crime and violence characterise these communities (Savahl & Adams, et al., 2015). Therefore, being a victim of violence causes children to be vulnerable to mental and physical health outcomes such as depression, anxiety and posttraumatic stress disorder. Essentially, poverty is a critical artefact of inequality within the country and is also one of the key determinants of children's standard of living and well-being. Action is required to enable an environment where children are well-nourished, protected from disease, have appropriate educational opportunities, feel safe, and live within a stress-free environment.

22.3 Importance of Researching Subjective Well-Being and *Quality of Life*

In recent years, many prominent political and intellectual leaders have indicated that improving and measuring QoL is crucial to ensuring that children become active members of their societies, communities, and families, which further contributes to general economic growth (Rees, Goswami, & Pople, 2013). Failure to promote and enhance the well-being of children has been linked to several negative outcomes namely, impaired cognitive development, lower levels of school achievement, that links to greater unemployment rates, reduced skill development, productivity, and earnings. Consequently, these outcomes place a greater burden on welfare systems, an increased prevalence of crime and antisocial behaviour, mental health related illness and an increase in drug and alcohol use that directly impact on health care costs and related services. Measuring child well-being is therefore essential to policy-making, the allocation of resources, advocacy, and the process of transparency and accountability (UNICEF Office of Research, 2013). While governments have made great strides in developing indicators to measure children's objective standards of living, researchers have pointed to obtaining children's subjective perceptions and experiences of their lives as critical in measuring overall QoL.

The nascent interest in children's well-being has expanded exponentially since the adoption of the UNCRC (Savahl & Malcolm et al., 2015). The propagation of the concept of well-being can be located in the work of Jahoda (1958), and more specifically the concept of positive psychological health, and is later evident in studies of QoL, and happiness (see Casas, 1997; Cummins, 1995), standard of living and health; as well as the field of social psychology. The conventional understanding of well-being was premised upon the absence of ill-health and disease. The history of the concept of well-being in the scientific research arena (in the health and social sciences), followed two distinct pathways both unfolding in the twentieth century (Ben-Arieh, Casas, Frønes, & Korbin, 2014). The foundations of well-being in the health sciences was premised upon a more positive conception, based on the World Health Organisations' (1946) preface of its initial articles of association, wherein it is defined well-being as "Health is a state of complete physical, mental and social well-being, and not merely the absence of disease or infirmity" (as cited in Vásquez, Hervás, Rahona, & Gómez, 2009, p. 16).

Within the social sciences, however, the foundations were fuelled by the 'social indicators movement' of the 1960s, consisting of an interconnected web of understandings and perspectives from academics across several disciplines. Social scientists as well as public officials in this 'movement' demonstrated that well-measured and coherent social indicators afford an approach to monitor and examine the circumstances of groups of individuals- in particular families and children (Land, 2000). Contemporary notions of well-being have envisaged developing an integrated model that amalgamates the treatment and prevention of problem behaviour and promoting strengths approaches. As Sandin (2014) critically notes:

> Consequently, well-being is also dependent on the definitions of childhood as shaped by gender, class, age definitions, and ethnicity, as well as on how care for children has been organized in different societies. It is intimately associated with how welfare surrounding children is historically understood, which, in turn, is also dependent on, among others, the definitions of the rights and social status of children and the legal role of the family. (p. 31)

Within the literature subjective well-being (SWB), QoL, and happiness are often used synonymously and present with substantial conceptual overlap (Camfield & Skevington, 2008; Medvedev & Landhuis, 2018). Diener (2000) in particular, considers SWB to be a key component of QoL. He defines SWB as an overarching concept that includes the cognitive and affective evaluations that individuals make about their lives, the circumstances influencing their lives, and the conditions in which they live (Diener, 2000, 2006; Diener, Lucas, & Oishi, 2005). The cognitive component refers to perceptions of global and domain-specific life satisfaction, while the affective component refers to the experience of positive and negative affect. Diener (2009) conceptualises these components as fitting on a 'tripartite' hierarchical structure that are conceptually aligned, moderately correlated, and with each making a unique contribution towards SWB. Theoretically, this model represents the first level deconstruction if regressed onto the single-item on life satisfaction: "How satisfied are you with your life as a whole"? (Cummins, 2000). Recently, some authors (Savahl, Casas, Adams, Gonzalez and Figuer, 2019) have revised Diener's model, instead proposing that the cognitive component, presents with two separate components – conceptualised as domain-specific and context-free components. They put forward an overall Quadripartite Model of SWB, consisting of domain specific and context-free cognitive components and positive and negative affect. Given the contention and lack of consensus around these constructs, the recent study by Medvedev and Langhuis (2018) sought to explore the relation between happiness, SWB, and QoL. These constructs were assessed using three widely used standardised scales to assess each aforementioned construct, namely the Oxford Happiness Questionnaire (Hills & Argyle, 2002), World Health Organisation Quality Of Life – BREF questionnaire (WHOQOL-BREF) (WHOQOL Group, 1998), Satisfaction With Life Scale (Diener et al., 1985), and the Positive and Negative Affect Scale (PANAS; Watson, Clark,

& Tellegen, 1988) among a sample of n = 180 university students in New Zealand. The results provide support for the 'interchangeable' utilisation of the constructs (happiness, SWB, and QoL). Ultimately, Medvedev and Langhuis (2018) emphasise the use of a global well-being construct that subsumes the three key constructs investigated.

Early emergence of the concept of SWB can be located in the *Social Indicators Movement* of the 1960s; more specifically in Wilson's (1967) *Correlates of avowed happiness* (as cited in Diener, Suh, Lucas, & Smith, 1999), Bradburn's (1969) *The structure of psychological well-being*, and is later evident in the work of Campbell, Converse, and Rodgers (1976) and Andrews and Withey (1976). Over the last three decades there has been a dramatic increase in studies focusing on SWB, driven largely by the *Social Indicators Movement* (Diener, 2013). Diener et al. (1999) contend that advancement in the field "reflects larger societal trends concerning the value of the individual, the importance of subjective views in evaluating life, and the recognition that well-being necessarily includes positive elements that transcend economic prosperity" (p. 276). Studies in SWB are premised on the notion that objective indicators only provide a partial explanation of QoL, and that what people think and feel about their lives are of critical importance (Savahl, Casas, & Adams, 2016).

Within child indicator and child well-being research, however, the interest has been less concerted, with the discipline largely pre-occupied with developing objective indicators of well-being largely in line with obligations imposed by the ratification of the UNCRC. Notwithstanding the languid start, research in subjective child well-being has experienced a substantial proliferation in recent years. In fact, within current international dialogue, it is highly unlikely to find commentary that disaffirms the significance of subjective perceptions of well-being, both in measuring and monitoring initiatives, as well as in assessing overall child well-being (Savahl & Adams et al., 2015). Early evidence of this shift was the inclusion of the domain of 'children's subjective well-being' in UNICEF's Report Card 7, a study that aimed to provide a comprehensive assessment of the lives and well-being of children and young people in 21 countries across 6 main dimensions namely, material well-being, health and safety, education, peer and family relationships, behaviours and risks, and young people's own subjective perceptions of their well-being (UNICEF Office of Research, 2007). Furthermore, the other domains reported on included children's subjective perceptions of various aspects of their lives; in particular their perceptions of their social relationships and safety.

Contemporary quantitative and qualitative studies on children's SWB suggest that the concept is often differentiated into a number of domains (see e.g. Fattore, Mason, & Watson, 2007; Land, Lamb, Meadows, & Taylor, 2007; Pollard & Davidson, 2001; Pollard & Lee, 2003; September & Savahl, 2009; Thornton, 2001; Zaff et al. 2003). Land et al. (2007) point out that the domains identified in these studies generally align to those identified in a systematic review conducted by Cummins (1996). Cummins (1996) concluded that the domains identified in the reviewed studies can be grouped into seven broad categories: economic and material well-being; health; safety; productive activity; place in community; intimacy; and emotional well-being. In their work on developing an index of SWB, Rees, Goswami and Bradshaw identified ten domains: family; friends; health; appearance; time use; the future; home; money and possessions; school; and amount of choice. In South Africa, research conducted by September and Savahl (2009) with children from two provinces identified five domains: protection and safety; basic needs and material resources; psycho-social well-being; social relationships; community resources and infrastructure.

22.4 Subjective Well-Being: The Methodological State of the Art

Given the fledging state of research into children's SWB, it is axiomatic that there would be limited large-scale studies using cross-national samples. The UNICEF's Report Cards, the Health Behaviour in School-Aged Children (www.hbsac.com) and the Programme for International Student Assessment study (Organisation for Economic Co-operation and Development, 2018), are examples of international cross-national surveys that have collected information on children's subjective perceptions of their lives. Recently, researchers aligned to the International Society for Child Indicators have initiated the Children's Worlds: International Survey on Children's Subjective Well-Being (see www.iscweb.org). The Children's Worlds Study represents the most ambitious attempt to collect substantive data on children's subjective perceptions and experiences of their lives, their time use, material well-being, and rights. Through three waves of data collection the study has generated substantial data allowing for comparisons across regions and countries.

When we ask children about their SWB, we are essentially asking them to appraise the extent to which they are satisfied with their lives in general, with certain aspects of their lives, and how they 'feel' about their lives, both in terms of positive and negative emotions (Savahl & Adams et al., 2015). This knowledge, policy-makers can use in conjunction with objective indicators to make more informed decisions in developing policies relevant to children that will ultimately have a direct impact on their lives. Two things are required. *Firstly*, a shift in thinking about children's cognitive capacity to provide valuable and meaningful knowledge about their lives. This essentially engenders an epistemological shift wherein childhood is regarded as a valid structural feature of society and children's perspectives acknowledged as valid, their experiences as real, with the capacity to meaningfully reflect on their lives (see James & Prout, 1990). While this epistemological shift is evident in the legislation governing children, it is not always reflected in every day decision-making. Part of the problem relates to the *second* requirement – developing appropriate methodologies to engage with children about their well-being. It is clear that the science related to engaging with children about their subjective perceptions of their well-being has not yet appropriately developed.

Researchers commenced with the use of standardised scales and measures, often adapted from adult versions, many of which demonstrated appropriate psychometric properties for use with specific populations, and some even showing evidence of cross-cultural comparison (Casas & Rees, 2015) (see also Proctor, Linley, & Maltby, 2009, for a review of life satisfaction measures developed for use with children and youth). When a measure is used in settings for which it was not originally developed, it has to be adapted from the original version to the language and culture of the target population. This process poses several challenges to ensuring that the measure continues to assess the same construct after it has been adapted and that the content remains the same in the adapted version.

Adaptation of research instruments is needed at a different level given that people who speak the same languages often have different cultural and life experiences that should be taken into account. The translation process itself is not simple as most languages have different dialects. Often the explicit differences, such as a different language are taken into consideration in the adaptation process, but the subtleties are not addressed. These include differences such as age, gender, educational background, SES, and even familiarity with response formats. If the concept engaged in the item is foreign to the new population, it is necessary to adapt the concept instead of just translating the words. Once a measure is translated, the developers also have to consider cultural, idiomatic, linguistic, and contextual aspects of the items.

Extensive research and consultation has been invested in developing guidelines for the adaptation of measures. The Standards for Educational and Psychological Tests (2013) include a chapter on testing for linguistic minority groups. Some of these standards are also applicable for cross-cultural testing. Sources of invalidity are addressed in different ways. Standard 6.2 states that a test has to be revalidated after major revisions have been made to the test while standard 13.4 states that the reliability and validity of an adapted test has to be addressed for its intended use, and standard 13.6 addresses the need to ensure the comparability of multi-lingual tests. Adaptation procedures have been improved over the years to include content and wording changes that consider cultural and contextual aspects of the construct being measured. The International Test Commission also developed a set of guidelines for test adaptation (van de Vijver & Hambleton, 1996). Failure to adhere to these guidelines can result in non-equivalent forms of a test.

When measures are adapted, the onus is on the developer to assess whether (1) it measures the same construct in the other population, (2) it is still useful once adapted, and (3) the scores mean the same that they did for the original target population. It is clear that measures have to be adapted for every new population. The validity and usefulness of a measure should be tested for each new population. However, many developers do not necessarily have the expertise to do as set out in the standards.

Results can only be compared across different populations once all these considerations have been taken into account. Thereafter, the tests have to be assessed to ensure that the content is maintained, the psychometric properties sound, and that the instrument is valid for the intended population. The advantage of adapting an existing instrument as opposed to developing a new instrument for each population is that the results can be compared across the groups, assuming that the adapted version is equivalent. Comparisons of this nature are important for large multi-national studies. The differences are however not only cultural, as indicated earlier, but could also include intersectionalities within a given culture such as gender, age, etc.

Developers who adapt measures for children have to proceed with caution. Children have even less exposure to outside cultures and different dialects of their languages. Children are also not a homogenous group and present with substantial variation in their cognitive capacity across age ranges. Measures that show good appropriate psychometric properties for older children, may not be applicable for use with younger children. It is thus necessary to ensure that there are no cultural and language biases in assessments for children as this will invalidate the results.

A second approach is founded on and promotes the theoretical and methodological stance of the 'new sociology of childhood' (see Adams & Savahl, 2017a; Fattore, Mason & Watson, 2012; Savahl & Malcolm et al., 2015). The emphasis in this approach is in locating the child centrally, (Fattore et al., 2012; Fattore, Fegter, & Hunner-Kreisel, 2016), with a focus on an in-depth exploration of what children think and feel about various aspects of their life. This is encapsulated in a range of qualitative research initiatives (see Adams & Savahl, 2017a; Fattore et al., 2007, 2012; Savahl & Malcolm et al., 2015; September & Savahl, 2009). For example, this mode of inquiry has been used both to solicit children's advice on improving subjective measures of well-being (see e.g. Casas, González, Navarro, & Aligué, 2012), as well as to determine children's perceptions of SWB, the nature of well-being domains, and how they make sense of and assign meaning to well-being (see e.g. Fattore et al. 2007, 2012; Savahl & Adams et al., 2015).

The Multinational Qualitative Study on Children's Understandings of Well-Being (CUWB), that encompasses a large-scale qualitative exploration between 12 countries, is further testament to the importance afforded to conducting qualitative research with children directly (Fattore et al. 2016). Notwithstanding this dichotomy, these two approaches advance a shared aim of including children in research as valid actors, possessing agency to reliably convey their subjective perceptions of their well-being. In this regard, Fattore et al. (2012) critically note the following:

> In viewing this dichotomy it is important not to confuse 'objectivist' and 'new sociology of childhood' approaches to research as different representations of method. It is important not to read each approach down as correspondingly 'quantitative' and 'qualitative'. The distinction that we present is not about the method employed or technique, but more fundamentally about the value position regarding knowledge acquisition (p. 426).

A key concept related to this approach is that of child participation that is evident in legislation relating to children, and has also recently become critical in research studies with children.

Child participation provides a critical framework for the inclusion of children in research, challenging the prior models of children's research controlled by privileged and powerful adults (Mason & Watson, 2014). It places the child centrally in the research process, with the aim of gaining a detailed understanding of their subjective experiences and meaning-making processes while taking into consideration the social, cultural, and historical contexts (Fattore et al., 2007). The researcher's role in child participation shifts from the adult-centric perspective, working instead as a collaborator in ways that enhance the power children have over their own lives (Langhout & Thomas, 2010). Grounded in the theoretical and methodological assertions of the 'new sociology of childhood', child participation research has its genesis in international legislation on children's rights, including the UNCRC. Article 12 of the UNCRC states that children have the right to freely express their opinion, to be heard, and have their opinions taken seriously on all matters that affect them (United Nations General Assembly, 1989a). Article 13 further supports child participation in the form of freedom of expression. This includes the right to seek, receive, or impart information and ideas through the child's preferred form of communication. Through the collaborative methodologies of child participation research, children have contributed valuable knowledge around issues relating to their lives, including children's experiences of the natural environment, self-concept, labour, schooling, play, gender, sexuality and spirituality, and developing indicators of children's well-being (Adams & Savahl, 2017b; Benninger & Savahl, 2016; Mason & Watson, 2014; September & Savahl, 2009).

However, Fattore, Fegter and Hunner-Kreisel (2018) warn that even though children's rights in general and participation rights in particular have become accepted within larger social discourse, the broader meaning and implication of these rights and enactments of participation are somewhat ambiguous. Furthermore, they the raise concern that if used without due consideration of context, then child participation runs the risk of being culturally insensitive and colonising. Similarly, Harcourt and Einarsdottir (2011) note that social context and social relations are often overlooked in child participation initiatives. The concept of child participation could then be perceived of as a normative construct rooted in a position of adult-child relations, that could potentially marginalise and alienate children who do not engender the norm. Part of these concerns raised by Fattore et al. (2018) could in some way be located in how early theoretical frameworks and conceptualisations of child participation were developed without a contextual grounding in and consideration of the diversity of childhoods, children's experiences, and socio-political 'lifeworlds' of children.

As Cuevas-Parra, Stephano, and Zhu (2016) note, the wealth of literature on child participation literature affords a number of models of child participation. Among these are "Hart's Ladder of Participation, Treseder's Degrees of Participation, Shier's Pathways to Participation, Lansdown's Model of Participation and Lundy's Model of Participation" (p. 8). More recently, McKendrick (2014) put forward a model Factors contributing to child well-being: A conceptual framework to situate place in context. This model is 'context-focused' and provides a conceptual framework to understand the influence of the neighbourhood on children's well-being. He developed a tool to expound the influence of place on children's overall well-being, in addition to his conceptual framework of place well-being. His tool, 'The impact of places on the well-being of children' is analogous to Hart's (1997) ladder of children's participation. It comprises a continuum ranging from the lowest rung, 'damaging' to 'transforming', the highest rung. Further, relevant to the South African context, Häkli and Kallio (2018) argue for the focus on children's 'political agency', by focusing on the 'phenomenologies of political action' rather than 'more elaborate ontologies of the political' (p. 3). Lundy (2007, p. 930) critically avers that, "There is a need for a greater awareness of the fact that respecting children's views is not just a model of good pedagogical practice (or policy making) but a legally binding obligation."

As Hultgren and Johannson (2018) contend, participation is considered necessary for citizenship, and alternatively is employed as a method to attain 'full citizenship'. In recent years, there has, however, been contention in relation to the operationalisation of child participation in varying cross-cultural contexts that have adopted the UNCRC (Ansell, 2016; Lundy, 2007; Rye & Vold, 2018; Skelton, 2010). The key premise of these debates is around the delineation of 'authentic participation' across different spheres that affect children's lives. At a more rudimentary level, the specific wording of Article 12 of the UNCRC has been a point of concern given the emphasis on children's participation being associated with their age, "Parties shall assure to the child who is capable of forming his or her own views the right to express those views freely in all matters affecting the child…". Clark and Richards (2017) thus note that participation is oft considered to be enacted by 'competent, responsible, reflexive individuals', essentially well-becomings (Ben-Arieh, 2008).

In relation to child participation in the research process, a critical deliberation is made by Fattore et al. (2018) in terms of the dearth of empirical endeavours exploring the hindrances in incorporating children's participation within the research process, particularly for children's well-being. Drawing on the work of Ben-Arieh (2005), Fattore et al. (2018) put forward crucial questions regarding children's participation, such as the aspect within the research process that children should participate, as well the way that children should be included in research regarding their well-being "…as part of the study design, as the source of information, as data collectors, as part of data analysis, or as partners in utilizing data?" In endeavouring to include 'ways of implementing participation' for young children in research, Hultgren and Johannson (2018) propose an alternative to the ladder-based models of participation. They put forward a model of participation comprising 'three interdependent levels, namely an ontological level, an ideological level, and an implementation level (Hultgren & Johannson, 2018). The consideration and integration of 'empowering research' (Holt, 2004) in this regard is critical, as it emphasises "participation as processual, observable and as happening in the meeting between people, places and things. Focus is on the process itself and the opening of lines of communication rather than on the outcomes of particular activities" (Hultgren & Johannson 2018, p.11).

22.4.1 Considerations for Method

Considering the fledging nature of research into children's SWB (Bradshaw, 2015), it is axiomatic that a greater investment in empirical research is required. Calls for large-scale population-based surveys are apposite and would allow much needed standardised data. However, the challenges related to cross-cultural measurement is heightened in the multicultural context of South Africa. Epistemological advancements and legislation foregrounding children's participation has fostered a greater interest in developing participatory methodologies, which are discussed below.

22.4.1.1 Mosaic Approach

As with foundations of several participatory methodologies, the Children's Mosaic Approach is premised on and advances the 'new sociology of childhood' with the child as an active contributor to knowledge. The Children's Mosaic Method (Clark & Moss, 2012) incorporates a number of different participatory visual and verbal data collection techniques (focus group interviews, community mapping, photovoice, and walking interviews). Each participatory technique employed forms part of the mosaic. Based on a framework of 'listening', the core components of the Children's Mosaic Approach incorporate a *multi-method* approach, advocating a *participatory* method, is *reflexive*, *adaptable*, and is *embedded into practice* (Clark, 2005).

The CUWB Study has incorporated a variation of the Children's Mosaic Approach (Clark, 2005), using "an ethnographic component documenting the fieldwork setting, and completion of two fieldwork stages each with core and optional modules" (Fattore, Fegter, & Watson, 2018, p. 14). The CUWB is an international project that aims to understand children's perceptions of well-being, between the ages of 11 and 14 years, and their daily lives using a qualitative perspective. The study endeavours to understand how children understand dimensions of well-being in a locally oriented, but multi-nationally comparative manner. The study currently includes 21 countries. Using a participatory approach, and children as agents and co-constructors of knowledge, the CUWB employs the use of interviews, community mapping, photovoice, and digital storytelling (short films) with participants involved in creating, editing, and finalising the short films reporting on their perspectives of their lives and well-being. More specifically, three modules are proposed, the first is centred on the thematic analysis of interviews conducted providing a basis for synthesising themes and posing subsequent questions to be explored; the second explicates children's subjective perceptions and experiences on domains of well-being; and the third includes the development of short films where children highlight key aspects of their life-worlds to share with children in other participating countries.

22.4.1.2 Photovoice

Photovoice, previously termed photo novella (Wang & Burris, 1994), has, in particular, been used to explore children's engagement with natural places (e.g. Castonguay & Jutras, 2009; Rasmussen, 2004). A systematic review of research focusing on children's environmental views by Adams and Savahl (2017b) found that the most commonly used data collection techniques across qualitative studies were drawings and mapping techniques (primarily with children between the ages of 5 and 7 years) (Kopnina, 2011; Malone & Tranter, 2003); observations (with children aged 7–18 years) (Malone & Tranter, 2003; Palmberg & Kuru, 2000); and interviews, both in-depth and focus groups (with children between the ages of 5 and 12 years) (Adams & Savahl, 2015; Hordyk, Dulude, & Shema, 2014; Kong, 2000). Among the photo-elicitation techniques, the participatory technique of photovoice in particular was used in the majority of these studies (Burke, 2005; Rasmussen, 2004), affording children the status of active participants within the research process. Through this participatory research method, children are considered as collaborators who possess agency, and are given a platform to present photo journeys of neighbourhood experiences. It is evident from the literature that photovoice as a participatory method has been increasingly employed with children across diverse contexts (e.g. Kopnina, 2011; Malone & Tranter, 2003; Sancar & Severcan, 2010; Strack, Magill, & McDonagh, 2004).

A study by Benninger and Savahl (2016) sought to explore children's constructions of the self across two urban communities in Cape Town, South Africa, using photovoice and community mapping. Similarly, a study by Malone (2016) explored children's encounters with place in La Paz, Bolivia, using the photovoice method. Additionally, a study by Adams, Savahl, and Fattore (2017) used the photovoice methodology to explore children's representations and perceptions of natural spaces. A key finding of the study was the influence of SES on children's understandings of well-being and concerns around safety. The significance of photovoice is captured in the conjecture by Wang and Redwood-Jones (2001, p. 560) that, "Photovoice is a powerful photographic technique that enables people to assess the strengths and concerns of their community and communicate their views to policy-makers". Delgado (2015) notes that it is significant to emphasize the distinctions between photo-elicitation and photovoice, as the former is a research method which may form part of "a wide variety of methodologies" (p. 7), while photovoice draws on participatory principles and is housed in methodology akin to community-based action research. With photographs being intricate, and interpretable in a number of ways (Radley, 2010), the use of photovoice provides the opportunity to explore the potential meanings behind children's representations with children directly.

22.4.1.3 Community Mapping

Community mapping is a visual data collection technique that provides unique representations of children's worlds. Amsden and VanWynsberghe (2005) note that community mapping may be utilised to not only document geographically significant spaces and places, but also additional varieties of abstract data. This abstract data and intricacies in children's maps are made sense of when children provide in-depth narratives for the detail therein. Widely considered as an empowering and child-centred technique, community mapping is foregrounded on "validating the knowledge and experiences of participants" (Amsden & VanWynsberghe, 2005, p. 361). Additionally, given the participatory nature of this technique, it is considered to address the issue of power dynamics and inequities present in the research-participant relationship. The use of community mapping is explicated in two participatory studies in the South African context with children exploring their perceptions of the 'self' and well-being (Benninger & Savahl, 2017) and of natural spaces and their SWB (Adams, et al., 2017). This data collection technique is often complemented by photovoice and focus group interviews in research studies.

22.4.1.4 The Children's Delphi

The Delphi technique is a flexible research approach, that entails an iterative multistage process designed to transform opinion into group consensus (Hasson, Keeney, & McKenna, 2000). The technique is intended to capture the collective opinions of experts who serve a consultative role on the Delphi panel (De Villiers, De Villiers, & Kent, 2005). The technique allows for the purposive selection of experts and does not require a representative sample of the population. In other words, the participants are selected to serve the purpose of applying their informed knowledge to a specific problem under investigation (Hasson et al., 2000). Traditionally, the Delphi 'experts' are academic, clinical, or field professionals who specialise in the area under investigation. Based on the epistemological position that children are knowledgeable experts and authorities on matters pertaining to their lives, Benninger and Savahl (2017) propose the use of the Children's Delphi as a means of engaging children in the research process around issues pertaining to their well-being. This position is supported by the growing use of child participation research that recognises children's rights to participate in matters affecting their lives and in the public sphere (Skivenese & Strandbu, 2006).

Unlike the traditional Delphi, the Children's Delphi places the child participants at the centre of the Delphi process, recognising their value as informed individuals on matters affecting their lives. Benninger and Savahl (2016) developed the Children's Delphi technique and employed it in a study that aimed to explore children's perceptions of the nature and content of intervention programmes aimed at improving children's self-concept within two impoverished communities of the Western Cape, South Africa. The Delphi technique was conducted with a group of ten children between the ages of 10 and 12 years who resided within the communities under investigation. The children's engagement in the Delphi process allowed them to represent a population (children in poverty) who are often excluded from decision-making processes. The final Delphi outcome was an agreed upon list of suggestions for intervention programmes which aimed to support the self-concept of children. This included a focus on safety, the provision of social support, the creation of opportunities for learning and for play and the provision of basic material needs.

The study provided a valuable contribution towards an understanding of the challenges faced by children in their communities and potential solutions for promoting a healthy self-concept. The study additionally supported child participation research and the value of engaging children in collaborative participatory processes. Further research utilising the Children's Delphi requires a flexible approach that caters to the participants' developmental level and resources, while maintaining the systematic rigor of the Delphi research process.

It is recommended that research investigating issues related to children's well-being consider including the Children's Delphi in the compendium of methods of data collection with children and young people. It is a research method aligned to the UNCRC, the 'new sociology of childhood' perspective, that encourages researchers to listen to children's perspectives and to view children as experts on their own lives (Langhout & Thomas, 2010). It advances the notion that children are the authentic knowers and authoritative experts of their lives and offers a structured framework for the meaningful inclusion of children's views in research.

22.5 Theoretical Perspectives

While there are limited child-specific theories on well-being, the literature abounds with seminal theories from both the hedonic and eudaimonic orientation. Prominent hedonic theories include the Adaptation Level Theory of Well-being (Brickman & Campbell, 1971; Diener, Lucas, & Scollon's 2006) Revision to the original Treadmill Theory, Cummins' Homeostasis Theory of Subjective Well-being (1995, 2003, 2010, 2014), The 3P Model (Durayappah, 2011), The Structural Model of Child Well-being (Minkkinen's, 2013) and Factors contributing to child well-being: A conceptual framework to situate place in context (McKendrick, 2014); while eudaimonic theories include Self-determination Theory (Deci & Ryan, 1985; Ryan & Deci, 2008a, 2008b), The Two Source Theory of Child Well-Being (Raghavan & Alexandrova, 2014), and more recently Flourishing Theory (Seligman, 2011), the Capability Approach (CA) (Fegter & Richter, 2014), and Child Standpoint Theory (Fattore, Mason, & Watson, 2017). Diener et al. (2010, p. 10) aptly note that "Seligman (2002), Ryff (1989), Ryff and Singer (1998), and Steger, Kashdan, Sullivan and Lorentz (2008) present arguments and data supporting the notion that purpose and meaning are beneficial to human functioning."

Although the field was developed on the perspectives of adult populations, the focus on the significance on children's SWB was advocated for with early efforts to elevate the status of children's self-reported well-being. Notwithstanding the role of key scholars in the paradigm shift from a focus on pathogenesis to salutogenesis, in particular the WHO (1946) was a key proponent with their definition of health which emphasised not only the absence of ill-health but also the physical, mental, and social components related to an individual's health. The influence of this shift was evident across numerous disciplines, which resulted in a changing focus of research and theory. Additionally, the ratification of the UNCRC (1989b) and the new sociology of childhood' (James & Prout, 1990) provided further momentum in espousing the rights of children. Considerations of children's lives across an array of domains were no longer sought from adults (such as parents or teachers) or guardians as proxies for children, but rather research was being conducted with children as social actors and no longer as subjects (Ben-Arieh, 2009, 2010).

One of the seminal theories of well-being, the Adaptation Level Theory of Well-being (Brickman & Campbell, 1971), has contributed greatly to the field. The original hedonic Treadmill Theory was developed and put forward by Brickman and Campbell (1971) which posited that people momentarily respond to good and bad events and revert to neutrality in a brief period; this theory formed the basis for Cummins' Homeostasis Theory of SWB (1995, 2003, 2010, 2014). However, continued analysis of the Adaptation Level Theory evinced several shortcomings. Amongst these is the notion that efforts to increase happiness are futile, and that after good and bad events people quickly revert to neutrality. In this regard Diener, Lucas, and Scollon (2006) proposed several revisions to the theory, based on empirical evidence. A crucial inference from Diener et al.'s (2006) article, is that evidence from early and key works in a field of study should not be blindly accepted, but instead continually engaged with, and analysed and re-analysed, with the use of large representative samples and longitudinal data to draw sound conclusions.

Cummins' Homeostasis Theory of SWB (1995, 2003, 2010, 2014) relates to the Adaptation Level Theory, in its notion of maintaining a 'normal' sense of well-being. Cummins (1995, 2003, 2010, 2014) theory, however, has been applied in a number of contexts with diverse samples, and has more recently been employed in research with children specifically (Cummins, 2010, 2014). Cummins (2014) indicated that the theory be used with children from 12-years old as they encompass the cognitive maturity for self-report. He posits further that data obtained when assessing children's well-being in the specified age cohort, when understood within SWB homeostasis, can illuminate the difficulties and supports they experience at this period in their lives; this provides a basis from which to tailor interventions for children.

More recently, McKendrick's (2014) conceptual model, *Factors contributing to child well-being: A conceptual framework to situate place in context*, shows how children's neighbourhoods play a pertinent role in their well-being, with key considerations of adequate resources, equal opportunities for all children and children's active participation; and more broadly family aspects (SES, parenting, and dynamics of family life). These considerations advance 'geographies of well-being' for children', and ultimately 'good places' for children that negate risk and promote children's QoL. As a cautionary note, McKendrick (2014) maintains that while evidence may show that some children attain an adequate level of well-being in spite of the impoverished neighbourhoods in which they live or an unsupportive family, this should not be used as a motivation to not address these inadequacies in these spheres. Low subjective SES has been found to be related to increased physical symptoms and psychological distress among adolescents, as well as a higher prevalence of children as victims of abuse, peer aggression, and community violence (Garbarino, 1999). This consideration is particularly crucial, as South Africa has one of the highest levels of inequality and violence in the world, that has resulted in children from different SES communities reporting distinct childhoods. Similar to the Adaptation Level and Homeostasis Theories, the 3P Model (Durayappah, 2011) shows that current life events influence happiness, however, the extent of this is escalated in the 3P Model which affirms that the memories of our experiences govern our feelings of SWB in temporal states (present, the past, and the prospect).

Two recent well-being theoretical frameworks that were developed specifically for children was the Structural Model of Child Well-being (SMCW) (Minkkinen, 2013) and the Two Source Theory (Raghavan & Alexandrova, 2014). While the former theory is based on that of Bronfenbrenner's Ecological Theory comprising concentric circles representing the domains of a child's life, the latter was based on philosophical theories of well-being, most notably Kraut's (2009) developmentalism. The SMCW (Minkkinen's, 2013) employed a multidisciplinary approach and used the WHO's (1946) definition of health. Minkkinen (2013) posits that children are affected by their own culture, but in turn contribute to and reproduce culture echoing the concept of interpretive reproduction as posited by Corsaro (1992, 2011, 2014). Minkkinen (2013) also considers the importance of social relationships, considered across all theories in this chapter and closely linked to the concept of social capital. Diener et al. (2010) indicate the work of Putnam (2000) and Helliwell, Barrington-Leigh, Harris, and Huang (2009) who proposed that social capital is rudimentary to the well-being of societies. While good social relationships were initially denoted as receiving support from others, Diener et al. (2010) show that contemporary research has demonstrated that people also need to support others (see Brown Nesse, Vinokur, & Smith, 2003; Dunn, Aknin, & Norton, 2008; Peterson et al., 1988; Scheier & Carver, 2003; Seligman, 2002).

The focus on enhancing well-being and QoL is also evident in the Capability Approach (CA) (Nussbaum, 1988, 2000; Sen, 1985, 1993, 2005, 2007). The CA has been developed over the past two decades by Sen (1985, 1993, 2005, 2007) and Nussbaum (1988, 2000), and focuses on participation, human well-being, and freedom as core components of development- merging ethics and economics (Comim, Ballet, Biggeri & Iervese, 2011). The emphasis of the CA is on the QoL that individuals are capable of achieving.

The key closely-related concepts that the framework proposes are functionings, capabilities, freedom, and agency (Dang, 2014). Handbooks and edited book series such as Children and the good life: New challenges for research on children (2010, edited by Sabine Andresen, Isabell Diehm, Uwe Sander, & Holger Ziegler), Children and the capability approach (2011, edited by Mario Biggeri, Jérôme Ballet, & Flavio Cummin), Handbook of Child Well-Being: Theories, Methods And Policies In Global Perspective (2014; edited by Asher Ben-Arieh, Ferran Casas, Ivar Frønes, & Jill E. Korbin) and Children's Rights and the Capability Approach: Challenges and prospects (2014, edited by Daniel Stoecklin & Jean-Michel Bovin) evince this growing focus on children's capabilities. Biggeri, Ballet, and Comim (2011) argue that children's development cannot be synonymous with reducing poverty and impoverishment, and further that well-being on a broad scale cannot solely consider material components of well-being. More recently, building on seminal qualitative research methods and theoretical considerations (see Fattore et al., 2007), Fattore et al. (2017) put forward Child Standpoint Theory wherein childhood is conceptualised as a structural phenomenon, that needs to be understood within the complexities of adult-child relations.

22.5.1 Considerations for Theory

Wells (2014) notes that a paradigm shift has ensued across disciplines since the WHO's (1946) definition of health focusing on salutogenesis, thus on the basis of health as opposed to pathogenesis. Paramount to these two fields is the 'future orientation' focus, to not only enhance feelings of well-being and happiness in terms of the interplay between the person and environment, but to strive toward aspirations, flourishing, and gain a sense of meaning in life, thus assimilating eudaimonia. This attention to 'future orientation' in turn feeds into discussions around positive behaviours. The theories of well-being display great dispersion, with former theories informing contemporary theories. Many theories of SWB borrow concepts from other theories, and in some way modify these concepts to align with proposed theories, from Brickman and Campbell (1971), Headey and Wearing (1989), and Cummins' (1995) Homeostasis Theory, to more contemporary theorisations of children's well-being (Minkkinen's Structural Model of Child Well-Being, 2013; Raghavan & Alexandro's Two Source Theory of Child Well-Being, 2014; Fattore et al.'s Child Standpoint Theory, 2017). While the significance of personality characteristics has been shown to be an important determinant of SWB, SES has become increasingly important as a determinant of SWB, particularly in developing countries with high levels of inequality.

A challenge when approaching the child well-being theory literature is the lack of delineation of a timeline of proposed theories. While some articles refer to other authors who have contributed to the field, the literature is quite disjointed. A gap in the literature is a recent, comprehensive review article that presents the various theories of SWB. While an extensive history of the concept of well-being is provided in The Handbook of Child Well-Being (Edited by Ben-Arieh et al., 2014), as well as journal articles by prominent scholars in the field (see Ben-Arieh, 2009; Ben-Arieh & Frønes, 2011), there is no such article summarising contemporary applications of the theories to children's SWB. Of the hedonic theories, those used most widely in the literature on children's SWB is Cummins' Homeostasis Theory of Subjective Well-being (2014), the CA (Fegter & Richter, 2014), and Child Standpoint Theory (Fattore et al., 2017). Diener et al. (2006) assert that researchers endeavouring to develop intervention programmes to improve happiness should have a thorough knowledge of theory (adaptation theory) to make sure that the impact is not merely transitory, but long-lasting. The relevance of the Homeostasis Theory to children is also evident in the recommendation that the theory can be used to pinpoint certain areas of difficulties children are experiencing in life, and thereby provide possible solutions to address this.

It is crucial to note that much of the research cited in this chapter, which provides support to the specific theories, have predominantly been conducted in developed contexts, with a few exceptions. Wang and Wang (2016) proposed that people residing in communities with varying SES display distinct levels of life satisfaction (see Dittmann & Goebel, 2010) and happiness (see Ludwig et al., 2012). In developed contexts, research often points to how people living in rural environments have higher SWB than those living in urban contexts. However, studies from impoverished rural communities in South Africa show that in this context rural communities are synonymous with low-SES, low-income, poor infrastructure and service delivery, high levels of crime and violence, and informal housing (Adams & Savahl, 2015; Parkes, 2007; Savahl, 2010). It is indicated by Wang and Wang (2016, p.) that "there are significant spatial differences in SWB at different levels of regions and various geographical factors have important effects on an individual's SWB. Specifically, the economic indicators, cultural differences, climate, urban facilities, neighbourhood environment and housing conditions all have important effects on SWB." While some theories have been applied and specifically developed for children, there is the necessity to test the applicability of these theories with children in diverse contexts, with more research required in developing countries, and further cross-national comparison studies. Contextually relevant theoretical frameworks, should, however, go beyond a consideration of space and an acknowledgement of diversity, to include a cautionary consideration to not reproduce western narratives of childhood and well-being (Fattore et al., 2018).

22.6 Subjective Well-Being, *Quality of Life*, and Social Policy

The influence of objective indicators of children's QoL on social policy is well-established. The development of measuring and monitoring systems, as an obligation to the UNCRC, and the subsequent investment in the collection of data on children has afforded policy-makers opportunities to develop 'evidence-based' policies relevant to improving children's overall QoL. There have also been dedicated initiatives aimed at developing indicators to monitor the various domains of well-being and QoL. Research advancing the 'new sociology of childhood', the UNCRC, the 'science of human capital formation' and 'social capital support' have contributed significantly in this regard (Lippman, Moore, & McIntosh, 2009). Willenberg, September and Savahl (2006) used the child participation approach to develop indicators from children's perspectives, while Dawes, Bray, and van Der Merwe (2007) have focused on developing a rights-based approach. As Dawes et al. (2007) note, the fundamental rationale for the development of indicators is to afford decision-makers the necessary and relevant information to influence the development of policy, allocation of resources, services, and advancing public awareness in terms of children's needs and contextual circumstances. Further, this enables the evaluation of policies, services, and programmes for children. Their right-based model presents five indicator types: child status indicators, family and household and environment indicators, service access indicators, and service quality indicators. Importantly, Dawes et al. (2007) contend that proposed indicator systems should be considered as 'live' and must be revised according to the needs of children. Notwithstanding this, the indicator system should also be boundaried to ensure that key indicators are maintained. Monitoring and evaluating indicator systems should therefore align and contribute to children's rights as enshrined in the UNCRC, United Nations Sustainable Development Goal of 'Good Health and Well-Being', and Africa's Agenda for children. It is crucial that these indicator systems are drawn on to evaluate and inform children's well-being and QoL using evidence-based empirical research. In relating social policy for well-being and QoL indicator research, Ben-Arieh et al. (2014) highlights that while pertinent to every citizen, social policy is particularly germane for children as it impacts on the various spheres of their lives (contextual and family environments, work, play, and overall well-being). A key motivation for this focus is based on the foundations of an individual's well-being and QoL life trajectory being largely determined by childhood (Ben-Ariehet al., 2014). More specifically, as Savahl et al. (2015) note, in South Africa SES has been found to directly influence children's QoL. Translating the policies into effective practices, however, requires further commitment and strategic investment, and remains a key challenge.

Providing support for the findings by Medvedev and Landhuis (2018), Ben-Arieh et al. (2014), and Dawes et al. (2007) highlight the need for the development of child QoL indicators to be 'interdisciplinary, multi-agency, and service cross-cutting'. While challenging, a good starting point is to consider international comparative research and indicators that entrench national and international child rights and legislations. Ben-Arieh et al. (2014) thus argues that child social policy must respect children and should be affixed to children's subjective experiences of their daily lives. Using school readiness social policy as an example, he maintains that while in the past the policy has focused on preparing the child for school; in future iterations instead the focus should be on 'preparing the schools for the children'. In essence, this does not merely suggest a shift in thinking on childhood, but more crucially encapsulates the changing nature of the concept of child well-being and the necessity of meaningfully incorporating children's subjective perceptions of their lives. As is poignantly noted "True child participation in this sphere can leverage the political power of children and enforce the politicians to hear them. This is especially important for democratic societies that want to include the opinions of all of their citizens in decision-making processes" (Ben-Arieh et al., 2014, p. 577).

A key consideration also relates to the extent to which SWB indicators can meaningfully contribute to and enrich understandings of children's QoL and ultimately influence programmes and policy; as reflected in a question posed by the National Research Council (2013):

> ...to what extent do results of subjective well-being (SWB) research go beyond the realm of the interesting and thought provoking...to a point that they might refocus policy or even directly inform it? (p. 87)

When applied to child SWB indicators, the concern is further exaggerated given that the capacity of children to meaningfully reflect on their lives is often questioned. Put differently, how do we motivate that children's subjective perceptions and evaluations of their lives be considered relevant for policy decisions?

Ben-Arieh (2010) points to the dynamic nature of child well-being indicators. He sketches the trajectory through nine major shifts in the child indicators movement over the preceding few decades, that is: from an earlier focus on child survival and well-becoming to well-being; from negative life outcomes to positive outcomes; a child rights perspective; from 'traditional' domains of child well-being to new interdisciplinary domains; from a focus on national geographic units to measuring various geographical units and cross-cultural research; increased development of several composite indices of children's well-being; with contemporary endeavours being directed by policy relevance; and finally from focusing solely on adult's perspectives to accentuating children's subjective perspectives. An important consideration in the context of the current chapter relates to the potential impact that indicators of SWB can have on social policy. The key question that arises is: how can we use children's subjective perceptions of their lives to influence social policy? Rees et al.'s (2010) recommendation for a composite index of children's SWB is intuitively appealing and provides the much-needed empirical evidence to advocate for social policy directives. Forgeard, Jayawickreme, Kern, and Seligman (2011) further to that, put forward the dashboard approach to the measurement of well-being wherein the measurement of well-being is assessed across a range of domains. The application of the dashboard approach would allow researchers and child advocates with a stronger base to identify more acutely the areas of children's lives policy initiatives are more likely to effect positive change. Ultimately, for child SWB indicators to meaningfully influence policy initiatives requires both the development of rigorous methodologies to collect information with children, and a consideration of how we translate findings of children's subjective perceptions into evidence that can be used by policy-makers. Fortunately, there is compelling evidence that objective indicators of well-being are strongly correlated with subjective indicators (Bradshaw, 2015). Using data from the UNICEF's Report Card 13, Bradshaw (2015) found higher levels of SWB in children who presented with higher levels of objective standards of living; all of which could be influenced by social policy. However, while some researchers have argued for the importance of grounding policy and planning initiatives in children's experiences (see Ben-Arieh & Goerge, 2006; Prout, 1997), there are no protocols or best practice models for how to achieve this. Ben-Arieh (2008) provides some advice in relation to child well-being indicators. He poses five questions that he believes should be considered in relation to developing policy initiatives. These five research questions are:

- What are the most salient outcome measures?
- How can indicators be used to maximise their influence on policy?
- How should indicators be packaged and marketed?
- How can indicators be used to shape public opinion?
- What are the most meaningful metrics for indicators?

Along with these, the critical question that arises is: How do we integrate indicators of SWB into the broader QoL indicator system? Part of the answer possibly lies in developing a 'rights-based' child well-being indicator system, premised on the core principles of non-discrimination, the child's best interests, survival and development, and participation (see Dawes et al., 2007). This is likely to result not only in civil society paying particularly close attention to the needs and well-being of children, but it also places the burden on policy-makers to consider children's voices and experiences as key factors in the development of policy initiatives. For this to materialise, researchers need to commit to the process of translating research evidence into effective practice, policies and social programmes.

22.7 Research Translation: From Evidence to Social Change

Research translation, defined here as the application of research-generated knowledge to drive social change and enhance QoL, has been declared a national imperative (Isobell, Lazarus, Suffla, & Seedat, 2016). However, despite the potential for research-based knowledge to inform practice, programmes, and policies, moving from evidence to action remains a key challenge (Palinkas & Soydan, 2012; Ssengooba et al., 2011). Translation processes are shaped by the methodological positioning of the researcher and have tended to promote participation of non-academics in parts of but not the full research process (Isobell et al., 2016). Furthermore, critique has also been levelled at academic researchers for communicating research in ways that are potentially inaccessible to non-academic audiences who may also be end-users (Isobell et al., 2016; Stuurman, 2002). When viewed from the lens of participatory methodologies, however, translation is an inherent part of the research process and outcome (Lazarus, Duran, Caldwell, & Bulbulia, 2012), supported by:

- Sustained participation through equal partnership with participants,
- Creation of spaces to hear from participants directly,
- Design and application of innovative and novel methodologies for engaging with participants
- Co-producing contextually relevant and responsive knowledge,
- Promotion of the agency and empowerment of participants, and
- Mutual knowledge-sharing within the research partnership (Isobell et al., 2016)

To optimise translation within participatory processes, researcher-participant power dynamics arising from gender, SES, education, race and, especially in the case of working with children, age, must also continually be examined and attended to (Isobell et al., 2016). Participatory researchers are urged to commit to participants and stakeholders beyond the usual academic research cycle (Lazarus et al., 2012) and when working with children, must ensure that their voices are heard alongside that of their families and the community if relevant knowledge and successful research translation is to occur (Cheng & Jenkins, 2009). Within this process, if the role of children is to be actively participative, then the role of the researcher is to prioritise outcomes over outputs and to afford child participants multiple opportunities for interaction to exert influence over intended social change processes. The envisaged outcome: benefits to funders and a greater commitment to mobilising and sustaining action (Isobell et al., 2016).

22.8 Conclusion

For policies to be effective, we need to reach consensus on what exactly constitutes SWB, and the best ways to measure it. There also needs to be more consideration of how indicators of SWB can be integrated into the broader QoL indicator system. Recent advances in contextually relevant theoretical models and the emergence of new participatory methodologies for collecting data with children offer new possibilities. However, the stakes are high. We need to invest heavily in refining participatory methodologies; particularly, we need to sharpen our skills as it relates to engaging with and obtaining information from children. Moreover, it is recommended that the agenda for research concerning children be set by the children themselves. This requires the foregrounding of children's agentic capacities and an investment by researchers to further develop these capacities. Given that children are not a homogenous group, especially in terms of their age-related cognitive capacity and cultural diversity, places an enormous burden on researchers and practitioners in the field. The greatest challenge, however, is the translation of the evidence into effective social policies. When one thinks of social policies related to children, it may be wise to think beyond traditional national policies and legislation, that is often curtailed by a lack of implementation. Targeting policies at the grass-roots level (e.g. municipal by-laws, school policies etc.) to consider children's voices and ultimately the implications of their subjective perceptions and experiences would have a greater and more relevant impact on their lives. Researchers should therefore think more broadly and target 'grass-roots policies' that are more connected to the daily lives of children.

References

Adams, S., & Savahl, S. (2015). Children's perceptions of the natural environment: A South African perspective. *Children's Geographies, 13*(2), 196–211.

Adams, S., & Savahl, S. (2017a). Children's discourses of natural spaces: Consideration for children's subjective well-being. *Child Indicators Research, 10*(2), 423–446, https://doi.org/10.1007/s12187-016-9374-2

Adams, S., & Savahl, S. (2017b). Nature as children's space: A systematic review. *Journal of Environmental Education, 48*(5), 291–321.

Adams, S., Savahl, S., & Fattore, T. (2017). Children's representations of nature using photovoice and community mapping: Perspectives from South Africa. *International Journal of Qualitative Studies on Health and Well-Being, 12*(1), https://doi.org/10.1080/17482631.2017.1333900

American Educational Research Association, American Psychological Association, National Council on Measurement in Education, Joint Committee on Standards for Educational and Psychological Testing (U.S.). (2014). *Standards for educational and psychological testing*. Washington, DC: AERA.

Andresen, S., Diehm, I., Sander, U., & Ziegler, H. (2010). *Children and the good life: New challenges for research on children*. Dordrecht, The Netherlands: Springer.

Andrews, F. M., & Withey, S. B. (1976). *Social indicators of well-being*. New York, NY: Plenum.

Ansell, N. (2016). From objects to subjects? Children and youth in development. In J. Grugel & D. Hammett (Eds.), *The Palgrave handbook of international development* (pp. 487–511). London, UK: Palgrave Macmillan UK.

Ben-Arieh, A. (2005). Where are the children? Children's role in measuring and monitoring their Well-being. *Social Indicators Research, 74*(3), 573–596.

Ben-Arieh, A. (2008). The child indicators movement: Past, present, and future. *Child Indicators Research, 1*(1), 3–16.

Ben-Arieh, A. (2009). From child welfare to children well-being: The child indicators perspective. In S. B. Kamerman, S. Phipps, & A. Ben-Arieh (Eds.), *From child welfare to children well-being: An international perspective on knowledge in the service of making policy* (pp. 9–22). Dordrecht, The Netherlands: Springer.

Ben-Arieh, A. (2010). Developing indicators for child Well-being in a changing context. In C. McCauley & W. Rose (Eds.), *Child Well-being: Understanding children's lives* (pp. 129–142). London: Jessica Kingsley Publishers.

Ben-Arieh, A., Casas, F., Frønes, I., & Korbin, J. E. (Eds.). (2014). *Handbook of child well-being: Theories, methods and policies in global perspective*. Dordrecht, The Netherlands: Springer.

Ben-Arieh, A., & Frønes, I. (2011). Taxonomy for child well-being indicators: A framework for the analysis of the well-being of children. *Childhood, 18*(4), 460–476.

Ben-Arieh, A., & Goerge, R. M. (Eds.). (2006). *Indicators of children's well-being: Understanding their role, usage and policy influence*. Dordrecht, The Netherlands: Springer.

Benninger, E., & Savahl, S. (2016). The children's Delphi: Considerations for developing a programme for promoting children's self-concept and well-being. *Child & Family Social Work, 22*(2), 1094–1103. https://doi.org/10.1111/cfs.12329

Benninger, E., & Savahl, S. (2017). A systematic review of children's construction of the self: Implications for children's subjective well-being. *Child Indicators Research, 10*(2), 545–569.

Biggeri, M., Ballet, J., & Comim, F. (Eds.). (2011). *Children and the capability approach*. United Kingdom: Palgrave Macmillan, UK.

Biko, S. (1978). Black consciousness and the quest for a true humanity. *UFAHAMU: Journal of the African Activist Association, 8*(3), 10–23.

Bradburn, N. M. (1969). *The structure of psychological well-being*. Chicago, IL: Aldine.

Bradshaw, J. (2015). Subjective well-being and social policy: Can nations make their children happier? *Child Indicators Research, 8*(1), 227–241. https://doi.org/10.1007/s12187-014-9283-1

Bray, R., Gooskens, I., Kahn, L., Moses, S., & Seekings, J. (2010). *Growing up in the new South Africa: Childhood and adolescence in post-apartheid Cape Town*. Cape Town: Human Sciences Research Council.

Brickman, P., & Campbell, D. T. (1971). Hedonic relativism and planning the good society. In M. H. Apley (Ed.) *Adaptation-level theory: A Symposium* (pp 287–302). New York, Academic Press.

Brown, S. L., Nesse, R. M., Vinokur, A. D., & Smith, D. M. (2003). Providing support may be more beneficial than receiving it: Results from a prospective study of mortality. *Psychological Science, 14*, 320–327.

Bulhan, H. A. (1985). Black Americans and psychopathology: An overview of research and theory. *Psychotherapy: Theory, Research, Practice, Training, 22*(2S), 370–378. https://doi.org/10.1037/h0085517

Burke, C. (2005). Play in focus: Children researching their own spaces and places for play. *Children, Youth and Environments, 15*(1), 27–53..

Camfield, L., & Skevington, S. M. (2008). On subjective well-being and quality of life. *Journal of Health Psychology, 13*(6), 764–775. https://doi.org/10.1177/1359105308093860

Campbell, A., Converse, P. E., & Rodgers, W. L. (1976). *The quality of American life: Perceptions, evaluations and satisfaction*. New York, NY: Russel Sage.

Casas, F. (1997). Children's rights and children's quality of life: conceptual and practical issues. *Social Indicators Research, 42*(3), 283–298.

Casas, F., González, M., Navarro, D., & Aligué, M. (2012). Children as advisors of their researchers: Assuming a different status for children. *Child Indicators Research*. https://doi.org/10.1007/s12187-012-9168-0

Casas, F., & Rees, G. (2015). Measures of children's subjective well-being: Analysis of the potential for cross-national comparisons. *Child Indicators Research, 8*(1), 49–69.

Castonguay, G., & Jutras, S. (2009). Children's appreciation of outdoor places in a poor neighbourhood. *Journal of Environmental Psychology, 29*, 101–109.

Cheng, T. L., & Jenkins, R. R. (2009). Health disparities across the lifespan: Where are the children? *Journal of the American Medical Association, 301*(23), 2491–2492.

Clark, A. (2005). Ways of seeing: Using the Mosaic approach to listen to young children's perspectives. In A. Clark, A. T. Kjørholt, & P. Moss (Eds.), *Beyond listening: Children's perspectives on early childhood services* (pp. 29–49). Bristol: Policy Press.

Clark, A. & Moss, P. (2012). *Listening to young children: The MOSAIC approach*. National Children's Bureau (2nd Revised edition).

Clark, J., & Richards, S. (2017). The cherished conceits of research with children: Does seeking the agentic voice of the child through participatory methods deliver what it promises? In I. E. Castro, M. B. Swauger, & B. Harger (Eds.), *Researching children and youth: Methodological issues, strategies, and innovations* (pp. 127–148). Bingley, UK: Emerald.

Comim, F., Ballet, J., Biggeri, M., & Iervese, V. (2011). Introduction-theoretical foundations and the Book's roadmap. In M. Biggeri, J. Ballet, & F. Comim (Eds.), *Children and the capability approach* (pp. 3–21). New York, NY: Palgrave Macmillan.

Corsaro, W. (1992). Interpretive reproduction in children's peer cultures. *Social Psychology Quarterly, 55*, 160–177.

Corsaro, W. A. (2011). *The sociology of childhood* (3rd ed.). Thousand Oaks, CA: Pine Forge Press.

Corsaro, W. A. (2014). Children's well-being and interpretive reproduction. In A. Ben-Arieh, F. Casas, I. Frønes, & J. E. Korbin (Eds.), *Handbook of child well-being: Theories, methods and policies in global perspective* (pp. 709–737). Dordrecht, The Netherlands: Springer.

Cuevas-Parra, P., Stephano, M., & Zhu, Y. (2016). *Unpacking gender equality approach to children and young People's participation.* World Vision.

Cummins, R. A. (2000). Objective and subjective quality of life: An interactive model. *Social Indicators Research, 52*(1), 55–72.

Cummins, R. A. (1995). *The comprehensive quality of life scale: Theory and development: Health outcomes and quality of life outcomes and quality of life measurement*. Canberra, Australia: Institute of Health and Welfare.

Cummins, R. A. (1996). The domains of life satisfaction: An attempt to order chaos. *Social Indicators Research, 38*, 303–328.

Cummins, R. A. (2003). Normative life satisfaction: Measurement issues and a homeostatic model. *Social Indicators Research, 64*(2), 225–256.

Cummins, R. A. (2010). Subjective wellbeing, homeostatically protected mood and depression: A synthesis. *Journal of Happiness Studies, 11*(1), 1–17.

Cummins, R. A. (2014). Understanding the well-being of children and adolescents through homeostatic theory. In A. Ben-Arieh, F. Casas, I. Frønes, & J. E. Korbin (Eds.), *Handbook of child well-being: Theories, methods and policies in global perspective* (pp. 635–662). Dordrecht, The Netherlands: Springer.

Dang, A. T. (2014). Amartya Sen's capability approach: A framework for well-being evaluation and policy analysis? *Review of Social Economy, 72*(4), 460–484.

Dawes, A., Bray, R. & Van der Merwe, A. (Eds). (2007). Monitoring child Well-being: A south African rights-based approach. Cape Town: HSRC Press.

Delgado, M. (2015). *Urban youth and photovoice.* New York, NY: Oxford University Press.

Department of Basic Education. (2018). *Education statistics in South Africa 2016*. Pretoria: Department of Basic Education.

De Villiers, M. R., De Villiers, P. J., & Kent, A. P. (2005). The Delphi technique in health sciences education research. *Medical Teacher, 27*(7), 639–643.

Deci, E., & Ryan, R. M. (1985). *Intrinsic motivation and self-determination in human behavior*. Berlin, Germany: Springer.

Diener, E., Emmons, R. A., Larsen, R. J., & Griffin, S. (1985). The satisfaction with life scale. *Journal of Personality Assessment, 49*(1), 71–75.

Diener, E. (2000). Subjective Well-being: The science of happiness and a proposal for a national index. *American Psychologist, 55*, 34–43. https://doi.org/10.1037//0003-066X.55.1.34

Diener, E. (2006). Guidelines for national indicators of subjective well-being and ill-being. *Journal of Happiness Studies, 7*, 397–404.

Diener, E. (2009). Subjective well-being. In E. Diener, *The science of well-being: The Collected works of Ed Diener* (pp. 11–58). Dordrecht, The Netherlands, Springer.

Diener, E. (2013). The remarkable changes in the science of subjective well-being. *Perspectives in Psychological Science, 8*, 663–666.

Diener, E., Lucas, R. E., & Oishi, S. (2005). Subjective well-being: The science of happiness and life satisfaction. In C. R. Snyder & S. J. Lopez (Eds.), *Handbook of positive psychology* (2nd ed., pp. 63–73). New York, NY: Oxford University Press.

Diener, E., Lucas, R. E., & Scollon, C. N. (2006). Beyond the hedonic treadmill: Revising the adaptation theory of well-being. *American Psychologist, 61*, 305–314.

Diener, E., Suh, E. M., Lucas, R. E., & Smith, H. L. (1999). Subjective well-being: Three decades of progress. *Psychological Bulletin, 125*(2), 276–302.

Diener, E., Wirtz, D., Tov, W., Kim-Prieto, C., Choi, D. W., Oishi, S., & Biswas-Diener, R. (2010). New well-being measures: Short scales to assess flourishing and positive and negative feelings. *Social Indicators Research, 97*(2), 143–156.

Dittmann, J., & Goebel, J. (2010). Your house, your car, your education: The socioeconomic situation of the neighborhood and its impact on life satisfaction in Germany. *Social Indicators Research, 96*(3), 497–513.

Dunn, E., Aknin, L. B., & Norton, M. I. (2008). Spending money on others promotes happiness. *Science, 319*, 1687–1688.

Durayappah, A. (2011). The 3P model: A general theory of subjective well-being. *Journal of Happiness Studies, 12*(4), 681–716.

Evans, G. W., Brauchle, G., Haq, A., Stecker, R., Wong, K., & Shapiro, E. (2007). Young children's environmental attitudes and behaviours. *Environment and Behavior, 39*(5), 635–659.

Fattore, T., Fegter, S., & Hunner-Kreisel, C. (2016). Child well-being and cultural contingency: A study of global child well-being. *ISA Sociology of Childhood Newsletter*.

Fattore, T., Fegter, S., & Hunner-Kreisel, C. (2018). Children's understandings of well-being in global and local contexts: Theoretical and methodological considerations for a multinational qualitative study. *Child Indicators Research. 12*(2), pp 385–407. https://doi.org/10.1007/s12187-018-9594-8

Fattore, T., Mason, J., & Watson, E. (2007). Children's conceptualisation(s) of their well-being. *Social Indicators Research, 80*(1), 5–29.

Fattore, T., Mason, J., & Watson, E. (2012). Locating the child centrally as subject in research: Towards a child interpretation of well-being. *Child Indicators Research, 5*, 423–435.

Fattore, T., Mason, J., Watson, E. (2017). Overviewing a child standpoint on well-being. In T. Fattore, J. Mason, and E. Watson, *Children's understandings of well-being: Towards a Child Standpoint* (pp. 45–62). Dordrecht: Springer.

Fegter, S., & Richter, M. (2014). Capability approach as a framework for research on children's well-being. In A. Ben-Arieh, F. Casas, I. Frønes, and J.E. Korbin (Eds.) *Handbook of child well-being* (pp. 739–758). Dordrecht, The Netherlands: Springer.

Forgeard, M. J. C., Jayawickreme, E., Kern, M. L., & Seligman, M. E. P. (2011). Doing the right hing: Measuring wellbeing for public policy. *International Journal of Wellbeing*, 1, 79–106. https://doi.org/10.5502/ijw.v1i1.15

Garbarino, J. (1999). The effects of community violence on children. In L. Balter & C. Tamis-LaMonda (Eds.), *Child psychology: A handbook of contemporary issues* (pp. 412–425). New York, NY: Psychology Press.

Häkli, J., & Kallio, K. P. (2018). On becoming political: The political in subjectivity. *Subjectivity, 11*, 57–73.

Harcourt, D., & Einarsdottir, J. (2011). Introducing children's perspectives and participation in research. *European Early Childhood Education Research Journal, 19*(3), 301–307. https://doi.org/10.1080/1350293X.2011.597962

Hall, K., Woolard, I., Lake, L., & Smith, C. (Eds.). (2012). *South African child gauge* (Vol. 2012). Cape Town: Children's Institute, University of Cape Town.

Hart, R. A. (1997). Children's participation: The theory and practice of involving young citizen's in community development and environmental care. New York, NY: UNESCO.

Hasson, F., Keeney, S., & McKenna, H. (2000). Research guidelines for the Delphi survey technique. *Journal of Advanced Nursing, 32*(4), 1008–1015.

Headey, B., & Wearing, A. (1989). Personality, life events, and subjective well-being: Toward a dynamic equilibrium model. *Journal of Personality and Social Psychology, 57*, 731–739.

Helliwell, J. F., Barrington-Leigh, C., Harris, A., & Huang, H. (2009). International evidence on the social context of well-being. In E. Diener, D. Kahneman, & J. F. Helliwell (Eds.), *International differences in well-being*. Oxford, UK: Oxford University Press.

Holt, L. (2004). The 'voices' of children: De-centring empowering research relations. *Children's Geographies, 2*(1), 13–27.

Hills, P., & Argyle, M. (2002). The Oxford happiness questionnaire: A compact scale for the measurement of psychological Well-being. *Personality and Individual Differences, 33*(7), 1073–1082. https://doi.org/10.1016/s0191-8869(01)00213-6

Hultgren, F., & Johansson, B. (2018). Including babies and toddlers: A new model of participation. *Children's Geographies*. https://doi.org/10.1080/14733285.2018.1527016

Isobell, D., Lazarus, S., Suffla, S., & Seedat, M. (2016). Research translation through participatory research: The case of two community-based projects in low-income African settings. *Action Research, 14*(4), 393–411.

Jahoda, M. (1958). *Current concepts of positive mental health*. New York, NY: Basic Books.

James, A., & Prout, A. (1990). *Constructing and reconstructing childhood. Contemporary issues in the social construction of childhood*. London, UK: Falmer.

Jamieson, L., Berry, L., & Lake, L. (2017). *South African child gauge 2017*. Cape Town: Children's Institute, University of Cape Town.

Kopnina, H. (2011). What is (responsible) consumption? Discussing environment and consumption with children from different socioeconomic backgrounds in the Netherlands. *Environmentalist, 31*, 216–226.

Kraut, R. (2009). *What is good and why: The ethics of well-being*. Cambridge, MA: Harvard University Press.

Land, K. (2000). Social indicators. In E. F. Borgatta & R. V. Montgomery (Eds.), *Encyclopedia of sociology* (pp. 2682–2690). New York, NY: Macmillan.

Land, K. C., Lamb, V. L., Meadows, S. O., & Taylor, A. (2007). Measuring trends in well-being: An evidence-based approach. *Social Indicators Research, 80*, 105–132.

Lippman, L. H., Moore, K. A. & McIntosh, H. (2009). *Positive Indicators of Child Well-Being: A Conceptual Framework, Measures and Methodological Issues*. Innocenti Working Paper No. 2009–21. Florence, UNICEF Innocenti Research Centre.

Langhout, R. D., & Thomas, E. (2010). Imagining participatory action research in collaboration with children: An introduction. *American Journal of Community Psychology, 46*(1), 60–66.

Lazarus, S., Duran, B., Caldwell, L., Bulbulia, S. (2012). Public health research and action: Reflections on possible challenges and possibilities of community-based participatory research. In J. Maddock (Ed.), *Public health* (pp. 309–324). Intech (Open Access Publisher). Available from http://www.intechweb.org

Ludwig, J., Duncan, G. J., Gennetian, L. A., Katz, L. F., Kessler, R. C., Kling, J. R., & Sanbonmatsu, L. (2012). Neighborhood effects on the long-term well-being of low-income adults. *Science, 337*(6101), 1505–1510.

Lundy, L. (2007). 'Voice' is not enough: Conceptualising article 12 of the United Nations convention on the rights of the child. *British Educational Research Journal, 33*(6), 927–942.

Malone, K., & Tranter, P. J. (2003). School grounds as sites for learning: Making the most of environmental opportunities. *Environmental Education Research, 9*(3), 283–303.

Malone, K. (2016). Reconsidering children's encounters with nature and place using posthumanism. *Australian Journal of Environmental Education, 32*, 42–56.

Mason, J., & Watson, E. (2014). Researching children: Research on, with, and by children. In A. Ben-Arieh, F. Casas, I. Frønes, & J. E. Korbin (Eds.), *Handbook of child well-being: Theories, methods and policies in global perspective* (pp. 2757–2796). Dordrecht, The Netherlands: Springer.

Mathews, S., & Martin, L. J. (2016). Developing an understanding of fatal child abuse and neglect: Results from the south African child death review pilot study. *SAMJ: South African Medical Journal, 106*(12), 1160–1163.

McKendrick, J. H. (2014). Geographies of children's well-being: in, of, and for Place. In A. Ben-Arieh, F. Casas, I. Frønes, and J.E. Korbin (Eds.) *Handbook of child well-being* (pp. 279–300). Dordrecht, The Netherlands: Springer.

Medvedev, O. N., & Landhuis, C. E. (2018). Exploring constructs of Well-being, happiness and quality of life. *Peer J, 6*, e4903. https://doi.org/10.7717/peerj.4903

Minkkinen, J. (2013). The structural model of child well-being. *Child Indicators Research, 6*(3), 547–558.

National Research Council. (2013). Subjective Well-being: Measuring happiness, suffering, and other dimensions of experience. Panel on measuring subjective Well-being in a policy-relevant framework. In A. A. Stone & C. Mackie (Eds.), *Committee on National Statistics, division of Behavioral and social sciences and education*. Washington, DC: The National Academies Press.

Nussbaum, M. C. (1988). Nature, function and capability: Aristotle on political distribution. *Oxford Studies in Ancient Philosophy, Supplementary Volume, 6*, 145–184.

Nussbaum, M. C. (2000). *Women and human development: The capabilities approach*. Cambridge, UK: Cambridge University Press.

OECD. (2017). *OECD economic surveys: South Africa 2017*. Paris: OECD Publishing.

Palmberg, I., & Kuru, J. (2000). Outdoor activities as a basis for environmental responsibility. *The Journal of Environmental Education, 31*(4), 32–46.

Palinkas, L. A., & Soydan, H. (2012). New horizons of translational research and research translation in social work. *Research on Social Work Practice, 22*(1), 85–92.

Parkes, J. (2007). The multiple meanings of violence: Children's talk about life in a South African neighbourhood. *Childhood, 14*(4), 401–414.

Pollard, E. L., & Davidson, L. (2001). *Foundations of child well-being* (UNESCO education sector monograph no. 18). Seattle, WA: Centre for Child Well-Being.

Pollard, E. L., & Lee, P. D. (2003). Child Well-being: A systematic review of the literature. *Social Indicators Research, 61*(1), 59–78.

Proctor, C., Linley, P. A., & Maltby, J. (2009). Youth life satisfaction measures: A review. *The Journal of Positive Psychology, 4*(2), 128–144.

Prout, A. (1997). Objective vs. subjective indicators or both? Whose perspective counts? *Eurosocial Reports, 62*, 89–100.

Putnam, R. D. (2000). *Bowling alone*. New York, NY: Simon & Schuster.

Radley, A. (2010). What people do with pictures. *Visual Studies, 25*(3), 268–279.

Raghavan, R., & Alexandrova, A. (2014). Toward a theory of child well-being. *Social Indicators Research, 121*(3), 887–902. https://doi.org/10.1007/s11205-014-0665-z

Rasmussen, K. (2004). Places for children-Children's places. *Childhood, 11*(2), 155–173.

Rees, G., Bradshaw, J., Goswami, H., & Keung, A. (2010). *Understanding children's Well-being: A national survey of young people's Well-being*. London: The Children's Society.

Rees, G., Goswami, H., & Pople, L. (2013). *The good childhood report*. London, UK: The children's society.

Ryan, R. M., & Deci, E. L. (2008a). A self-determination theory approach to psychotherapy: The motivational basis for effective change. *Canadian Psychology, 49*, 186–193.

Ryan, R. M., & Deci, E. L. (2008b). From ego-depletion to vitality: Theory and findings concerning the facilitation of energy available to the self. *Social and Personality Psychology Compass, 2*, 702–717.

Rye, S. A., & Vold, S. (2018). International development aid and young people's participation in societal development of the global south. *Children's Geographies*. https://doi.org/10.1080/14733285.2018.1497139

Ryff, C. D., & Singer, B. (1998). The contours of positive human health. *Psychological Inquiry, 9*, 1–28.

Sandin, B. (2014). History of children's Well-being. In A. Ben-Arieh, F. Casas, I. Frones, & J. E. Korbin (Eds.), *Handbook of child Well-being: Theories, methods and policies in global perspective* (pp. 31–86). Dordrecht: Springer.

Savahl, S. (2010). *Ideological constructions of childhood*. Unpublished doctoral thesis. University of the Western Cape. Bellville.

Savahl, S., Casas, F., & Adams, S. (2015). Validation of the Children's Hope scale amongst a sample of adolescents in the Western cape region of South Africa. *Child Indicators Research, 9*, 701–713.

Savahl, S., Casas, F., & Adams, S. (2016). Children's subjective Well-being: Multi-group analysis among a sample of children from two socio-economic status groups in the Western cape, South Africa. *Child Indicators Research, 10*(2), 473–488. https://doi.org/10.1007/s12187-016-9392-0

Savahl, S., Adams, S., Isaacs, S., September, R., Hendricks, G., & Noordien, Z. (2015). Subjective well-being amongst a sample of South African children: A descriptive study. *Child Indicators Research, 8*(1), 211–226.

Savahl, S., Casas, F., Adams, S., Gonzalez, M. &, Figuer, C. (2019). Considering a Quadripartite Model of Subjective Well-Being in Adolescents. Paper presented at the International Society of Child Indicators Conference (27th-29th August 2019).

Savahl, S., Malcolm, C., Slembrouk, S., Adams, S., Willenberg, I. A., & September, R. (2015). Discourses on well-being. *Child Indicators Research, 8*(4), 747–766.

Scheier, M. F., & Carver, C. S. (2003). Self-regulatory processes and responses to health threats: Effects of optimism on well-being. In J. Suls & K. A. Wallston (Eds.), *Social psychological foundations of health and illness* (pp. 395–428). Malden, MA: Blackwell.

Seligman, M. E. (2011). Flourish: A visionary new understanding of happiness and well-being. *Policy, 27*(3), 60–61.

Seligman, M. E. P. (2002). *Authentic happiness: Using the new positive psychology to realize your potential for lasting fulfillment*. New York, NY: Free Press.

Sen, A. K. (1985). Well-being, agency and freedom: The Dewey lectures 1984. *Journal of Philosophy, 82*(4), 169–221.

Sen, A. K. (1993). Capability and well-being. In M. Nussbaum & A. Sen (Eds.), *The quality of life* (pp. 30–53). Oxford, UK: Oxford University Press.

Sen, A. K. (2005). Human rights and capabilities. *Journal of Human Development, 6*(2), 151–166.

Sen, A. K. (2007). Children and human rights. *Indian Journal of Human Development, 2*(1), 1–12.

September, R. L., & Savahl, S. (2009). Children's perspectives on child well-being. *Social Work Practitioner Research, 21*(1), 23–40.

Skelton, T. (2010). Taking young people as political actors seriously: Opening the borders of political geography. *Area, 42*(2), 145–151.

Skivenese, M., & Strandbu, A. (2006). A child perspective and children's participation. *Children Youth and Environments, 16*(2), 10–27.

South African Police Service (SAPS). (2017). *Addendum to the SAPS annual report: Annual crime report 2016/2017.* Pretoria: SAPS.

Ssengooba, F., Atuyambe, L., Kiwanuka, S. N., Puvanachandra, P., Glass, N., & Hyder, A. A. (2011). Research translation to inform national health policies: Learning from multiple perspectives in Uganda. *BMC International Health and Human Rights, 11*(1), S13.

Statistics South Africa. (2014). *General Household Survey 2013.* Pretoria, South Africa: Statistics South Africa.

Steger, M. F., Kashdan, T. B., Sullivan, B. A., & Lorentz, D. (2008). Understanding the search for meaning in life: Personality, cognitive style, and the dynamic between seeking and experiencing meaning. *Journal of Personality, 76,* 199–228.

Stoecklin, D., & Bonvin, J. (Eds.). (2014). *Children's rights and the capability approach challenges and prospects.* Dordrecht, The Netherlands: Springer.

Stuurman, M. (2002). Research translation in South Africa. *Science & Technology Libraries, 23*(2–3), 145–150. https://doi.org/10.1300/J122v23n02

The African Child Policy Forum. (2016). The African report on child wellbeing 2016: Getting it right: Bridging the gap between policy and practice. Addis Ababa, Ethiopia: The African Child Policy Forum (ACPF).

Thornton, A. (2001). Introduction and overview. In A. Thornton (Ed.), *The well-being of children and families: Research and data needs* (pp. 3–27). Ann Arbor, MI: University of Michigan Press.

UNICEF. (2017). *State of the world's children: Children in a digital world.* New York, NY: UNICEF.

UNICEF Office of Research. (2007). *Child poverty in perspective: An overview of child well-being in rich countries, Innocenti report card 7.* Florence, Italy: UNICEF Office of Research.

UNICEF Office of Research. (2013). *Child well-being in rich countries: A comparative overview* (Innocenti report card 11). Florence, Italy: UNICEF Office of Research.

United Nations General Assembly. (1989a). *Adoption of the convention on the rights if the child.* New York, NY: United Nations.

United Nations General Assembly, *Convention on the Rights of the Child.* (1989b). United Nations, Treaty Series, vol. 1577, p. 3, available at: http://www.refworld.org/docid/3ae6b38f0.html. Accessed 6 Mar 2016.

van de Vijver, F., & Hambleton, R. K. (1996). Translating tests. *European Psychologist, 1*(2), 89–99.

Vásquez, C., Hervás, G., Rahona, J. J., & Gómez, D. (2009). Psychological Well-being and health: Contributions of positive psychology. *Annuary of Health and Clinical Psychology, 5,* 15–27.

Wang, C., & Burris, M. A. (1994). Empowerment through photo novella: Portraits of participation. *Health Education Quarterly, 21*(2), 171–186.

Wang, C. C., & Redwood-Jones, Y. A. (2001). Photovoice ethics: Perspectives from Flint photovoice. *Health Education & Behavior, 28*(5), 560–572.

Wang, F., & Wang, D. (2016). Place, geographical context and subjective wellbeing: State of art and future directions. In D. Wang & S. He (Eds.), *Mobility, sociability and wellbeing of urban living* (pp. 189–230). Publisher: Springer-Verlag, Berlin.

Watson, D., Clark, L. A., & Tellegen, A. (1988). Development and validation of brief measures of positive and negative affect: The PANAS scales. *Journal of Personality and Social Psychology, 54*(6), 1063.

Wells, N. M. (2014). The role of nature in children's resilience: Cognitive and social processes. In K. G. Tidball & M. E. Krasny (Eds.), *Greening in the red zone: Disaster, resilience and community greening* (pp. 95–110). Dordrecht, The Netherlands: Springer.

WHO. (1946). Constitution of the World Health Organisation. Basic Documents, Supplement 2006. https://www.who.int/governance/eb/who_constitution_en.pdf. Accessed 20 Aug 2012

Willenberg, I., September, R., & Savahl, S. (2006). *Towards the development of child Well-being indicators from children's perspectives.* Cape Town: CYRTP.

World Bank. (2018). South Africa overview. https://www.worldbank.org/en/country/southafrica/overview

World Health Organization Quality of Life (WHOQOL) Group. (1998). Development of the World Health Organization WHOQOL-BREF quality of life assessment. *Psychological Medicine, 28*(3), 551–558.

Zaff, J. F., Smith, D. C., Rogers, M. F., Leavitt, C. H., Halle, T. G., & Bornstein, M. H. (2003). Holistic wellbeing and the developing child. In M. H. Bornstein, L. Davidson, C. L. M. Keyes, & K. Moore (Eds.), *Well-being: Positive development across the life course* (pp. 23–32). Mahwah, NJ: Lawrence Erlbaum.

An Outsider in South Africa: Critical Reflections on Ubuntu

23

Sheila Trahar

Abstract

This chapter is about being – or feeling myself to be – an outsider in South Africa. My relationship with South Africa began 10 years ago but, in the chapter, I focus mainly on the past 3 years during which I have visited the country three or four times each year in connection with two projects with which I have been involved. I weave anecdotes of remembered events, including critical reflections on my involvement with the two research projects, together with my reading of literature on Ubuntu, on decolonization and decoloniality. I employ different voices in the writing as I braid together myriad threads of experience and insight, occasionally, scholarly insight. The chapter is, therefore, not intended to be a neat, linear account. It is a story – or several stories – of being an outsider. "The thing about stories is that they are like bindweeds that have to wind round and round and creep all over the place before they get to the top of the pole" (de Bernieres, Birds without wings. Secker & Warburg, London, p 141, 2004). My stories 'wind round and round and creep all over the place' but, whether or not they 'get to the top of the pole', wherever that might be, I leave it to you, the reader, to judge.

S. Trahar (✉)
University of Bristol, Bristol, UK
e-mail: s.trahar@bristol.ac.uk

23.1 Introduction

I was surprised when I was invited to contribute a chapter to this Handbook. I mused on whether I would accept the invitation and, if so, how I, as a complete outsider to the African context, could craft a chapter that would have a place in a Handbook of Quality of Life in African Societies. On impulse, I proposed that I could offer an account of how I experienced South Africa as an outsider, reflecting critically on how those experiences related to Ubuntu. Naively, I thought that I 'knew' something about Ubuntu because I was involved, as a methodological consultant, in an Ubuntu research project. My involvement in that project, albeit on the periphery, meant that I had heard myriad accounts of Ubuntu, accounts that challenged my initial understanding of it, an understanding developed through my first encounters with the philosophy when I embarked on my PhD some 18 years ago. In addition, over the past 3 years, I have visited South Africa several times. I am beginning to feel more familiar with the country and am developing a fondness for it, yet still, I feel that I am an outsider.

I am an adherent of writing as inquiry (Richardson & St Pierre, 2005). I write in order to learn or understand something that I did not understand previously. Writing can enable me to understand a complex concept or situation, to understand myself. I decided, therefore, to write the chapter as a stream of consciousness, to write

I. Eloff (ed.), *Handbook of Quality of Life in African Societies*, International Handbooks of Quality-of-Life, https://doi.org/10.1007/978-3-030-15367-0_23

what I wanted to write and then to strive to frame it into something comprehensible to a reader. Sometimes the words tumbled easily onto the page, at other times I would be struggling to show the links between my experiences, impressions and Ubuntu and quality of life. Throughout the chapter, I recount anecdotes, interweaving them with my reading of literature on Ubuntu, on decolonization and decoloniality together with critical reflections on my involvement with the two research projects based in South Africa. An anecdote is defined as an "account of something interesting" or a "humorous incident" (Gallop, 2002, p. 2), often criticized for being "diametrically opposed to the seriousness implicit in theory" (Larrain, 2013, p. 149) yet it can be "used to generate new knowledge and produce theory with a better sense of humour" (ibid). I endeavour to provide interesting accounts of incidents, and to articulate my developing understanding of the 'theory/ies' of Ubuntu and its/their place in South Africa today making connections with quality of life wherever I can. My aim is not to "produce theory" but it is to "generate new knowledge", if only for and/or about myself and my relationship with South Africa although my accounts may resonate with others who are positioned similarly.

As I began to write about my experiences in South Africa, I traced so many connections, connections with my past life, relationships and work. I realized that I could detect links with my research and teaching, informed by the integration of the two interdependent concepts of internationalization of higher education and of social justice in higher education and my use of narrative inquiry and autoethnography. I began to see how connections could be made with decolonization, decoloniality and curricular justice, issues that are to the fore not only in higher education in South Africa but also in the UK. This chapter is, therefore, a series of stories, a meander through several events, making connections and catching some 'theory' along the way.

> It is telling that in 1994 the government of South Africa, the last country on the continent to gain its independence, promised a 'better life' to meet its newly enfranchised black citizens' aspirations for housing, running water, and electricity. Some twenty years later, there is still a marked difference between what determines happiness among black and white South Africans. Economists report that better access to infrastructure and public goods increases happiness among black South Africans, while determinants of the happiness among wealthier white South Africans mirror those typically found in Western developed research settings (Moller, Roberts, Tiliouine, & Loschky, 2017, pp. 87–88)

What constitutes a better life for people in South Africa? Does lessening spatial inequality result in improved quality of life? As an outsider, to what extent can I make judgements on such matters? Following a discussion of insider/outsider, the chapter develops as a series of recollections about experiences in South Africa, and discussion of my involvement in the two research projects. These recollections are interlaced with encounters with Ubuntu, decolonization and decoloniality and, as appropriate, their relationship with 'quality of life'.

23.2 Insider/Outsider

I resist "essentialist dualisms such as the insider/outsider" (McNess, Arthur, & Crossley, 2015, p. 298). I recognize that I am not "fixed, stable and coherent, but constantly shifting, incomplete, fragmented and contradictory in relation to both collective and personal existence" (ibid). I move constantly, restlessly, between insider/outsider positions and can vacillate between them in the same context. I can feel as if I am an outsider in what might be perceived to be my own milieu because I feel that I do not belong. A poignant example is that of being an academic in an elite university that would not have accepted me as an undergraduate because of my poor A level grades.[1] I believe that, if one desires to do so, as I do, one can subvert and transform elite, dominant systems more effectively from the inside rather than hovering on the periphery and deliberately

[1]The 'A' level refers to the Advanced Level examinations that, in the UK, are the main determinant of university entry.

marginalizing oneself by taking an outsider position. Indeed, I have experienced some success in doing so. Nonetheless, I continue to suffer from imposter syndrome. One day someone will discover that I am an imposter, an intruder in a world in which I have no place; that I am not an insider at all. Intellectually, I know that making such a statement is abhorrent. It contradicts all of the beliefs about equality of access and social justice that I hold but, emotionally, that is how I can feel. In contrast, I have realized that I was more of an insider in a context in which I might be perceived as an outsider when I worked regularly in Hong Kong. On one of my visits, I was accompanied by a colleague. It was her first time in the Far East and she would comment on situations and behaviours that she found to be different from the UK. I found myself bemused by her observations, as I did not see that these behaviours and situations were at all different. Gradually, it occurred to me that I no longer noticed these differences, as they had become a part of me. I was an outsider and an insider. In some other contexts, for example, when I was working on a project in Israel, I felt like an outsider all of the time. Although I argued that this gave me some licence to ask awkward questions in this conflicted society, I rarely felt comfortable as it was as if being an outsider meant that I was prohibited from proffering my perspective on the 'political situation' as the ongoing conflict with the Palestinians is referred to. As I write these words, I am in Australia and I realise that many behaviours that I did not even think about when I lived here, I now notice as different and, in doing so, somewhat truculently, position myself deliberately as an outsider. I am an outsider when I respond "Fine" in answer to "How are you?" rather than "Good, thanks". Is this something that I do in order to confirm my status as an outsider? I could so easily reply in ways that I know to be the protocol, yet I choose not to, to not pretend to be an insider in what is a very familiar context.

In the Ubuntu project, which I discuss later in the chapter, I was wary of continuously asking questions, feeling that people would get bored of explaining things to me. It is difficult when one is becoming more and more intrinsic to a project – moving to becoming an insider – yet often not understanding the nuances of the conversation or being unfamiliar with many of the people spoken about – politicians, for example. I gradually gathered confidence to ask provocative questions, questions that baffled me, as an outsider, about South Africa. I wanted to try and understand the way things were, or why they seemed to be that way or why, if Ubuntu was so significant, many people behaved towards one another in ways that appeared to contravene the essence of Ubuntu, as I understood it. Holding to an outsider position, while shifting to becoming much more of an insider, enabled rich conversations to take place, conversations that were a source of learning for all of us.

I may seem to be creeping all over the place but my intention is to establish that, although I use 'outsider' in the title and, in many ways continue to feel like an outsider in South Africa, I can shift constantly between being an insider and an outsider in other contexts, including that of my own. Does this outsider position entitle me to comment on quality of life in South Africa? As the chapter unfolds, I will reflect on this question. Through the process of writing, I may begin to feel that I am more of an insider than I thought.

23.3 Some South African Stories

23.3.1 Johannesburg April 2018

It is 10 years since I first came here although my first visit was to Cape Town. I am missing my son's birthday again as I did 10 years ago. On the plane, I calculated the number of trips I had made since July 2015 when I first went to Pretoria in connection with the Ubuntu project. It was 10 – so this is my 12th trip in total and 11th in 3 years. As soon as I arrive, or at least leave the airport, everything looks familiar. As always, I am overwhelmed by the space. We arrive at the guesthouse and I see the barbed wire on top of the security fencing that surrounds it. We discuss whether we will walk to a restaurant to eat this evening, whether we will walk back. We feel frustrated that we have to ponder on whether or not to take a 10-minutes walk that, at home, we would not even think about doing. Deciding that we ought to play safe, we book an Uber. Inevitably, I start to think about whether I have witnessed any changes in 10 years. Are there successes to celebrate? Has the quality of life improved for the majority of people? As an outsider, am I really in a position to comment? I cast my mind back to April 2008 and arriving in Cape Town…

23.3.2 Cape Town, April 2008

> The first sight for many visitors to Cape Town is a ribbon of shack settlements leading from the airport right up to the suburbs nestled under the city's landmark Table Mountain. (Moller, 2007, p. 187)

I was met at Cape Town airport by a driver who chatted all the way to the University of Cape Town (UCT), which was where I was staying. As we were driving away from the airport, on the left hand side, I saw something, the like of which I had never seen before, even when travelling in areas of huge deprivation in India and other parts of sub-Saharan Africa. This was an extensive collection of buildings that seemed to be made from corrugated iron. The driver pointed it out to me much as a tourist guide would indicate a site of interest, telling me the name of it. Crossroads. I was shocked by it. Entering the UCT campus, I saw black students and white students, but not walking together. I was shown the statue of Cecil Rhodes, expressing surprise that it was still there. I remember the student who told me how she and other black students were ignored by their white lecturers. I recall the opulent wealth of the suburb where we had dinner every night. But were these really my first impressions? Memory plays tricks on us of course and so is what I am remembering what I am choosing to for the purposes of this chapter? Am I shaping those memories so that they fit into the kind of narrative that I want to present? Maybe, maybe not. And, even if I were, would it matter?

As my first week in South Africa progressed, I felt more and more uncomfortable. I could not wait to get home. I remember telling a colleague on my return that I was never going to South Africa again. She retorted that, if people did not visit the country, what would that achieve? Having now visited the country so many more times, I believe that she was right. I have learned from experience that it is through visiting and, preferably, working in a context that enables me to make a more informed judgment about its complexities. Perhaps, therefore, I am earning the right to comment, as an outsider, on the complexities of life in South Africa?

23.3.3 Pretoria July 2015

Once again I was collected at the airport but this time by a driver who did not speak one word to me on the drive to Pretoria. I was greeted at the guesthouse by the owner, a charming white woman who served me coffee in the garden. I had lunch with Grace, who I had not seen since my first visit in 2008. We drove to a restaurant where she paid a man to look after her car. I had never paid anyone to look after a car and so I asked her why she did it. She explained that it was common in South Africa, the people only expected a few ZAR but looking after parked cars was a way that they could earn money. We finished our meal and Grace asked for the food that we had not eaten to be bagged up. I assumed that she was taking home this 'doggy bag' but she told me that she was giving it to the man who was looking after her car. I felt ashamed, ashamed because I would never have thought of doing that, ashamed because it did not occur to me that he might be hungry. I experienced double discomfort. I was in turmoil. Not only was she giving someone our leftovers, about which I felt very uncomfortable, but also such a gesture, a really kind one, was totally outside my frame of reference. What must his quality of life be like? Is Grace's behaviour an example of Ubuntu?

> "Don't go out on your own", Grace said. "You may be rather conspicuous as a foreigner and you need to avoid places where you might be in danger. You're OK to go to the Mall but, try not to have anything visible."

"But, if I go out, I may need to buy something. I'll have to take my money. How am I supposed to carry that"?

"Well, don't have it visible".

Is that Ubuntu? To feel fear? To feel that I am restricted in the places that I can visit alone? Even in daylight?

As I write now about that very enjoyable lunch with Grace, I remember having dinner with her in Cape Town on my first visit in 2008. She took me to a restaurant with great music and food and a wonderful ambiance. My relationship with her has always been robust and I recall how, on that evening, we talked about apartheid and how people continued to identify, 14 years after its end, according to the categories ascribed to them. Grace identified – and identifies – as black but, because her skin is fair, others ascribe the 'coloured' label to her. She explained to me that, no matter how she identifies herself, others mark her as coloured. This marker shapes her daily experiences and it is difficult for her to navigate social and political spaces without the marker and identifier acting as a filter. She then pointed out to me those people in the restaurant that I was convinced were white but who she insisted were coloured. This warm, crazy, wine fuelled conversation was like a game that we were playing 'Guess how people identify and are identified'. It illustrated for me how insidious it was to make judgements about people's identities on the basis of skin colour. Intellectually and emotionally, I was, of course, aware of this, but our conversation drove it home to me more powerfully and poignantly than reading about it ever could.

23.3.4 Johannesburg April 2018

I decided that, as I was in the process of writing this chapter, I would keep a diary during this visit, an account of what I noticed and experienced, in order to 'test' some of my other recollections. My intentions were good but, unfortunately, I ended up keeping it only for a couple of days and so this account is a combination of diary entries and hindsight.

It was warm and reasonably sunny when we arrived. It was nice to be staying somewhere where I had stayed previously, even with its idiosyncrasies. I recognized the guesthouse employees, it was still difficult to operate the room safe AND it was 2 days after Winnie Mandela's death. References to Ubuntu proliferated.

23.3.5 April 2018 University of Johannesburg Soweto Campus

The students have travelled 20 hours by coach, overnight, so that they can be here, they can meet each other and they can meet us. There are about 60 of them, student co-researchers in our SARiHE project that I discuss later in the chapter. They are from Rhodes University, the University of Fort Hare and the University of Johannesburg. This is the first time that the majority of them have visited Johannesburg. They are beautiful and confident. They disagree with each other but in ways that are so articulate and respectful. They ask us questions about the SARiHE project. Why have we not involved all universities in South Africa? Why could more people not have been involved? Our answers, though entirely legitimate, seem woeful. The funding was limited, the time was limited. There are external constraints on any funded research. This research is about them, their lives. We revel in the spontaneous singing and dancing at the end of our 2 days together, yet we remain on the periphery, watching with our stiff and awkward white bodies, embarrassed by our lack of movement, not knowing whether we should join in. They are singing in a language that we do not understand. One of our South African colleagues tells us that they are singing the praises of the SARiHE project, what it is striving to achieve and their role in it. So – is this Ubuntu? They seem to us to be the future of South Africa. We feel optimistic.

23.3.6 April 2018: Snippets of Conversations

"I refuse to talk about decolonization", he said.

"These people" she said, as if somehow she was surprised that 'these people' were capable of anything, let alone high academic achievement.

"Why should our graduation ceremonies be formal and stilted"? he said. "Why do we not have ululating"?

"Why don't you?" I replied. '

"Because we continue to follow a dominant Eurocentric model". I nodded in agreement.

We spent the week-end at an expensive, luxury game lodge in Pilanesburg, driven there and back by a man whose services had cost us a lot of money and who we imagine will not see very much of it. On the way back to Johannesburg, we drive past an accident. The others were dozing but I realized that someone had been killed as I saw a body at the side of the road, covered in gold foil. There was nobody near it. Why was nobody near her or him? I have driven along this road before and it is impossible to cross it without dodging the traffic. There are communities on either side, people living in poor housing who cannot get from one side to the other without risking their lives. "If these were white communities, there would be a bridge or an underpass", I find myself thinking as I gaze out of the window.

We gasped in horror at the sight of the dead rhino, poached, the 12th we are told, since January.

"How terrible", we say in our first world angst.

"They can get ZAR 200,000 for that horn", the tracker said.

"Well, if you have nothing, I can see the temptation", I say.

"No, no", some of the others cry, "That's no excuse". Isn't it? Who are we to judge? We who have no need to kill animals in order to eat, to feed our families.

Where is Ubuntu?

23.3.7 21 April Bristol

I have been back at home for a week and I realize that all of my good intentions to keep a diary have come to nothing. So, I am relying, once more, on memories, although they are very recent memories. What bubbles up to the surface as I write? The driver who took me to Oliver Reginald Tambo (ORT) airport for my flight home and who, to avoid the late afternoon traffic, took a series of back roads, none of which I had ever been on before. In taking these roads, we passed through neighbourhoods that I do not recall seeing on any of my visits to Johannesburg. The properties are dilapidated and people are wandering around with those looks of desperation, resignation, hopelessness. I did not want to see them, to be reminded of how so many people in this country are forced to live and whose quality of life seems to me to continue to be extremely low, 24 years after the end of apartheid. I think about my comfortable life in a country that is, of course, also not without its problems and racial tensions. This week we commemorate 25 years since the racist murder of the black teenager, Stephen Lawrence, in London. I find myself consumed by the three television programmes "Stephen: the murder that changed a nation" that deal in horrific detail with the corruption, with the racism of the police, with the abominable treatment of the Lawrence family. I have seen The Colour of Justice in the theatre, the play that was produced entirely from the transcripts of the inquiry into Stephen's murder; I have been to hear Doreen Lawrence, Stephen's mother, speak so eloquently and movingly. The TV critic in The Guardian newspaper considered that there ought to have been a question mark following the words "the murder that changed a nation". I agree. Did his murder really change a nation? I read about Cyril Ramaphosa returning to South Africa, cutting short his visit to the Commonwealth Leaders' summit because of riots in Mahikeng in the North West province. I look at where Mahikeng is on a map. "Boiling frustration over lack of housing, health services and jobs… Shops owned by foreigners were looted". This seems familiar…

Ubuntu highlights the interconnectedness of human beings, with the implication that people should treat others as part of the extended human family. However, the ongoing violence against foreign migrants suggests that certain groups may be excluded from the scope of its benefits. Ubuntu is simultaneously present and absent in the community

> and its members. Concrete acts of goodness are juxtaposed with the darkness of violence and murder, locating both sets of actions within the same people and exploring what this tells us about Ubuntu. (Muller, Eliastam, & Trahar, 2019, p. 8)

So, what or where is Ubuntu? Is that still an appropriate or useful question?

The driver tells me that he is from Zimbabwe and has lived in South Africa for 13 years. His family are at home in Zim. He asks me how easy it is to find work in the UK. He tells me that he is a landscape gardener. I do not know what to say. I mumble something about the 'living wage', trying to avoid getting into conversation about our draconian attitudes to immigration, knowing or being fairly certain that he would not stand a chance of entering the UK to work. On arrival at the airport, I push a few notes into his hand. He is so grateful for the tip. Once again that dis-ease washes over me. Do I do this to quell my conscience? To assuage my guilt at my comfortable life? A life whose quality is higher than his?

> "You people need to up your game", she said, after the fourth time of asking for the bill in the airport café where we meet. I realize that I would never dare to say that even though I might share her frustration. But she is black and so I feel she can. I feel sorry for them. It is not their fault. It is clear that they have not had proper training. Excuses, excuses, excuses…
> Where is Ubuntu?

23.3.8 May 2018 Australia

I have no intention of engaging in a comparative study of Australia and South Africa but there are similarities between the two countries – or at least there are for me – especially in the vastness of their landscapes. But, being here now, I cannot discern many similarities. Australian spaces seem so much larger, the soil so much redder and we are driving through Western Australia but see hardly any Aboriginal people. When I first went to South Africa 10 years ago, I remember thinking that Cape Town was like Sydney. They are both located in beautiful, natural settings, both display enormous wealth – and poverty – but maybe the similarities end there. In so far as I am aware, houses in Sydney are not surrounded by high, barbed wire fences and I have always felt safe walking around alone. And yet, and yet:

> There's evidence everywhere of the whitefella siege mentality – the high chain-link fences and padlocked gates around their houses, the alarms and locking devices on their cars, the welded steel cage around the petrol browser. (Mahood, 2016, p. 19)

The word 'whitefella' is a clue but the words refer, not to Sydney, but to Balgo in Western Australia. They are taken from the book "Position doubtful: mapping landscape and memories" that I read while in Australia in May 2018. This book is written by a white Australian woman who spends months at a time with the Aboriginal people in the part of Western Australia where she grew up, mapping the territory using methods that are respectful to indigenous ways. I am gripped by this book, even though I am uncomfortable, occasionally, with some of the activities in which Mahood and her friend Pam engage in the name of art. But Mahood spends much of her time listening to stories and some of the ways in which she describes these stories really resonate with me.

Why am I telling this story about a recent trip to Australia? What does it have to do with a chapter that I am writing about Ubuntu and South Africa? Are the links too tenuous? A key focus of Mahood's book is space and land and its appropriation by white settlers and the way of existing together, often still very uncomfortable, that people have learned. In South Africa, space is also a deeply political matter due to the displacement effects of apartheid. The relationship between race, geography and land is highlighted by Gordon (2015) who refers to a "geography of race" in which "white populations have [e] more geographical space than people of colour" (p. 163). It seems that I feel connected to vast landscapes in countries that were colonized by the UK, in which land was appropriated and over which there continues to be controversy. So – where – and what is Ubuntu?

23.4 Ubuntu: First Encounters

My first encounters with Ubuntu occurred when I began my PhD research in 2000. The initial focus of my PhD was the learning experiences of a group of 'international' postgraduate students undertaking a Master's degree in what was then the Graduate School of Education – it is now a School of Education- at the University of Bristol where I was employed as a lecturer and where I continue to be employed. I have written elsewhere and in different ways about how the doctoral process began for me (see, for example, Trahar, 2011, 2013, 2015, 2019) and of how that, before too long, I realized that I needed to include all of the students in the group in my study, irrespective of from where they came. In addition, it seemed disingenuous to be inviting these students to share with me their experiences as learners in our academic environment and to reflect deeply on those experiences, comparing them with previous ones, if I did not engage in similar, in depth reflections on my own learning experiences and, importantly, on my approaches to teaching.

I was very clear about the philosophies that informed my student centred approach to teaching but I had never thought about interrogating the roots of those philosophies. For example, the humanistic philosophy of Carl Rogers (see, for example, Rogers, 1994) that I admired and strove to emulate was grounded in views of the world and of the people in it that, although congruent with mine, may not have been congruent with those of many of the students. Subsequently, I developed an obsession with philosophy, realizing that I – and others- are always operating from a philosophical position even though we may not be aware of what that might be. My avid reading led me to the concept of epistemological racism (Scheurich, 1997; Stanfield, 1993, 1994) and to a critique of the appropriateness of the dominant paradigms in social science, in particular to inform the intercultural research in which I was engaged. Those paradigms are rooted in Eurocentric philosophy yet are inflicted on – and often adopted by – those from contexts with very different worldviews. I viewed this as continuing to perpetuate colonialism. I revelled in ideas that appeared to contradict theories with which I was more accustomed, delighting in disrupting what seemed to be the status quo in philosophical positioning, in the School and in the field of international higher education at the time. Ubuntu – or the definition of it that I read then, "I am because we are" – spoke to me because it seemed to subvert the individualist "I think therefore I am" of Descartes, with which I was more familiar and which underpins the individualism of humanistic philosophy in its search for self-actualization and the "true self".

> Ubuntu directly contradicts the Cartesian conception of individuality in terms of which the individual or self can be conceived without thereby necessarily conceiving the other...The Cartesian individual exists prior to, or separately and independently from the rest of the community or society...Ubuntu *defines* the individual in terms of his/her relationship with others...individuals only exist *in* their relationships with others (Louw, 1998, p. 4, emphasis in original)

My training as a counsellor had introduced me to humanistic philosophy and, much later to narrative therapy and I grappled with the inappropriateness of locating my research within paradigmatic perspectives that were alien to many of those who participated in it. My critiques of Eurocentric perspectives have continued, influenced by those such as Tuhiwai Smith (2012), Connell (2007, 2017), Swadener and Mutua (2008), Zeleza (2012) and, more recently, Mbembe (2015, 2016), Ndlovu-Gatsheni (2014), de Sousa Santos (2012), and Motsa (2017). Such ongoing critical reflection informs my research, writing and teaching, and my supervision of doctoral researchers from all over the world. I now realize that the issues of decolonization of the curriculum, decoloniality and epistemicide, foregrounded by Mbembe (2015, 2016), Ndlovu-Gatsheni (2014), and Motsa (2017) are informing every dimension of my work and have their roots in my earlier encounters with Ubuntu.

My own, profound PhD experiences challenged my thinking in many ways and, subsequently, enabled me to challenge others to ask similar, difficult questions of themselves. Encountering Ubuntu, a totally different way of thinking about the world, and myself, was, therefore, an important step on this journey. It was one of the many ideas or philosophies that challenged and enabled me to confront – or start to confront – my own identities as a white, British woman working in environments with people who were from former colonies (see, for example, Trahar, 2011, 2019) and, indeed, as a woman who was often working in former colonies in which the vestiges of colonialism were still visible. As I wrote earlier, I had been aware of the philosophical concepts that underpinned my preferred approaches to learning and teaching but was much less cognizant of the extent to which they were culturally mediated. Engaging in such dialogue with myself led to the doctorate developing strong autoethnographic dimensions, including, intense reflection on my "whiteness". I held Ubuntu up as a philosophy to aim for, one that I believed challenged the Eurocentric status quo.

23.5 The Ubuntu Project: Re-encountering Ubuntu

I now move on to discuss how I re-encountered Ubuntu some 4 years ago and the significance that it has had for me since then. In the summer of 2014, I received an email from Professor Julian Muller from the University of Pretoria. His son and family lived in Bristol and Julian had found our (then named) Narrative Inquiry Centre, of which I was a member, on the University of Bristol website. Julian, a narrative therapist, asked whether we could meet and we did so in September of that year during his visit to Bristol. We connected with each other immediately, finding that we thought and felt the same way about many things, including our approaches to research, which were located firmly within narrative inquiry and autoethnography. During that meeting, Julian told me about what I refer to throughout this chapter as the Ubuntu project, the full title of which is "The meaning and value of Ubuntu in human and social development in Africa". This was a 3 year (2014–2017) research project, involving researchers from the Faculties of Humanities, Law and Theology at the University of Pretoria and funded by the Templeton World Charity Foundation. Its aims were to locate the concept of Ubuntu within broader, intellectual debates of self and community and to demonstrate its intellectual and philosophical value and theoretical grounding in known practices throughout Africa. The project explored Ubuntu from the myriad perspectives of the four research clusters of African literature, law, political science and theology. At that first meeting, Julian asked whether I would like to be a member of the project's Advisory Board. I agreed – and thought no more about it. Some 6 months later, I received an email from him, inviting me to South Africa to participate in a meeting of all of the researchers involved in his theology cluster. He felt that I would be well placed to advise the group on their use of narrative inquiry in their research. I was flattered by the invitation but at the same time felt some tension. Did I really did want to go to South Africa again, 7 years after my troubled experiences in Cape Town? On the other hand, 7 years had passed and maybe the country had changed. I was interested in the project and my curiosity got the better of me. I went.

Prior to the meeting, Julian sent a list of questions from each of the researchers in his group. They had been asked to pose methodological – including ethical – and contextual questions of the people attending the meeting. I felt confident in responding to the methodological and ethical questions but very uncertain about the contextual ones. I found myself researching meanings of Ubuntu, anxious not to appear ignorant. I really enjoyed meeting the Ubuntu researchers and the other people who joined us who had written about Ubuntu and/or were familiar with narrative inquiry. I was fascinated by the research that those in the group were doing and I had many of my stereotypes shattered, in particular those of the white, male Afrikaner farmer. One of the group members who identified as such shared the research he was conducting with his black farm manager and how he was struggling with addressing the ethical complexities inherent in his study. I was extremely moved by his insightfulness, by his sensitivity and integrity.

At that meeting, as people spoke about their research, I realized that fictionalization was a possible method of re-presenting the narratives, especially those that were more controversial, painful and difficult to re-tell. I believe that fictionalization can be a "device…to bring to the awareness of readers complex situations that may be difficult to do otherwise" (Trahar & Yu, 2015, p. xvii) and that it can be a way of telling a story that is "based on 'real' events to produce a version of the 'truth' as [the author] sees it" (ibid, p. xviii). I was unsure about whether to suggest the use of fictionalization, however, as I did not want to be seen as an 'expert'. I was an outsider and, moreover, from a country that has had a troubled history with South Africa. I did, however, suggest it to one of the group members as I felt that her research really lent itself to fictionalization in the re-presentation of the narratives. I recall that my suggestion was greeted politely but with a look of puzzlement.

Following that first meeting, Julian invited me to join the group on several occasions and I began to realize that my contributions were welcomed and considered carefully by everyone. At one of the earlier meetings, Julian encouraged the researchers to use a chapter from one of my books (Trahar, 2011) as a guide to being reflexive about their methodologies. This is another example of the tension that I described earlier in this chapter. I was pleased that he valued my work but also embarrassed, concerned that it might have no relevance for the group, anxious that I, an outsider, might be seen to be imposing my perspectives on narrative inquiry on them. We then decided to re-introduce the idea of fictionalization to the group. We proposed that each researcher fictionalize one of the narratives that s/he had gathered through her/his research in ways that were similar to how I had used fictionalization in reporting elements of my research. There followed several iterations of writing, reading that writing aloud to the group, receiving feedback and more writing. I participated fully in these activities, sharing my writing in the group, writing that reflected many of the insider/outsider ambivalences that I share in this chapter, writing that asked provocative questions, in particular of Ubuntu. This process of writing and sharing it with each other engendered trust within the group, enabling people to challenge and question others' writing but always with respect. I was astounded by the creativity and power of the fictionalized narratives that were produced, narratives that have been collected together into a book "Unfolding narratives of Ubuntu in Southern Africa" (Muller et al., 2019). The ways in which we depended on each other for this edited collection to come to fruition is, as we claim in the book, an example of Ubuntu at work.

23.6 Southern African Rurality in Higher Education (SARiHE)

A year or so after my first visit to Pretoria, two colleagues and I, together with a group of people from three South African universities were successful in gaining a research grant from the UK's Economic and Social Research Council (ESRC)/Newton Fund to investigate how students from deep rural areas in South Africa negotiated the transition to higher education and their subsequent journeys through it. This project is now known as Southern African Rurality in Higher Education (SARiHE). It seemed serendipitous to me that, after having had such ambivalent feelings towards South Africa, I was now involved in two projects that meant that I would be continuing to visit and work in the country until March 2019. My involvement in SARiHE, together with the Ubuntu project, is what has led me to engage with critiques of Ubuntu and with decolonization and decoloniality. Even as I write those words, I cannot help but muse on whether the projects have initiated those critiques or whether I have been engaging with these concepts ever since I embarked on my PhD and probably before then but have used different language to define them. I referred earlier in the chapter to some of these terms such as inclusivity in learning and teaching and cultural mediation of learning, teaching and assessment and their tentative relationship to Ubuntu, as I understood it. Later in the chapter, I articulate how they connect to decolonization and decoloniality. But, before doing so, I want to offer a more scholarly discussion of Ubuntu.

23.7 What Is Ubuntu?

Ruth Hayhoe, whose work I admire greatly, draws a link between Confucian educational values and Ubuntu. Why am I beginning this critical analysis of Ubuntu by mentioning Confucianism? For some 15 years I worked regularly on the School of Education's programmes in Hong Kong, directing the Master of Education (MEd), now MSc, there for 7 years, teaching on the Doctor of Education (EdD) and supervising doctoral researchers. As I wrote earlier, beginning to work with students from different parts of the world and embarking on my PhD had challenged me to interrogate my approaches to learning and teaching and to understand how they were culturally mediated. A significant part of this process was developing insight into what informed learning and teaching in other contexts, including Confucian heritage contexts (CHC). My work in Hong Kong dovetailed very nicely into this developing understanding as I became familiar with how Confucian values influenced – and continue to influence – education. Hayhoe (2017) draws on the work of Li (2015) in writing about the "synergies between core Confucian values and the moral orientation of *Ubuntu*" that suggest "a shared commitment to justice, morality and practicality as well as an embrace of diversity at the needs of the individual student as well as the community and society" (Hayhoe, 2017, p. 23, emphasis in original). The values that Hayhoe lists reflect my own values and, therefore, I welcomed the synergies that she drew between Ubuntu and conceptualizations of learning in CHC. My involvement in the Ubuntu project, however, and the stories that I heard from the researchers told to them by their participants, together with the conversations in our group, had begun to test my views of Ubuntu. I mused on whether my understanding was sepia tinted and nostalgic. Perhaps, originally, I had found Ubuntu so seductive because of its challenges to Descartes and to European philosophies, because of Tutu's and Mandela's adherence to it and also perhaps because I perceived it to be "a Rainbow Humanism…in which Ubuntu is sentimentally reduced to everything nice" (Praeg, 2017, p. 296). The stories that were retold by the researchers in the Ubuntu project were most definitely not all positive with some asserting that Ubuntu no longer existed or that it was irrelevant.

> Many participants in the myriad projects struggled to produce a clear and comprehensive definition of Ubuntu, pointing us, instead, to examples of embodied action in their contexts. They told us stories; these stories not only exemplified Ubuntu but also described it in a manner that was both nuanced and evocative. The telling of such rich stories convinced us that to strip Ubuntu of its storied nature and to try to present it as some kind of abstract philosophy would be to divorce it from its African worldview – and possibly to violate it. (Muller et al., 2019, p. 12)

Divorcing Ubuntu from its 'African worldview' seemed anathema to me and I began to engage in rather more critical reflection in much the same way as when I had engaged more deeply with European philosophies.

> Since the advent of democracy in South Africa, there has been a concerted effort at reviving the notion of Ubuntu. Variously conceived, it is seen as the authentic African ethical concept, a way of life, an authentic mode of being African, an individual ideal, the appropriate public spirit, a definition of life itself and the preferred manner of conducting public and private business. (Matolino & Kwindingwi, 2013, p. 197)

They refer to Ubuntu as the "narrative of return", "an attempt to restore the dignity of the African person" (p. 198) but their critique of this includes the claim that these "narratives of return" are "failed projects" (p. 199) and, moreover, that "advocates of the narrative of return take it to be the case that they give an authentic representation of African life" and "shut down space for the possibility of other interpretations of modes of being African that could be at variance with their preferred narrative" (ibid). As a narrative inquirer and one who leans towards postmodernism, these words resonated with me because of their challenge to the notion of dominant narratives. I was intrigued and wanted to learn more about these other modes of being African. Somewhat similarly, Louw (1998) believes that the "Ubuntu desire for consensus also has a potential dark side in terms of which it demands an oppressive conformity and loyalty to the group" (p. 3). He continues, more optimistically, by claiming that "The process of nation-building in post-apartheid South Africa does not, for example, require universal sameness or oppressive communalism. What it does require is true Ubuntu" (ibid). He then quotes Van der Merwe's 1996 translation of *ummuntu ngumuntu ngabantu* as "To be human is to affirm one's humanity by recognizing the humanity of others in its infinite variety and form.... This translation of Ubuntu attests to a respect for particularity, individuality and historicality, without which decolonization cannot be" (ibid). I realize that this is a definition with which I am familiar and more comfortable and, importantly, he has established a link between Ubuntu and decolonization, which I discuss in the following section.

23.8 Decolonization and Decoloniality

The SARiHE project team have been challenged to consider much more critically, the appropriateness of the use of the term decolonization, in particular by Emmanuel Mqwashu, the lead co-investigator at Rhodes University. His view is that decolonization is a political expression that denotes the removal, either through negotiation (for example, in South Africa, Lesotho, Botswana) or by force (for example in Zimbabwe, Mozambique) of the former colonizers, with very little benefit to the people of those former colonies. Decoloniality, on the other hand, focuses on dealing definitively with colonial vestiges in knowledge generation traditions and knowledge itself, together with the sense of unworthiness that continues to be engendered in the colonized through colonial institutions such as schools and universities (Ndlovu-Gatsheni, 2014). In the SARiHE project, therefore, we are striving to frame the lack of attention given to indigenous knowledge systems in higher education in South Africa within decoloniality. Our analysis is set against a background of the continuing dominance of the Global North, western models of academic rigour and what counts as powerful or even relevant knowledge.

Connell (1992) claims that higher education curricula need to address the marginalization or discrediting of cultural, religious and linguistic traditions. Current student demands in South Africa and internationally, call for a critical interrogation into curricula and the development of curricula that are more relevant to the changing student constituency. We relate this not only to decoloniality but also to "epistemicide", the concept that the realities of the Global South are ignored in most epistemologies – the ways in which "knowledge" is understood (de Sousa Santos, 2012). For Motsa (2017, p. 30) these realities/knowledge systems "have been perceived as pagan, mystic, non-scientific, incompetent, irrelevant and downright non-existent" and not worth including in curricula. Valuing cultural diversity and different forms of knowledge in universities enables more inclusive and socially just higher education systems, with the potential to transform the lives of those who participate and their ability to act as global citizens. In the SARiHE project, we are striving to extend our shared understanding of these issues, to further the research agenda in addressing how to move beyond the grand narrative of decolonization. This will include how higher education in South Africa can address the continuing and intransigent ways in which colonized knowledge and knowledge from the North maintains its hold and, thus, hopefully contribute to improving the quality of life for many people.

I wrote earlier that, when I embarked on my PhD some 18 years ago, one of my earliest actions was to interrogate the philosophies that informed my approach to teaching. Interrogating these philosophical ideas led me to interrogating philosophies more broadly and encountering epistemological racism. I wanted to position my research within philosophies that were more congruent with the worldviews of the participants but I struggled to determine what they might be. Seehawer (2018), in her paper that explores Ubuntu as a foundation for research methodology, describes a process very similar to the one in which I engaged:

> The point was not to establish Ubuntu as necessarily oppositional to conventional qualitative methodologies, but to emphasise a way of researching that builds on the epistemologies of the research participants and that contributes to their own purposes. (p. 11)

My involvement in the SARiHE project has led me to grapple, more specifically, with writing on African philosophy in order to ensure that our research is positioned appropriately:

> While German sociologist Max Weber advanced the notion of an autonomous citizen within Western democratic states, different philosophical and cultural assumptions operate in South Africa, where the individual is not separate from, but, rather embedded in, the community into which one is born. (Kubow, 2017, p. 1)

What are these 'different philosophical and cultural assumptions'? Ubuntu?
Dladla (2017) writes:

> The question of whether these exists an African philosophy or not derived its legitimacy from the fact of it being asked and not itself interrogated… the question would not come from indigenous Africans themselves. Meaning that to ask this question one necessarily would have to be situated outside the cultures' own precincts and effectively viewing the African from the outside. (p. 351)

I do not find those words very helpful. If the question would not come from an African, then that suggests to me that an African would know what an African philosophy was. This seems to me to constitute some form of academic trickery/chicanery. I am positioned as the one asking the question because I do not have an answer and those who have answers are not going to yield them up. If I were an African, an insider, I would not be asking the question? Is this an example of keeping the Global North guessing? Excluding those of us who are from the Global North? Positioning us as outsiders and never permitting us to be insiders? Am I back where I started? That seems somewhat negative. Perhaps it is more that, as I look back, I am more able to identify how to move forward. More twists and turns…

23.9 Back to Ubuntu

Praeg (2017, p. 292) claims that:

> Any Ubuntu theorist has to …avoid the twin seductions of being either a contemporary variant of an outdated ethnophilosophy, or an ahistorical analysis of Ubuntu that remains oblivious to the historicity of the concept.

I am not an 'Ubuntu theorist' and I am writing this critical commentary as an outsider. What can I know about Ubuntu as a white, British woman? Am I indulging in an academic exercise for the purposes of this chapter? Do I have any right to pronounce on Ubuntu? Several of the participants in the Ubuntu project claimed that white people cannot 'have' Ubuntu, yet Assie-Lumumba (2016, p. 11) writes that "the worldview it [Ubuntu] encompasses is neither specific to this subregion or exclusively African". Gade, however, writing in 2012, indicates that, "before the 1950s, all written sources mentioning *ubuntu* were authored by people of European descent"(p. 486) and, moreover, that in the South African Journal of Philosophy "a leading journal on *ubuntu*: to date 22 articles…contain the term '*ubuntu*', but only four of these are authored by Africans" (ibid, original emphasis). But, when I look at the names, I wonder whether he is referring to black Africans, as it seems apparent to me that the authors are African. I then turned to Oviawe (2016, p. 7) who writes that "The *ubuntu* paradigm seems to be a way forward to create convergence between the indigenous and the Western, reminiscent of the African philosophy of *sankofa,* which proposes looking at the past to reclaim the future" (emphasis in original). I learn that "The Sankofa Bird is not stuck in the past as it keeps moving forward while looking back to take stock" Assie-Lumumba (2016, p. 10). It is a "mythical bird through which individuals, groups and, communities are reminded to look back in order to reposition themselves to more strategically move forward" (ibid). Perhaps that is what the process of writing as inquiry is helping me to understand, that, like the Sankofa bird, I am *looking* back, not *moving* back, in order to move forward.

23.10 From the Global North: Truly an Outsider?

One of the complexities of the SARiHE project is the funding and the way in which the funding model is a form of re-colonization (Noxolo, 2017). The money emanates from the UK and funding for the UK researchers' time is intrinsic to the model. This does not necessarily mean that they are able to take that time i.e. to use the funding to employ others to do aspects of their work so that they can give the requisite time to the project but the funding in South Africa is filtered through the National Research Foundation (NRF) whose policy is not to pay for staff time. This means that our South African colleagues have conducted the research with the student co-researchers without receiving any allocation of time or financial recompense for doing so. The study has been designed collaboratively by the UK and South African teams but the South Africans have done the work on the ground – and we are very conscious of this. We have striven to surface these tensions and to reflect on them critically as a team but, it is inescapable that the Global North is funding research that, we hope will be of value to the Global South. More tensions.

I now describe an incident that, for me, illustrates these tensions and that confirmed my/our outsider status. The event was a conference in South Africa. There were several papers on decolonization of the curriculum at the conference and, as indicated earlier, as questions about the curriculum are intrinsic to our SARiHE study, my colleague and I felt that it was important that we hear what South African academics had to say about this matter. We had read extensively about decolonization and decoloniality but to hear how people were grappling with such issues in more practical ways in the context would, we thought, be very valuable. During one of the sessions, a member of the audience asked whether the Global North was also engaging with decolonization – or whether they were ignoring it. I had bitten my lip at many of the derogatory comments that had been made about the Global North but, on hearing this question, I decided to respond. I asked whether anyone in the room – I should add that almost everyone was South African – was aware of the 'why is my curriculum white' initiative in the UK that had begun in 2015 (see, for example, https://www.nusconnect.org.uk/articles/why-is-my-curriculum-white-decolonising-the-academy). It became apparent that others were not aware of this initiative and the person who had posed the question showed some interest in hearing more about it. The presenter interrupted him by saying, "The Global North can do what it wants. It has the resources to do so. We don't want to hear what happens there". I was shocked by this riposte. Not only had I never been silenced in such a way at an academic conference – I had been challenged, yes but not silenced – that I felt, subsequently, that I had no desire to be there. My colleague and I shared this incident with the South Africans on our team who expressed disappointment and who appeared to agree that, unless we can debate such issues, we are never going to progress. We acknowledged, however, that we were the 'outsiders' and maybe that did not give us the right to speak? We are white and British, does that mean that we cannot have a voice? We also acknowledged how salutary it was to be silenced in such a way, the ways in which others, in particular black Africans, have been silenced for years. But, is it only South Africans who can speak about South Africa? If this is the case, then it is deeply disappointing and, potentially, renders international collaborations pointless. It also makes a mockery of Ubuntu – and of this chapter!

23.11 A Being White Anecdote

Earlier in this chapter, I wrote of how my PhD developed autoethnographic dimensions and, in particular, challenged me to reflect on what it means to me to be white. I have alluded to that whiteness throughout the chapter but have not interrogated it in ways that I have done elsewhere (see for example, Trahar, 2011, 2013, 2019). Inevitably, however, I do feel that I am positioned in particular ways in South Africa because I am white and I resist that positioning. I am especially resistant to the assumption that I will agree with comments that are racist because my skin is the same colour as the perpetrator.

> "Do you know", she said, "Some of them have never seen a muffin". She laughed, clearly expecting us to laugh too as if never having seen a muffin was a signifier of being uncivilized.
>
> "Do you know", I said "If you asked each one of us here to tell you what a muffin was, you would get 4 different answers".
>
> She looked at me. "What do you mean"?
>
> "Coming from the North of England, a muffin, to me, is a type of bread roll. That meaning differs from yours and from the others here".
>
> We silenced her.

23.12 Finally...

> Language speaks place; place speaks language. Humans organise themselves through a series of sounds that describe their relationship to those places and storytelling evolves. The mapping of thoughts and ideas, the creation of stories to carry the meanings of place, becomes a vehicle to carry the meanings of being human. (Mahood, 2016, p. 195)

I cannot claim to have written as eloquently as Mahood but, her words encapsulate what I have been striving to do in this chapter that is to use language – "a series of sounds"- to describe my relationship with, in the main, South Africa, and to show how, through stories, the meanings of that place and of some other places are carried for me. As ever, in writing the chapter, I have come to know something that maybe I did not know before, or at least did not recognize overtly, and that is the connections that I have traced through what at first sight appear to be a series of random events. I do not claim to have developed 'theory' through retelling the anecdotes but I have become more familiar with critiques of Ubuntu and how it relates to decolonization and decoloniality. As I reach the end of the chapter, however, I continue to be ambivalent about my right to comment on quality of life in South Africa. I can only comment on what I observe and experience – as an outsider. Many of the events that I have described give a rather negative impression but, at the same time, I hope that you, the reader, can glimpse the increasing optimism that I feel.

An author whose work I came to admire when I was doing my PhD while, at the same time, finding it very challenging was Trinh T. Minh-ha, who identifies as a Vietnamese filmmaker, writer, literary theorist, composer and professor. I used her work liberally in my doctoral thesis and even constructed a chapter where I had an imaginary conversation with her, a conversation that was, essentially, about analyzing data. I used the following words of hers to end the Prologue to my thesis:

> The story never really begins nor ends, even though there is a beginning and an end to every story, just as there is a beginning and an end to every teller... The story never stops beginning or ending. It appears headless and bottomless for it is built on differences. Its (in) finitude subverts every notion of completeness and its frame remains a non-totalizable one. (Trinh, 1989, pp. 1–2)

And so, the story – or stories – does not, do not and cannot end here. My relationship with South Africa and her people continues and will do so now, forever, even though my visits will stop or become less frequent. Whether or not I will ever feel as though I am an insider, well, who knows? Perhaps I – and the country – are like the Sankofa bird. We have to look back, not in the more negative sense of taking backward steps, but in order to move forward positively to a future that is more informed and thus better for the majority.

Acknowledgements The Southern African Rurality in Higher Education (SARiHE) project is funded by the Economic and Social Research Council (ESRC) and the Newton Fund. The grant reference number is ES/ P002072/1.

References

Assie-Lumumba, N.'. D. T. (2016). The Ubuntu paradigm and comparative and international education: Epistemological challenges and opportunities in our field. *Comparative Education Review, 61*(1), 1–21.

Connell, R. (1992). Citizenship, social justice and curriculum. *International Studies in Sociology of Education, 2*(2), 133–146.

Connell, R. (2007). *Southern theory: The global dynamics of knowledge in social science*. Cambridge, UK: Polity Press.

Connell, R. (2017). Southern theory and world universities. *Higher Education Research and Development, 36*(1), 4–15.

De Bernieres, L. (2004). *Birds without wings*. London, UK: Secker & Warburg.

De Sousa Santos, B. (2012). Public sphere and epistemologies of the South. *African Development, XXXVII*(1), 43–67.

Dladla, T. (2017). Archie Mafeje and the question of African philosophy: A liberatory discourse. *South African Journal of Philosophy, 36*(3), 350–361.

Gade, C. B. N. (2012). What is *Ubuntu?* Different interpretations among South Africans of African descent. *South African Journal of Philosophy, 31*(3), 484–450.

Gallop, J. (2002). *Anecdotal theory*. Durham, NC: Duke University Press.

Gordon, L. (2015). Race and justice in higher education: Some global challenges with attention to the South African context. In P. Tabensky & S. Matthews (Eds.), *Being at home: Race, institutional culture and transformation at South African higher education institutions*. Pietermaritzburg, South Africa: UKZN Press.

Hayhoe, R. (2017). China in the center: What will it mean for global education? *Frontiers in Education in China, 12*(1), 3–28.

Kubow, P. K. (2017). Exploring Western and non-Western epistemological influences in South Africa: Theorising a critical democratic citizenship education. *Compare, 48*(3), 349–361.

Larrain, V. (2013). Catalan teacher meets Chilean researcher. (De) constructing subjectivities through the interplay of textual narrative. In S. Trahar (Ed.), *Contextualising narrative inquiry: Developing methodological approaches for local contexts* (pp. 140–157). Abingdon, UK: Routledge.

Li, J. (2015). When Confucianism meets Ubuntu: Rediscovering justice, morality and practicality for education and development. *International Journal of Comparative Education Development, 17*(1), 38–45.

Louw, D. J. (1998). *Ubuntu: An African assessment of the religious other*. Philosophy in Africa downloaded from https://www.bu.edu/wcp/Papers/Afri/AfriLouw.htm. (01/11/2017).

Mahood, K. (2016). *Position doubtful: Mapping landscapes and memories*. Brunswick, Australia: Scribe Publications.

Matolino, B., & Kwindingwi, W. (2013). The end of Ubuntu. *South African Journal of Philosophy, 32*(2), 197–205.

Mbembe, A. (2015). *Decolonizing knowledge and the question of the archive*. Aula magistral proferida.

Mbembe, A. (2016). Decolonizing the university: New directions. *Arts and Humanities in Higher Education, 15*(1), 29–45.

McNess, E., Arthur, L., & Crossley, M. (2015). 'Ethnographic dazzle' and the construction of the 'Other': Revisiting dimensions of insider and outsider research for international and comparative education. *Compare, 45*(2), 295–316.

Moller, V. (2007). Quality of life in South Africa – the first ten years of democracy. *Social Indicators Research, 81*(2), 181–201.

Moller, V., Roberts, B. J., Tiliouine, H., & Loschky, J. (2017). Waiting for happiness in Africa. In J. Helliwell, R. Layard, & J. Sachs (Eds.), *World happiness report* (pp. 84–121). New York, NY: Sustainable Development Solutions Network.

Motsa, Z. (2017). When the lion tells the story: A response from South Africa. *Higher Education Research and Development, 36*(1), 28–35.

Muller, J., Eliastam, J., & Trahar, S. (Eds.). (2019). *Unfolding narratives of Ubuntu in Southern Africa*. Abingdon, UK: Routledge.

Ndlovu-Gatsheni, S. J. (2014). Global coloniality and the challenges of creating African futures. *Strategic Review for Southern Africa, 36*(2), 181.

Noxolo, P. (2017). Decolonial theory in a time of the re-colonisation of UK research. *Transactions of the Institute of British Geographers, 42*, 342–344.

Oviawe, J. O. (2016). How to rediscover the Ubuntu paradigm in education. *International Review of Education, 62*(1), 1–10.

Praeg, L. (2017). Essential building blocks of the Ubuntu debate; or: I write what I must. *South African Journal of Philosophy, 36*(2), 292–304.

Richardson, L., & St Pierre, E. (2005). Writing: A method of inquiry. In N. K. Denzin & Y. S. Lincoln (Eds.), *The sage handbook of qualitative research* (3rd ed., pp. 959–978). Thousand Oaks, CA: Sage.

Rogers, C. R. (1994). *Freedom to learn* (3rd ed.). Upper Saddle River, NJ: Merrill.

Scheurich, J. J. (1997). *Research method in the postmodern*. London, UK: Routledge, Falmer.

Seehawer, M. K. (2018). Decolonising research in a Sub-Saharan African context: Exploring Ubuntu as a foundation for research methodology, ethics and agenda. *International Journal of Research Methodology*. https://doi.org/10.1080/13645579.2018.1432404

Stanfield, J. H. (1993). Epistemological considerations. In J. Stanfield II & D. M. Rutledge (Eds.), *Race and ethnicity in research methods* (pp. 16–36). Newbury Park, CA: Sage.

Stanfield, J. H. (1994). Ethnic modeling in qualitative research. In N. K. Denzin & Y. S. Lincoln (Eds.), *The handbook of qualitative research* (pp. 175–188). Thousand Oaks, CA: Sage.

Swadener, B. B., & Mutua, K. (2008). Decolonizing performances: Deconstructing the global postcolonial. In N. K. Denzin, Y. S. Lincoln, & L. Tuhiwai Smith (Eds.), *Handbook of critical and indigenous methodologies* (pp. 31–43). Thousand Oaks, CA: Sage.

Trahar, S. (2011). *Developing cultural capability in international higher education: A narrative inquiry*. London, UK: Routledge.

Trahar, S. (2013). Autoethnographic journeys in learning and teaching in higher education. *European Educational Research Journal, 12*(3), 367–375.

Trahar, S. (2015). Learning and teaching on transnational higher education programmes in Hong Kong. *Learning and Teaching, 8*(1), 95–112.

Trahar, S. (2019). Snow White, a mirror and whiteness: Entangling thoughts in metaphors. In S. Farquhar & E. Fitzpatrick (Eds.), *Innovations in narrative and metaphor – Methodologies and practices* (pp.149–166). Singapore, Singapore: Springer.

Trahar, S., & Yu, W. M. (Eds.). (2015). *Using narrative inquiry for educational research in the Asia Pacific* (pp. xii–xxvii). Abingdon, UK: Routledge.

Trinh, T. Minh-ha (1989). *Woman, native, other: Writing postcoloniality and feminism*. Bloomington, IN: Indiana University Press.

Tuhiwai Smith, L. (2012). *Decolonizing methodologies: Research and indigenous peoples* (2nd ed.). London, UK: Zen Books.

Zeleza, P. M. (2012). *Internationalization in higher education: Opportunities and challenges for the global south*. Keynote address for Sarua Leadership Dialogue on Building the capacity of higher education to enhance regional development, Maputo, Mozambique 21–22 March 2012. Available online at http://www.sarua.org/files/Internationalization%20of%20Higher%20Education%20Final%20Paper%20-%20Prof%20Paul%20Tiyambe%20Zeleza.pdf. Accessed 15 Nov 2017.

Narratives of *Quality of Life* in Africa: A Kaleidoscope of Hope

24

Irma Eloff

Abstract

Narratives about Quality of Life have to depict the comprehensivity of Quality of Life indicators. By definition, Quality of Life studies need to indicate the large-scale descriptions of what constitutes our Quality of Life as human beings and as nations. It describes the life satisfaction, happiness and perceptions of life and the trends that this present over time. Yet, within these descriptions, the *details* of what Quality of Life means at the very personal level can easily be neglected. This chapter seeks to present mini-narratives from across the continent of Africa that can complement the existing discourses about Quality of Life in Africa. It acknowledges the vast challenges within the realm of the search for Quality of Life, but it focuses on personal narratives where Quality of Life has been supported, or is in the process of being supported, by means of agency, collective partnerships and collaboration. The chapter argues that these kaleidoscopes of hope, present important vehicles to understand the complexities of Quality of Life in African communities.

I. Eloff (✉)
Faculty of Education, University of Pretoria, Pretoria, South Africa
e-mail: irma.eloff@up.ac.za

24.1 Introduction

Do we really need more stories about Africa? We listen to stories about Africa constantly and we tell and repeat stories on a daily basis. We continuously create grand narratives about people and places and we supplement these stories with visuals that confirm, support or challenge these master narratives. So, at the conclusion of a book on Quality of life in Africa, what more is there to say?

In this chapter, I share a number of mini-narratives that emanated from a wide variety of African initiatives that is supporting Quality of Life. The invitations to share stories for this chapter were similar to the invitations to the chapter authors: Please share narratives that offer views in, of and from Africa that might challenge some of the master narratives about Africa, with specific reference to Quality of life in Africa. By "master narratives" I meant the frequently found deficit discourses that showcase need and dysfunction as the only conceptual parameters within which to understand Africa. Even though this notion was a risky notion to insert into an invitation to generate mini-stories, I did not need to explain that to even one of the story-writers. They immediately understood what I was asking. Their main concern was more about the timeline on which the mini-stories needed to be completed.

For this chapter therefore, researchers and practitioners from a variety of scientific

I. Eloff (ed.), *Handbook of Quality of Life in African Societies*, International Handbooks of Quality-of-Life, https://doi.org/10.1007/978-3-030-15367-0_24

backgrounds were asked to create a 'mini-narrative' or a 'mini-story' that presents a "picture" of Africa where Quality of Life has been impacted or improved. I was not prescriptive on the theme or the context. It could be a story about anything that shaped the Quality of Life of Africans.

There were stories from Sierra Leone, Kenya, Botswana, Zimbabwe, Rwanda, Ghana, Tanzania, South Africa, as well as multi-country stories.

What these stories share are ideas that address seemingly insurmountable challenges. It also shares an ingrained pragmatism – a pragmatism that adapts as time goes by. It is stories of ambition, but it is also stories of realism.

According to Bruner (2002) there is something about the subtlety of narrative structures that enhances our understandings of the world. He states (Bruner, 2002: p. 9) that it is "only when we suspect we have the wrong story do we begin asking how a narrative may structure (or distort) our view of how things really are. And eventually we ask how story, *eo ipso*, shapes our experience of the world".

As an African, I have often been frustrated about the ways in which our lives (and therefore our *quality of life)* are portrayed in both popular and scientific literature. Not so much the deficit-paradigms of many portrayals, but rather the frequent uni-dimensionality. Living a life in Africa is all, but one-dimensional. We live lives that are simultaneously simple and complex, excruciating and delightful, often thoughtless and even more often deeply thoughtful. We are not defined by what is missing. The Quality of Life of some can be regarded as privileged by some indicators, but those very same lives can be disadvantaged in many other ways. In turn, lives that may be regarded as disadvantaged, may also have embedded rewards (Mpofu, 2016). Fortunately, there are also multiple examples in the literature where these complexities *have* been captured. The South African Quality of Life Trends project, for instance, is probably the most comprehensive study of subjective well-being in South Africa (Møller, 2013). The study portrays findings from a large, representative sample of the country population, it is cross-sectional and it collected data on wellbeing indicators repeatedly over time. The study also connects to political and social transitions at the time and presents the shifts in current life satisfaction, future life satisfaction, happiness, the "life you are living now", and participants' "living conditions as compared to the past". Møller (2013: p. 936) raises the multi-generational question on whether future generations "will see their life chances differently from their parents and grandparents". To think about Quality of Life, is to think beyond individual lifetimes. But how do we capture this?

With the mini-stories presented in this chapter, we wish to share referents of supplementary 'truths' about Quality of Life in Africa. This is what Bruner (2002: p. 11) calls the intention to cultivate "illusions of reality, to "subjunctivize" the self-evident declaratives of everyday life. Quality of life literature predominantly provides broad pictures. As it should. This chapter, however, zooms in in the minutiae of quality of life: a bakery at a school, an entrepreneurial programme for job creation, the introduction of technology to enhance educational experiences at the tertiary level. These "zoomed-in" stories provide what Clandinin and Connelly (2000: p. 19) call "life as it is experienced in the here and now but also with life as it is experienced on a continuum – people's lives, institutional lives, lives of things".

Each mini-story will be presented, and then some reflections on how this story connects with Quality of Life in African communities will be shared. The intention is to *show*, rather than to tell, how Quality of Life manifests on the continent of Africa. In weaving together these stories, I am concurrently the writer and the reader. I am writing the chapter, but I am reading the stories of others as I do so. In each instance, the writer of the mini-story will be introduced in the first line of the story. In doing so, the nuances of the stories as it plays and presents in the minds and lives of African individuals will be distilled. The assumption is therefore, that by recognising the individual story-teller, within the broader Quality of Life narratives, a space would be created for the intricacies of Quality of Life to be captured. Each story is concluded by my own reaction to the story.

24.2 Zimbabwe: The Zunga School Bakery

The writer of this story is John Charema, Director of Education: Mophato Education Centre, Botswana.

Eleanor Tachiona was born of a peasant farmer in Gomana village Chibi in the Zunga area. She and five others are part of the African success story turning obstacles into opportunities through innovation, to live a positive life in a country that experiences hardships and limited resources. From 2005 wheat products in Zimbabwe sometimes become scarce. Having noticed the need for bread and other related wheat products, six women came to the rescue of the community. The bread making bakery was initiated in September 2005 by a team of spirited Zimbabwean rural women in a poor village in Chibi 80 km from Fort Victoria (now Masvingo) the oldest town in Zimbabwe. The bakery is located near a prominent Missionary School, Zunga. Led by Mrs. Eleanor Tichaona, six women put their heads together and underwent training for baking and cooking after which they formed a bakery where they make bread, buns, scones and a few other related products. The bakery services the local rural shops, boarding schools, farming areas and the surrounding community. Typically the bakery became well known and very popular during the acute shortages of bread and flour in 2008, like the present time October 2018. Apart from difficulties in securing the required ingredients, the bakery is doing very well.

However, after some time, due to the dwindling resources of fire wood, the group used their initiative to invent biogas from cow dung which they used for baking, cooking, lighting and heating. They mixed an equal amount of cow dung and water, thoroughly and then poured the mixture into the plastic containers. The containers were fitted with the necessary pipes and other fittings for easy and safe use. Excess waste was utilized as organic fertilizer to grow plants.

The formation of the bakery and the adoption of biogas, capture the enterprising spirit of African innovation. It is a reflection of the resourcefulness with which African people find local solutions to local challenges. This demonstrates how Africa's challenges can be turned into opportunities by those who think positively.

Paradoxically, despite the prevailing challenges of inadequate resources, poor technological development and lack of modern infrastructure, innovation in Africa continues to develop. Africa relies on extensive supply of ideas nursed within the minds of its educated and unemployed youth guided by the wise elderly who think of and employ suitable African solutions that include among others, entrepreneurship, to solve widespread African problems. Typically, the use of biogas in the African rural communities indicates that innovation stems from the need to find sustainable solutions for critical problems that threaten to hinder progress and development. Biogas is used in many rural African countries, with Kenya using it to service rural dairy farmers.

Biogas is a type of biofuel. When organic waste decomposes, it can be captured within a system of pipes and containers, with inlets and outlets that can generate the biofuel. Waste products, such as food, garden and animal waste can be broken down in an anaerobic environment (e.g. an environment without oxygen) to release a blend of gases, often consisting of methane, carbon dioxide and other trace gases. This creates an eco-friendly, low cost technology that can be used in developing contexts as a healthy cooking alternative.

This is interesting. But what is even more interesting from this story, is the way how this group of women has taken a national challenge (food shortages), to generate long-term solutions that contributed to the Quality of Life of their community. What is also interesting, is that this was not a once-off occurrence, because when the next challenges arose (lack of firewood for cooking), they reinforced the ethos of rising above challenges by utilising the resources within their environment.

24.3 Kenya: Employing Academics and Entrepreneurship to Improve *Quality of Life*

The writer of this story is Sahaya G. Selvam from the Tangaza University College, Nairobi.

E4Impact combines academics and social entrepreneurship to deliver some of the Sustainable Development Goals. Currently, partnering with universities in eight countries across Africa (Kenya, Ghana, Sierra Leone, Uganda, Côte d'Ivoire, Senegal and Ethiopia), the project delivers a Master of Business Administration (MBA) degree in social entrepreneurship (http://e4impact.org/). It was initiated by ALTIS – Graduate School of Business and Society of the Catholic University of the Sacred Heart in Milan, Italy.

Informed by the Social Teaching of the Catholic Church, the initiative trains potential entrepreneurs to be sensitive to the social wellbeing of their fellow-citizens while creating jobs and generating income through small and medium sized enterprises (SMEs). Quality of life here, is not understood in profit-oriented economic development, but as a holistic development that bridges the gap between the rich and poor.

Social enterprises have a clear social and/or environmental agenda, generate majority of income through trade, reinvest a large portion of their profits back into the business for sustainability, and are governed by principles of social ethics. They operate their businesses with high standards of transparency, accountability, fairness, respect for creation, and providing equal opportunity to all.

Almost 33% of the entrants to the E4Impact programme are active entrepreneurs, but by the time they graduate 73% of them have a business in place. The academic programme is run in blocks of six 3-day sessions and three 7-day bootcamps. Between the blocks, the candidates are mentored and helped to fine tune their business idea into a business model, and eventually into a business plan. E4Impact is a competency-based education.

The alumni, now numbering 662, of whom 33% are women, have created over 3500 jobs. In some countries, the alumni have gone ahead to form an Association of Social Enterprises (see for example: http://www.socialenterprise.or.ke/) with an aim of being agents of social entrepreneurship in the country.

The approach of E4Impact is ideal for Africa in that it is led by the Ubuntu-philosophy. It respects social, religious and cultural sensibilities of the local communities. At the same time, it creates jobs and generates income, thus contributing to poverty eradication. It is quality of life at its best.

(Note: Tangaza is one of the partners of E4Impact)

The partnerships between churches and education initiatives span centuries. The *E4Impact* is a "zoomed-in" story, but it serves as an example of hundreds of similar initiatives across the continent where educational organizations, churches, networks and partner universities have come together to create socially responsive initiatives that address specific contextual needs. In doing so, Quality of Life of individuals and broader communities are positively impacted. Of note, is the compound effect of partnership initiatives being consistently applied over time. There are hundreds of alumni from this one initiative. They are not only reaping the benefits of the initiative themselves, but they are serving as examples to the younger generation who have the opportunity to witness their entrepreneurial skills on a daily basis. With this, patterns are changed and Quality of Life is improved by tangible measures.

24.4 Rwanda: Umuganda for Education

The writer of this story is Etienne Ntawigira, Communications Advisor for VVOB in Kigali, Rwanda.

In 2003, the Rwandan government abolished school fees to encourage universal basic education. This led to a big increase in the number of learners completing primary education, putting pressure on secondary education institutions. As a result, some learners never transitioned to secondary education or dropped out without finishing, leaving them insufficiently skilled to already take up their roles in society.

To somewhat mitigate the high repetition and dropout rates, the government introduced a policy of 9-year basic education (9YBE) in 2009, eventually extended to 12YBE. The next pressing issue surfaced: an immediate need for thousands of additional classrooms. Umuganda, a community practice introduced by the Rwandan government in the sixties after the country's independence, was the key.

But what is umuganda? Once a month, the residents of a village come together to build up their community: bridges are repaired, roads cleaned, trees planted, and so on. Community members contribute their time and hands, and use locally available resources such as stones, sand, water and wood to repair and build public facilities. Umuganda also serves as a platform for community members to discuss any issues they face and ways forward. While the government still offers support where necessary, this approach saves the country a lot of money that can be directed to other development activities.

For the whole of 2009 and 2010, all umuganda activities were concentrated on building new classrooms. I was part of that process. Fresh out of university, I helped prepare terrains, carry bricks, stones and sands. In the end, more than 6000 new classrooms and close to 15,000 latrines were constructed to accommodate at least hundreds of thousands of children in need.

To complement the infrastructural side of the 9YBE policy, the curriculum and content of the taught courses in basic education were realigned, and teacher training strategies were adopted, among many others. The government's partners in education were brought on board to support the improvement of the education system, among them VVOB – education for development, for which I work.

VVOB's purpose is to develop the capacity of ministries of education and their institutions, so these important actors can improve the quality of education in their countries. VVOB has been working in Rwanda since 2003. Today, VVOB is still working alongside the government for quality education, focusing on effective school leadership and induction of newly qualified teachers in basic and secondary education.

I'm proud to say I contribute to the country's development, both through umuganda and VVOB.

Driving and walking through the streets of Kigali, the effects of the spirit of Umuganda are noticeable. This small African country, where natural resources are more limited than in other African countries, is, however, improving the Quality of Life of its citizens. Even though the remnants of a violent history are still present, the country is utilising its natural beauty to grow its tourism industry. New financial systems are being developed and the levels of corruption are low in comparison to other African countries. In this "country of a thousand hills", Kigali is the ninth safest city in the *world* (at the time of writing) and the national government is one of only two in the world where females hold the majority of the seats.

Umuganda as a community practice is a classic example where available resources are identified and mobilised for greater good, e.g. in this instance, opening up opportunities for resources to be redirected to other initiatives. The implicit message of umuganda is however, also one of collective responsibility, a sense of community and the hope for a brighter future.

24.5 Botswana: Ipelegeng Program

This story was written by an anonymous writer.

Ipelegeng is a Government programme in Botswana that was initiated by the former president, Seretse Khama Ian in 2008 and is being implemented by the Ministry of Local government. Before 2008, the program was called 'food for work'. The aim of the programme is to provide short term employment for unskilled citizens, in addition to developing essential projects that may have been identified and given priority in government planning processes so as to alleviate poverty and improve citizens' quality of Life (QOL). The communities, with assistance from local authorities initiate the projects which are then approved by the Ministry of Local government, dependent on availability of funds.

Project implementation is supervised by the Local Authorities through Programme Coordinators and the programme is implemented country wide, in both urban and rural areas. Any citizen 18 years and above may apply for an opportunity to be engaged in the programme as long as they have a valid Identity card (Omang). Recruitment is done by the Village or Ward Development Committees at the village court (Kgotla). The projects done are mainly: maintenance of drift fences, schools, government and health facilities; desilting of dams and storm water drains, vegetation control (bush clearing and grass cutting in public spaces and along public roads) and many others.

Workers are paid P550 per month as casual labourers and P634 as supervisors (personal communication). The wages are not regarded as payment, but as stipends, although some of the workers, particularly young adults, may not have any other source of income. Employment is not on permanent basis because all beneficiaries must apply monthly and are engaged on rotational basis with preference given to those who were not engaged previously thereby spreading the opportunities and benefits. Workers are also given food when at work so that they do not work when hungry. The monetary benefits do not suffice but beneficiaries say they socialize as they work and thus alleviating social isolation and loneliness, particularly older people, thereby improving their wellbeing.

During research on Influences on Quality of Life of older people in Botswana (anonymous), *a female caregiver had this to say "My pension and the food basket I get from government is not enough for all of us here so at times I apply for Ipelegeng. As we work, we discuss our problems and share best practices. It really helps as I get to know that I am not alone. When I get home after work, I have no time to brood as I will be tired. Manual work also serves as a form of exercise, making us live longer and healthier. It is also a form of social integration, serving as support groups, and networking, thereby increasing my sense of worth and wellbeing."*

More background on the Ipelegeng programme in Botswana can be found on the government portal of the Republic of Botswana by searching for the keyword ipelegeng programme.

Similar to the collective efforts that are evident in the Umuganda activities in Rwanda, the Ipelegeng programme articulates the need for shared responsibilities when it comes to job creation in Africa. The rotation basis in this programme, showcases the communal ethos needed to improve Quality of Life.

24.6 South Africa: The Kgolo Mmogo Project

This story was written by Michelle Finestone, Project Director, Kgolo Mmogo project.

The Kgolo Mmogo project was a 5 year scientific study in the early 2000s that focused on the resilience of mothers and children affected by HIV/AIDS. Apart from investigating the factors that influenced the resilience of HIV-positive mothers and their children, the intention was to develop a low-cost intervention that could be implemented by careworkers who were working with affected populations at the grassroots level on a daily basis.

With inadequate health support services, and scant psychological support services available to support HIV-positive mothers and their children, the need for more accessible psychological support was evident. At the time, many interventions were tried and tested, but very few were based on clinical evidence from a randomised control trial and even fewer were conducted over an extended time period.

This longitudinal randomised control trial study was the first study that demonstrated the benefits of a theory-based, manual-led intervention that was specifically designed to promote resilience among young children of HIV-positive mothers. The intervention was designed in an African context for an African context and was designed to benefit large numbers of children and their mothers.

The team of researchers, primarily from Yale University and the University of Pretoria, decided to publish the manual for the intervention in open access, so that careworkers in a variety of contexts could utilise the material.

This extensive intervention consists of 24 structured intervention sessions. Initially, there are 14 sessions for the mothers and 14 sessions for the children. These are conducted separately. The series of 14 sessions are then followed by a combined 10 sessions, which consists of collaborative sessions between the mothers and their children. The intervention sessions for the mothers include themes such as "the emotional experience of having HIV", "knowing and understanding myself as a parent" and "knowing and understanding my child". For the children, the themes include "identifying strengths within myself", "problem-solving", "social skills" and "identifying meaning, purpose and future orientation". The collective sessions have themes such as "creating a legacy", "let's have fun", "let's dream together" and "let's celebrate life".

The Intervention Programme for the Enhancement of Children's Resilience is available at: http://tinyurl.com/KgoloMmogoInterventionManual

When the Kgolo Mmogo project was conducted in the early 2000s the long-term effects of the HIV-pandemic was still unknown. Yet, the potential impact of the pandemic on individuals, families and communities was estimated to be astronomical. The mental health of those affected most intimately, as well as their concurrent Quality of Life, was of particular concern. Since then, social support structures have been developed around vulnerable populations and large-scale interventions have been implemented in African countries affected by HIV. It has been one of the fields where the canyons between science and the realities of lived experiences have been most effectively bridged. The accessibility of the Kgolo Mmogo manual to support mothers and children affected by HIV, is one of many examples, where science have impacted on Quality of Life in tangible ways.

24.7 Ghana: Using Educational Technology in Higher Education

This story was written by Albert Amoah Saah, KNUST, Kumasi.

Kwame Nkrumah University of Science and Technology (KNUST), Kumasi had been a dual mode higher education institution in Ghana for more than a decade. There had been some success of being a nationwide educational institution and also by going offshore to Nigeria and United Arab Emirates. However, the educational technology inertia experienced in Quality Higher Education at the Institute of Distance Learning, remained a challenge. A strategy that would overcome this inertia was therefore sought. In order to understand the scope of the challenge a survey study was conducted. Data was collected by means of questionnaires, interviews and document analysis. Due to the focus of the study the sampling was nonrandom. A non-probability technique was used to collect data from 195 learners' whose perceptions were measured and analyzed with descriptive statistics, comparing means and correlations.

Perceptions of Educational Technology application in enhancing quality higher education among degree students were assessed. The results from the study showed that perceptions were positively correlated significantly, at the 0.01 level (2-tailed) for variables of employment ($\rho = 0.249$) and gender ($\rho = 0.121$). Teaching and learning transactions ($\overline{x} = 4.4335$), Teaching and learning materials ($\overline{x} = 4.3092$), ICT Integration skills and learning strategy (Ave. $\overline{x} = 4.1358$), and Tools and techniques of technology ($\overline{x} = 4.1008$) were all rated high in their contribution to the effect of Educational Technology Application on Quality Higher Education. The study therefore concluded that an E-Learner centred problem based learning approach had the potential to achieve higher educational technology application for quality higher education experiences. This, in turn, could contribute toward continuing professional development.

Subsequent to the exploratory study, KNUST exercised a robust ICT integration policy and TQM framework. An institutional Distance Education and IT policy were also developed. The Teaching and Learning ICT integration Technology usage strategy, enhanced the quality of higher education at the Institute of Distance Learning, KNUST, Kumasi.

Distance education has arguably improved the Quality of Life of many individuals and families across Africa. Gaining access to tertiary education remains a challenge in most African countries. Strategies where technologies are leveraged to improve access to university programmes are critical to overcome these challenges. However, one of the most frequently reported factors that hinder the implementation of distance/hybrid/dual mode programmes, are the inertia of tertiary education staff towards the use of technology. The KNUST strategy, to approach the challenge by gaining deeper insights into the complexities of this challenge by means of scientific investigation, is commendable. It deepened understandings of the dynamics of technology use to support the academic project. It also provided a platform for future planning.

24.8 Becoming a Teacher: Female Empowerment in Rural Sierra Leone

This story was written by Freda Wolfenden, Open University, UK

'Teaching is quite exciting, it makes you even have time to study with your own children, I look at my children, their books… I say, come and sit by me, then you're teaching… even my own sister I take such a look' Teaching Assistant, Sierra Leone, March 2017.

Teachers are recognised to play a pivotal role in post-conflict (and post-Ebola) reconstruction but in rural areas of Sierra Leone there is a shortage of qualified teachers and women teachers are scarce. Teachers, particularly female teachers, are often reluctant to move to these areas – far from family, friends and commercial centres and with limited transport options.

Since 2012 rural communities in five districts in Sierra Leone have been working with the Forum for African Women Educationalists (FAWE) and the Open University UK (OU) to design, develop and implement a programme to address community education needs and contribute to gender equity in education in a sustainable manner. This 4 year 'Learning Assistant' programme prepares young women in rural communities to take on teaching roles within their own communities. Participants are selected by the community from young women (18–25) who did not complete the full cycle of secondary education and who aspire to become teachers. Around 50% are mothers and almost all had no formal employment prior to enrolment on the programme. Their re-integration into the educational system is initially through supported distance study in Maths and English in preparation for the Teachers' College entrance exam. Simultaneously the Learning Assistants undertake mentored work experience in their local primary school supporting pupil learning.

To date over 800 young women have participated in the programme and 450 have now progressed to study on the distance Teaching Certificate at local Teachers' Colleges. Whilst enrolled at the Teachers' College they continue their 'apprenticeship' at their local primary school, supported by an experienced mentor.

Evaluation data reveals multiple benefits from the scheme; in schools teachers value their assistance with administrative and teaching tasks and for pupils they serve as role models.

Becoming educationally active has been personally transformative for many of the Learning Assistants. They have gained in self-esteem, self-organisation and in confidence to speak, study and successfully negotiate new experiences, 'No-body asks you to talk to pupils, you become bold' (LA, 2017).

And the benefits of the programme have extended beyond the school and individual transformation to micro-system changes within the communities. Perceptions of these young women have been disrupted and shifted in response to their changed role, supporting their developing identity as members of the teaching profession,

'Now they call us teacher in the community, before we were nothing', 'Everyone says my life has changed... we have a space in the community now... they call us teachers, they encourage us to be part of it' (LAs, 2017).

More background about this work can be read at: http://www.open.ac.uk/about/international-development/projects-and-programmes/gate-girls-access-education

The GATE (Girls' Access to Education) project supports two of the sustainable development goals directly, e.g. quality education (SDG4), as well as gender equality (SDG5). At the same time, it is responding to an emerging discourse about the education workforce in the world. The Education Workforce Initiative (EWI, 2018) is investigating and rethinking the global education workforce. It calls for innovation and reform around the world, in order to ensure that learning is optimised. By creating opportunities for young women to become Learning Assistants, the education workforce is improved in innovative ways and learning is supported for children in the classrooms. When girls are supported, families are supported. When girls are supported to improve their qualifications, entire families benefit for lifetimes to come; and when families benefit, Quality of Life improves.

24.9 Zimbabwe: A Tale of Two Minerals

This story was written by Tanaka Chiromo Master's Degree student in Electronic Engineering at the University of Pretoria.

The turn of the twenty-first century marked the beginning of a period that would see a promising young Zimbabwean Republic endure one of the worst economic meltdowns ever recorded in modern history. This was characterised by an underperforming local industry, high unemployment rates, high costs of living, meagre salaries, underdevelopment, corruption, high rates of inflation, a cash crisis that led to the subsequent abandonment of the local currency and a lot more characteristics of a dying economy.

Despite the economic crunch, two interesting industries were arguably borne out of this murky environment. By the year 2006, rumours of the discovery of diamonds in the country were circulating among the general populace. Battered with a litany of poverty related shortcomings, a legion of Zimbabweans flocked to the Marange regions in the Eastern parts of the country in search of this precious mineral. It only took a bit of prospecting by this group of hopefuls to provide evidence that indeed there was a deposit of diamonds existing in the country. In fact, as was later realised, Zimbabwe actually had one of the largest deposits of diamonds in the world!

Even though it was later reported that the De Beers mining company had long since been exploiting the fields, to the ordinary Zimbabwean, the existence of diamonds was practically a new discovery that they hoped would go a long way in alleviating their problems. Eventually the government took over mining activities from both the De Beers company, whose license had expired and chased away the multitude of illegal miners that had populated the area. To date, diamonds from the Marange fields worth millions of US dollars have been sold.

In another tale of an unknown mineral; following a controversial deposing of a sitting President in November 2017, the new government sought ways in which to improve the persistently poor performing economy. In February of 2018, the nation was to hear that the government was going to be involved in the extraction of lithium worth billions of US dollars. This report was brought to the attention of the nation the fact that there was yet another mineral in existence that had the potential of generating a lot of revenue for the country. As with the case of diamonds, little had been known by the general populace of the existence of this mineral.

Even though the actual exploitation of lithium is still in its infancy, the rising global demand for lithium as a key raw material in the manufacturing of modern electronic batteries almost guarantees huge rewards if this sector is handled correctly.

These two minerals would inevitably have been exploited at a time in the future one way or the other. However, it is worthwhile to note that the interest in these two minerals was somewhat due to the prevailing decaying economic conditions in the country. How the current government exploits its newly found source of potential wealth remains to be seen. The extent to which these two industries will alleviate poverty of everyone up to the poorest Zimbabwean citizen will also remain to be seen. At the moment, however, what has been seen is the birth of two potentially lucrative industries in the country.

[Tanaka Chiromo holds an Honours Degree in Electronic Engineering from NUST in Zimbabwe, an Honours Degree in Electronic Engineering from the University of Pretoria in South Africa and is currently pursuing a Master's Degree in Electronic Engineering at the University of Pretoria. His key research areas include Machine Learning, Computer Vision and Data analytics].

Narratives about Zimbabwe frequently circle around the political situation in the country. Until recently, the former president frequently made international headlines and reports of corruption and social decay permeated discussions about the country. Yet, at the same time, this country, formerly known as Rhodesia, or "the breadbasket of Africa" remains one of the countries which are most rich with natural resources. This particular story is different from the others presented in this chapter, in that it is pointing towards opportunities *not yet realized*. This "tale of two minerals" is a story of potential, a story that tentatively presents the delicate hopes for a future that may improve the Quality of Life of the most vulnerable Zimbabweans.

24.10 Conclusion

This chapter provides kaleidoscopic views of Quality of Life in Africa. In many instances it simultaneously presents the fragility and the tenacity of individuals and organizations who are working to provide hope against the odds. Individuals who are resourceful, connected to one another and future-focused. Organizations that are deeply committed to improving lives in Africa.

These narratives are presented through lenses that are *zoomed in*. It is narratives about specific places, specific people and specific plans to cultivate better futures. Does it communicate important, or even relevant, views? In this regard, I align with Bruner (2002: p. 89), when he says, "for all that narrative is one of our evident delights, it is serious business". We shape the world by the stories we tell, we understand the world by the stories we choose to hear and we improve our world by creating avenues for new stories to emerge.

References

Bruner, J. (2002). *Making stories – Law, literature, life*. Cambridge, MA: Harvard University Press.

Clandinin, D. J., & Connelly, F. M. (2000). *Narrative inquiry*. San Francisco, CA: Jossey-Bass.

Møller, V. (2013). South African quality of life trends over three decades, 1980–2010. *Social Indicators Research, 113*, 915–940.

Mpofu, E. (2016). The evolution of quality of life perspectives in the developing world. In R. L. Schalock & K. D. Keith (Eds.), *Cross-cultural quality of life: Enhancing the lives of persons with intellectual disability* (2nd ed., pp. 175–180). Washington, DC: American Association on Mental Retardation.

The Education Workforce Initiative. (2018). Accessed on: 29 Nov 2018. http://educationcommission.org/education-workforce-initiative/

Printed by Printforce, the Netherlands